CRAM'S INTRODUCTION TO
Surface Electromyography

SECOND EDITION

Edited by

ELEANOR CRISWELL, EdD

Director, Novato Institute for Somatic Research and Training
Professor Emeritus, Sonoma State University

JONES AND BARTLETT PUBLISHERS
Sudbury, Massachusetts
BOSTON   TORONTO   LONDON   SINGAPORE

World Headquarters
Jones and Bartlett Publishers
40 Tall Pine Drive
Sudbury, MA 01776
978-443-5000
info@jbpub.com
www.jbpub.com

Jones and Bartlett Publishers
Canada
6339 Ormindale Way
Mississauga, Ontario L5V 1J2
Canada

Jones and Bartlett Publishers
International
Barb House, Barb Mews
London W6 7PA
United Kingdom

Jones and Bartlett's books and products are available through most bookstores and online booksellers. To contact Jones and Bartlett Publishers directly, call 800-832-0034, fax 978-443-8000, or visit our website, www.jbpub.com.

Substantial discounts on bulk quantities of Jones and Bartlett's publications are available to corporations, professional associations, and other qualified organizations. For details and specific discount information, contact the special sales department at Jones and Bartlett via the above contact information or send an email to specialsales@jbpub.com.

The authors, editor, and publisher have made every effort to provide accurate information. However, they are not responsible for errors, omissions, or for any outcomes related to the use of the contents of this book and take no responsibility for the use of the products and procedures described. Treatments and side effects described in this book may not be applicable to all people; likewise, some people may require a dose or experience a side effect that is not described herein. Drugs and medical devices are discussed that may have limited availability controlled by the Food and Drug Administration (FDA) for use only in a research study or clinical trial. Research, clinical practice, and government regulations often change the accepted standard in this field. When consideration is being given to use of any drug in the clinical setting, the health care provider or reader is responsible for determining FDA status of the drug, reading the package insert, and reviewing prescribing information for the most up-to-date recommendations on dose, precautions, and contraindications, and determining the appropriate usage for the product. This is especially important in the case of drugs that are new or seldom used.

Production Credits
Publisher: David Cella
Associate Editor: Maro Gartside
Production Director: Amy Rose
Associate Production Editor: Julia Waugaman
Marketing Manager: Grace Richards
Manufacturing and Inventory Control Supervisor: Amy Bacus
Composition: Cape Cod Compositors, Inc.
Cover and Title Page Design: Scott Moden
Photo Research and Permissions Manager: Kimberly Potvin
Assistant Photo Researcher: Emily Howard
Cover Image: © gulsev/ShutterStock, Inc.
Printing and Binding: Malloy Incorporated
Cover Printing: Malloy Incorporated

Library of Congress Cataloging-in-Publication Data
Criswell, Eleanor.
   Cram's introduction to surface electromyography / by Eleanor Criswell.—2nd ed.
      p. ; cm.
   Rev. ed. of: Introduction to surface electromyography / Jeffrey R. Cram. 1998.
   Includes bibliographical references and index.
   ISBN-13: 978-0-7637-3274-5 (pbk.)
   ISBN-10: 0-7637-3274-5 (pbk.)
   1. Electromyography.   I. Cram, Jeffrey R. Introduction to surface electromyography.   II. Title.   III. Title:
Introduction to surface electromyography.
   [DNLM: 1. Electromyography.   WE 500 C933c 2011]
   RC77.5.C73 2011
   616.7'407547—dc22
                                                                                        2009042383
6048
Printed in the United States of America
14 13 12 11 10   10 9 8 7 6 5 4 3 2 1

In memoriam

Jeffrey R. Cram

March 30, 1949 – March 2, 2005

Dedicated to Shannon, Heidi, and Maya

Brief Contents

Contents

Foreword to the First Edition

The privilege of reading the manuscript of a book by distinguished authors before its publication is always a thrilling experience. When the material is as sparkling as in this book, one feels truly privileged and honored to be asked to write the foreword. This is a fine book that will meet the needs of many scientists and clinicians in a wide range of specialties. Both those who directly employ surface electromyography for any purpose and those who have to understand its consequences will be ever grateful to the authors.

This book is written in an astute style that clearly informs *all* readers, even such as this grizzled veteran. Only after a while will the novice reader awaken to the fact that, *mirabile diciu*, a profound learning experience has happened without the use of a computer or TV screen. Few scientific or clinical books today succeed in this game of seizing and holding the reader's interest in spite of the level of sophistication of either the reader or the subject matter.

Not only are the style and organization complete and well integrated, the choices of words and phrases are friendly and beckoning without annoying those readers who are more comfortable with scientific and clinical jargon. In this book, a spade is called a spade, but it is a shiny, well-used spade and not an "automated excavating system" used by over-anointed writers.

To summarize, it is simple and accurate to say this is a very fine book and I am happy to have read it before its birth. Moreover, I expect to refer to it *ad lib* after publication and to recommend it to others.

John V. Basmajian, DC, MD, FRCP, FRCPS
Professor Emeritus
McMaster University
Hamilton, Canada

Preface

The muscles of the body are critical to almost every form of human behavior. In fact, without muscle activity there would be no observable behavior or skilled actions that we come to expect in behavior. [1] (p. 229)

[Surface electromyography] is a very interesting area in which to work, because the same end organ (the muscle) is under the command of three masters: gravity (posture), emotions, and movement. [2] (p. xiii)

What is surface electromyography? Surface electromyography (SEMG) is a field specializing in the use of electronic devices to measure the energy of the muscles, to analyze the data, and to display the results. Surface electromyography rests on the practitioner's understanding of anatomy, physiology, and the instrumentation. It is an example of applied psychophysiology: the use of psychophysiological knowledge and skills in the evaluation and treatment or training of individuals presenting with psychophysiological complaints or goals. Surface electromyography is a multidisciplinary field that encompasses contributions from electronics, medicine, anatomy, physiology, psychology, psychophysiology, physical therapy, occupational therapy, ergonomics, and so forth.

Surface EMG has many applications, including assessment, treatment planning, evaluation of progress and outcomes, rehabilitation, worksite ergonomic design, sports training, and research. This technology helps differentiate between beliefs about muscle function and actual function, and is used in evaluation and rehabilitation. Surface electromyography is used with patients and clients by physical therapists, occupational therapists, psychologists, dental professionals, biofeedback trainers, stress management consultants, corporate safety consultants, sports psychologists, arts medicine practitioners, ergonomics consultants, and somatics

educators/practitioners, among others. The feedback provided by this technique works best when combined with other therapies. Regardless of how SEMG is being used, a solid foundation in the principles of SEMG is necessary to be effective.

There were 14 chapters in the first edition of this book; there are 17 chapters in this second edition. In the second edition, 13 of the original chapters, the SEMG atlas, and the appendices remain. Chapter 14, "Surface Electromyography Past, Present, and Future," has been rewritten to reflect progress in the field. New chapters by Jeffrey R. Cram, Maya Durie, Eleanor Criswell, and Marek Jantos have been added as well. An emphasis on somatics has been included in the second edition at Jeffrey Cram's request.

Part I provides information on the basics of surface electromyography, including the history of SEMG; the advantages and disadvantages of SEMG; anatomy and physiology; instrumentation; electrodes and site selection strategies; general assessment considerations; static assessment and clinical protocol; emotional assessment and clinical protocol; dynamic assessment; treatment considerations and protocols; and documentation. Part II features chapters titled "The History of Muscle Dysfunction and Surface Electromyography" by Jeffrey R. Cram and Maya Durie, "Somatics and Surface Electromyography" by Eleanor Criswell,

"Electromyographic Assessment of Female Pelvic Floor Disorders" by Marek Jantos, "Surface Electromyography Past, Present, and Future" by Eleanor Criswell, and the conclusion. Part III features the Atlas for Electrode Placement developed by Jeffrey R. Cram and Glenn S. Kasman with Jonathan Holtz, the electrode atlas overview, and electrode placements for key muscles. An expanded glossary of terms appears at the back of the book; the answers to the chapter questions can also be found there.

The cornerstone of this book remains the electrode atlas found in Part III. "Knowing the map of the territory—where to place the surface electromyography (SEMG) electrodes and what to expect to see during a given movement—will greatly assist the practitioner in understanding the energy that the muscle gives off."[2(p. xiii)] The atlas of electrode placement covers 69 electrode placement sites. Along with illustrations showing electrode placement sites, information is provided about each muscle in question: its action or purpose, clinical uses (such as for specific presenting complaints), origin and insertions of the muscle, innervation of the muscle (nerve supply to the muscle), as well as information on joint considerations, location of electrodes, behavioral tests to determine the type of placement (general or specific), the accuracy of the electrode placement, comments about the tracings, volume conduction, other sites of interest, possible artifacts, and benchmark measures. Surface EMG tracings, photographs, tables, graphs, and drawings throughout the book demonstrate the concepts under discussion. The discoveries by Cram, Kasman, and others are highly useful gems scattered throughout the book.

Since the first edition of this book was published, a tremendous amount of research has been conducted using surface EMG. This research has taken place all over the world (see Chapter 14). In these studies, many aspects of human behavior have been assessed using SEMG, including work performance, sports performance, rehabilitation, and movement analysis. The second edition reflects that research.

Who can benefit from *Cram's Introduction to Surface Electromyography*? Designed to introduce the reader to the principles and practices of SEMG, this book is suited to both beginners in the field—upper-division university students, master's and PhD students, beginning professionals, and educated laypersons—and advanced professionals who want to deepen their SEMG knowledge. This book will prove useful for physical therapists, occupational therapists, biofeedback trainers, behavioral medicine practitioners, psychologists, dentists, chiropractors, biomedical engineers, exercise physiologists, and complementary and alternative medicine practitioners. The reader who learns more about SEMG will be more effective in his or her work.

Physical and occupational therapists will benefit greatly from SEMG objective measures that can show chronic muscle contractions, postural difficulties, inadequate activation of muscles, and the like. They have a great need for such data in their assessments, evaluations of patient progress, and discharge planning. In situations where objective data are highly valued, such as with third-party payers, SEMG recordings are invaluable. Nevertheless, the information in this book is useful regardless of whether the reader plans to use SEMG directly or indirectly in his or her work. This modality is an important means of gathering data about human functioning: it offers a clear measure of the mind-body connection. The SEMG data are particularly understandable because people are used to contracting muscles to engage in movements to achieve their goals. For this reason, SEMG is finding a home in mind-body medicine.

Surface electromyography is valuable for somatics educators of all disciplines who seek a deeper understanding of the mind-body connection, for the training of somatics practitioners/educators, and as a means of enhancing the effectiveness of the somatics approaches. For somatics educators using SEMG, it is valuable to see what is happening inside the client during somatics practices; for SEMG biofeedback practitioners, it is valuable to use the somatics disciplines to complement the adjunctive procedures, such as progressive relaxation, that are typically employed.

Although the use of SEMG equipment can be learned through manuals and online instructions, the reader is strongly urged to get thorough training in the use of SEMG through an established training program with highly trained, experienced SEMG professionals in the field. Certification by the Biofeedback Certification Institute of America in general biofeedback, which includes SEMG, is important for using this technology in a clinical setting.

Accuracy in SEMG recordings is essential. The old computer-related saying, "Garbage in, garbage out," is very apt here. In other words, if the recordings are not accurate, the data will not be accurate. Reliability and validity of the data are always important. Inaccurate data are always worse than worthless, because the practitioner and the patient may draw conclusions from the data that are not warranted. Accuracy is particularly important in SEMG research. Research design and description of the procedures, equipment, data gathered, conclusions, and so forth need to allow for replication. This book provides detailed step-by-step methods for ensuring accurate SEMG recordings.

The reader already knowledgeable about SEMG may want to read those sections that are most relevant to his or her needs first; those new to the field may wish to start at the beginning. Another approach is to begin with the instrumentation chapter, practice using the equipment, and then go on to acquire more detailed knowledge from the chapters devoted to anatomy and physiology, neurophysiology, and the like over time, reading the rest of the chapters in Part I and referring to Part III as needed. For continued SEMG study, a variety of professional training programs and university-based programs include SEMG as part of their general biofeedback offerings. (Contact the Association of Applied Psychophysiology and Biofeedback [AAPB] and the Biofeedback Certification Institute of America [BCIA] for information about relevant programs.)

The term *patient* is used throughout this book, except in Chapter 12, because SEMG is most commonly used in rehabilitation and other medical settings. The term *client* is used in the "Somatics and Surface Electromyography" chapter because in the somatics world the participant is called a client and the practitioner is called an educator or practitioner. Somatics is a client-centered educational process. Many biofeedback (SEMG) settings are client centered as well.

The SEMG field continues to have enormous potential. The professionals and organizations that serve it continue to expand the knowledge, skills, and application areas through professional meetings, journals, seminars, conferences, and networking. For example, SEMG research has appeared in more than 42 journals worldwide in the last 10 years. Key organizations in the field are the Association for Applied Psychophysiology and Biofeedback (AAPB) (the Surface EMG Society of North America is now the Surface EMG division of AAPB), the Biofeedback Foundation of Europe, and the International Society of Electrophysiological Kinesiology (ISEK) (formerly the International Society of Electromyography and Kinesiology).

Surface electromyography is an exciting and growing field with huge potential for teaching people how to grow healthily; age successfully; take care of neuromuscular complaints that develop over time due to accident, injury, illness, repetitive use, and the like; and actualize more of their somatic potential for optimal performance. Manufacturers of SEMG equipment can be found throughout the world. Research, clinical applications, and new technology are all fostering the growth of this field. Neuroimaging in relationship to motor performance is a valuable development in the understanding of SEMG. Telemetry systems and other technological innovations will continue to expand what is possible with SEMG and its contribution to enhanced human functioning.

ACKNOWLEDGMENTS

I would like to acknowledge and offer my deep thanks to the following individuals: Marsha Calhoun, the copy editor for the second edition, whose work on this edition was invaluable; Wendell Hanna, for her research assistance; Satri Pencak, for assistance with the Hanna photograph; Jeffrey Cram, Glenn Kasman, and Jonathan Holtz for their fine earlier edition; Jeffrey Cram for his invitation to bring somatics into this edition and finally to assume editorship; Shannon Cram, Heidi Cram, and Maya Durie for their help and encouragement; Allegra Hiner and Sam Hiner, key staff members, and Phil Shenk and Susan Koenig, Hanna Somatic Education Core Teachers of the Novato Institute for Somatic Research and Training, for their ongoing support; my advisors Richard Stone, Belinda Scrimenti, and Neil Russack; Charles Merrill, Stephen Sideroff, Jone Bondoc, Elaine Leeder, Dennis and Deborah Reis, and Kara Knack for their friendship and encouragement; our care team of Marianne Locke, Jerry Moore, Conrad Knudsen, Marsha Harrison, and Lyman Spencer; my long-time colleagues at the Biofeedback Society of California, the Association for Applied Psychophysiology and Biofeedback, and the Biofeedback Certification Institute of America; Steve Wall and Katee Wynia of the Bio Research Institute for our many years of shared biofeedback explorations at Sonoma State University (SSU) and beyond; the students in the Professional Biofeedback Training Sequence at SSU over the past 25 years from whom I learned so much; the chair, Gerryann Olson, and faculty and staff of the Psychology Department at SSU for their appreciation and support of the biofeedback program over the years; and the staff from Jones and Bartlett Publishers, especially Maro Gartside, Julia Waugaman, and Teresa Reilly, for their understanding and able assistance. Above all, I would like to thank my husband, Pernell Roberts, for his deep understanding and caring.

Preface to the First Edition

The cornerstone of this book is the electrode atlas found in Part II. Knowing the map of the territory—where to place the surface electromyography (SEMG) electrodes and what to expect to see during a given movement—will greatly assist the practitioner in understanding the energy that the muscle gives off. Indeed, many times during the collection of tracings for a particular set of muscles, I found myself and others asking, "What happens if we do x?" Then we tried x and were either pleasantly surprised or confused and disappointed. Some-times the system worked as we had been told it would by others. Sometimes it was far too complex to see what we expected to see, given the simple tools and procedures we were using. Capturing a valid SEMG tracing is sometimes associated with a subtle event. For example, I was duly impressed by the changes in recruitment patterns as we instituted small postural or positional requirements on the limbs or torso. To this day, I remember my amazement at how a simple sternal lift could facilitate the recruitment of lower trapezius. There are literally dozens of gems like this sprinkled throughout this book. The tracings in this book illustrate what can be seen using the SEMG technology. We hope that they stimulate the reader's curiosity and that readers explore the movement of their own patients while measuring muscle energy patterns.

The static and dynamic assessment chapters provide the background and protocols in detail for almost all of the current assessment procedures. This is a very interesting area in which to work, because the same end organ (the muscle) is under the command of three masters: gravity (posture), emotions, and movement. Muscle scanning is a method for assessing the neuromuscular aspects of posture; stress profiling is the method to quantify the emotional component; dynamic SEMG procedures provide the basis for assessing movement. Practitioners need to think in this three-dimensional manner if they want to find successful solutions when something goes wrong.

Part I reviews the basic tenets of the treatment of musculoskeletal and pain-related disorders and provides a few examples of these approaches. Additional information is found in the companion book *Clinical Applications in Surface Electromyography: Chronic Musculoskeletal Pain*. I highly recommend that readers study this very scholarly, yet pragmatic review of what we know about the use of SEMG in treating a variety of conditions.

History, anatomy, physiology, and instrumentation are the foundations upon which the clinical practice of SEMG rests. Every practitioner who uses electromyography should have a sound understanding of what is behind the SEMG screen displays. Chapters 1 through 3 provide this information in an easy-to-understand fashion. For those who are new to the area of SEMG and are just learning the jargon, we have included a glossary

(Appendix A) to provide definitions of some of the basic concepts.

Surface EMG is seen as an emerging technology. We have just begun to scratch the surface of its clinical potential. Chapter 11 provides some glimpses into where SEMG may be moving as it unfolds.

As is true for all manuscripts, literally hundreds of people have helped bring this book into print. The greatest contributors to this book were the many students in my workshops, whose curiosity and enthusiasm led me to seek out the "essence" of a given muscle, for a given movement, while exploring electrode placement strategies. Four of these students became dear friends, colleagues, and eventually my teachers. Will Taylor, Stu Donaldson, Jonathan Holtz, and Glenn Kasman helped to create the boundaries and channels into which this introductory volume on SEMG flowed, but it was Glenn Kasman's commitment to work on this book that set it in motion. And, once under way, it was the substantive editing of Steven Wolf that provided the basis for course corrections, and the buff and polish of Glenn Kasman, Blair Schular, Diana Huff, and Maya Cram that made it intelligible.

Many people made the tracings for the electrode atlas possible. With minds like those of Glenn Kasman and Jonathan Holtz, the power and beauty of SEMG recordings began to emerge as we intensively studied a few individuals. Some of those individuals, who spent hours or days with us and allowed us to place electrodes here and there while we asked them to move this way or that, deserve special recognition. Specifically, the efforts of David Rommen, Dennis Harmoo, Mark Woodburn, Carrie Hall, Paula Holtz, and Maya Cram helped to make the atlas possible. Finally, this book has hundreds of graphics contained within its pages. Many of these were created by Bella and Dave Bingham and Heidi Cram.

Jeffrey R. Cram, PhD

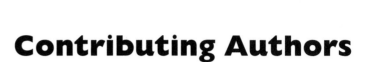

Contributing Authors

Jeffrey R. Cram, PhD
Director, Sierra Health Institute
President, Clinical Resources
Nevada City, California

Maya Durie, MEd, CMT
Massage Therapist and Movement Educator
Mill Valley, California

Jonathan Holtz, MA, PT
Santa Cruz, California

Marek Jantos, PhD
Director of the Behavioural Medicine Institute
Adelaide, Australia

Glenn S. Kasman, MS, PT, FACHE
Vice President of Professional Services and Business
 Development
MultiCare Good Samaritan Hospital
Puyallup, Washington

The Basics of Surface Electromyography

Jeffrey R. Cram and Glenn S. Kasman

Introduction

"Electromyography is the study of muscle function through the inquiry of the electrical signal the muscle emanates."[1]

THE HISTORY OF SURFACE ELECTROMYOGRAPHY

The history of surface electromyography (SEMG) has to do with the discovery of electricity and the development of the ability to see through the aid of instruments things that cannot be seen, felt, or touched with the normal senses. It is also the story of the emergence of a new paradigm for assessing and treating the energy of the muscles—a form of "energy medicine," in which the emphasis is on the energy of the body rather than its form. (In this paradigm, form is not unimportant, but it is only of secondary interest.) As is true for all paradigm shifts, many individuals are reluctant to give up their investment in the old paradigm. For example, many practitioners still prefer clinical palpation and observation over measurement of the energy of the muscle, even though each technique may tap into a different domain of information.

The theme of the development of SEMG can be traced back to the mid-1600s, when Francesco Redi[2,3] documented that a highly specialized muscle was the source of the electric ray fish's energy. By 1773, Walsh had been able to demonstrate clearly that the eel's muscle tissue could generate a spark of electricity. It was not until the 1790s that Galvani obtained direct evidence of the relationship between muscle contraction and electricity; he conducted a series of studies that demonstrated that muscle contractions could be evoked by the discharge of static electricity.[4] In 1792, Volta[5] initially agreed; he later concluded that the phenomenon Galvani had seen did not emanate from the tissue itself, but rather was an artifact of the dissimilar metals touching the muscle tissue. Galvani rebutted Volta's criticism and was able to demonstrate the firing of the muscle by contracting it with a severed nerve rather than metal. This finding, however, went unnoticed for four decades because of Volta's popularity. Volta had developed a powerful tool that could be used both to generate electricity and to stimulate muscle. The technique of using electricity to stimulate muscles gained wide attention during the nineteenth century, and some people exploited this novel technique for research purposes. In the 1860s, Duchenne[6] conducted the first systematic study of the dynamics and function of the intact muscle, using electrical stimulation to study muscle function.

It was not until the early 1800s that the galvanometer, a tool for measuring electrical currents and muscle activity, was invented. In 1838, Matteucci used the galvanometer to demonstrate an electrical potential between an excised frog's nerve and its damaged muscle. By 1849, Du Bois-Reymond[7] provided the first evidence of electrical activity in human muscles during voluntary contraction. In his classic experiment, Du Bois-Reymond placed blotting cloth on each of his subject's hands or forearms and immersed them in separate vats of saline solution, while connecting the electrodes to the galvanometer. He noted very minute but very consistent and predictable deflections whenever the subject flexed a hand or an arm. He deduced that the magnitude of the current was diminished by the impedance of the skin. After removing a portion of the subject's skin, Du Bois-Reymond replaced the electrodes and noted a dramatic increase in the magnitude of the signal during wrist flexion.

By the early 1900s, Pratt[8] had begun to demonstrate that the magnitude of the energy associated with muscle contraction was due to the recruitment of individual muscle fibers, rather than the size of the neural impulse. In the 1920s, Gasser and Newcomer[9] used the newly invented cathode ray oscilloscope to show the signals from muscles. This feat won them the Nobel Prize in 1944.

As a result of continuing improvements in EMG instrumentation beginning in the 1930s and continuing through the 1950s, researchers began to use SEMG more widely for the study of normal and abnormal muscle function. During the 1930s, Edmund Jacobson, the father of progressive relaxation, used SEMG extensively to study the effects of imagination and emotion on a variety of muscles.[10] He also used SEMG to study systematically the effects of his relaxation training protocol on muscle activity.[11]

In the 1940s, researchers began to use SEMG to study dynamic movement. For example, Inman and his colleagues conducted a highly regarded study on the movements of the shoulder.[12] In the late 1940s, Price and her colleagues[13] studied clinical populations of back pain patients and noted that the SEMG activation patterns began to migrate away from the site of original injury. Their work was the first documentation of antalgic (painful) postures or protective guarding muscle patterns. Floyd and Silver,[14] in the early 1950s, presented an exceptionally strong study of EMG and the erector spinae muscles. They clearly demonstrated that as a person goes through forward flexion of the trunk, the back muscles shut off as the trunk goes out onto ligamental support.

During the late 1950s and the 1960s, George Whatmore,[15] a student of Jacobson, used SEMG to study and treat emotional and functional disorders. His work was summarized in a very unusual book, *The Physiopathology and Treatment of Functional Disorders*,[15] in which he used SEMG to augment the basic progressive relaxation technique he had learned from Jacobson. In addition, he coined the term *dysponesis* to describe

"bad" muscle energy patterns that can be observed using SEMG instrumentation.

During the 1960s, the technique of biofeedback was born. Basmajian's[16] work on single motor unit training provided some of the impetus for research on biofeedback (see Figure 1–1). Although this type of training entailed the use of fine-wire electrodes rather than surface electrodes, it clearly demonstrated that EMG feedback could be used to train the neuromuscular system down to its most basic element—the single motor unit. Elmer Green[17] first used SEMG with biofeedback at the Menninger Clinic, where he modified Basmajian's single motor unit training paradigm for general relaxation training. A few years later, Budzynski and colleagues[18] began using SEMG feedback to treat muscle contraction headaches. From there, the biofeedback arena began to expand rapidly.

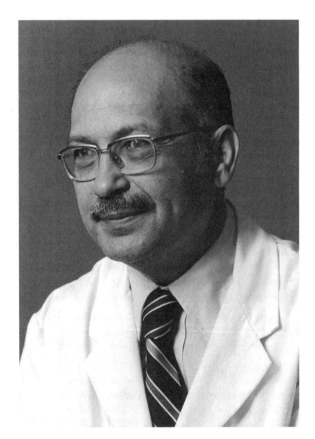

Figure 1–1 John Basmajian, the father of surface electromyography.
Source: Courtesy of Faculty of Health Sciences, McMaster University.

Clinical use of SEMG for the treatment of more specific disorders began in the 1960s. Hardyck and colleagues[19] were among the first practitioners to use SEMG. They used SEMG to teach students not to subvocalize during silent reading, which accelerated students' reading development. Booker and colleagues[20] demonstrated retraining methods for patients with various neuromuscular conditions, and Johnson and Garton[21] used SEMG to assist in the restoration of function of hemiplegic patients. Wolf et al.[22,23] were among the first to use SEMG biofeedback techniques in the assessment and treatment of low-back pain. For a comprehensive review of the history of SEMG and low-back pain through the early 1990s, see the work of Sherman and Arena[24] or an earlier review article by Dolce and Raczynski.[25]

In the early 1980s, Cram and Steger[26] introduced a clinical method for scanning a variety of muscles using a handheld SEMG sensing device; a few years later, Cram and Engstrom[27] presented a normative database of 104 normal subjects, which they used to guide their clinical work. Using the scanning tool, they rapidly sampled the right and left aspects of as many as 15 muscle sites for patients in both the sitting and standing postures. This level of analysis of the postural elements of muscle led to the differentiation of three clinical concepts: (1) site of activity, (2) impact of posture, and (3) degree of symmetry.

Donaldson and Donaldson[28] took the concept of symmetry and made it dynamic. They studied the degree of symmetrical recruitment during symmetrical and asymmetrical movement patterns in both normal subjects and patients. From this work, they concluded that 20% asymmetry is acceptable during symmetrical movements; levels greater than this are considered pathognomonic. Conversely, asymmetrical movements should bring about asymmetrical recruitment patterns. Donaldson popularized the concept of *cocontractions* as an abnormal finding in asymmetrical movements.

During the 1980s, Will Taylor[29] introduced the concept of measuring synergy patterns in the upper and lower trapezius during abduction. Following the work of Karol Lewit,[30] Taylor noted that myalgias in the upper quarter were commonly associated with postural muscles doing the work of their phasic counterparts. Here, the upper trapezius dominated the stabilizing muscular action associated with abduction to 90 degrees, even though the lower trapezius should have been doing the stabilizing. Thus, Taylor saw the hyperactivity of the upper trapezius as being facilitated by the inhibition of the lower trapezius. Susan Middaugh and colleagues[31] have also clearly delineated the role of a hyperactive upper trapezius in headache and neck and shoulder pain. They concluded that almost all of the dysfunctional patterns in the upper back involve hyperactivity of the upper trapezius.

Scholarly research on SEMG has also flourished. During the early 1960s, Basmajian conceived of an international forum to share information on SEMG, and in 1965 the International Society of Electrophysiological Kinesiology (ISEK) was formed. The organization still exists today, publishing one of the only journals that specifically addresses issues pertaining to SEMG (*The Journal of Electromyography and Kinesiology*). The American and European academic communities (especially the Scandinavian researchers) have provided a strong fundamental basis for understanding EMG in general and SEMG in particular. Space limits the ability to acknowledge the many contributors to this field, but the influence of Carlo DeLuca and his colleagues at the Neuromuscular Research Institute in Boston cannot be overlooked. Much of their work on spectral analysis and muscle fatigue[32] has shed light on the physiology of muscle and methods of measuring it. The work of Scandinavian researchers on tension myalgia in the workplace is very impressive,[33-38] and has clearly added to our understanding of dysfunctions in the workplace. In addition, an excellent summary of the use of SEMG in the occupational setting may be found in a book by Soderberg.[39]

THE ADVANTAGES AND DISADVANTAGES OF SURFACE ELECTROMYOGRAPHY

The use of SEMG has many advantages. Surface EMG recordings provide a safe, easy, and noninvasive method that allows objective quantification of the energy of the muscle. It is not necessary to penetrate the skin and record from single motor units to obtain useful and meaningful information regarding muscles. Rather, one can "see" synergies in the energy patterns that cannot be seen with the naked eye. The technique allows the observer to see the muscle energy at rest and changing continuously over the course of a movement. With the use of multiple sensor arrays, it becomes possible to differentiate how different aspects of muscles do different things. Although palpation skills, muscle testing, and visual observation of posture and movement should never be discarded, they have their limitations. By adding SEMG recording information to the practitioner's fund of knowledge about the muscle function of a particular patient, the practitioner begins to blend valuable information concerning how the nervous system participates in the orchestration of the muscle function. By using SEMG, practitioners may be able to answer the following questions: Is the resting tone congruent with the palpation exam? Do the muscles fire early or late in a recruitment pattern? Does a particular exercise actually activate the muscle it is intended to, or is a substitution pattern present? Does the muscle turn off following a given movement, or does it show irritability following movement?

The tracings and numerical printouts associated with SEMG provide information to clinicians and researchers alike regarding mechanisms of muscle function and dysfunction; they also suggest methods to improve treatment approaches. The objective tracings and data from SEMG recordings allow clinicians to communicate with one another and to insurance carriers about their findings. In the Western world, such objective findings are considered essential. Finally, the biological information obtained via SEMG methods can be fed back to the patient, providing a basis for neuromuscular reeducation and for self-regulation. Such information can fine-tune the response of the patient's nervous system to the therapist's verbal instructions. When the therapist asks the patient to relax the muscle between movements, the patient can actually see whether he or she has "let go" of the recruitment pattern or if it is necessary to "let go" again. As the patient learns to recruit a particular muscle, the initial attempts may be compared to the current attempts. This type of information provides feedback and motivation for the patient's therapeutic efforts. It may also become an important source to demonstrate to third-party payers that the prescribed treatment is having the desired effect.

The weakness of SEMG is inherent in the anatomy we study, the instruments we use to study it, and the methods or procedures we choose to use. It is important that clinicians acknowledge and understand these limitations. One key limitation is our ability to monitor only a few muscle sites. The neuromuscular system is very rich and complex, and to reduce it to one or two channels of SEMG information is very limiting. At a minimum, a four-channel SEMG instrument allows one to study the right and left aspects of two opposing groups. At this level, the information becomes much more meaningful and practical. Scanning multiple sets of muscles in their resting state may help the practitioner to decide which regions of the musculature might be of further interest. Another possible shortcoming of SEMG recordings has to do with muscle substitution patterns. The neuromus-

cular system may express the same movement using different muscle groups. When this occurs, the naive practitioner may believe that SEMG recordings are either inconsistent or unreliable. Thus, it is important for practitioners to understand the "normal" case, so that they can interpret recordings with greater confidence. To that end, this book contains an atlas of tracings for many movement patterns (see Part III).

Another difficulty with SEMG is the possibility of "crosstalk," a phenomenon where energy from one muscle group travels over into the recording field of another muscle group. When this happens, problems may arise in the specificity of SEMG recordings. It may make it difficult or even impossible to isolate the SEMG recordings from a specific muscle. Some electrode placement sites have greater specificity than others. The electrode atlas grades the electrode sites according to their specificity. Three grades are used: general, quasi-specific, and specific. An additional limitation to SEMG is that, to date, there are only a few published guides to electrode placement[35,40–42] and two video presentations.[43,44] Unfortunately, none of these guides has become the standard. Thus, an upper trapezius recording from one clinic or study may not represent the same energy pattern recorded in another clinic because of differences in electrode placement. The atlas in this volume should be complete and comprehensive enough to encourage a more standardized method for SEMG electrode placement. Use of a standardized method strengthens the interpretation of SEMG recordings at a given muscle site.

The practitioner should remember that SEMG is not a measure of force, nor is it a measure of strength, or of the amount of effort given, or of muscle resting length. It is simply a measure of the electrical activity given off by the muscle. Practitioners must be cautious about how they interpret the SEMG findings, being careful not to overinterpret them. For example, under normal circumstances, one should not compare the SEMG amplitudes recorded from one muscle (e.g., upper trapezius) with that of another muscle (e.g., lower trapezius). Differences in the SEMG amplitudes during dynamic procedures may simply be due to differences in the amount of muscle mass present for each muscle, rather than to differences in how hard the muscles are working. To compare across muscle groups, one must normalize the SEMG data first (see Chapter 3). For example, clinicians might normalize the activity of the upper trapezius to lower trapezius as a ratio, or they might reference muscle groups to a maximum voluntary isometric contraction (MVIC) and work with the percentage of MVIC.

A final shortcoming is that SEMG electrodes are not totally unobtrusive. The electrodes and leads can potentially encumber a movement pattern or make the patient feel self-conscious about a posture or movement. Thus, the SEMG recordings may not perfectly reflect the customary patterns of use for the patient. Practitioners are encouraged to have several different kinds of electrodes on hand so that they can choose the correct type of electrode for the muscle and movement pattern they wish to study.

Readers are encouraged to keep the previously discussed strengths and limitations of SEMG in mind as they read this book. By learning what SEMG can and cannot do, clinicians will be able to serve their patients better.

REFERENCES

1. Basmajian JV, DeLuca C. *Muscles Alive*. 5th ed. Baltimore, MD: Williams & Wilkins; 1985.
2. Redi F. *Esperienze intorno a diverse cose naturali e particolarmente a quelle che ci sono portate dalle Indie*. Florence, Italy: 1617:47–51.
3. Wu CH. Electric fish and the discovery of animal electricity. *Am Scientist*. 1984;72:598–607.
4. Galvani L; Green RM, trans. *Commentary on the Effect of Electricity on Muscular Motion*. Cambridge, MA: 1953.
5. Volta A. Mommoria prima sull' elettricita animale. In *Collezione dell'Opere, II*. Florence, Italy: G. Piatti; 1792.
6. Duchenne GB; Kaplan EB, trans. *Physiology of Movement*. Philadelphia, PA: WB Saunders; 1949.
7. Du Bois-Reymond E. *Untersuchungen ueber thiersiche electricitae* (vol 2, second part). Berlin: Teimer-verlag; 1849.
8. Pratt FH. The all or none principle in graded response of skeletal muscle. *Am J Physiol*. 1917;44:517–542.
9. Gasser HS, Newcomer HS. Physiological action currents in the phrenic nerve: an application of the thermionic vacuum tube to nerve physiology. *Am J Physiol*. 1921;57:1–26.
10. Jacobson E. Electrical measurement concerning muscular contraction (tonus) and the cultivation of relaxation in man: Relaxation times of individuals. *Am J Physiol*. 1934;108:573–580.
11. Jacobson E. *You Must Relax*. New York, NY: McGraw-Hill; 1976.
12. Inman VT, Saunders JB, Abbott LC. Observations on the function of the shoulder joint. *J Bone Joint Surg*. 1944;26: 1–30.
13. Price JP, Clare MH, Ewerhardt RH. Studies in low backache with persistent spasm. *Achiev Phys Med*. 1948;29:703–709.
14. Floyd WF, Silver P. The function of the erector spinae muscles in certain movements and postures in man. *J Physiol*. 1955;129:184–203.
15. Whatmore G, Kohli D. *The Physiopathology and Treatment of Functional Disorders*. New York, NY: Grune & Stratton; 1974.
16. Basmajian JV. Control and training of individual motor units. *Science*. 1963;141:440–441.
17. Green EE, Walters ED, Green A, Murphy G. Feedback techniques for deep relaxation. *Psychophysiology*. 1969;6:371–377.
18. Budzynski T, Stoyva J, Adler C, Mullaney DJ. EMG biofeedback and tension study. *Psychosomatic Med*. 1973;35:484–496.
19. Hardyck CD, Petrincovich LV, Ellsworth DW. Feedback of speech muscle activity during silent reading: rapid extension. *Science*. 1966;154:1467–1468.
20. Booker HE, Rubow RT, Coleman PJ. Simplified feedback in neuromuscular retraining: an automated approach using EMG signals. *Arch Phys Med*. 1969;50:621–625.
21. Johnson HE, Garton WH. Muscle re-education in hemiplegia by use of electromyographic device. *Arch Phys Med*. 1973;54:320–322.
22. Wolf S, Basmajian JV. Assessment of paraspinal electromyographic activity in normal subjects and chronic back pain patients using a muscle biofeedback device. In: Asmussen E, Jorgensen K, eds. *International Series on Biomechanics, VI-B*. Baltimore, MD: University Press; 1978.
23. Wolf S, Nacht M, Kelly J. EMG feedback training during dynamic movement for low back pain patients. *Behav Ther*. 1982;13:395–406.
24. Sherman R, Arena J. Biofeedback for assessment and treatment of low back pain. In: Basmajian JV, Wolf S, eds. *Rational Manual Therapies*. Baltimore, MD: Williams & Wilkins; 1994:177–197.
25. Dolce JJ, Raczynski JM. Neuromuscular activity and electromyography in painful backs: psychological and biomechanical models in assessment and treatment. *Psychological Bull*. 1985;97:502–520.
26. Cram JR, Steger JC. Muscle scanning and the diagnosis of chronic pain. *Biofeedback Self-Regul*. 1983;8:229–241.
27. Cram JR, Engstrom D. Patterns of neuromuscular activity in pain and non-pain patients. *Clin Biofeedback Health*. 1986;9:106–116.
28. Donaldson S, Donaldson M. Multi-channel EMG assessment and treatment techniques. In: Cram JR, ed. *Clinical EMG for Surface Recordings, II*. Nevada City, CA: Clinical Resources; 1990:143–174.
29. Taylor W. Dynamic EMG biofeedback in assessment and treatment using a neuromuscular re-education model. In: Cram JR, ed. *Clinical EMG for Surface Recordings, II*. Nevada City, CA: Clinical Resources; 1990:175–196.
30. Lewit K. *Manipulative Therapy in Rehabilitation of the Locomotor System*. Boston, MA: Butterworth Heinemann; 1991.
31. Middaugh SJ, Kee WG, Nicholson JA. Muscle overuse and posture as factors in the development and maintenance of chronic musculoskeletal pain. In: Grzesiak RC, Ciccone DS, eds. *Psychological Vulnerability to Chronic Pain*. New York, NY: Springer; 1994:55–89.

32. DeLuca C. Myoelectric manifestations of localized muscular fatigue in humans. *CRC Crit Rev Biomed Eng.* 1984;11:251.

33. Hagberg M. Occupational musculoskeletal stress disorders of the neck and shoulder: a review of possible pathophysiology. *Int Arch Occup Environ Health.* 1984;53: 269–278.

34. Hagberg M. Muscular endurance and surface EMG in isometric and dynamic exercise. *Arch Phys Med.* 1981; 60:111–121.

35. Jonsson B. Kinesiology: With special reference to electromyographic kinesiology. *Cont Clin Neurophysiol EEG Suppl.* 1978;34:417–428.

36. Mathiassen SE, Winkel J, Hagg GM. Normalization of surface EMG amplitude from the upper trapezius muscle in ergonomic studies: a review. *J Electromyogr Kinesiol.* 1995;5:199–226.

37. Veiersted KB, Westgaard RH, Andersen P. Electromyographic evaluation of muscular work pattern as a predictor of trapezius myalgia. *Scand J Work Environ Health.* 1993;19:284–290.

38. Winkel J, Mathiassen SE, Haag GM. Normalization of upper trapezius EMG amplitude in ergonomic studies. *J Electromyogr Kinesiol.* 1995;5:195–198.

39. Soderberg GL, ed. *Selected Topics in Surface Electromyography for Use in the Occupational Setting: Expert Perspective.* Washington, DC: U.S. Department of Health and Human Services; 1992. U.S. Department of Health and Human Services publication NIOSH 91–100.

40. Basmajian JV, Blumenstein R. Electrode placement in electromyographic biofeedback. In: Basmajian JV, ed. *Biofeedback: Principles and Practice for Clinicians.* Baltimore, MD: Williams & Wilkins; 1989:363–377.

41. Cram JR. *Clinical EMG for Surface Recordings, I.* Poulsbo, WA: J&J Engineering; 1986.

42. Fridlund AJ, Cacioppo JT. Guidelines for human electromyographic research. *Psychophysiology.* 1986; 23:567–598.

43. Cram JR, Holtz J. *Introduction to Electrode Placement* [videotape]. Nevada City, CA: Clinical Resources; 1995.

44. Wolf S. *Anatomy and Electrode Placement: Upper Extremities; Face and Back; Lower Extremities* [videotape]. Nevada City, CA: Clinical Resources; 1991.

Anatomy and Physiology

BASIC OVERVIEW OF THE NEUROMUSCULAR SYSTEM

To consider the human musculature outside the context of a complex and interdependent system such as the human body is probably not fair. Without the connective tissue providing the "sacks" for the muscle fibers, the muscles would neither be organized into meaningful directions of pull, nor would they be anchored to the bones, and their actions would not produce movement of the body. Without a digestive system, there would be no glucose available for the body to burn. Without the lungs, there would be no oxygen to fan the flames of cellular respiration and produce the gasoline for the muscle—adenosine triphosphate (ATP). Without a circulatory system, these vital substances would not find their way to each and every cell, nor would the waste products of muscular metabolism (lactic acid) be carried away. Finally, without the nervous system, the muscle cells would not know when to fire or how to orchestrate their firings with other muscle cells.

Huxley states that the muscle is truly the primary organ of the human body, the dominant tissue of animal life.[1] After all, 70% to 85% of gross body weight is typically muscle. (Exceptions to this rule occur with extreme obesity.) Muscle is the largest consumer of energy in the body. The metabolic needs of muscle increase radically as a function of work, while the needs of the other organ

systems increase to only a small degree. In the human body there are literally millions of tiny muscle cells called myofibrils. These muscle cells do their work through shortening their resting lengths via a process of ratcheting myosin fibers against the actin fiber. Without an adequate supply of oxygen and glucose to form APT, along with the removal of lactic acid, muscle fatigue sets in and the muscle ceases to function.

It is essential to understand the connective tissue and bones if we are to understand muscle function. Connective tissue is found throughout the human body and is essentially responsible for "gluing" it all together. For muscles, it provides the sacks or fasciae that house and organize the muscles. More than 600 of these muscle compartments exist, each of which is systematically placed under the direction of the genetic code. Not only does connective tissue form the boundaries of each and every muscle, but the connective tissue known as tendons also connects the muscles to the bones and provides a series of anchors or pulleys through which the forces of muscle action work. When this connective tissue develops tears, shortenings, or other irregularities, the organization of the muscles in the immediate area may become disordered.

The bones provide the rigidity needed for erect posture and movement of the extremities. Without the bones, our muscles would pool as a quivering mass on the floor, unable to do any work. Muscles are affected by asymmetrical growth patterns in the bones. Leg-length discrepancies of more than one-half inch, for example, cause faulty posture. Ligaments, another type of connective tissue, secure bone to bone. They also provide the needed limitations in range of motion, while adding stability to the bones themselves. In fact, all of the bones in the body are knit together with ligaments. This lends a certain coherence to the support that the bones provide. The spine and pelvis are very clear examples of this phenomenon.

Mother Nature would much prefer that we rest on our bones and ligaments as the means of holding ourselves erect in the neutral posture against the gravitational field, thereby sparing the metabolic consequences of using muscle to do the same task. But what happens to our muscles when we habitually defy the well-aligned posture? In essence, they overwork and often eventually ache. It is as if Mother Nature is using the ache to beckon us back into stacking our weight on our bones and ligaments.

What happens if we fall or otherwise tear the connective tissue from around the bones? Such microtears are not uncommon in spinal flexion/extension injuries associated with motor vehicle accidents. This ligament laxity may create disorder in associated muscles. The muscles tend to increase their tonus around the injured joint, as if to provide an internal splint to the bones. Although this splinting may provide an effective short-term solution to a weakened joint, the long-term consequence is usually pain.

If there is asymmetry in the nature of connective tissue associated with a particular joint, this imbalance usually leads to an asymmetrical recruitment of the muscles associated with that joint. For example, if the left temporomandibular joint (TMJ) has ligament laxity while the right aspect of the joint has normal ligamental support, an asymmetrical recruitment of motor units will be seen in surface electromyography (SEMG) recordings from homologous muscles during a symmetrical movement (e.g., opening the mouth). Surface EMG monitoring can help clinicians interpret information about the joints (end range of motion or joint play) and can help manual therapists demonstrate the effects of mobilization of the joint. The postmanipulation effects on SEMG should yield normalized recruitment patterns ($\pm 20\%$) during symmetrical dynamic movements. In addition, feedback and retraining of the newly mobilized joint may help prevent the movements and postures of life from creating the same limitation in the future.

If the fasciae provide the sacks for the muscles, and the bones provide the rigidity needed for an erect posture, then it is the muscle bulk (along with other connective tissue) that gives the body its final shape. In addition, muscles provide stability to the bones. The skeleton cannot stand erect by itself. It is the muscles that give us our posture—our stance toward life. This stance relies on both mechanical (gravitational) and emotional contributions. It is the muscles that give us the dynamic movement we associate with life itself.

The recruitment of muscle would not happen were it not for the nervous system. The *motor unit* is the final common pathway of the alpha motor system's outflow to the end plates located on the muscle fibers. The lower motor neuron associated with the motor unit resides in the ventral horn of the spinal cord. Hundreds or even thousands of interneuronal connections converge upon that motor neuron (see **Figure 2–1**). The segmental interplay of the spinal reflexes is driven by excitatory and inhibitory potentials: The stretch receptors of the muscle spindle place an excitatory valence on the lower motor neuron, while the Golgi tendon organs provide the reflex-driven inhibitory potentials. These two inputs function as sensory motor integrators that deal with gravity, the mass of everyday life, and our efforts to interact with the world. They keep us up and moving and inform the rest of the nervous system of the instantaneous length of each muscle and the force it is exerting.

The lower motor neuron is also regulated by upper motor neurons. Some of these come directly from the cortex, carrying out fine motor intentions. The thought behind a movement originates in the frontal lobes. It then passes through the prefrontal cortex to pick up the general body position in space needed for the movement. Then it goes through the motor strip to pick up the final details of any fine motor aspects of the movement. Some of the cortical outflow goes directly to the lower motor neuron via the pyramidal tracts. Some travel via the extrapyramidal tract, which synapses with lower centers of the brain. Here the intended movement is integrated with the internal (kinesthetic) and external senses, and is blended with motor patterns associated with given and acquired reflexes. The cerebellum monitors the whole affair, fine-tuning the final act.

When examining muscles, clinicians tend to study each compartment for its own function. Manual muscle testing is routinely taught as a method to isolate the strength of a given muscle. To test muscles correctly, one must know how to position the limb, where to resist it, how to coach the subject to exert effort, and how to

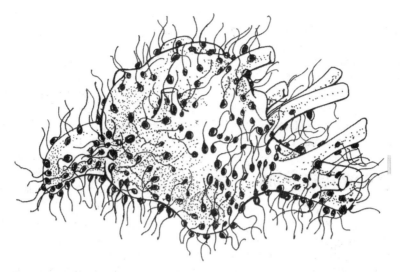

Figure 2–1 A reconstructed model of a spinal motor neuron showing the large number of small presynaptic knobs from other neurons terminating on it.

Source: Reproduced from J. Mishlove. *The Roots of Consciousness.* Random House, 1975. Illustration by Sherry Hogue. Scan provided courtesy of Jeffrey Mishlove.

grade the strength of the resulting effort. These tests are far from natural movement patterns. Rather, they are more like slices of unique movement patterns, taken out of a normal muscle contraction context and frozen in time. They are relevant only to the extent that the information gained can be placed within a more functional context.

A single, discrete muscle rarely works on its own in a real and varied life situation. The nervous system has more than 600 muscles from which to choose and an area as large as the human form with which to work. Many muscles need to serve the three functions of posture, emotions, and motions. To think of testing one muscle is entirely too simplistic. Instead, the only way in which muscle testing works is to have a theory of dysfunction that involves areas of effort up and down the kinetic chain of movement. Then, in the process of determining which muscles are weak or strong in that chain, all or part of the chain might be tested.

When testing muscles, the clinician should assess muscle grouping such as agonists (prime movers), synergists (helpers), and antagonists (opposing muscle groups). In addition, as the tests move toward real and varied life activities, it becomes necessary to address issues of timing. Surface EMG as an assessment tool, like muscle testing, begins to make sense only when it is viewed in a much broader perspective. Along with muscle testing, SEMG can be used to monitor the muscles

involved or suspected to be involved in a particular movement. In this way, clinicians can assess not only the muscles' strength, but also their synergy with other muscles.

This type of thinking is illustrated by simple abduction of the left arm. Imagine that the subject is standing with arms at his or her sides. The intention is to raise the left arm out from the side to a horizontal 90-degree posture. The muscle fibers of the middle deltoid act as the primary mover. The anterior and posterior aspects of the deltoid assist in a synergistic fashion. The upper fibers of the trapezius, along with the deeper supraspinatus, also assist in this movement. The middle and lower fibers of the trapezius, serratus anterior, and others stabilize the scapula to anchor the weight of the 15-pound arm against the chest wall. Because this is an asymmetrical action, the erector spinae muscles on the contralateral (right) side begin to activate to stabilize the cantilevered effect of gravity's pull on the torso. This places a strain on the pelvis, which is stabilized by the gluteus medius and tensor fasciae latae. The left leg bears a greater weight, and muscles are slightly activated in various aspects of the thigh, calf, and foot. In addition, it is necessary to superimpose the waves of respiration in the abdominal and intercostal area upon this holding pattern. Place a little bit of emotional arousal into the situation, and the overall tone is increased by, say, 10%. Place a 10-pound weight in the outstretched hand, and the recruitment pattern along the entire kinetic chain increases dramatically. Such a weight can be held at this height for only a short period of time, because the more distal muscles begin to fatigue much faster than the more proximal postural muscles. Within the first minute, the volley of activity to the middle deltoid has increased and synchronized to counter the fatigue factor. Within 4 minutes the failure point is reached, the arm gives way to the gravitational pull, and the posture is recalibrated.

MUSCLE FIBERS AND HOW THEY WORK

To understand how muscles work, it is helpful to examine a muscle from a macroscopic level to a microscopic level. On a macroscopic level, muscle fibers are grouped together and traditionally identified by their line of action, their direction of pull, and their origins and insertions. A closer examination of this arrangement, however, reveals that the muscle really consists of compartments. Rather than being one massive muscle, some muscles are really a series of smaller compartments that run in the same direction or in slightly different directions. Each compartment provides a subtly different pull on the lever arm. Researchers have demonstrated "compartmentalization" for the biceps,[2,3] extensor and flexor carpi radialis,[4,5] soleus,[6] and gastrocnemius.[7] Researchers are beginning to understand the compartmentalization of muscles better, and compartmentalization may soon come to replace the more macroscopic view of origins and insertions that is presently taught in educational programs as the primary level for understanding muscle function.

Each muscle compartment contains muscle fibers (see **Figure 2–2**). These fibers may be clustered together into narrow subcompartments separated by a thin septum of connective tissue that holds the muscle cells together in their parallel arrangements. These individual fibers may be broken down into clusters of individual *myofibrils*, which are tiny, hairlike strands. Under a microscope, myofibrils appear to be braided in light and dark bands. Each myofibril consists of aggregates of *myosin* and *actin* filaments. The basic anatomical structure from which all muscles are made is called a *sarcomere*. It is defined as a single unit of overlapping myosin and actin filaments from one *Z* line to the next *Z* line in the muscle. These dark lines reflect the attachment of actin fibers. Within the sarcomere, there are areas where only actin resides (*I* bands), areas where only myosin resides (*H* bands), and areas where myosin

overlaps the actin fibers (*A* bands). The *A* band is where all of the work of the cross-bridging takes place.

The actin filament is a thin fiber with two negatively charged molecules that spiral around each other. The myosin filament is a much thicker filament with "globular heads" on it. These filaments are also negatively charged. In the resting state, these two filaments lie next to each other, mutually repelled by their negative charges. In the 1950s, Huxley[8] proposed a "ratchet" or sliding filament model that describes the generation of active tension. In this model, each globular head of the myosin fiber has one ATP molecule attached to it, which is negatively charged.

The nerve action potential from the lower motor neuron causes a release of acetylcholine (ACh) at the neuromuscular junction. This sends a charge through the transverse tubules (**Figure 2–3**) that, when it reaches the sarcoplasmic reticulum, allows pores to be opened and calcium ions to flood the space where the myosin and actin fibers are located. Each calcium ion has a very strong positive charge to it, and it bonds instantly with the actin filament. At this point, the negatively charged myosin filament with its ATP molecule is strongly attracted to the now positively charged actin filament (**Figure 2–4**). As these two filaments are pressed against each other by the chemically induced electromagnetic attraction, the globular heads are forced to flatten out; the resulting ratchet effect forces the two filaments to move past each other. The force of the bending of the globular heads, however, causes the ATP molecule to be released. The energy associated with this release provides the energy needed to free the calcium ion from the actin fiber and pumps it back to the sarcoplasmic reticulum. Simultaneously, the myosin and actin filaments separate from each other, being held slightly apart by the two negative charges. Immediately, another ATP molecule attaches to the globular head on the myosin filament and the cycle is ready to begin all over again. Thus, the globular heads of the myosin act as cross-bridges for the actin chains. Through successive activations and cross-bridging, the muscle twitches while it shortens and work is done.

The metabolized ATP molecule, now known as adenosine diphosphate (ADP), is reconstituted in the mitochondria. Using the Krebs cycle, the mitochondrion rebuilds the ADP back into ATP, using the glucose and oxygen provided by the circulation system. The byproducts of this process include lactic acid, free hydrogen ions, and carbon dioxide. These by-products need to be

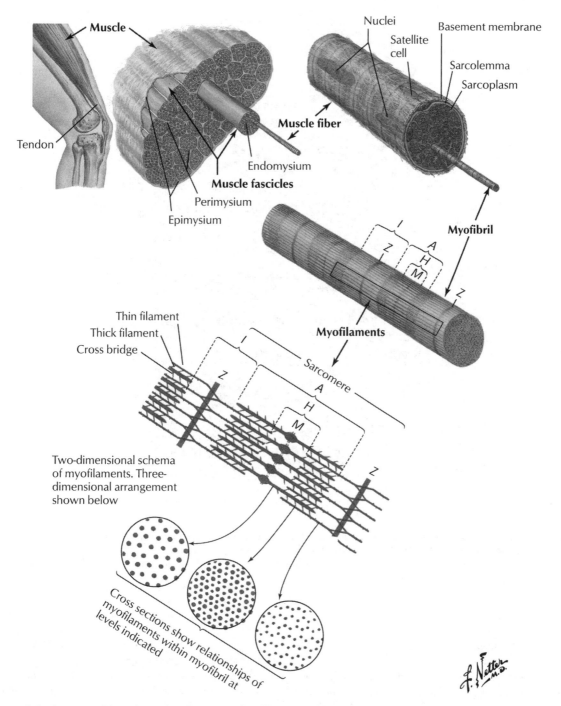

Figure 2–2 The composition of muscle cells, muscle fascicles, muscle fiber, myofibril, myofilaments, sarcomere, thick and thin filaments.

Source: Netter Anatomy Illustration Collection, © Elsevier, Inc. All Rights Reserved.

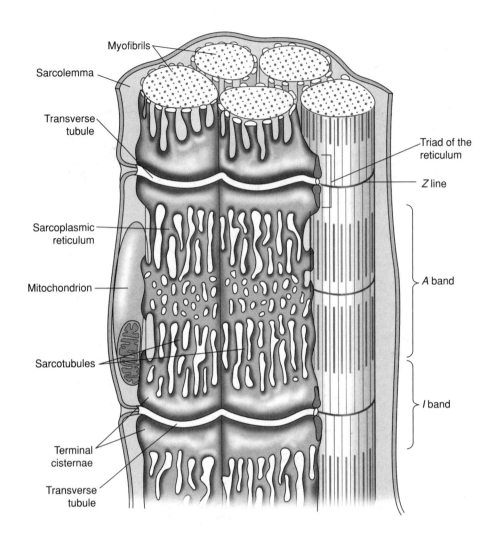

Myofibrils

Sarcolemma

Transverse tubule

Triad of the reticulum

Z line

Sarcoplasmic reticulum

Mitochondrion

A band

Sarcotubules

I band

Terminal cisternae

Transverse tubule

Figure 2–3 The system of transverse tubules in a section of muscle cell. Transverse tubules create an intricate, three-dimensional maze, surrounding every bundle of myosin and actin filament.

Source: Adapted from W. Bloom and D.W. Fawcett, *A Textbook of Histology*, © 1970, Chapman & Hall.

removed and transported away from the muscle cell via the circulatory system.

The strength of the contraction is greater when the muscle is elongated to about its midpoint of the filament sliding range. This phenomenon has to do with the structure of the myosin and actin fibers. **Figure 2–5** illustrates the relationship between strength (percentage of maximum tension) and degree of myosin–actin overlap. Strength is lost when there is very little overlap of the two fiber types and when the overlap is complete.

Strength is found in the middle range, where a number of myosin-actin cross-bridges can be formed.

Muscle fibers can be divided into three broad categories based on appearance, speed of contraction, and fatigability:

- Slow-twitch muscles take more than 35 milliseconds to complete a depolarization/repolarization cycle and are reddish in appearance. These muscles twitch

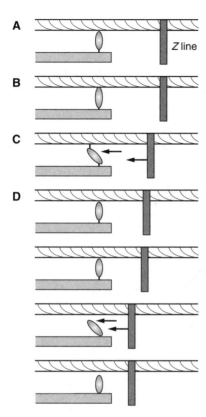

Figure 2–4 The ratchet effect. (A) Prior to the calcium bonding, the myosin heads with their negative ATP molecule are held away from the negative actin filament. (B) After calcium bonding, the negative ATP myosin heads attach to the now positive actin. This positive bond is also attracted to the negative myosin shaft. (C) The myosin head folds downward, pulling the actin chain forward one notch. (D) The ATP myosin bond breaks under the stress of the folding and releases the myosin filament from the actin chain, allowing the globular head to stand upright again. Immediately, another ATP molecule attaches to it. As the muscle fibers depolarize, ratchet themselves to a shorter resting length, and repolarize, they undergo one motor unit action potential (MUAP) or twitch.

cycle and are whitish in appearance. These are classified as Type II, fast-twitch fibers. Fast-twitch fibers twitch at a rate faster than 25 twitches per second, which is typically between 30 and 50 Hz.

A classic example in the human body of fast- and slow-twitch muscles is found in the calf of the leg. The soleus consists of predominantly slow-twitch fibers and is reddish in color, while the gastrocnemius consists primarily of fast-twitch fibers and is a paler color. The morphological differentiation of the fiber type is determined by the type of motor nerve that activates the fibers. Small, slow nerve fibers develop slow-twitch muscles; large, fast nerve fibers develop fast-twitch muscles. Most muscles contain a mixture of fast- and slow-twitch fibers.

The distinctions made between the two types of muscle fibers—slow, fatigue-resistant versus fast, fatigable—represent a gross oversimplification; in reality, a gradation along a continuum for the attributes given later in this section would better represent the types of fibers. In general, however, Type I fibers are smaller in size and produce less tension. They are innervated by small, slow-moving neuronal axons. They are fairly resilient to fatigue and are more amenable to anaerobic glucolysis. They have a low reflex threshold from the muscle spindle and Golgi tendon organ and generally tend to maintain a tonic repetitive discharge. In contrast, Type II fibers have a low reflex threshold and respond reflexively with short burst patterns. In general terms, the Type I fibers appear ideal for postural activities and the Type II fibers seem best suited for phasic movement.

Not only do different fiber types perform different types of work, but the same muscle fiber types can do work in different ways. Three clearly identifiable types of muscle contractions are distinguished: isometric, concentric, and eccentric. The SEMG patterns observed during dynamic protocols may differ, depending upon which type of contraction one is studying.

Isometric contractions are muscle contractions in which a constant muscle length is maintained. Technically, the contractile force does not exceed the force of resistance and, therefore, there is no change in muscle length. These contractions are used in postural control and for stabilization of axial body parts during extreme movements. They are also used during manual muscle testing. Surface EMG recordings are typically greatest under isometric testing conditions.

fewer than 25 times per second, usually around 10 to 20 Hertz (Hz—a unit of frequency equal to one cycle per second).

- Fast-twitch, fatigue-resistant muscles are pale in appearance and, like the slow-twitch muscles, have a considerable ability for aerobic metabolism. These are classified as Type I, fast-twitch fibers.

- Fast-twitch, fatigable muscles take less than 35 milliseconds to complete a contraction or twitch

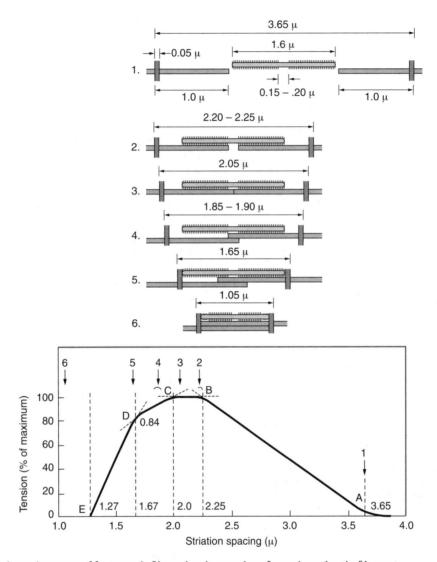

Figure 2–5 Length-tension curve of frog muscle fiber related to overlap of myosin and actin filaments.

Source: Reprinted with permission from the *Journal of Physiology*, Vol. 184, pp. 170–192, © 1966, The Physiological Society.

Concentric contractions occur when the muscle shortens during the contraction. Technically, a concentric contraction is defined as a contraction with enough force to overcome the external resistance, thereby allowing the muscle to shorten. During concentric contractions, the moving body part usually accelerates. This type of contraction is the action taken by a prime mover during the active phase of a movement pattern. A classic example of concentric contractions is biceps activity during elbow flexion associated with lifting a weight. The amount of muscular energy available is greater during an isometric contraction than during a concentric contraction, because 20% of the energy efficiency of the movement is lost during concentric contraction due to the shortening of the muscle. Thus, the greatest load that a concentric muscle contraction can carry is only 80% of the load carried by maximum isometric contraction.

Eccentric contractions occur when the muscle lengthens during a contraction. Technically, eccentric contractions occur in an already shortened muscle where the external force is greater than the tension created by the muscle contraction. Here, the muscle acts as a braking agent as a load is manipulated. The classic example of eccentric contraction is biceps activity as the weight is slowly lowered during elbow extension. Eccentric contractions are extremely common. In fact, every movement in the direction of gravity is controlled by an eccentric contraction. Other examples include sitting, squatting, lying down, bending forward or sideways, and going down stairs. The amount of energy expended during an eccentric contraction is always less than that observed during a concentric contraction for the same muscle. The amount of metabolic work associated with eccentric contractions is one-third to one-thirteenth the work of concentric contractions. In SEMG recordings, the microvolt amplitude of a concentric contraction is always larger than it is for the eccentric contraction, given the same amount of weight. For example, the erector spinae of the low back work harder and show higher levels of recruitment when returning from a flexed position than when going down into forward flexion from the neutral position. Researchers believe that the eccentric contractions require less SEMG activity because much of the work has to do with "breaking" existing cross-bridges rather than building new cross-bridges.

Another form of contraction is isotonic contraction, a subset (special class) of the concentric and eccentric contractions. Isotonic contractions occur when constant muscle force is employed as the muscle either shortens or lengthens. This type of force is studied most commonly on instruments in which the force is controlled over the range of motion.

Surface EMG recruitment patterns may differ when they are observed in an open versus closed kinetic chain. In an *open kinetic chain*, the distal segment is free to move—as in the case where a person is not bearing weight in the lower extremities. The open kinetic chain entails a movement that is not resisted manually or through weight bearing. Movement of one joint does not necessarily cause movement in other joints. In a *closed kinetic chain*, the distal segment is fixed, as in weight bearing for the lower extremities. Movement at one joint induces movement at another joint. For example, in sitting with the leg hanging over the edge of the table (open kinetic chain), a person can move the ankle without moving the knee or hip. But when the person stands (closed kinetic chain), he or she cannot move the ankle without affecting other joints. Surface EMG recruitment patterns are typically greater under the conditions of a closed kinetic chain compared to those observed under the conditions of an open kinetic chain. For example, the level of SEMG activity from rectus femoris during a squat (closed kinetic chain) is greater than when the muscle is contracted from the seated position and the knee extends without resistance (open kinetic chain).

SENSORY MOTOR INTEGRATION

Initially, researchers thought that muscles were relatively insensitive structures. They derived this conclusion from the observation that a surgeon could cut and probe muscle tissue with the patient experiencing little or no pain. More recently, however, researchers have discovered that muscle is actually quite rich and sophisticated in its sensory apparatus. Of the sensory organs found within the muscle, the two major sensory systems are the *muscle spindle* and the *Golgi tendon organ*.

The muscle spindle is the stretch receptor. It contains specialized nerve endings that provide the nervous system with information concerning the instantaneous resting length of the muscle and velocity (or rate) of change. The output of the muscle spindle is transmitted to the cord and terminates on an excitatory alpha motor neuron. This arrangement assists in the fine calibration of alpha motor output and the resulting muscle contraction at a local or spinal level. If the output from the muscle spindle is strong or sharp enough, it may result in alpha motor output, causing the extrafusal fibers that surround the muscle spindle to contract, thereby causing the muscle in which it is located to shorten (see **Figure 2–6**). In addition, the muscle spindle simultaneously transmits information to the reticular core and basal ganglia to help modulate the descending motor pathways. Because spindle activity is not projected to the cortex, it is not consciously perceived.

These tiny stretch receptors are associated with *intrafusal muscle fibers*, which are scattered among and run parallel to the large extrafusal muscle fibers in which they are housed (see **Figure 2–7**). The intrafusal muscles are much smaller (5 to 10 fibers) and shorter (4 to 10 mm) than the extrafusal muscle fibers. The extrafusal fibers are innervated by the *alpha motor system* and are designed to do the work of moving bones; the intrafusal fibers are innervated by the *gamma motor system* and are designed to adjust the calibration of the stretch receptor. Because muscles are constantly changing their length as they do work, and because the stretch receptors inform the central nervous system (CNS) of the instantaneous length and velocity of the muscle fibers, it is vitally important to continually adjust the tonus on the stretch receptor. Perhaps that is why nearly one-third of the descending efferent motor nerve fibers are associated

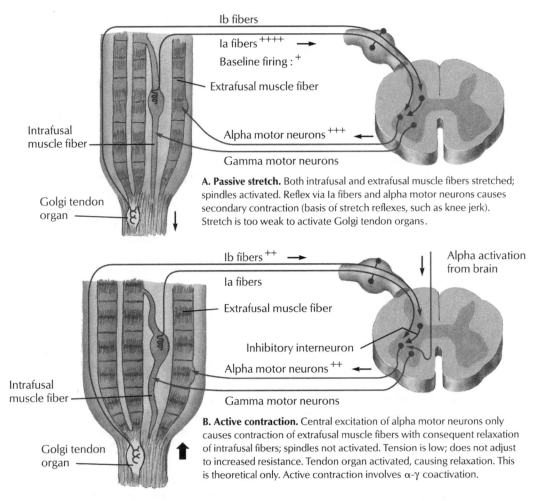

Figure 2–6 Relationship of muscle spindle and Golgi tendon organ to extrafusal muscle fibers. (A) Spindle (located within the intrafusal muscle fiber) is parallel to the muscle fibers so that passive muscle stretch causes a secondary contraction or stretch reflex. (B) Muscle contraction slackens tension on the spindle. Golgi tendon organ is in series with the muscle fibers (resides between the muscle fibers and their bony attachments) so that both passive and active contractions of the muscle cause the receptor to become active.

Source: Netter Anatomy Illustration Collection, © Elsevier, Inc. All Rights Reserved.

with the gamma motor system. These gamma motor nerves are smaller and have slower conduction velocities than the alpha motor nerves. The gamma motor system primarily emerges from the lower centers of the brain, while the alpha motor system originates primarily from the cortex. There is commonly a CNS linkage or coactivation of the alpha and gamma motor systems—a relationship that was first observed by Hunt and Kuffler[9] in the 1950s, and elaborated upon by Vallbo[10] in the 1980s.

The primary purpose of the muscle spindle, then, is to regulate the muscle length, make postural adjustments, and maintain a predicted muscle length and ve-

locity. An artificial example of this functionality is the knee jerk. When the patella tendon receives a swift blow, the quadriceps muscle is unpredictably and suddenly elongated, and the muscle spindle is stretched. This leads to excitatory outflow to the motor neuron, which results in the contraction of the quadriceps muscle. This, in turn, quiets the muscle spindle. The briskness of this response is commonly graded in neurological examinations. On a functional level, the briskness of the response is determined by the output of the gamma motor system. Edmund Jacobson[11] conducted studies on progressive relaxation procedures, in which he was able to demonstrate a substantial diminution (if

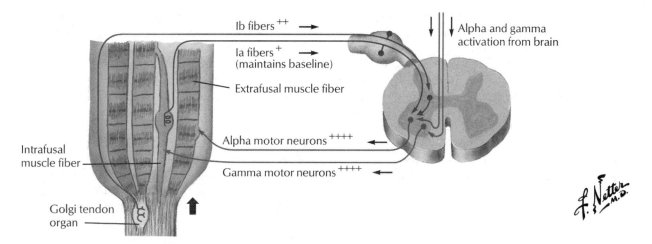

Figure 2–7 Relationship of alpha and gamma motor neurons to muscle spindles and Golgi tendon organs. The alpha and gamma motor systems must coordinate to maintain the correct tension on the muscle spindle.

Source: Netter Anatomy Illustration Collection, © Elsevier, Inc. All Rights Reserved.

not frank absence) in the knee jerk in patients who were deeply relaxed. Thus, one can learn to alter and control the sensitivity of the stretch receptor through alterations in the level of gamma motor activity through deep relaxation.

In real-life situations, the muscle spindle monitors the effects of the gravitational field upon a person's posture and helps keep the person erect. For example, when a person walks along an uneven surface, the muscle spindle constantly adjusts the tone of the muscle (excitatory input to the alpha motor neuron) to compensate for the unpredicted stretches upon the muscle. The resting tone of the gamma motor system is especially important for an athlete. If the muscle tone is too high or too low, the timing and effort of the athletic performance can be thrown off. Researchers have recently found that the muscle spindle responds to emotional arousal.[4] Perhaps this response explains why professional and Olympic athletes work on their emotions and attitudes toward their performances just as much as on their motor coordination skills.

Recently, the muscle spindle has been suggested as a potential site for the *trigger point*.[12] Trigger points are anatomical locations that, when activated by pressure or movement, refer pain to the immediate area or a distant site.[13] Dynamic SEMG studies[14] have reported that during a symmetrical movement (i.e., forward flexion of the head), muscles that have an active trigger point tend to contract at a higher level of activation than do the contralateral muscles without trigger points. This find-

ing suggests that an active trigger point in a muscle tends to alter the sensitivity of muscle spindles for the involved muscle, making it more sensitive to changes in its length.

Another important sensory organ within the muscle is the Golgi tendon organ (see Figures 2–6 and 2–7), which is found at the muscle tendon junction and runs in series with the muscle. It is exquisitely sensitive to the tension placed on the tendon, and it perceives the effort given out by the muscle. On its most basic level, the output from the Golgi tendon organ loops through the cord and inhibits the alpha motor neuron for the 5 to 10 motor units that are pulling on it. In essence, the inhibitory influence of the Golgi tendon organ protects the muscle from tearing itself loose from its attachments. On a more subtle level, the Golgi tendon organ informs the CNS of the effort that is under way and facilitates the necessary inhibition needed for learning. For example, when a piano student is learning to distinguish between playing the piano softly and playing it loudly, the student must learn to press on the keys in soft and hard fashion. While the ear can readily hear the difference, the Golgi tendon organ can feel the difference; it provides the proprioceptive basis for knowing when the key has been pressed just hard enough. The output of the Golgi tendon organ terminates in the lower centers of the brain (i.e., basal ganglia). This output does not reach the cortex, so we are unconscious of its presence. Yet it is through the interaction of the information supplied by the Golgi tendon organ with the information provided by higher centers that we acquire basic and refined motor skills. Like the spindle apparatus, the Golgi tendon organ makes our muscular efforts more efficient.

Two other sense organs are found inside the muscle itself. The first is the *pacinian corpuscle*, which is capable of measuring the deep, internal pressure within the muscle. The second is the *free nerve ending*, which is sensitive to nocioception or pain. The afferent pain travels via the lateral spinothalamic tract, reaches the cortex, and is consciously perceived. This pain receptor is activated by a change in the acidity of muscle or by chemical changes associated with swelling, edema, and inflammation.

When the muscle does work, the metabolic by-product of this process is a substance called *lactic acid*. When lactic acid is retained in the muscle due to the lack of adequate circulation (associated with a sustained muscle contraction), the free nerve ending is activated. For example, when a person makes a very tight fist and holds it for several minutes, he or she begins to feel a dull ache in the forearm muscles. This dull ache emanates from the free nerve ending and is associated with the disturbance of the microcirculation in the muscle itself and the resultant buildup of lactic acid. Usually this type of pain follows a prolonged activation pattern in fairly close temporal sequence.

In contrast, pain associated with inflammation usually lags behind the activating event by several hours. Inflammation can be brought about by the overuse of muscles, but because of fluid transport issues, it simply takes longer to develop. For example, a person who is out of shape and goes skiing for the first time of the season will probably tire from time to time but might not experience pain during the skiing because of adequate perfusion of the tissue associated with the rhythmic use of the muscles. On the ride home or the next day, however, that person might feel the muscle soreness associated with the overuse of the muscles. This overuse may be associated with microtears in the muscle tissue and is accompanied by inflammation. The afferent from the free nerve endings (nociception) loops through the cord, placing an excitatory bias on the lower motor neuron and forming the basis for the withdrawal reflex. In addition, this afferent interfaces with the gamma motor system, potentially providing the basis for muscle *splinting*—Mother Nature's way of providing a muscular "cast" for an injured area.

Another source of information about muscle function is found in the *joint receptors* (e.g., Ruffini endings). Such apparatus is found in each and every joint. It is sensitive to one degree of arc, and never habituates (turns off). It continuously provides the nervous system with information concerning joint angle and position. One of the important aspects of this sensory system is that we are conscious of it. Although we are not conscious of the level of tension in our muscles, we are readily aware of our limb and joint position. For example, it may make more sense to talk to a patient about how high the shoulders are than to talk about how tense the upper trapezius muscles might be. Similarly, it is easier for patients to respond to the request to lower the shoulders than to a request to relax them. This terminology simply makes more sense to patients, because they can be consciously aware of joint movements yet consciously blind to their tension levels.

The sensory network of the muscles provides a wealth of information to the central nervous system concerning muscle function. Some of these influences are excitatory, some are inhibitory, some reach the cortex and are conscious, and some terminate in the lower brain and are not consciously perceived. All pass through the cord and influence the segmental intelligence of the total system.

NERVOUS SYSTEM CONTROL

The nervous system's control of the neuromuscular system can be roughly broken into three levels, which are organized both hierarchically and in parallel. The lowest level is the spinal reflex, with its segmental and suprasegmental organization and intelligence. This level is primarily associated with survival and the mechanical work humans do against gravity. The middle level is represented by the lower brain. This level includes some of the prewired reflexes, some of the acquired reflexes, postural reflexes aided by the semicircular canals, the fine-tuning of movements by the cerebellum, and the limbic system that controls the emotional aspect of muscle. At the highest level is the cortex, where three-quarters of all nerve cells reside. It is here that intentionality of movement occurs, along with learning, associations, and thought.

If a person wants to touch a finger to the nose, the following events will more than likely take place. At a cortical level, the frontal lobes create the plan; the plan passes through the premotor cortex to organize how the body, as a whole, will fit into the plan; the motor strip integrates the fine movements of pointing the finger. Some of this information passes directly to the motor units associated with the fine motor control of the upper extremity. Other aspects of the cortical information connect with the basal ganglia to pick up the reflexes (acquired) needed to assist in this movement and to integrate the other sense organs, such as the eyes, into the movement. As the plan for the postural tone necessary to conduct the movement is initiated, the gamma motor system is engaged. It is important for the person not to be thrown off balance as he or she moves off the center of gravity to conduct the movement. The cerebellum becomes engaged to monitor the movement and assist in the final touchdown, so that the person does not stop short or move the hand too far and break the nose. At a spinal level, the alpha motor neurons for the prime movers and stabilizers are activated, along with the gamma motor neurons, to set the right muscle tone. As the act of touching the nose is put into motion, the muscle spindles inform the nervous system about the instantaneous length of muscle and its velocity of change, the Golgi tendon organs inform the nervous system about the amount of effort they perceive, the joint receptors inform the nervous system about the movements at the joint, and the cerebellum monitors the whole affair and orchestrates a perfect touchdown. Given all the complexity involved, it is no wonder that the police use this test to determine whether alcohol has affected a driver's neuromuscular system.

The Spinal Reflexes

The spine controls simple reflexes. Simple reflexes are hard-wired and obligatory movements. Another basic reflex is the *withdrawal reflex*, in which the muscle moves the body part away from the source of pain. If a person touches something hot, the hand is reflexively moved away before the person is even aware of the sensation. If the stimulation is strong enough, it can create a *flexion/cross-extension reflex*. This polysynaptic reflex excites the flexor group and inhibits the extensor group on the ipsilateral side of pain, while simultaneously exciting the extensor group and inhibiting the flexor group on the contralateral side. The *scratch reflex* is an example of a polysynaptic suprasegmental reflex, where the stimulus evokes a motor response several vertebral segments away that has an action directed toward eradicating the stimulation of the original segment.

During the early stages of human development, one can observe a number of primitive and very predictable reflexes in the infant. For example, the *tonic labyrinthine reflexes* are stimulated by the effects of body or head position on the labyrinthine receptor (part of the semicircular canals). Following is a description of these reflexes:

- Labyrinthine righting reflex: Stimulation of the labyrinthine receptor evokes contractions of the neck muscles that orient the head in relationship to the gravitational force.
- Body-on-head reflex: Asymmetrical stimulation of the skin receptors from the supporting surface leads to contraction of the trunk, limb, and neck muscles that lift the head into an upright position.
- Neck righting reflex: Proprioception from the joints of the neck bring about contractions of the trunk and limbs to bring the head in alignment with the body.
- Body-on-body righting reflex: Asymmetrical stimulation of the skin receptors causes contraction of the trunk muscles, which raises the body toward the upright position.
- Visual righting reflex: Visual feedback is used to orient the head and body correctly with the environment.

Neck reflexes result from stimulation of the joint receptors in the cervical spine, particularly when the head is moved forward or backward, or rotated. These *tonic neck reflexes*, which are described here and illustrated in **Figure 2–8**, are present from birth until approximately the age of 6 to 8 weeks:

- Head ventriflexed (flexion): Evokes upper extremity flexion and lower extremity extension.
- Head dorsiflexed (extension): Evokes extension of the upper extremities while lower extremities are flexed.
- Head rotation: Rotation of the head to the left evokes extension and abduction of left upper and lower extremities, while the right upper and lower extremities are adducted and flexed. The reverse pattern is true when the head is rotated to the right.

As humans mature, they begin to integrate these reflexes into new patterns of behavior. Learning, then, is essentially the integration of reflexes. However, this does not mean that these reflexes go away. Consider the person who spills a water-filled ice tray as a result of these reflexes. The tray is full of water; the person is ready to slip it into the freezer, momentarily looks away, and spills a small amount. The tonic neck reflexes more

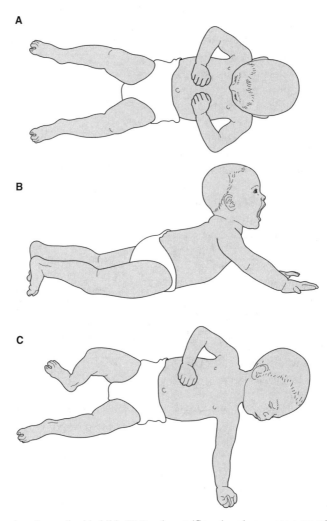

Figure 2–8 Tonic neck reflexes in a 7-month-old child. (A) Head ventriflexed evokes upper extremities flexed and lower extremities extended. (B) Head dorsiflexed evokes upper extremities extended with lower extremities flexed. (C) Head rotation to the left evokes left upper and lower extremities to be abducted and extended, while the right upper and lower extremities are adducted and flexed.

than likely caused a slight flexion or extension of the upper extremity as the person rotated the head one way or the other. Or consider a youngster who is learning how to dive into a swimming pool for the first time. The labyrinthine righting reflex can cause the young diver to belly flop because he or she raises the head due to the loss of balance. When the nervous system is compromised, these primitive reflexes may return. This effect is clearly seen in stroke patients, and, in a more subtle way, in patients with carpal tunnel syndrome. Using SEMG to study carpal tunnel syndrome, researchers have demonstrated that in a majority of these patients, head rotation is associated with recruitment in the forearm musculature.[15] Researchers believe that this reflexively driven activation of the forearm muscles leads to the inflammation of the synovial lining of the carpal tunnel. In addition, it has been demonstrated that when the tonic neck reflexes are integrated again, the forearm firing subsides and the conduction velocities at the carpal tunnel improve.

The Subcortex

The lower centers of the brain are where the cell bodies of the gamma motor system are most densely organized. The brain stem is both phylogenetically and ontogenetically the oldest part of the brain and is commonly referred to as the "reptilian" brain. The brain stem controls arousal levels and consciousness, and is responsible for regulating the heart and breath. It also contains all of the ancient knowledge contained in the obligatory reflexes mentioned in the prior section. It helps to integrate the senses by allowing eye movements to precede head turn, allowing head position to follow sound, extending an upper extremity in the direction of the head turn, and so forth.

The hypothalamus regulates body temperature, body weight, libido, hunger, and thirst. This regulation is accomplished by the integrated action of the reticular formation, the basal ganglia, the thalamus, the limbic system, and the cerebellum.

The *reticular formation* is responsible for our level of arousal. It wakes us up in the morning and turns off so we can drift off to sleep. The seat of human consciousness, it alerts the cortex of incoming information.

The *thalamus* acts as a relay station between the reticular formation and specific areas of the cortex. It signals the cortex, preparing it to receive the upcoming sensory-based information. From a muscular point of view, the reticular formation regulates whether movements are calm, trembling, or sluggish.

The *basal ganglia* help to orchestrate the neuromuscular system's response to sensory stimulation. They contain some of the reflexes described previously and regulate the sequence and timing of muscle contraction. Basal ganglia consist of multiple parts, each of which addresses a different aspect of movement. The *substantia nigra* is particularly responsible for the interpretation and coordination of the overall sensory information coming from the muscle spindles and Golgi tendon organs. When this part of the basal ganglia is damaged, coordination is seriously affected. The classic example is Parkinson's disease, which grossly affects the substantia nigra.

The *globus pallidus* interprets the incoming sensory information so that humans can appropriately brace certain parts of the body to support the prime movers. It fixes body parts into position to facilitate movement. For example, the lower trapezius and serratus anterior must be activated to support the anterior, middle, and posterior deltoid's movement of the arm up into abduc-tion or forward flexion. The *striate body* initiates and monitors a wide range of stereotyped movement patterns—from individual movements that have common utility, to movements that encompass the synchronized background motions necessary for limb movements, to movements that communicate emotional intentions (e.g., sexual arousal, docility, fear, anger, sadness, disgust, and joy).

Although these lower centers of the brain are imbued with the ancient knowledge of human reflexes, they are also open to the acquisition of new habits. The learning associated with the integration of reflexes is partially stored here. Through hundreds or thousands of repetitions, the ancient and acquired reflexes begin to blend. In addition, it is in the lower brain that some of the human's unique, individual stances toward life are recorded and stored.

As well as taking into account all of the motor control directed toward movement and postural tone, one needs to factor in the *limbic system*, the seat of the emotions. This system communicates with the frontal lobes concerning the emotional valence of perception. When one sees a bear, for example, the limbic system recognizes the danger of the situation and alerts the frontal lobes of the condition of fear. The frontal lobes then lay down the plan of response (e.g., run, climb a tree, shoot a gun), which is then carried out through the total orchestration of the neuromuscular system. In essence, the limbic system is also responsible for the lines on our faces: The emotional displays that humans exhibit and receive from the faces of others are directed by the limbic system. Negative emotions tend to affect the upper face more than the lower face, and the left side of the face more than the right side of the face.[16] Notice how common it is for the lines on the left side of people's faces to be much more developed than those on the right side.

The limbic system also plays a major role in setting the overall muscular tone. One of the channels of outflow of the limbic system goes to the hypothalamus and then onto the ascending reticular system. Whatmore and Kohli[17] have described a situation in which the incoming afferent of muscular bracing may also play a role in activating the limbic system.

In addition to the basal ganglia and limbic system, the centers of muscular organization in the midbrain include the *cerebellum*, where the fine-tuning of sensory motor integration occurs. The cerebellum processes neural information 10 times faster than cortical processing. It receives sensory input from all of the senses (e.g., visual, auditory, vestibular, proprioceptive). It receives input from all of the muscle spindles and Golgi tendon organs as well as a large portion of the extrapyramidal output from the cortex and gamma motor output from the basal ganglia. No alpha or gamma motor responses originate from the cerebellum, but almost all of them pass through its influence. This part of the brain is highly organized and mapped, just like the cortex, with its own sensory and motor homunculus. It sends out information to the reticular formation, the basal ganglia, the thalamus, the motor cortex, and the spine. Its basic job is to take the cortical plan for movement and compare the incoming sensory information with the descending alpha and gamma motor information and fine-tune the final output so that the movement is smooth and coordinated.

The Cortex

Control of the neuromuscular system is quite complex and involves three major divisions—cortex, brain-stem, and spinal cord—which operate in a hierarchical arrangement as well as in parallel. **Figure 2–9** illustrates a dynamic systems approach in which there is a very strong interrelation between the various levels. Thus, the motor areas of the cortex can influence the spinal cord both directly or through systems descending through the brain stem. All three levels of the motor sys-tem receive sensory information and are under the influence of two independent subcortical systems: the basal ganglia and the cerebellum. Both the basal ganglia and cerebellum act on the cerebral cortex through the relay nucleus of the thalamus.

The cortex plays an important role in neuromuscular control. The cortex is the location where all new learning takes place. Its surface area is highly differentiated, with different parts taking on different functions. **Figure 2–10** shows the basic cortical layout. The premotor (including the supplemental) and motor areas are most important for muscle control. The premotor and supplemental area is just anterior to the motor area. It is here that the gross motor plan for movement is formed. This information is then passed to the motor area, where fine motor coordination is set forth. The motor area is laid out in a highly differentiated fashion, as seen in the anatomical map shown in **Figure 2–11**. In this figure, the size of the icon for a particular body part represents the amount of cortical space allocated to that region. It is clear that the face and hand consume most of the neurons. From the motor area, nearly 60% of the fibers travel in a finely differentiated fashion directly to the lower motor neurons via the pyramidal tracts. The other 40% synapse along the way in the basal ganglia and the brain stem to receive fine-tuning from the cerebellum and to integrate some of the higher-order reflexes.

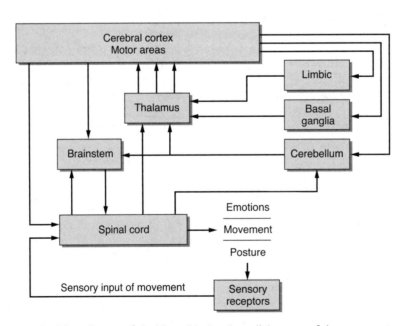

Figure 2–9 A highly schematized flow diagram of the hierarchical and parallel aspects of the motor system.

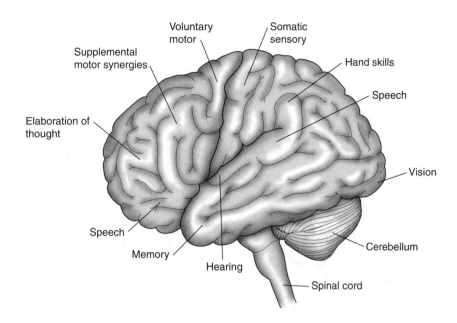

Figure 2–10 Functional areas of the human cerebral cortex.

The extrapyramidal system has three distinct descending tracts, each with its own function:

- The vestibulospinal tract primarily has to do with righting reflexes, postural stabilization, and the facilitation of extensors and inhibition of flexors that assist in maintaining the upright posture
- The reticulospinal tract primarily mediates the facilitation or inhibition of the gamma motor system
- The rubrospinal tract carries the fine-tuning information coming out of the cerebellum

All of these tracts carry information that ultimately modifies the inherited reflexes, usually by inhibiting the obligatory responses in favor of some learned pattern.

It would appear that we have two very different sensorimotor systems: the alpha and gamma motor systems. Each has its own muscles, motor neurons, and principles of organization. The *gamma motor system*, whose origins lie primarily in the basal ganglia, carries out the "ancient knowledge." It controls the resting length of the stretch receptors, thereby passing on our species-specific postures and behaviors through control of our reflexes. These reflexes have been selected and passed down through thousands of generations; they are fixed and obligatory and there is no danger of forgetting them. Yet, they are modifiable with enough repetitions of a new posture or movement. In contrast, the *alpha motor system*, whose origins lie in the cortex, provides us with the opportunity to acquire and use new knowledge. It primarily modulates or inhibits the obligatory reflexes we inherited. While the gamma motor system provides us with the wisdom of our ancestors, the alpha motor system allows us to adapt to the ever-changing aspects of our world. Together, these two systems provide us with the best of both worlds.

It is important to recognize that the neuromuscular system is extremely complex and that it involves more than just these two motor systems. The neuromuscular system is, in fact, a very interactive and dynamic, multilayered system that operates in both hierarchical and parallel modes. No one part of the system is more important than any other. In fact, for the system to survive successfully as a whole, all of the various parts are linked together through feedback and feedforward loops that must be integrated at any given movement.

Pyramidal System

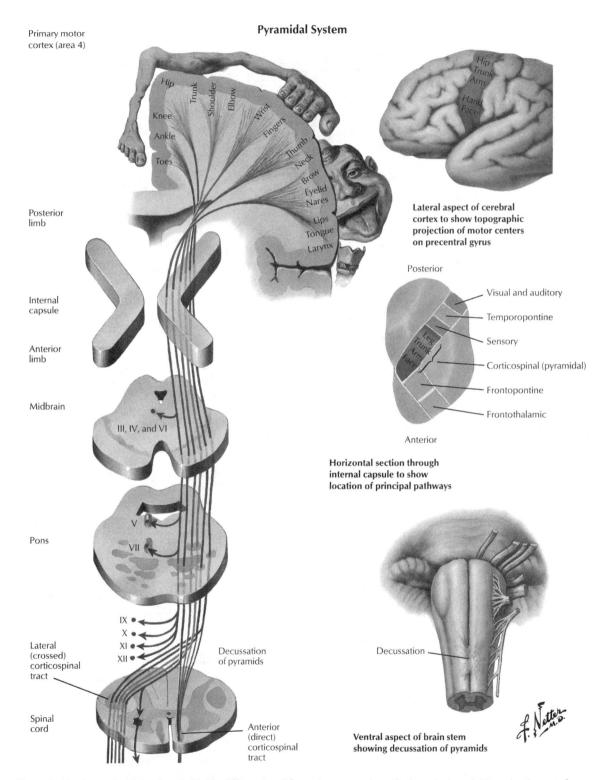

Primary motor cortex (area 4)

Hip
Trunk
Shoulder
Elbow
Wrist
Fingers
Hip
Knee
Ankle
Toes
Thumb
Neck
Brow
Eyelid
Nares
Lips
Tongue
Larynx

Posterior limb

Internal capsule

Anterior limb

Midbrain

III, IV, and VI

Pons

V

VII

Lateral (crossed) corticospinal tract

IX
X
XI
XII

Decussation of pyramids

Spinal cord

Anterior (direct) corticospinal tract

Hip
Trunk
Arm
Hand
Face

Lateral aspect of cerebral cortex to show topographic projection of motor centers on precentral gyrus

Posterior

Visual and auditory
Temporopontine
Sensory
Corticospinal (pyramidal)
Frontopontine
Frontothalamic

Leg
Trunk
Arm
Face

Anterior

Horizontal section through internal capsule to show location of principal pathways

Decussation

Ventral aspect of brain stem showing decussation of pyramids

Figure 2–11 The pyramidal system is highly differentiated from the cortex through the spinal cord. Note the degree of cortical representation of the various body parts.

Source: Netter Anatomy Illustration Collection, © Elsevier, Inc. All Rights Reserved.

THE MOTOR UNIT

The basic level of nervous system organization of the muscle is the motor unit, along with its associated alpha motor system—that is, the lower motor neuron, its axon, and the muscle fibers it innervates. The number of muscle fibers per motor unit varies greatly in the human body. The muscles of the face represent the highest level of innervation, with the extraocular muscles having an innervation ratio of 3 to 1, the highest level of innervation in the human body. The lowest innervation ratio (2000 to 1) is found in the gastrocnemius muscle of the leg. The higher innervation ratios are excellent for fine motor tasks, whereas the lower innervation ratios are ideal for strength production.

The lower motor axon branches so that it can attach itself to the muscle fiber at the motor end plate, creating neuromuscular synapses. When a nerve action potential travels down the axon, it reaches the neuromuscular synapse and releases acetylcholine (ACh), which causes the breakdown of the ionic barrier of the muscle tissue and sends the signal throughout the entire system via the transverse tubules. This creates the motor unit action potential, and the muscle con-

tracts. The depolarization runs in both directions from the motor end plate to the tendinous attachments at both ends.

Extracellular recording of this energy exchange provides the basis for electromyography. For specific details concerning the genesis of action potentials, consult a basic physiology text.[18] Action potentials are associated with a sudden increase in the cell membrane's permeability to sodium ions (Na^+; depolarization). This causes a sudden influx of Na^+ into the muscle fiber that is associated with a measurable change in the resting potential of the cell. Near the peak of this influx, a rapid efflux of potassium ions (K^+) causes a rapid repolarization of the cell (see **Figure 2–12**).

The motor unit has a number of branches and innervates a number of muscle fibers. Because the branching nerve fibers that extend to each muscle fiber vary in their length and diameter, the time at which the nerve action potential reaches the motor end plate varies, resulting in an asynchronous activation of the muscle fibers belonging to a given motor unit. A single muscle fiber receives input from only one motor unit. However, different motor units tend

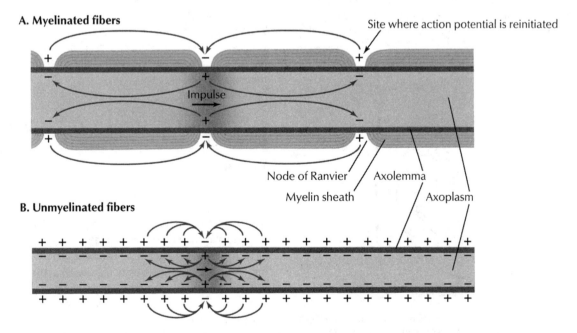

Figure 2–12 Mechanisms of conduction in unmyelinated axon (B). (A) shows the action potential propagating from left to right. The arrow shows the direction of the current flow in front of the action potential.

Source: Netter Anatomy Illustration Collection, © Elsevier, Inc. All Rights Reserved.

to overlap their fiber territories spatially (see **Figure 2–13**). The action potentials from each of the muscle fibers spatially and temporally summate to form a *motor unit action potential*. When motor unit action potentials are recorded using an indwelling electrode, the magnitude of energy recorded is in the millivolt range. With surface sensors, clinicians tend to record from populations of motor units (rather than single motor units), with the magnitude of energy recorded being in the microvolt range. This reduced amplitude is due to the loss of energy associated with the impedance of the body tissue. In essence, the tissue absorbs some of the electrical potential from the muscle as it makes its way to the surface of the skin.

MOTOR UNIT RECRUITMENT PATTERNS

Muscle tone represents a state of low-level contraction that is characteristic of muscles at rest. It represents the resting volley of central nervous system activity sent down the motor units to the muscle. Its function is to stabilize the skeletal structure and to keep the joints from slipping apart. Muscle tone provides the basis for resistance to gravity's pull, emotional tone, and movement. The pull of gravity is ubiquitous, and the muscles must respond to this call. This is, in fact, a normal part of muscle function. Without it, the muscle cells would not thrive (this relationship is why astronauts who return from extended stays in outer space exhibit

muscle atrophy). Conversely, if muscle fibers fired continuously to counter this force, they would soon become exhausted. This predicament is handled by asynchronous stimulation of the motor units. In other words, the central nervous system rotates the motor units that are firing within a given muscle group. In this way, the postural load of a muscle is transferred from one motor unit to another in a smooth and continuous fashion.

In addition to its mechanical work, muscle tone provides the basis for emotional tone. Anxiety or fear tends to take up the general slack of the neuromuscular network. George Whatmore[17] called this "bracing." In laypersons' terms, it is referred to as "being uptight."

Finally, movements are superimposed upon the resting tone of muscle. In our daily lives, as well as in athletic competitions, it is important to have the correct tone for the task at hand. Too much or too little tone, and the timing of actions becomes distorted.

When a muscle contraction occurs, motor unit recruitment is based on the size principle. Here, the smallest muscle fibers and motor units are recruited first, with larger muscle fibers and motor units being called into play as the synaptic drive continues to increase. The firing rate of muscle fibers is usually in the range of 8 to 50 Hz. As the exertional demands increase, the firing rate moves from slower to higher frequencies. In addition, the motor unit recruitment strategy can move from an asynchronous pattern to a synchronous pattern. All of these mechanisms result in higher SEMG readings.

FACTORS THAT AFFECT MUSCLE TENSION OR FORCE

Fatigue

If the contraction of a muscle is sustained with enough force for a long enough period, the conduction velocities of the action potentials along the muscle fibers begin to slow down and the muscle begins to discharge or twitch less frequently. This outcome can be seen during 1 to 5 minutes of continuous muscle contraction at 11% of maximum voluntary contraction.[19] The effects of this muscle fatigue are associated with inadequate perfusion of the tissue, the depletion of energy sources, and the buildup of metabolites (excessive hydrogen ions) in the muscular tissue.[20] Researchers believe that it is the buildup of excessive hydrogen ions that slows

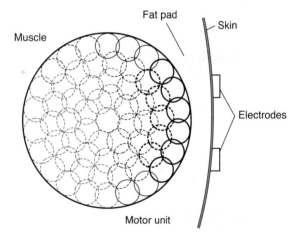

Figure 2–13 Motor unit territories relative to surface EMG electrodes. The motor unit recruitment territories are represented by the small, overlapping circles. Only the heavy, dark motor unit pools contribute substantially to the SEMG recordings.

down the wave form of the motor unit action potential. This phenomenon can be regarded as intracellular "rush hour" traffic, in which the ion channels simply get jammed up. Thus, two electrophysiological events are often associated with fatigue prior to the failure point: (1) increased amplitude associated with synchronization of the motor unit pools and (2) a reduction of the median frequency of the muscle energy.

During a muscular contraction, an internal pressure develops that is associated with the shortening of the muscle fibers. At 10% to 50% of the maximum voluntary contraction, the amount of internal pressure developed is substantial enough to collapse the small arteriole walls of the vessels that are feeding the muscle.[21,22] During rhythmic muscular contractions, the pressure waves of the contraction actually assist the muscle in distributing the metabolic resources and removing the resulting metabolites. In contrast, during a sustained contraction, the muscle is deprived of its nutrients and sustains the buildup of toxic wastes. Perhaps this is why it is essential for the muscle to have interspersed or "micromomentary" (less than 0.5 second) rest periods as part of its activity cycle. Researchers have reported that workers who do not demonstrate "SEMG gaps" or micromomentary rest periods in their work activities tend to develop tension myalgias.[23]

Force-Amplitude Relationships

In general, SEMG amplitude does not equal force. But how well does SEMG activity reflect the amount of force developed by a muscle? This topic has been studied extensively, and an excellent review of this topic can be found in Basmajian and DeLuca's book.[20] A synopsis of the findings appears here.

First, there appears to be a high level of individual variability in the findings. In a population of subjects, the contraction force has a dispersion equal to approximately 25% of the mean value. This may reflect different levels of muscle conditioning across the subjects studied. Deconditioned individuals may display higher levels of SEMG activity while exerting the same amount of force exerted by someone with a well-conditioned muscle.

Second, the force curve relationship varies according to the muscle studied. This can be seen in **Figure 2–14**, where multiple isometric contractions are normalized to the maximum voluntary contraction and plotted as a percentage of maximum voluntary contraction. During isometric contractions of the smaller, first dorsal interosseous muscle, there is a quasi-linear relationship between force and SEMG. The larger muscles such as the biceps, however, take on a curvilinear relationship. The differences between the large and small muscles

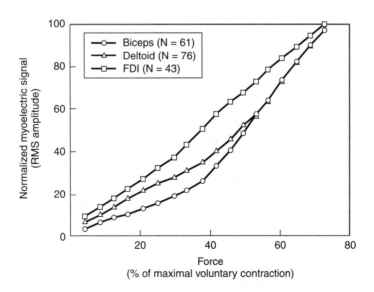

Figure 2–14 Effects of muscle on SEMG signal-force relationship. FDI = first dorsal interosseous muscle. N = average number of isometric contractions for each muscle group.

Source: Reprinted with permission from J. H. Lawrence and C. DeLuca, Myoelectric signal versus force relationship in different human muscles. Figure 1. *Journal of Applied Physiology,* © 1983, The American Physiological Society.

may possibly reflect the differences in the firing rates of the muscles (slow versus fast), their recruitment properties (which fibers recruit as a function of the strength of the contraction), and other anatomical and electrical considerations. In general, muscles that consist of predominantly one fiber type tend to have a more linear relationship between force exerted and SEMG. In muscles of a mixed fiber type (fast- and slow-twitch fibers), the relationship appears to be more curvilinear, with the breaking point at approximately 50% of maximum voluntary contraction.

Length–Tension Relationships

The amount of effort or force that a muscle can put forth depends on the resting length of the muscle. As was noted in an earlier section of this chapter, the length-tension relationship is mediated by the degree of overlap of the sarcomeres (see Figure 2–5). In essence, when there is either too little or too much overlap of the actin and myosin fibers, the number of potential cross-bridging sites diminishes, causing the strength of the contraction to diminish. **Figure 2–15** illustrates the relationship between muscle tension and percentage of resting length in an isolated muscle. Both the passive elastic properties of the muscle while being stretched (curve 1) and the total tension exerted by the

actively contracting muscle (curve 2) are depicted. Curve 2 represents the sum of both the elastic force contribution and the contribution made by the contraction of the muscle. Curve 3 subtracts the force exerted by the elastic properties of the muscle, thus representing the amount of tension generated by the contraction itself.

Several facts can be discerned from this graph. First, the muscle is unable to exert any tension whatsoever when it is at less than 50% of its normal resting length. In general, most muscles have the capacity to shorten 50% of their muscle length, and the ability of a muscle to exert force is reduced as it is placed in a shortened position. At its normal resting length, the amount of tension produced by the contraction of the muscle (curve 3) is greatest. However, the total tension of the muscle is augmented by the elastic properties of muscle when it is stretched (curve 2). Thus, at 120% of its resting length, the total tension possible (contraction + elastic properties) reaches its peak. This length coincides with the length of the muscle when the joint is in the relaxed position.[24] Beyond that point, the force attributable to muscle contraction begins to fall off rapidly. By 200% of its resting length, all of the tension in the muscle has transferred exclusively to the elastic properties of the muscle itself.

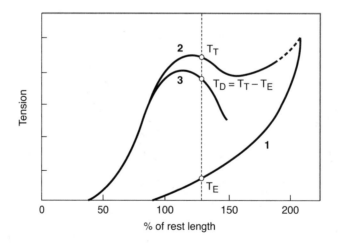

Figure 2–15 Tension-length curves for isolated muscle. Curve 1 = passive elastic tension T_E in a muscle passively stretched to increasing lengths. Curve 2 = total tension T_T exerted by muscle contracting actively from increasing initial lengths. Curve 3 = developed tension T_D calculated by subtracting elastic tension values on curve 1 from the total tension values at equivalent lengths on curve 2 ($T_D = T_T - T_E$).

Source: Reprinted with permission from B. Gowitzke and M. Milner, *Scientific Bases of Human Movement*, 3rd edition, © 1988, Williams and Wilkins.

Force–Velocity Relationships

The contraction velocity of a muscle also affects the amount of tension or force that a muscle produces.[25] This is clearly seen in **Figure 2–16**. The speed at which a muscle can contract is primarily limited by the rate at which the cross-bridging can be manifested at the sarcomere level. Under conditions in which there is no change in the velocity of the contraction (i.e., an isometric contraction), cross-bridges are built more rapidly when the resistance to the contraction is low. Therefore, the amount of time it takes to reach a given tension level is determined solely by the amount of tension to be developed. Lower tension levels are reached more quickly than higher tension levels.

In the case of concentric contractions, the amount of tension generated is moderated by the velocity of the contraction. In situations where different velocities of contractions are conducted using the same amount of resistance, contractions that require higher speeds build fewer cross-bridges than those conducted at slower speeds. This results in the generation of less force during faster concentric contractions than during slower concentric contractions. In the case of eccentric contractions, however, the amount of force or tension created by the muscle actually increases as the velocity of the eccentric contraction increases.

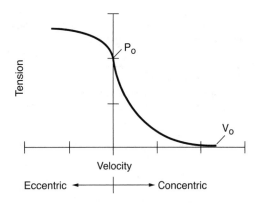

Figure 2–16 Velocity-active tension relationship for muscle.

Source: Reprinted from G. Soderberg, *Selected Topics in Surface Electromyography for Use in the Occupational Setting: Expert Perspective*. DHHS (NIOSH), Publication No. 91-100, Washington DC, NIOSH, 1992.

Surface EMG amplitudes do not equal muscle tension or force. The relationships described previously refer only to force and tension, not SEMG amplitudes. For example, the SEMG amplitudes of a concentric contraction are greater than those of an eccentric contraction when lifting or letting down the same weight.

REFERENCES

1. Huxley HE. The mechanism of muscular contraction. *Sci Am*. December 1965.
2. Brown JMM, Solomon C, Paton M. Further evidence of functional differentiation within biceps brachii. *Electromyogr Clin Neurophysiol*. 1933;33:301–309.
3. Haar Romeny BMT, Denier van der Gon JJ, Gielen CC. Relation between location of the motor unit in the human biceps brachii and its critical firing levels for different tasks. *Exp Neurol*. 1984;85:631–650.
4. McNutty W, Gevertz R, Berkoff G, Hubbard D. Needle electromyographic evaluation of a trigger point response to a psychological stressor. *Psychophysiology*. 1994;31:313–316.
5. Riek S, Bawa P. Recruitment of motor units in human forearm extensors. *J Neurophysiol*. 1992;68:100–108.
6. Jorgensen K, Winkel J. On the function of the human soleus muscle. In: Jonsson B, ed. *Biomechanics, X*. Champaign, IL: Human Kinetics; 1987:259–264.
7. Wolf S, LeCraw D, Barton L. Comparison of motor copy and targeted biofeedback training techniques for restitution of upper extremity function among patients with neurologic disorders. *Phys Ther*. 1988;69:719–735.
8. Huxley AF. Muscle-structure and theories of contraction. *Prog Biophys*. 1957;7:255–318.
9. Hunt CC, Kuffler SW. Stretch receptor discharges during muscle contraction. *J Physiol (Lond)*. 1951;113:298–315.
10. Vallbo AB. Basic patterns of muscle spindle discharge in man. In: Taylor A, Prochazka A, eds. *Muscle Receptors and Movement*. London, UK: MacMillan; 1981.
11. Jacobson E. Electrical measurement concerning muscular contraction (tonus) and the cultivation of relaxation in man: relaxation times of individuals. *Am J Physiol*. 1934;108:573–580.
12. Hubbard D, Berkoff G. Myofascial trigger points show spontaneous needle EMG activity. *Spine*. 1993;18:1803–1807.
13. Travell J, Simons D. *Myofascial Pain and Dysfunction: A Trigger Point Manual, I and II*. Baltimore, MD: Williams & Wilkins; 1983.

14. Donaldson S, Skubick D, Clasby R, Cram J. The evaluation of trigger-point activity using dynamic EMG techniques. *Am J Pain Manage.* 1994;4:118–122.
15. Skubick D, Clasby R, Donaldson CCS, Marshall W. Carpal tunnel syndrome as an expression of muscular dysfunction in the neck. *J Occup Rehab.* 1993;3:31–43.
16. Sackeim HA, Gur RC, Saucy MC. Emotions are expressed more intensely on the left side of the face. *Science.* 1978; 202:434–436.
17. Whatmore G, Kohli D. *The Physiopathology and Treatment of Functional Disorders.* New York, NY: Grune & Stratton; 1974.
18. Guyton AC. *Textbook of Medical Physiology.* 6th ed. Philadelphia, PA: WB Saunders; 1981.
19. Chaffin DB. Localized muscle fatigue-dimension and measurement. *J Occup Med.* 1973;15:346–354.
20. Basmajian JV, DeLuca C. *Muscles Alive.* 5th ed. Baltimore, MD: Williams & Wilkins; 1985.
21. Hagberg M. Occupational musculoskeletal stress disorders of the neck and shoulder: a review of possible pathophysiology. *Int Arch Occup Environ Health.* 1984;53: 269–278.
22. Mortimer JT, Kerstein MD, Magnusson R, Petersen H. Muscle blood flow in the human biceps as a function of developed muscle force. *Arch Surg.* 1971;103:376–377.
23. Veiersted KB, Westgaard RH, Andersen P. Electromyographic evaluation of muscular work pattern as a predictor of trapezius myalgia. *Scand J Work Environ Health.* 1993;19:284–290.
24. Butchthal F, Guld C, Rosenfalch P. Multi-electrode study of the territory of a motor unit. *Acta Physiol Scand.* 1978;39: 83–103.
25. Hill AV. The heat of shortening and the dynamic constants of muscle. *Proc R Soc London (Biol).* 1938;243: 136–195.

CHAPTER QUESTIONS

1. The connective tissue associated with muscle is known as:
   a. fascia
   b. tendons
   c. ligaments
   d. all of the above
2. Without muscles, would the bones and ligaments provide enough stability to allow the skeleton to stand on its own against gravity?
   a. yes
   b. no
3. How many muscles are in the human body?
   a. 200
   b. 400
   c. 500
   d. 600+
4. The two main molecules that make up a muscle fiber are:
   a. myosin and Golgi
   b. Golgi and spindle
   c. actin and myosin
   d. spindle and Ruffini
5. A sarcomere is made up of which of the following bands?
   a. *A, Z, G, I*
   b. *A, Z, I, H*
   c. *H, G, I, J*
   d. *A, I, K, Z*
6. The sarcoplasmic reticulum stores:
   a. glucose
   b. calcium
   c. potassium
   d. myosin
7. It is proposed that muscles do their work through a process that involves:
   a. cross-bridging
   b. hatcheting
   c. the Krebs cycle
   d. minicontractions
8. How large a voluntary contraction does it take to create a disturbance in the microcirculation of muscle?
   a. 5–10% of maximum voluntary contraction
   b. 10–50% of maximum voluntary contraction
   c. 70–80% of maximum voluntary contraction
   d. 90+ % of maximum voluntary contraction
9. Which of the following does not describe the fast-twitch muscle fiber type?
   a. great fatigability
   b. large size, high tension
   c. rich capillary supply
   d. high glucose stores
10. Which of the following is not an element of the motor unit?
    a. upper motor neuron
    b. lower motor neuron
    c. axon
    d. muscle fibers
11. Which muscle tends to have the highest innervation ratio (3 to 1) of muscle fibers to motor units?
    a. trapezius
    b. extraocular muscles
    c. biceps
    d. quadriceps
12. Which of the following sensory mechanisms runs parallel to the muscle fibers?
    a. muscle spindle
    b. Golgi tendon organ
    c. Ruffini endings
    d. free nerve ending
13. Which of the following sensory mechanisms runs in series to the muscle fibers?
    a. muscle spindle
    b. Golgi tendon organ
    c. Ruffini endings
    d. free nerve ending

14. The gamma motor system controls the:
    a. extrafusal fibers
    b. intrafusal fibers
    c. motor unit
    d. none of the above

15. When the muscle spindle is activated by a stretch, it causes the muscle that it is located within to:
    a. relax
    b. become inhibited
    c. contract
    d. undergo flexion/cross-extension

16. It is speculated that trigger points are located in the:
    a. extrafusal fibers
    b. intrafusal fibers
    c. muscle spindle
    d. dermatome

17. The Golgi tendon organ is sensitive to:
    a. amount of muscle tension or effort
    b. joint position
    c. instantaneous muscle length
    d. velocity of muscle

18. The gamma motor system regulates:
    a. movement
    b. posture
    c. coordination
    d. all of the above

19. Free nerve endings are sensitive to:
    a. nociception
    b. too much lactic acid retention
    c. inflammation and swelling
    d. all of the above

20. The Ruffini endings sense:
    a. muscle tension
    b. joint position
    c. velocity of contraction
    d. pain

21. Which of the following muscle sense organs is consciously perceived?
    a. muscle spindle
    b. stretch receptor
    c. Golgi tendon organ
    d. joint receptors

22. Which of the following reflexes is suprasegmental?
    a. stretch reflex
    b. withdrawal reflex
    c. flexion/cross-extension reflex
    d. scratch reflex

23. Which part of the brain controls arousal?
    a. ascending reticular formation
    b. basal ganglia
    c. cerebellum
    d. cortex

24. The basal ganglia stores:
    a. primitive reflexes
    b. acquired reflexes
    c. postures
    d. all of the above

25. Which part of the brain conducts/processes information the fastest?
    a. cortex
    b. cerebellum
    c. spinal cord
    d. pyramidal tract

26. Which part of the brain has as its primary purpose the final execution and refinement of each and every movement?
    a. cortex
    b. cerebellum
    c. spinal cord
    d. extrapyramidal tract

27. What percentage of the motor neurons exiting the motor strip stops off in the lower brain before going down to the lower motor neuron?
    a. 10%
    b. 20%
    c. 40%
    d. 60%

28. When a muscle shortens during a contraction, this is called a(n):
    a. concentric contraction
    b. eccentric contraction
    c. isometric contraction
    d. mesocentric contraction

29. When a person in a standing position squats down and comes back up, this is called a(n):
    a. open kinetic chain
    b. closed kinetic chain
    c. isometric contraction
    d. ergonomic chain

30. In SEMG, which of the following can be expected to show the largest recruitment pattern?
    a. eccentric contraction
    b. concentric contraction
    c. isometric contraction
    d. flexion relaxation

31. Which type of contraction do we primarily use when we go down stairs?
    a. eccentric contraction
    b. concentric contraction
    c. isometric contraction
    d. reflexive contraction

32. Which muscles tend to show a quasi-linear relationship between force and SEMG amplitudes?
    a. small fine motor
    b. large gross motor
    c. soleus muscle
    d. erector spinae

33. At which point of muscle resting length would one expect to see the greatest strength?
    a. 50%
    b. 75%
    c. 90%
    d. 125%

34. What is the relationship between force and velocity?
    a. The faster the contraction, the greater the force.
    b. The slower the contraction, the greater the force.
    c. Force and velocity are independent of each other.
    d. none of the above

35. In general, is it reasonable to think that SEMG amplitude equals the amount of muscle force generated?
    a. yes
    b. no

Instrumentation

INTRODUCTION

The energy that is generated by the muscle has a very small value and is measured in millionths of a volt (microvolts). It is necessary to use very sophisticated and sensitive instruments to amplify this signal so that it can be seen and heard. In essence, a surface electromyograph is nothing but a very sensitive voltmeter.

In the early days of surface electromyography (SEMG), the amplifiers that were used were easily contaminated by other electromagnetic energy in the recording environment. Thus, SEMG recordings were commonly conducted in a "copper room." These rooms were sometimes merely copper screens. The copper screen caught the electrical noise in the room and sent it to "ground," thereby eliminating it from the recording environment.

During the 1950s, biomedical engineering introduced the differential amplifier. This amplifier essentially eliminated the need for the copper rooms, and SEMG recordings moved out of the realm of researchers and into the realm of clinicians. Because of the advances in instrumentation, clinical SEMG began to flourish. Clinical SEMG was initially used by psychologists for biofeedback, but later spread to other specialties such as chiropractic, physical therapy, physical medicine, neurology, and urology.

This chapter seeks to familiarize the practitioner with the basic concepts behind the instrumentation of SEMG. It covers the fundamentals of the electronics behind what is seen on the screen, the different types of SEMG displays and ways in which the SEMG signal can be processed, ways to identify noise and artifact, and ways to set specifications for an SEMG instrument. **Figure 3–1** shows a block diagram of the various components of SEMG instrumentation. Each of the elements in this diagram will be addressed in this chapter. For more in-depth reading on this topic, consider Peek's excellent chapter for clinicians,[1] Basmajian and DeLuca's more technical discussion in *Muscles Alive*,[2] or a book edited by Soderberg.[3] For a broader view of the topic, see the work of Cacioppo, Tassinary, and Fridlund.[4]

THE SOURCE OF THE ELECTROMYOGRAPHIC SIGNAL

Let us begin with the first element of the diagram in Figure 3–1, the source of the SEMG signal, and work through the subelements leading up to differential amplification. The tissue and electrode elements are depicted in **Figure 3–2**. The source of the SEMG signal is the motor unit action potential (MUAP). Action potentials are given off by each of the motor units activated during

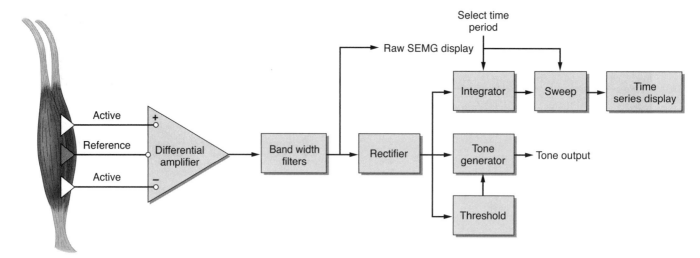

Figure 3–1 Block diagram of SEMG instrument with several options.

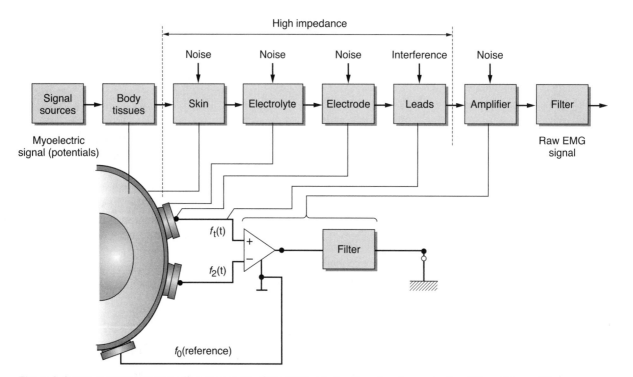

Figure 3–2 The components that affect the source of the EMG signal as it makes its way to the differential amplifiers.

Source: Reprinted from G. Soderberg, *Selected Topics in Surface Electromyography for Use in the Occupational Setting: Expert Perspective.* DHHS (NIOSH), Publication No. 91-100, Washington DC, NIOSH, 1992.

a given contraction. In any given recruitment pattern, populations of motor units are activated in an asynchronous pattern. This asynchronous pattern of activation provides the possibility of smooth movement. It is the sum of the activity that constitutes the volume conducted signal, which is picked up at the electrodes and amplified by the SEMG instrument.

In **Figure 3–3**, each small circle represents the fiber's territory associated with one motor unit recruitment area. Note how they slightly overlap. The solid circles closest to the surface of the skin and, therefore, closest to the recording electrodes make the greatest contributions to the SEMG signal. The fainter the circle, the farther away it is from the recording electrodes and the less likely it is to contribute to the SEMG recording. The farther the signal needs to travel through body tissue before reaching the recording electrodes, the more resistance it encounters. This resistance absorbs the energy, so that less of the original energy reaches the surface electrode. In addition, the body tissues tend to absorb higher-frequency components of the signal, allowing slower frequencies to pass through more readily. In this way, the body tissue is considered to provide a low pass filter for the signal.

In addition, if adipose tissue exists between the muscle and the recording electrodes, more of the signal will be absorbed. This fatty layer acts like an imperfect electrical insulator between the muscle and the recording electrodes. An insulator stops the flow of electrical current, much like the plastic coverings that surround extension cords. Because it is an imperfect insulator, the thicker the layer of adipose, the smaller the amount of signal reaching the electrodes. For example, given the same movement and electrode placement strategy (e.g., monitoring the upper trapezius during abduction), it is not uncommon to see higher resting and peak amplitudes of SEMG activity in a thin person than in a person with a thick layer of fat beneath the recording electrodes. Even within an individual, the amplitude of SEMG is likely to be greater over areas with thin layers of fat compared to areas with thicker layers of fat. For example, amplitudes recorded from the extensors of the forearm muscles are typically much greater than those from the gluteal muscles. Because the gluteus maximus has a much larger muscle mass than the forearm extensors, one might expect to see much larger SEMG amplitudes from this area—but this is not the case. The attenuating effects of adipose tissue cannot be overlooked. We have observed that the correlation between skin-fold thickness at the electrode site (an indication of adipose thickness) and SEMG amplitude values are higher ($r \sim -0.5$) in the resting state than during an active recruitment pattern ($r \sim -0.25$). This evidence indicates that the fatty layer plays a larger role in the interpretation of resting SEMG values than in dynamic SEMG recordings.

IMPEDANCE

Once the energy from the muscle reaches the skin, it is sensed by the electrodes. The interface between the sensing electrode and the skin is a delicate matter. For example, the impedance of the skin, also described as resistance to a direct current [DC], may vary as a function of the moisture of the skin, the superficial skin oil content, and the density of the horny, dead-cell layer. In addition, some sort of electrolytic medium is commonly used to provide a cushion between the surface of the electrode and the surface of the skin. This usually hypersalinic medium potentiates the SEMG from the skin to the electrode. If no electrolyte is used (a dry electrode), the skin senses the presence of the foreign object (the electrode) and eventually begins to produce sweat, thereby providing its own electrolytic medium. In SEMG, it is important to keep the impedance of the skin at the electrode site as low as possible and balanced for the two recording electrodes. This is commonly accomplished by abrading the skin vigorously with an alcohol pad. For research purposes, the impedance at the electrode site should be less than 5,000 to 10,000 Ohms. In

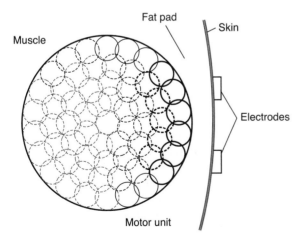

Figure 3–3 Visual depiction of motor unit activity in relation to the recording electrodes.

some research settings, the experimenter may actually puncture the skin at the site of the electrode to ensure a low impedance at the site. Although this practice is too rigorous for most clinical purposes, the practitioner needs to get the impedance low enough to provide a clean signal.

When the impedance at the electrode skin interface is too high or too imbalanced, the common mode rejection of the SEMG amplifier is defeated. In turn, the amplification process is affected by the 60-cycle interference from the energy in the room. This outcome is explained in greater detail in a later section.

How low should the impedance at the skin be to allow a valid and meaningful clinical recording? The answer to this question depends on the SEMG instrument. One attribute of the SEMG amplifier is its input impedance. The interface of skin impedance and input impedance must be matched in certain ways, as shown schematically in **Figure 3–4**. The input impedance of the preamplifier (represented as I_i) essentially absorbs the muscle energy that has reached the electrode–skin interface, thereby providing a basis for amplifying the small signal. Oscillating voltages can be measured only as a function of impedance. This is based on Ohm's law: E = IR (voltage = current × impedance). Thus, the SEMG amplification system puts out a known input impedance to absorb the energy that it wishes to quantify. For this fancy voltmeter to work, it is important that the impedance of the skin (I_s) is less than that of the input impedance of the preamplifier (I_i). *The input impedance of the SEMG preamplifier should be 10 to 100 times greater than the impedance at the electrode–skin interface.* Thus, if an SEMG instrument has an input impedance of 1 megOhm (1 million Ohms), then it will tolerate impedance at the electrode–skin interface of up to 10,000 Ohms. However,

if the SEMG instrument has an input impedance of 1 gigaOhm (1 billion Ohms), the preamplifier can tolerate impedance at the electrode-skin interface of 10 million Ohms (or 10 megOhms).

As a general rule, the greater the input impedance of the SEMG preamplifier, the better. Higher input impedance makes the SEMG more robust to poor electrode skin connections. The latter amplifier certainly will provide a nice basis for clinical work. However, one should not be seduced into thinking that because the SEMG will allow resistance at the electrode–skin interface of 10 megOhms, it is not necessary to abrade or otherwise prepare the skin for the electrode; dry, horny skin or oily skin can easily exceed an impedance of 10 megOhms.

Surface EMG amplifiers, regardless of their input impedance, are still sensitive to imbalances in the impedance at the two recording electrode sites. Differences in impedance may occur when one electrode is placed on a slightly hairy portion of the body, while the other electrode is not. One should avoid placement on hairy areas whenever possible. In addition, imbalances may occur when one electrode loses good adhesion to the skin during a dynamic evaluation or treatment session. In any event, SEMG amplifiers can usually tolerate up to a 20% discrepancy in the impedance between the two sites. Differences greater than 20%, however, lead to faulty elevations in the signal amplitude. **Figure 3–5** shows what can happen to an SEMG recording when one electrode temporarily comes loose during a dynamic study. The rhythmic quality of the poor recording reflects the ringing of the amplifier as it attempts to compensate electronically for the imbalance in the impedance between the two electrodes. This phenomenon may be seen in both raw and processed SEMG recordings.

Two other elements can moderate the impedance of the signal. The first element is the electrode itself, as explained in greater detail in Chapter 4. In general, the size of the electrode and the material it is made of can make a difference. Today, most electrodes are made of silver chloride. The second element is the cable that exists between the electrode and the amplifier itself. This cable is actually one of the most vulnerable parts of the SEMG system; it usually breaks and must be replaced at some point during the lifetime of the instrument. If a lead does break, the resulting infinite resistance will totally saturate the amplifier. It is best to keep these cables as short as possible and to inspect them from time to time.

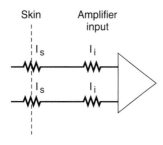

Figure 3–4 The interface of skin impedance and input of SEMG preamplifier. I_i represents input impedance of the preamplifier. I_s represents impedance of the skin.

Source: Courtesy of Will Taylor, Portland, Oregon.

A

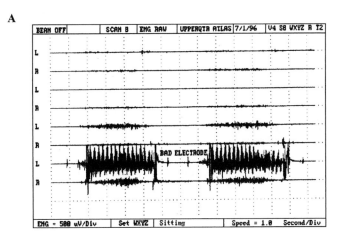

B

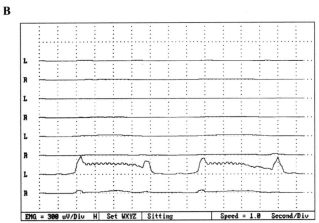

Figure 3–5 (A) Raw SEMG recording during a dynamic protocol in which one of the recording electrodes periodically comes loose. (B) Processed root mean square (RMS) tracing of (A). The "ringing" of the circuit is associated with excessive 60-Hz noise.

Source: Copyright © Clinical Resources, Inc.

DIFFERENTIAL AMPLIFICATION AND COMMON MODE REJECTION

Once the action potential from the muscle has crossed the electrode–skin interface, it passes through the process of differential amplification and common mode rejection. During amplification, the size of the biological signal is "boosted" or made larger. This outcome is referred to as *gain*. The amount of gain or amplification determines how large or how small the SEMG appears on the visual display.

The development of *differential amplification* and *common mode rejection* brought SEMG out from behind the copper cage and into the clinic. In differential amplification, three electrodes are necessary: two recording electrodes and one reference electrode. The recording electrodes are placed over the muscles, with the reference electrode simply making good contact somewhere on the body. The biological energy that reaches both recording electrodes is then compared to the reference electrode. Only the energy that is unique to each recording electrode is passed on for further signal conditioning and display. This system works because the energy given off by a muscle follows the course of the muscle fibers from the motor end plate to the tendinous insertions at both ends. When the recording electrodes are placed parallel to the muscle fibers and slightly off the center of the muscle belly, where the highest density of motor end plates can be found, the action potential given off from the fiber travels to and reaches the two recording electrodes at different times.

Thus, this energy is unique to each electrode and is passed on for further amplification. In contrast, the energy that is common to both recording electrodes—the common mode—is eliminated by this process. The common mode signal typically comes from external electromagnetic noise, such as the 60-cycle current that powers lights and computers.

Sometimes the use of an analogy helps to clarify a concept. Peek[1] uses a sound metaphor with some clarity—monitoring the amplitude of bird songs in the field (see **Figure 3–6**). Using the differential amplifier model, two large microphones are set up to record the bird songs. As the birds fly toward the two microphones, each microphone receives a slightly different sound, because the birds are closer to one microphone than the other. The differential amplifier simply subtracts the level of song on one microphone from that of the other, presenting the difference as the index of loudness. The louder the birds sing, the larger the difference and the higher the loudness meter. Now suppose that a thunderstorm in the area produces a roll of thunder. The thunder moves out in all directions, eventually reaching the microphones. Because the thunder comes from a distant source, it reaches the microphones at nearly the same time and the same intensity. The microphones pass on both the thunder roll and the bird songs to the differential amplifier. Because of common mode rejection, the thunder roll that is common to both microphones is subtracted out of the signal, leaving only the bird songs to be passed on to the loudness meter.

The degree to which a differential amplifier is successful at common mode rejection is described by the common mode rejection ratio (CMRR). This ratio is calculated by dividing the amplification of the common mode signal (A) by the amplification of the differential mode signal (B), and finally multiplying this quotient by $20 \log_{10}$ to achieve a value termed dB. Mathematically, the expression looks like this:

$$20 \log_{10} (A/B) = CMRR\ dB$$

The higher the CMRR dB, the better. It is typically between 90 and 140 dB.

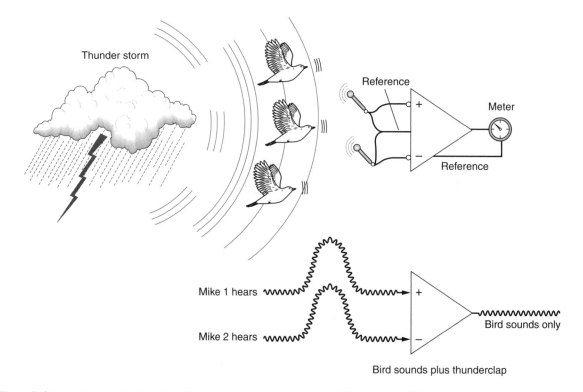

Figure 3–6 Analogy using bird songs to illustrate noise subtraction in a differential amplifier.
Source: Reprinted with permission from Schwartz, *Biofeedback*, p. 55, © 1987, Guilford Publications, Inc.

FILTERING THE ELECTROMYOGRAPHIC SIGNAL

Once the SEMG signal has been boosted by the differential amplifiers, it is then processed in some way. The first level of processing is known as filtering. Most SEMG instruments contain a 60-Hz notch filter. This filter may be found in the electronic circuitry of the SEMG instrument (an analog filter) or in the software it uses (a digital filter). A *notch filter* is a band reject filter that is typically very narrow in width (59–61 Hz) and has a very steep slope to the filter. The purpose of this notch filter is to eliminate any of the electrical noise (60 Hz) from the recording environment that exceeds the capabilities of the common mode rejection scheme. In other words, it rejects (does not let through) any energy that is between 59 and 61 Hz. Unfortunately, these filters are not perfect: If the noise levels are too great, they readily saturate out the filter. **Figure 3–7** represents such a phenomenon. The rhythmic beats seen in the third and seventh tracings represent the ringing of the amplifying circuits due to the presence of too much 60-Hz noise.

The next essential filter for SEMG is the *band pass filter*. This filter passes on only a certain frequency range of energy for further quantification and display. For example, a typical band pass filter might let through all of the energy above 20 Hz and then close the gate at 300 Hz. The lower cutoff point assists the practitioner by eliminating much of the electrical noise associated with wire sway and miscellaneous biological artifacts associated with slow-moving DC potential shifts. The upper cutoff point eliminates the tissue noise at the electrode site.

Selecting the filters for SEMG recordings is something of an art, because certain filters are better for some applications than others. For example, for SEMG recordings from the face, a 25- to 500-Hz band pass filter is preferable because the muscles of the face readily emit frequencies up to the 500-Hz range. This range is determined by the innervation ratio of the muscles of the face, along with their repetitive firing patterns. The 100- to 200-Hz or 100- to 500-Hz filter is effective for eliminating heart rate artifact but may be insensitive to fatigued muscles, because the frequency spectrum of muscles shifts to the slower range during fatigue. **Figure 3–8** illustrates the difference in processed SEMG recordings from the upper trapezius site using a 100- to 200-Hz

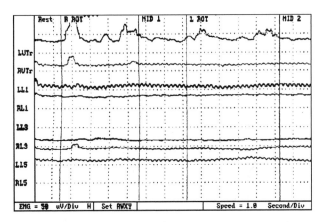

Figure 3–7 Surface EMG example of the ringing of the amplifiers due to the presence of too much 60-cycle noise. This ringing can be seen in the third and seventh channels.

Source: Copyright © Clinical Resources, Inc.

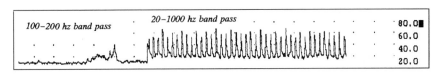

Figure 3–8 Elimination of ECG artifact from upper trapezius lead by using a narrow 100- to 200-Hz filter (left side) and a 20- to 1000-Hz filter (right side).

filter (left side) and a 20- to 1000-Hz filter (right side). The 100- to 200-Hz filter essentially eliminates the electrocardiogram (ECG) artifact. In addition to changing the visual presentation of the tracing, these filters alter the values yielded during the quantification of the SEMG. The wider band pass sample has the large ECG spikes and yields an amplitude of approximately 30 microvolts RMS (root mean square), while the narrower band pass filter yields a much smaller signal with a much smaller amplitude of approximately 15 microvolts RMS.

SPECTRAL ANALYSIS, FATIGUE, AND BAND PASS FILTERS

The energy from muscles has a frequency spectrum. Much like the rainbow colors seen with light refracted through a prism, the SEMG signal can be displayed so as to reveal its range of frequencies. "Power spectral density" curves plot the frequency components of the SEMG signal as a function of the probability of their occurrence. To do so, spectral analysis uses a mathematical technique called *fast Fourier transform* (FFT) to decompose the signal into its various frequency components.

The SEMG signal that reaches the differential amplifier consists of the sum of many motor units firing. Consider a case in which only three sources of energy simultaneously reach the preamplifier. **Figure 3–9A** shows the three independent signals whose frequencies are 0.5, 1.0, and 1.5 Hz. **Figure 3–9B** shows a composite of the three signals. In SEMG recordings, the amplifiers always see the composite. Were an FFT spectral analysis to be conducted on this composite signal, it would decompose the energy into the spectral graph shown in **Figure 3–10**, which illustrates that the composite signal is composed of three frequencies at 0.5, 1.0, and 1.5 Hz.

The power spectral density of the SEMG for a muscle shows the height of the curve at any given frequency and indicates how prevalent the muscle energy is at that frequency. For example, when a muscle is contracted, a 20- to 300-Hz filter might represent nearly all of the energy in the spectrum of the muscle. If one were using a 100- to 200-Hz band pass filter, however, only a portion of the energy of the muscle would be observed.

The relationship of muscle energy represented by the two filters described above could shift under various conditions. For illustrative purposes, consider work versus fatigue. Imagine a graph of the raw and processed SEMG of a first dorsal interosseous muscle once it has been passed through a 20- to 300-Hz band pass filter. The top line of the graph would represent the amount of force exerted over time. The amount of force eventually declines at a point referred to as the *failure point*. Just prior to that point, the RMS amplitude increases briefly. You can see the power spectral density curves computed at the beginning of the contraction and just before the failure point. During the initial part of the contraction, the median frequency of the spectrum (the 50th percentile) might reside slightly above 100 Hz. During muscle fatigue, there might be a downward shift in the shape of the power

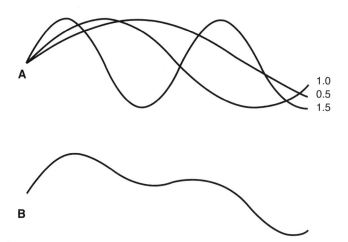

A

1.0
0.5
1.5

B

Figure 3–9 (A) Three independent signals of 0.5, 1.0, and 1.5 Hz and (B) their composite signal.

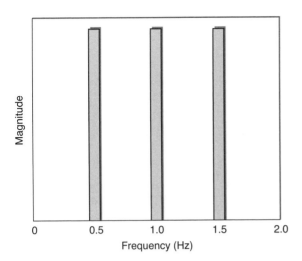

Figure 3–10 Power spectral density of the composite signal shown in Figure 3–9.

density such that the median frequency would then reside at about 55 Hz. In fatigued muscles, the shape of the frequency spectrum changes such that there is a diminution of the higher frequencies and an augmentation of the lower frequencies. This downward shift in the median frequency could be attributed to the synchronization of motor unit recruitment patterns, a slowing of the conduction velocities of the muscle fibers, a shift in dominance from fast-twitch fiber to slow-twitch fiber as a result of the fatigability of the fast-twitch fibers, or a combination of all of these factors.

To quantify the spectral shift secondary to fatigue, however, one must ask the patient to exert a steady isometric contraction at approximately 80% of maximum voluntary contraction (MVC) for a period of 1 minute. Such an analysis can be quite powerful. Researchers who studied the back muscles in this way in control subjects and patients with back pain reported that the initial shift in the median frequency and its course of recovery after 1 minute showed a sensitivity and specificity of 88% to 100%.[5] This type of specificity and sensitivity may be useful in distinguishing patients with true back pain from malingering patients. The work of DeLuca[6] and Roy et al.[7,8] provides more information on this topic.

An understanding of spectral analysis and band pass filters will help practitioners interpret their clinical findings. The spectral analysis presented in **Figure 3–11** is from a recording from a normal latissimus dorsi at 75%

MVC for a 6-second epoch. A 1.7-second sample is taken from the middle of the contraction (marked by the vertical lines) and submitted for analysis. Two spectral analyses are observed: one for the right aspect and one for the left aspect of the muscle. The 60-Hz notch filter is seen in each, with the power of the spectrum dropping sharply at the 60-Hz point. The median frequency of the spectrum is 92.2 Hz for the left aspect and 92.7 for the right aspect.

Figure 3–12 shows a raw SEMG tracing using a 20- to 450-Hz band pass filter, along with the power spectral density curve observed during a resting baseline on a 17-year-old woman during an intense headache. The RMS microvolt level for the 15-second recording was 74.7 microvolts. Upon examining the power density curve, one can easily see that almost all of that energy resided below 40 Hz. Perhaps this is an indication of chronic muscle fatigue. Had the practitioner selected a 100- to 200-Hz filter during this examination (note the amount of energy present between 100 and 200 Hz on the spectral analysis), the findings would have yielded a normal SEMG tracing.

Clearly, it is important to know the filter characteristics of the SEMG instrument so that clinicians can interpret the signals correctly. If the SEMG instrument has selective filters, it is important to choose the correct filter for the task at hand. We recommend using a narrow 100- to 200-Hz band pass filter when noise or artifact is problematic for interpretation and cannot otherwise be eliminated. A wider 20- to 300-Hz filter is generally preferred to display the SEMG signal most accurately. This level of band pass is sensitive to muscle fatigue, while the high pass (100- to 200-Hz) filter is not.

TYPES OF SURFACE ELECTROMYOGRAPHY VISUAL DISPLAYS

Once the SEMG signal has been amplified and filtered, it is prepared for visual display and quantitative presentation. Four primary types of SEMG visual displays are distinguished: raw SEMG, processed SEMG, spectral analysis, and probability amplitude histogram. Each style of presentation has both benefits and disadvantages.

The Raw Surface Electromyography Display

The raw SEMG display is the oldest form of SEMG presentation. It presents an unprocessed, peak-to-peak oscilloscopic display of the SEMG signal. As the MUAPs

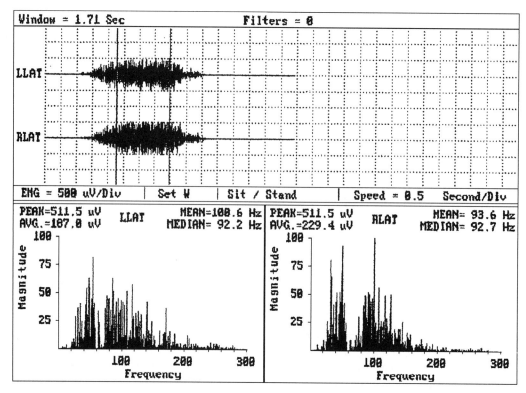

Figure 3–11 Power spectral analysis of an SEMG tracing from a normal contraction of latissimus dorsi. The upper panel shows the raw SEMG recording with the lines in the center representing the portion of the recording submitted for spectral analysis. The lower panel shows the spectral analysis of the SEMG signal.

Source: Copyright © Clinical Resources, Inc.

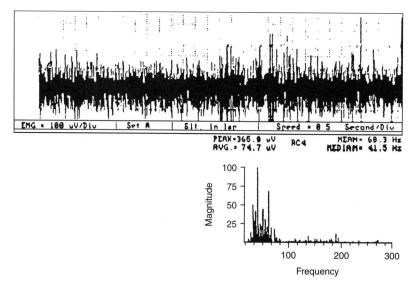

Figure 3–12 Surface EMG recording from cervical paraspinals during intense headache.

Source: Courtesy of Will Taylor, Portland, Oregon.

sum and reach the skin, the small SEMG potentials are amplified and their sinusoidal nature is presented as they oscillate between the positive and negative poles.

As **Figure 3-13** illustrates, the SEMG signal oscillates in both the positive and negative directions, and also varies in its thickness and height. The thickness of the tracing represents the amplitude or strength of the contraction. The thicker the tracing, the stronger the SEMG signal and the stronger the contraction. In this example, the muscle goes from approximately 2 microvolts (peak to peak) at rest to approximately 200 microvolts (peak to peak) during the contraction. The unit of measurement for raw tracings is microvolts peak to peak (commonly referred to as pp), which represents the thickness of the tracing.

The advantage of the raw SEMG tracing is that it contains all of the information from the SEMG signal. None of it is processed out. One can readily see the various forms of artifact in the signal. These artifacts, which are explored in greater depth later in this chapter, include 60-cycle noise, ECG artifact, and movement artifact. In addition, raw SEMG tracings allow clinicians to see post-

movement irritability in a muscle that harbors a trigger point. **Figure 3-14** demonstrates this phenomenon in a recording taken from the upper trapezius muscle following abduction. Before the movement, the muscle is quiet. During the movement, the SEMG activity rises appropriately and becomes thicker. However, following the cessation of the movement, the SEMG activity level does not return to the resting baseline level. Not only does it remain thicker, but it contains hairlike elements in the left upper trapezius (LUT; top tracing) portion that extend above the majority of the tracing on a somewhat irregular basis. The right upper trapezius (RUT; second tracing) also does not return to the baseline levels, but it lacks the hairlike elements. The LUT site contains an active trigger point, and the RUT site does not. The lack of return to premovement baseline levels and the hairlike elements seen in the postrecruitment pattern may represent a disturbance in the muscle spindle secondary to the presence of a trigger point. The assessment of trigger points is reviewed in Chapter 8.

The primary drawback of the raw SEMG display is that the additional information may make it more difficult

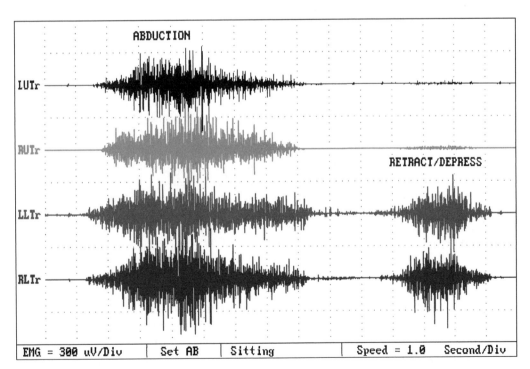

Figure 3-13 Raw SEMG tracing from the trapezius site during abduction and retraction. The signal goes from thin (low activity) to thick (high activity).

Source: Copyright © Clinical Resources, Inc.

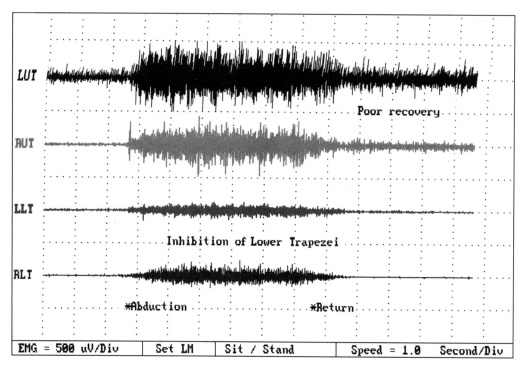

Figure 3–14 Activation and poor recovery for recordings taken from the upper and lower trapezius during abduction and recovery. The left upper trapezius (LUT) (upper tracing) contains an active trigger point. This is noted not only by the lack of recovery of amplitude during the recovery phase, but also by the presence of hairlike elements on the tracing.

Source: Copyright © Clinical Resources, Inc.

for the patient to interpret the signal. This complication becomes relevant during biofeedback training sessions, in which the SEMG signal is presented to the patient as a means to guide the use of muscle. Teaching symmetry of movement, for example, may be easier if the two channels of SEMG are overlaid on top of each other so that the patient can see which muscle activity is higher or lower. In addition, when using a template to teach the patient a particular recruitment pattern, the processed signal is easier to use. An SEMG system that allows both processed and raw displays would be ideal.

The Processed Signal

The manufacturers of SEMG instruments process the SEMG signal in several different ways. For example, this processing may be done either electronically by the resistors, capacitors, and integrated circuits (ICs) that follow the amplifier or digitally by computer software. Researchers have developed ways to process the SEMG signal as a means to make the signal easier to under-

stand, read, and interpret. Because the very nature of muscle activity is a random, staccotic firing of groups of muscle fibers, finding ways to reduce the variability of muscle activity makes it a little easier to understand. As noted previously, this consideration may be especially important when the SEMG instrument is used to train patients in how to control their muscle function. The simpler and easier the SEMG display is to understand, the better the training effects.

Although the processing of the signal may result in a variety of quantities (e.g., RMS, integral average), initially they all begin with a common series of steps. The first step in the process entails rectifying the signal. That is, the portion of the signal that resides below the 0 point (the negative electrical potential) is made positive and artificially placed above the 0 crossing line, as illustrated in **Figure 3–15**.

The next step entails smoothing out the signal in some way. This is frequently done mathematically, and is commonly referred to as *digital filtering*. For example, rather than displaying every point of the rectified signal,

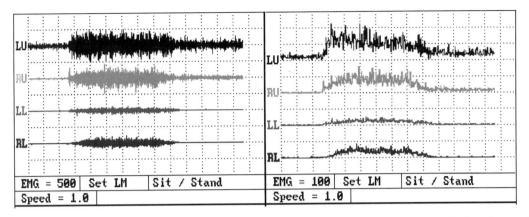

Figure 3–15 The raw SEMG signal of Figure 3–14 is placed side by side with its rectified and averaged display. The raw data points are averaged across every six data points and then drawn to the screen. The amount of upward deflection represents SEMG activity. The moment-to-moment amplitude of the SEMG varies considerably.

Source: Copyright © Clinical Resources, Inc.

an average of every 6 data points of SEMG data may be plotted—a scheme referred to as *integral averaging*. By plotting the average of every 6 data points, the variability of the SEMG is reduced by a factor of 6. By increasing the number of samples in the average (e.g., going from 6 samples to 20 samples), the amount of spontaneous variability in the SEMG signal is reduced. The "odd" SEMG value would get diluted by the 19 other values surrounding it.

Visually, the smoothing process is represented by taking the bumps out of the signal—by reducing its variability. It can be compared to putting shock absorbers on a car so that passengers do not feel every bump in the road. Figures 3–15 and **Figure 3–16** visually represent three levels of smoothing the data. Figure 3–15 shows the rectified tracing with very little in the way of smoothing (every 6 points are averaged and then plotted). Figure 3–16 shows higher degrees of averaging, with graph A representing an averaging of every 12 data points and graph B representing an averaging of every 24 points. The SEMG tracing becomes progressively less jagged as the level of processing increases. Instrument manufacturers refer to this phenomenon using different terms. Some call it *filtering*, because it is a form of digital filtering. Some call it a *time constant*, a term that dates from the age of resistors and capacitors and refers to the amount of time it takes for an RC circuit to discharge its stored charge. Others refer to the process as *smoothing*.

QUANTIFICATION OF THE SURFACE ELECTROMYOGRAPHIC SIGNAL

Along with the visual presentation of information related to SEMG amplitude, SEMG information is processed quantitatively. This process yields numbers that describe the amount of muscular energy expended. Because the SEMG signal oscillates between a positive and negative value or voltage, it is not possible to simply sum up all of the voltages to determine a quantity: All of the positive values would cancel out all of the negative values, and the resulting sum would be zero. For this reason, there are three ways in which SEMG values are commonly derived: peak to peak, integral averaging, and RMS.

Peak to peak is used in raw SEMG recordings. This quantity represents the amount of muscle energy measured from the top to the bottom of the tracing, or its width. Usually the peak-to-peak measurement is summed and averaged over a period of time. Peak-to-peak values in a normal resting muscle might range between 2 and 10 microvolts, depending on the spacing of the electrodes, the degree of body fat below the sensors, the muscle being monitored, the posture of the patient during the recording period, and the particular amplifier characteristics of the SEMG instrument.

Integral average (μv/sec) is used with the processed SEMG signals. It represents the simple arithmetic mean of the rectified SEMG over a given unit of time. The plus and minus signs of the raw SEMG data are ignored (to

A

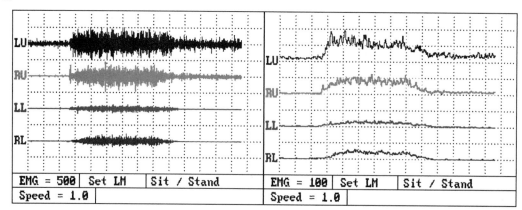

B

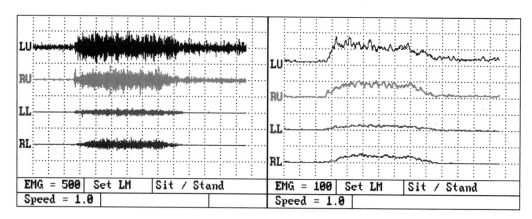

Figure 3–16 The effects of digital filtering or smoothing on the SEMG signal. (A) represents an averaging of every 12 data points; (B) represents an averaging of every 24 data points.
Source: Copyright © Clinical Resources, Inc.

yield the absolute value). These values are summed over the period of time defined and then divided by the number of values observed. This average would represent 0.637 of one-half of the peak-to-peak value. The mean of the SEMG data is represented by the following mathematical equation:

$$\mu v/sec = I\{|m(t)|\} = 1/T \int_{t}^{t+T} |m(t)| dt$$

where T is the time period of integration.

RMS approaches the quantification of the SEMG signal by squaring the data, summing the squares, dividing this sum by the number of observations, and finally taking the square root. For technical reasons having to do with cancellation effects, this method of quantifying SEMG information is more commonly used than the in-

tegral averaging technique. It is thought to provide less distortion, because it converts an analog signal to a digital form. RMS represent 0.707 of one-half of the peak-to-peak value. The RMS conversion is represented by the following mathematical equation:

$$RMS = \{|m(t)|\} = 1/T [\int_{t}^{t+T} m^2 (t) dt]^{1/2}$$

where T is the time period of integration.

COMPARISON OF QUANTIFIED SURFACE ELECTROMYOGRAPHY VALUES ACROSS INSTRUMENTS

Each SEMG instrument handles the amplification, filtering, and quantification of the SEMG signal differently. For this reason, it is impossible to compare directly the values obtained on one SEMG instrument with the values obtained on an instrument from another manufacturer. **Table 3–1** helps clinicians with this comparison process by providing a benchmark basis for comparison. When colleagues want to share findings from different SEMG instruments, they can establish some rough equivalences of the findings from their various instruments. The major weakness of such a comparison is that it is not exact. In fact, it is difficult to make comparisons for SEMG signals in general. One should not directly compare, for example, isometric contractions to concentric contractions, or an activity done by one muscle to the same activity done by another muscle. Clinicians should always exercise caution when making comparisons. Note that Table 3–1 does not list all of the SEMG instruments that are commercially available, and that new SEMG instruments are added over time. In addition, inclusion in this list is not meant as an endorsement by the authors for any of the products listed.

Table 3–1 Conversion Table for Benchmark

Instrument	Ratio
Benchmark	1.00
Davicon (30–300 Hz)	1.67
DMS 4000 (25–450 Hz)	1.17
Flexiplus (100–1000 Hz)	1.07
J&J M-53 (100–200 Hz)	1.00
J&J M-501 (100–200 Hz)	1.00
J&J M-501 (25–1000 Hz)	1.41
J&J I-410 Myoamp (software controlled)	1.31
Norodyne 8000 (25–450 Hz)	1.67
Physiotech 4000 (25–450 Hz)	1.17
SRS: Orion (100–1000 Hz)	1.07
SRS: Gemini (100–1000 Hz)	1.65
SRS: Gemini (25–1000 Hz)	2.31
SRS: Gemini (100–200 Hz)	1.08
SRS: Aries (100–200 Hz)	0.90
SRS: Aries (25–1000 Hz)	1.53
Thought Technology: Myotrac (100–200 Hz)	1.27
Thought Technology: Myotrac (20–500 Hz)	1.75
Thought Technology: Myotrac2 (100–200 Hz)	1.21
Thought Technology: Myotrac2 (20–500 Hz)	1.74
Thought Technology: Flexcomp (100–200 Hz)	1.21
Thought Technology: Flexcomp (20+ high pass)	1.76
Thought Technology: Procomp (100–200 Hz)	1.13
Thought Technology: Procomp (20–500 Hz)	1.60
Verimed Myo2 Dual Channel (20–1000 Hz)	1.22
Verimed VStim 2 (20–1000 Hz)	1.26
Verimed Myo3 Dual (20–1000 Hz)	1.23
Verimed Myo2 (20–1000 Hz)	1.09

The ratios presented in Table 3–1 were derived using the following procedure. Each instrument was provided with a standard input device (a signal generator), whose output provided a pink noise generator with frequencies within the typical range of muscle function and whose amplitudes averaged around 5 microvolts (J&J M-501 benchmark). Such a signal generator has been described as a "synthetic muscle." This output was sent to the amplifiers of the particular SEMG instruments. Five RMS values displayed by the instrument were recorded and averaged to determine the value for the particular SEMG instrument. A mathematical ratio was then calculated that compares all of the SEMG instruments to the J&J M-501 SEMG amplifier. The formula was

$$\text{Ratio} = \text{Test Instrument} / \text{J\&J M-501}$$

This ratio allows the provider to convert the RMS values listed for a particular instrument to a value that is comparable to other instruments. To make this comparison, the practitioner finds the conversion factor for his or her particular instrument, and multiplies the SEMG values by that ratio to obtain a standardized RMS value. The same procedure is used on the second instrument. The resulting values are then roughly equivalent.

COMPARISON OF QUANTIFIED SURFACE ELECTROMYOGRAPHY VALUES ACROSS MUSCLES AND INDIVIDUALS

Comparison of SEMG values both within and between individuals is potentially fraught with problems. Anthropomorphic differences between different recording sites and between individuals suggest that such comparisons should be approached cautiously. Some of the factors that might affect these comparisons include thickness of subcutaneous adipose tissue, muscle resting length, velocity of contraction, muscle mass/cross-sectional area, fiber type, age, sex, subtle changes in posture, interelectrode distance, and impedance of the skin. The effects of the various anthropomorphic moderating variables on comparisons made between individuals are reviewed in some depth in Chapter 5. The bottom line is that it is possible to compare RMS values across muscle sites for the resting baseline conditions only. Population statistics for the sites of comparison are extremely valuable. During dynamic movements, however, comparison of amplitude measurements alone (i.e., peak RMS) across muscle groups can be very misleading if one does not first normalize the SEMG data.

Researchers and practitioners have attempted to deal with these issues. One technique used to control for these variables is *normalization*.[9] Several forms of normalization exist, each of which uses some sort of an anchor related to SEMG amplitudes. Each method calculates all other activity as a percentage of that anchor. The most common method is the *maximum voluntary isometric contraction (MVIC)*.[10] Here the patient is asked to make approximately three MVICs for the muscle group of interest. The middle 2 seconds of a 6-second contraction are recorded and then averaged over three trials of the MVIC. All subsequent recordings are then referenced back to the strongest effort observed as percentage of MVIC (%MVIC). All SEMG data points are divided by the MVIC value, representing a percentage between 0 and 100%. There are no absolute microvolt values, only a relative comparison to a maximal effort. Thus, all muscle function can be reduced to this common feature of percentage of MVIC, and comparisons between muscles and individuals become possible.

For example, to compare the level of SEMG activity of the upper trapezius to that of the lower trapezius, one might ask the patient to make a resisted maximum contraction of the upper trapezius during shoulder elevation, along with maximum contraction of the lower trapezius during shoulder retraction and depression using a manual muscle-testing procedure. These values can then be used to calculate a percentage of MVIC for each muscle to compare the work done by the lower trapezius to that of the upper trapezius. Because of the differences in cross-sectional area for the two muscles, it would not be accurate to compare the peak RMS contraction of the lower trapezius directly to that of the upper trapezius during a task such as abduction versus flexion.

Unfortunately, this solution is not without its flaws. The primary problem with the technique is that it relies on a voluntary component. How do we know whether the person has given his or her maximal effort? Is this maximal effort replicable for this individual across time? The illusion of objectivity of the technique should be placed into the context of a subjective, voluntary effort. Working with patients who have pain complicates this even further, because they may choose not to give a maximal effort either because it will hurt or because they want to protect themselves from hurting in the future. Restrictions in the range of motion of the patient may also create problems. The motivation of the patient may also be suspect in some cases. For example, a ma-

lingering patient may not put forth his or her best effort because it may hurt a claim or litigation.

Some of these objections may be overcome by requesting that the individual conduct a submaximal voluntary contraction. Here, the practitioner might ask the patient to exert a quantifiable force using a dynamometer, at 50% of what would commonly be seen for that muscle and that movement. Alternatively, the practitioner might ask the patient simply to conduct an abduction of the arm to 90 degrees as the standardized reference contraction for the upper and lower trapezius muscles. In either case, the practitioner might ask the patient to hold the position for 15 seconds, taking the middle 5 seconds as reference data. Averaging the middle 5 seconds over four repetitions provides a stable reference value. The reference anchor is used to calculate the percentage of reference voluntary contraction (%RVC). This type of normalization method has a higher reliability across testers compared to the maximum voluntary isometric contraction method.[10]

The next most common method is to record contractions as a function of a dynamic movement cycle, such as walking. Yang and Winter[9] and Knutson, Soderberg, Ballantyne, and Clarke[10] have studied the submaximal contraction values for the *peak* of the contraction. This method provides a reliable anchor point when at least four repetitions of a movement have been conducted.[11] As a variation of using peak values for a single muscle, one could use the average of several muscles that are being monitored during the same movement as the anchoring point. Like %MVIC, the %RVC is now anchored to the peak or mean value observed during the dynamic movement, and percent values are derived from this. In the case of peak values, the %RVC is usually less than 100%. In the case of the mean value, the %RVC could exceed 100%. An example of this type of normalization might entail monitoring of the soleus, gastrocnemius, tibialis anterior, hamstrings, rectus femoris, gluteus maximus, gluteus medius, and tensor fasciae latae muscles during walking. The peak values of each muscle are obtained during at least four gait cycles. The average of the four peaks for each muscle is then used to determine the specific %RVC for each muscle during the gait cycle. In this way, one can compare the activation pattern of one muscle to another during the gait cycle. It is possible to compare not only the peak values, but also the minimum values (rest) as well as the slopes for recruitment and derecruitment of each muscle.

Although the two previously described techniques are not perfect reflections of a muscular effort, researchers have studied them extensively and know a great deal about them.[10-13] Both the maximal and relative contraction anchors appear to have reasonable test–retest reliability in the upper trapezius (11% to 15% coefficient of variation). The %MVIC appears to be more sensitive to contractions that require more effort and loses its sensitivity at low levels of effort. The %RVC is most appropriate when lower levels of activation are to be studied or assessed. When these measures were studied on the gastrocnemius muscle for their reliability and relevance to knee-related problems, for example, the %MVIC measure provided more reliable and reproducible data compared to the %RVC measures.[10] Thus, it is not possible to select one normalization technique for all occasions. One must choose the best normalization method for the muscle and task to be studied.

Another strategy that can be used to avoid anthropomorphic issues is to study the percentage of asymmetry of a submaximal contraction between homologous muscle groups during a dynamic movement such as forward flexion of the head. The formula for this quantity reflects the difference between the peak of contraction for the right and left aspects of homologous muscles as a ratio of the highest peak:

%asymmetry = (high peak – low peak)/high peak

Donaldson[14] has reported that this normalization procedure can differentiate between normal patients and patients with pain during forward flexion of the head and torso. In addition, he has presented data that indicate whether a trapezius or sternocleidomastoid (SCM) muscle has a trigger point. Donaldson has proposed a 20% cutoff point during the peak of concentric contraction to separate the two groups. In reviewing Donaldson's data, it appears that the 40% to 50% range shows greater specificity. The main criticism of this technique is that the percentage of asymmetry may be attributable to mechanical problems, differences in range of motion, or posture, rather than to muscle function. For example, a person may deviate the head slightly to the right during forward flexion because of a facet restriction, thereby bringing about a recruitment asymmetry due to mechanical limitations rather than problems in muscle function per se. Careful observation—if not actual measurement of range of motion—should be factored into this type of measurement system. This would more clearly identify possible mechanical reasons for asymmetries. In addition, because this type of assessment requires movement, the asymmetries or levels of activation could possibly

change with repetitions. Donaldson has reported that the correlation between the first movement and all other movements is exceptionally poor (personal communication). In contrast, the correlation between the second repetition and subsequent repetitions is much higher. Thus, the practitioner might discard the first percent asymmetry score (deeming it a practice movement), and rely more heavily on the third to fifth repetitions. Data from the first and second trials are always discarded.

AMPLITUDE PROBABILITY DISTRIBUTION FUNCTION

The amplitude probability distribution function is a relatively new graphing technique for the SEMG signal, introduced by Jonsson in 1978.[15] Although this style of visual presentation is fairly new, the conceptual framework behind it is not. The curves presented in **Figure 3–17** illustrate a way of plotting the variance of the signal. The range of amplitudes is plotted across the bottom of the graph, instead of along the side. The percentage of time spent at a given amplitude is plotted along the side. When the histogram shows a high value, a large amount of time was spent at that given amplitude. In Figure 3–17, a person has engaged in a very light activity (e.g., writing with a pencil) for 10 minutes. The amount of time spent at the continuum of RMS amplitudes is plotted. The high levels at the left side of this curve indicate that a fairly large amount of time was spent at rest (defined as less than 5 microvolts RMS). In the middle of the graph, another broader elevation indicates the amount of time that work was done. These plots show the probability of a given RMS amplitude—thus the term *amplitude probability distribution function*.

During rest or relaxation-oriented therapies, one would expect the distribution to take on the shape of the curve on the left side of Figure 3–17. The curve would have a very narrow distribution located only at the low end of the amplitude spectrum, with perhaps a right-tailed kurtosis (flat tail) as the physiology of the muscle activity runs into the "cellar" of its ability to become more quiet. Cram[16] noted that perhaps it was the reduction of variability that was the "active ingredient" in relaxation-based biofeedback therapies, rather than the reduction in the actual amplitude of the signal. In Cram's study, headache sufferers were offered a relaxation-based biofeedback program or one that taught them to discriminate +/– 10% of the

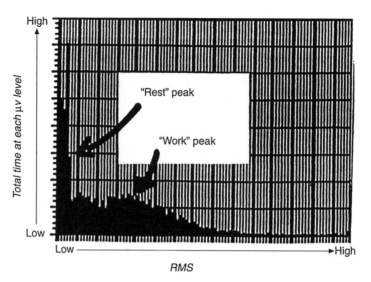

Figure 3–17 Amplitude probability distribution function during light work (writing with a pencil for 10 minutes). The range of SEMG amplitudes is along the *x*-axis, while the probability of any given amplitude is plotted along the *y*-axis.
Source: Courtesy of Will Taylor, Portland, Oregon.

baseline values observed during their baseline condition. At the end of treatment, only the subjects in the relaxation group had learned to lower their general levels of SEMG amplitude for the frontal muscles, but both groups showed reductions in the variability of the SEMG signal. At the end of treatment, both groups showed a significant decrease in headache activity, and at 6-month follow-up the discrimination training group had not just maintained their gains but improved on them. The probability amplitude modulation curves allow the practitioner an opportunity to examine the variability of the SEMG signal.

Clinically, amplitude probability distribution function curves also allow one to examine the distribution of the SEMG signals for the occurrence of interspersed rest during a work period. Researchers[17,18] have observed that the distribution of the RMS amplitudes during work should be bimodal, as opposed to being unimodal or normally distributed. There should be one peak associated with the effort, and a second peak associated with micromomentary or interspersed rest. Again, an example of this type of configuration is noted in the work distribution of Figure 3–20. In several studies, workers who did not show the rest peak have tended to develop muscle pain or tension myalgias in those muscles.[15,17] Usually, rest is defined as SEMG activity below the 5th percentile of either the %MVIC or the %RVC

during a work cycle. Using the J&J M-501 benchmark framework, this point is approximately around the 5-microvolt RMS level.

One can actually calculate the percentage of time spent below such an anchor point. **Figure 3–18** illustrates a work pattern of the right and left upper trapezius during a light typing task that was performed over a 10-minute period by a patient with a tension myalgia on the right aspect of the shoulder/neck. The tracing for the left upper trapezius (LUT) shows a fairly typical distribution. The work amplitudes are relatively low, and a clearly defined rest peak is present. The percentage of time below the 5-microvolt RMS level is 12.2%. Compared to LUT, the right upper trapezius (RUT) graph has a smaller distribution range for the *y*-axis (160 compared to 250). In addition, the RUT graph shows a significantly greater dispersion of RMS amplitudes, with the highest peak being farther to the right on the graph. The rest peak is greatly diminished compared to the LUT graph; only 3.8% of the time is spent below 5 microvolts RMS. Some clinicians believe that the percentage of time for rest below the 5-microvolt range should be greater than 5%. When the percentage of time below 5 microvolts RMS is less than 5%, pain is commonly experienced with prolonged exertion. This was the case for the patient whose data appear in Figure 3–18.

A

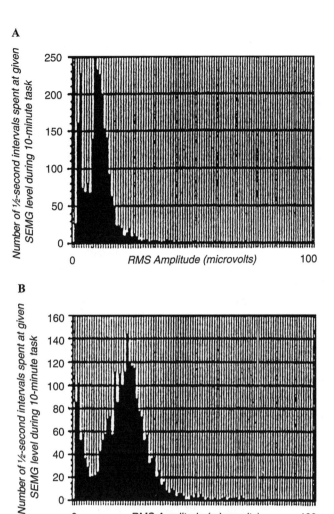

B

Figure 3–18 Amplitude probability distribution function for the left (A) and right (B) upper trapezius during a 10-minute typing task. The *x*-axis represents 0-100 microvolts RMS. The *y*-axis represents the number of half-second periods of time spent at a given RMS amplitude. Note that the scale for these counts differs for the graphs (A) and (B). The peak rest and work values for (A), the normal side of the patient, are around 2 and 10, respectively. The rest and work peaks for (B), the painful side of the patient, are around 2 and 23, respectively.

Source: Courtesy of Will Taylor, Portland, Oregon.

AUDITORY DISPLAYS

The discussion to this point has focused on visually oriented displays. Many SEMG instruments also have auditory capabilities. Some of the instruments allow the observer to listen to the raw SEMG signal. This feature is always incorporated in needle EMG systems and provides some of the clues that guide diagnosis. In SEMG, the raw signal sounds like white noise or the ocean. When it is contaminated with 60-cycle interference, one can hear a distinct hum. Many biofeedback instruments convert the SEMG signal into a variety of tones or "musical instruments." For example, the pitch may go higher as the SEMG amplitude goes higher.

Audio tones are commonly linked to thresholds. Here, the practitioner sets an amplitude level, and whenever the SEMG exceeds that amplitude, a special tone is played. These thresholds may be used to "shape" the patient's SEMG signals to higher or lower levels. Shaping is a process in which the practitioner gradually increases (or decreases) the threshold as the patient shows improvement in obtaining the threshold goal.

ISSUES REGARDING NOISE AND ARTIFACT

Noise and artifact are functionally defined as anything contained in the SEMG signal that the practitioner does not want. One attribute of an SEMG amplifier is its signal-to-noise ratio. The ideal amplifier has a very high signal-to-noise ratio—all signal and no noise. This section describes some of the primary examples of noise and artifact that pertain to the internal noise of the electronic circuitry of the instrument. Noise from outside the instrument may also be a problem.

A common source of noise for the electromyographer is the *ECG artifact*. The ECG is very coherent and much larger than that of the muscles. It is clearly picked up on nearly all of the sites located on the torso. It is primarily seen on the left side of the body and, therefore, may lead to asymmetrical RMS values during rest. This artifact is clearly shown in both the raw and processed SEMG tracings from the left serratus anterior (LSer) in **Figure 3–19**. It is also commonly seen in the left lumbar area. ECG artifact is not commonly seen in the extremities, except when wrist-to-wrist or ankle-to-ankle leads are used. This type of artifact can be minimized by placing the electrodes close together and using a 100- to 200-Hz band pass filter. Many practitioners, however, readily accept the ECG artifact as a fact of life and merely educate their patients about this phenomenon. As a side benefit, one could use the ECG as an index of arousal by observing changes in the patient's pulse rate.

Movement artifact is seen as direct current (DC) shifts and/or massive deflections in the SEMG potentials of the raw SEMG recording. This occurs because the electrode slips around on the surface of the skin, generating an electrical potential of its own. The upper panel of Figure 3–19 shows this slippage in the raw SEMG for the left serratus anterior site as a distortion in the DC levels around which the SEMG signal oscillates. In this particular instance, a momentary slippage of the electrode occurs as a function of skin distortion (stretch) as the patient moves his or her arms out of abduction and into shoulder elevation. When this tracing is then converted to the processed mode (Figure 3–19B), however, the movement artifact simply appears as an upward deflection. With the process mode, it is difficult to differentiate the movement artifact from the real SEMG signal. Only

in the raw mode can the practitioner discriminate this artifact from the real SEMG recruitment. Movement artifact can be reduced by using floating electrodes rather than direct-contact electrodes. The cushion of paste between the skin and the electrode can absorb the electrode slippage and greatly reduce this type of artifact. An additional strategy involves taping the electrodes to the body of the patient so the patient does not sway or pull on the electrodes.

Another major source of noise is *60-cycle energy*—the type of energy that we use to power lights, offices, and the computers used to monitor the SEMG. This phenomenon is such a significant source of noise that nearly all SEMG instruments have a special notch filter to try and eradicate it. Poor electrode connections can easily provide the medium by which the 60-cycle noise exceeds the capacity of the notch filter to eliminate it, so that it spills over into the visual and quantitative displays. A 60-cycle artifact may be seen in the oscillating pattern in Figure 3–8. It is represented in a more subtle way in the left upper trapezius in **Figure 3–20A**. This type of artifact is typically easier to see with a raw SEMG display than with a processed one. **Figure 3–20B** shows the spectral analysis of a 1-second epoch of the tracing in Figure 3–20A. Here, one can see that the 60-Hz portion of the signal has successfully been eliminated. Unfortunately, the harmonics of 60-cycle energy have not been filtered out and contribute heavily to the signal. This artifact is seen as "telephone poles" in the spectral analysis at 120 Hz, 180 Hz, and 240 Hz.

If clinicians observe a 60-cycle artifact, they should begin troubleshooting by replacing the electrodes along with a vigorous abrade. They should reduce the possibility that the electrode leads are acting like antennae that pick up the noise. Single-stranded leads should be twisted tightly together, and the length of the leads should be shortened if possible. Shielded leads can be tried instead. Clinicians may also want to eliminate any possible sources of 60-cycle noise in the recording environment. One common source of this noise is the computer monitor; to avoid this type of interference, the patient should be as far away from the computer as possible (a minimum of 3 feet).

Respiration is another biological artifact commonly seen in SEMG recordings. This artifact is most commonly seen in the upper torso and neck. Specifically, placements on the upper trapezius, scalene, and sternocleidomastoid muscles may show SEMG potentials associated with breathing. This is shown for the scalene

A

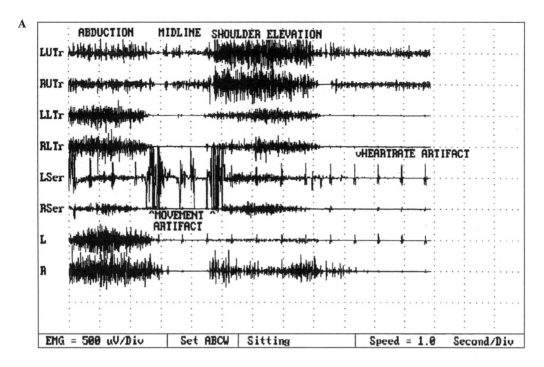

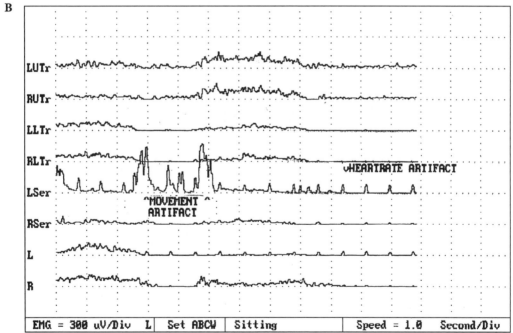

Figure 3–19 (A) Raw and (B) processed SEMG tracings with clear ECG and movement artifact. The ECG artifact is clearly seen as rhythmic deflections in the serratus anterior (LSer) for both the raw and processed tracings. The movement artifact is seen in the DC shifts in the LSer for the raw tracing. Note how it is difficult to discern the movement artifact in the LSer track of the processed EMG recording.

Source: Copyright © Clinical Resources, Inc.

A

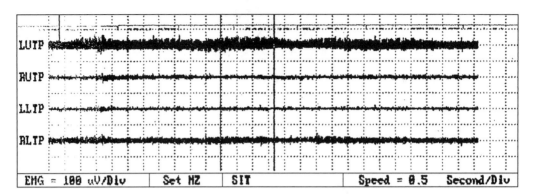

B

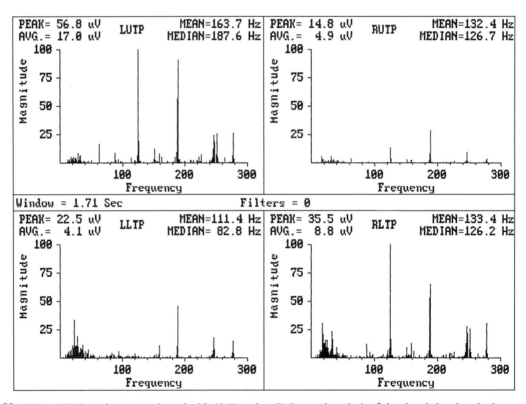

Figure 3–20 (A) Raw SEMG tracing contaminated with 60-Hz noise. (B) Spectral analysis of the signal showing the harmonics of 60-Hz noise.

Source: Copyright © Clinical Resources, Inc.

muscles in **Figure 3–21**. Both sets of these muscles are considered ancillary muscles of respiration, and they are invoked when the patient needs to raise the ribs to facilitate breathing into the upper lobes of the lungs. This movement is very common in high-demand situations such as running. During quiet sitting, however, it is highly unusual to see large recruitment patterns associated with respiration in these muscles. The major exceptions to this rule are patients with chronic obstructive pulmonary disease or patients who breathe in a para-

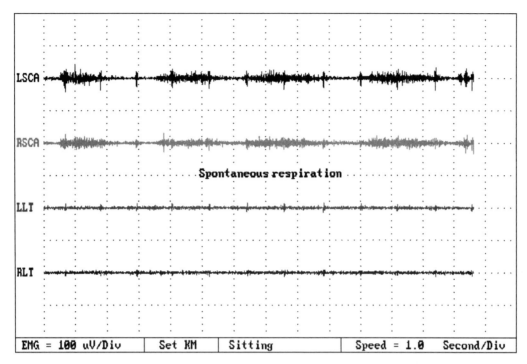

Figure 3–21 Surface EMG recordings from scalene (LSCA and RSCA) and lower trapezius (LLT and RLT) muscles. The scalene muscles show a clear respiration artifact.

Source: Copyright © Clinical Resources, Inc.

doxical fashion. When this artifact is noted, biofeedback training for the correct respiratory pattern is indicated.

Another artifact that may occasionally be encountered is caused by radio frequency (RF). Here, the signals from a local radio station are picked up by the antenna effect of the electrode leads and fed into the amplifiers. This phenomenon is fairly rare but does happen. It can be observed most dramatically on SEMG instruments with a raw SEMG audio option, when the radio can be heard on the speaker. Using only the visual display in a processed or raw mode, the practitioner would note large, spontaneous changes in the SEMG signal that had nothing to do with the patient's movements. If RF noise is suspected, it is necessary to move the SEMG instrument into another room or to the other side of the building. Moving the recording environment is the only solution to RF noise.

One other biological artifact is cross-talk, which occurs when the energy from a distant muscle reaches the electrodes placed over another muscle site. Although it is the bane of dynamic SEMG, it really does not matter for relaxation-oriented protocols. A very clear example of cross-talk is seen in frontal SEMG recordings when the patient clenches the teeth. An example may be seen in **Figure 3–22**, which illustrates the specificity of the frontal recording site during an eyebrow flash. Cross-talk occurs when the energy of the masseter and temporalis muscles that are recruited during a clench is picked up by the frontal leads.

Careful placement of closely spaced electrodes is the only hope for limiting the cross-talk artifact. It is important to recognize its presence and to monitor from those potentially offending distant muscles.

HOW TO CHECK SPECIFICATIONS OF SURFACE ELECTROMYOGRAPHIC INSTRUMENTS

Not all SEMG instruments are made alike. In a review of 11 SEMG instruments, Rugh and Schwitzgebel[19] noted tremendous variability in several key features. It is important for practitioners to know what to look for in the SEMG instruments they are currently using or planning to acquire. The purpose of this section is not to compare one SEMG system directly with another, but rather to recap the instrumentation issues presented in this chap-

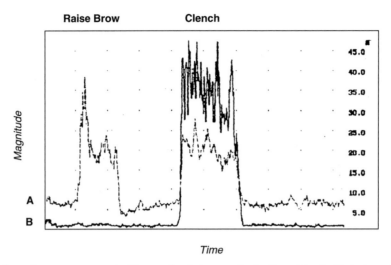

Figure 3–22 Cross-talk from the masseter muscle (A) may clearly be seen in the frontal leads (B) during a jaw clench.

ter so that practitioners can note their own instruments' strengths and weaknesses or make an informed choice in an equipment purchase. **Table 3–2** reviews the different attributes of SEMG instruments.

As an aid to the practitioner, a checklist is provided that lists all of the attributes of an SEMG instrument (**Exhibit 3–1**). This form can be used to organize all of the information available on an instrument.

Table 3–2 The Specifications of Surface Electromyographic Instruments

Concept	Desirable Range	Comments
Input impedance	100 kilohm 1 gigaohm	Most commercial machines have 1 megOhm input impedance or better. This is more than adequate for medical uses.
Common mode rejection (CMR or CMMR)	70–180 dB	This determines the ability of the SEMG amplifier to eliminate external noise from the environment, such as noise from energy used to power lights and computers. In general, the higher this value, the better.
Instrument noise level	0.1–1.0 μV	This represents the lowest level of SEMG an instrument can pick up. It is, in essence, the noise level of the SEMG amplifier: The lower, the better. Most commercially available instruments allow detection of 0.5 μV or higher.
Band pass filter width		Most of the SEMG energy resides between 20 and 300 Hz. The facial muscles are exceptions; because they are closer to the surface, are smaller, and have a
General case	20–1000 Hz	high innervation ratio, they can be monitored up to 600 Hz. The band pass
Relaxation training	100–200 Hz	width also determines the nature of the noise that is let in. ECG artifact can
Musculoskeletal assessment and rehabilitation	20–300 Hz	be all but eliminated by using a 100–200 Hz filter. If the SEMG instrument allows the user to set the band pass filter width, it provides more degrees of freedom. The filter width should be selected to fit the type of work. When
Facial muscle recordings	20–600 Hz	working with musculoskeletal dysfunction or soft-tissue injury, where the muscle may have a fatigue component, the practitioner should make sure that the lower end of the band pass is around 20 Hz. On the other hand, the 100–200 Hz filter width should work fine with relaxation-based work.

(continues)

Table 3–2 *(Continued)*

Concept	Desirable Range	Comments

Range/gain
  General case
  Dynamic
    movement
  Relaxation
	
	0–1000 RMS µV
	0–1000 RMS µV
	
	0–100 RMS µV
		Range represents the amplitude that can be monitored using a particular SEMG instrument. For dynamic SEMG recordings, the general case of amplitude should be possible. If the SEMG instrument has a range of 0–500 µV and the practitioner is studying events that exceed that amount, the amplifiers would simply saturate at the top end of the scale and potentially valuable information would be lost. For relaxation-oriented work, one would not expect to see amplitudes over 100 µV. It is best if the instrument allows the practitioner to select from several ranges so that the recording can be sensitive to what is being studied or treated.

Smoothing options	0.1–10 second time constant	The smoothing option on an SEMG instrument may or may not be specified as a time constant. Usually it is necessary to turn a dial or increment a number on a computerized system. Sometimes this feature is referred to as a filter, which refers to digital filtering or smoothing.[20] It is highly desirable for instruments to allow the practitioner to choose how much smoothing or processing of the signal is done.
Visual displays		The visual display is the practitioner's link to the SEMG information. It should be easy to read.
Meter	Linear versus logarithmic	Meters commonly come in two varieties: linear and logarithmic. With linear meters, there is an equal spacing between each number. This is the most common type of meter. Logarithmic meters give more space to the low end than to the high end of the scale. We have more precision in how we use our muscles at the low microvolt level than at the high microvolt level. The logarithmic meter makes more sense for relaxation work.
Digital		Digital displays are highly desirable so that the practitioner can see the quantified SEMG as it changes from moment to moment. It is always nice to be able to control how frequently the digital value updates.
Computer	Raw and processed	Computer displays allow the practitioner to see time-series scrolls of the SEMG information. Instruments that allow the practitioner to choose between the raw and processed signals offer the greatest versatility. In general, raw SEMG provides greater diagnostic information, while processed visual displays are easier for the patient to understand.

Audio displays
  Raw SEMG
    audio
  Thresholds
  Binary versus
    analog
	Raw
	feedback
		The audio portion of the SEMG should be considered. A raw SEMG channel yields valuable diagnostic information to the trained ear. The audio feedback features of an SEMG instrument are essential for retraining purposes. This feedback may be in the form of an analog tone—one that simply varies in pitch. Alternatively, it may come in the form of a binary tone that comes on only when the patient is above or below a preset threshold. With today's multimedia computer capabilities, it is possible to play music or complex tones or even have the computer talk to the patient.

Exhibit 3–1 Surface EMG Unit Worksheet for Physical Medicine Practitioners

Check User Priorities Criteria	Unit Name/Model			
____ Stand-alone (SA), personal computer (PC), both (B)	SA/PC/B	SA/PC/B	SA/PC/B	SA/PC/B
____ Special computer requirements				
Power source/safety				
____ 3-Prong plug, optical isolation	yes/no/NA	yes/no/NA	yes/no/NA	yes/no/NA
____ Battery type/life	NA	NA	NA	NA
Electrode compatibility				
____ Any (A), manufacturer's electrode only (M)	A/M	A/M	A/M	A/M
____ Electrode system	active/passive	active/passive	active/passive	active/passive
____ Electrode distance	fixed/modifiable	fixed/modifiable	fixed/modifiable	fixed/modifiable
Lead wires				
____ Electrode connectors	snap/alligator	snap/alligator	snap/alligator	snap/alligator
____ Shielding, general quality	sturdy/okay/flimsy	sturdy/okay/flimsy	sturdy/okay/flimsy	sturdy/okay/flimsy
____ Quality of amplifier connectors	sturdy/okay/flimsy	sturdy/okay/flimsy	sturdy/okay/flimsy	sturdy/okay/flimsy
____ Ground lead	integral/separate	integral/separate	integral/separate	integral/separate
____ Lead length				
Amplifier				
____ Input impedance				
____ **CMRR (common mode rejection ratio)**				
____ Total gain				
Frequency filter				
____ Band width limits/roll-off	/	/	/	/
____ 60-Hz notch filter/roll-off	yes/no	yes/no	yes/no	yes/no
____ **Sampling rate**				
____ **Time constant/smoothing range**				
____ **Microvolt quantification**				
____ RMS, integral average, other				
____ **Adequate noise suppression**	always/not always	always/not always	always/not always	always/not always
Visual display output				
____ Display type	video/crystal/LED	video/crystal/LED	video/crystal/LED	video/crystal/LED
____ Display type	linear/log/both	linear/log/both	linear/log/both	linear/log/both
____ Optional raw display	yes/no	yes/no	yes/no	yes/no
____ Digital	yes/no	yes/no	yes/no	yes/no
____ Moving line, oscilloscope-like	yes/no	yes/no	yes/no	yes/no
____ Variable sweep speed	yes/no	yes/no	yes/no	yes/no
____ Bar graph	yes/no	yes/no	yes/no	yes/no
____ Motor templates	yes/no	yes/no	yes/no	yes/no
____ Games, others				
Audio output				
____ Modulating	pitch/click/other	pitch/click/other	pitch/click/other	pitch/click/other
____ Optional raw audio	yes/no	yes/no	yes/no	yes/no
Audio yoking to signal				
____ Above goal	yes/no	yes/no	yes/no	yes/no
____ Below goal	yes/no	yes/no	yes/no	yes/no
____ Between dual goals	yes/no	yes/no	yes/no	yes/no

(continues)

Exhibit 3–1 *(Continued)*

Check User Priorities Criteria	Unit Name/Model			
Sensitivity	manual/auto only/	manual/auto only/	manual/auto only/	manual/auto only/
____ Adjustment	manual & auto	manual & auto	manual & auto	manual & auto
____ Adequate low-end response range	yes/no	yes/no	yes/no	yes/no
____ Adequate high-end response range	yes/no	yes/no	yes/no	yes/no
____ Choice of sensitivity ranges	okay/limited	okay/limited	okay/limited	okay/limited
____ Ease of adjustment	easy/okay/difficult	easy/okay/difficult	easy/okay/difficult	easy/okay/difficult
____ Scale offset available	yes/no	yes/no	yes/no	yes/no
Thresholds/goals				
____ Easy to see	easy/okay/difficult	easy/okay/difficult	easy/okay/difficult	easy/okay/difficult
____ Ease of adjustment	easy/okay/difficult	easy/okay/difficult	easy/okay/difficult	easy/okay/difficult
EMG channels				
____ Number				
____ Modular additions possible	yes/no	yes/no	yes/no	yes/no
____ **Graphic print capability**	yes/no	yes/no	yes/no	yes/no

Comments regarding print functions/report generation

____ **EMG data storage capacity**				
____ **Statistical management**	max/min/avg/rng	max/min/avg/rng	max/min/avg/rng	max/min/avg/rng
	ratio/% diff	ratio/% diff	ratio/% diff	ratio/% diff
____ Event counter	yes/no	yes/no	yes/no	yes/no
____ Frequency spectral analysis	yes/no	yes/no	yes/no	yes/no
____ Download to statistics package	yes/no	yes/no	yes/no	yes/no
Software: general				
____ Overall ease of operation	easy/okay/difficult	easy/okay/difficult	easy/okay/difficult	easy/okay/difficult
____ Labeled/dedicated keys	yes/no	yes/no	yes/no	yes/no
____ Menu driven	yes/no	yes/no	yes/no	yes/no
____ Mouse drag and click	yes/no	yes/no	yes/no	yes/no
____ Ability to store patient files	yes/no	yes/no	yes/no	yes/no
____ Playback ability	yes/no	yes/no	yes/no	yes/no
____ Other special software features				
____ Software upgradable	yes/no	yes/no	yes/no	yes/no
External relay for neuromuscular				
electrical stimulation	yes/no	yes/no	yes/no	yes/no
____ Ease of EMG-NMES software	easy/okay/difficult	easy/okay/difficult	easy/okay/difficult	easy/okay/difficult
Cost				
____ Finance/lease arrangements				
____ **Warranty period**				
After-purchase services				
____ Area representative	yes/no	yes/no	yes/no	yes/no
____ Educational support	yes/no	yes/no	yes/no	yes/no
____ Trade-ins for upgrades	yes/no	yes/no	yes/no	yes/no
____ Other				
____ **Other comments**				

Source: Courtesy of Movement Systems, Inc., Seattle, Washington.

REFERENCES

1. Peek CJ. A primer of biofeedback instrumentation. In: Schwartz M, ed. *Biofeedback: A Practitioner's Guide.* New York, NY: Guilford Press; 1987:45–95.
2. Basmajian JV, DeLuca C. *Muscles Alive.* 5th ed. Baltimore, MD: Williams & Wilkins; 1985.
3. Soderberg GL, ed. *Selected Topics in Surface Electromyography for Use in the Occupational Setting: Expert Perspective.* Washington, DC: U.S. Department of Health and Human Services; 1992. U.S. Department of Health and Human Services publication NIOSH 91-100.
4. Cacioppo JT, Tassinary G, Fridlund AJ. The skeletalmotor system. In: Cacioppo JT, Tassinary G, eds. *Principles of Psychophysiology.* New York, NY: Cambridge University Press; 1990:325–384.
5. Kessler M, Cram JR, Traue H. EMG muscle scanning in pain patients and controls: a replication and extension. *Am J Pain Manage.* 1993;3:20–28.
6. DeLuca C. Myoelectric manifestations of localized muscular fatigue in humans. *CRC Crit Rev Biomed Eng.* 1984;11:251.
7. Roy SH, DeLuca CJ, Casavant DA. Lumbar muscle fatigue and chronic back pain. *Spine.* 1989;14:992–1001.
8. Roy SH, DeLuca CJ, Snyder-Mackler L, et al. Fatigue, recovery and low back pain in elite rowers. *Med Sci Sports Exerc.* 1990;22:463–469.
9. Yang JF, Winter DA. Electromyographic amplitude normalization methods: improving their sensitivity, as a diagnostic tool in gait analysis. *Arch Phys Med.* 1984;65:517–521.
10. Knutson LM, Soderberg GL, Ballantyne BT, Clarke WR. A study of various normalization procedures for within day electromyographic data. *J Electromyogr Kinesiol.* 1994;1:47–59.
11. Mathiassen SE, Winkel J, Hagg GM. Normalization of surface EMG amplitude from the upper trapezius muscle in ergonomic studies: a review. *J Electromyogr Kinesiol.* 1995;5:197–226.
12. Attebrant M, Mathiassen SE, Winkel J. Normalizing upper trapezius EMG amplitude: comparison of ramp and constant force procedures. *J Electromyogr Kinesiol.* 1995;5:245–250.
13. Bao S, Mathiassen SE, Winkel J. Normalizing upper trapezius EMG amplitude: comparison of different procedures. *J Electromyogr Kinesiol.* 1995;5:251–257.
14. Donaldson S, Donaldson M. Multi-channel EMG assessment and treatment techniques. In: Cram JR, ed. *Clinical EMG for Surface Recordings, II.* Nevada City, CA: Clinical Resources; 1990:143–174.
15. Jonsson B. Kinesiology: with special reference to electromyographic kinesiology. *Cont Clin Neurophysiol EEG Suppl.* 1978;34:417–428.
16. Cram JR. EMG biofeedback and the treatment of tension headaches: a systematic analysis of treatment components. *Behav Ther.* 1980;11:699–710.
17. Veiersted KB, Westgaard RH, Andersen P. Electromyographic evaluation of muscular work pattern as a predictor of trapezius myalgia. *Scan J Work Environ Health.* 1993;19:284–290.
18. Veiersted KB, Westgaard RH. Work related risk factors for trapezius myalgia. *Int Arch Occup Environ Health.* 1990;62:31–41.
19. Rugh J, Schwitzgebel R. Variability in commercial electromyographic biofeedback devices. *Behav Res Methods Instrum.* 1977;9:281–285.

CHAPTER QUESTIONS

1. The tissue of the human body acts like:
   a. a high-pass filter
   b. a low-pass filter
   c. a notch filter
   d. an amplifier
2. A differential amplifier:
   a. amplifies the difference of two separate muscle sites
   b. finds the difference between two muscles
   c. amplifies everything that is common to the recording electrodes
   d. amplifies everything that is unique to the recording electrodes
3. Which of the following would represent a band reject filter?
   a. 100- to 200-Hz band pass filter
   b. 60-Hz notch filter
   c. 35-Hz low-pass filter
   d. 20-Hz high-pass filter
4. Which of the following amplifiers is considered to have the best common mode rejection?
   a. 70 dB
   b. 50 μv
   c. 140 dB
   d. 10 megOhm
5. How much larger should the impedance of the electrode to skin interface be than the input impedance of the amplifier?
   a. 2 times greater
   b. 5 times greater
   c. 10 to 100 times greater
   d. equal to the input impedance of the amplifier
6. How would the SEMG recordings of an obese individual compare to the SEMG levels of a very thin individual?
   a. They would be the same.
   b. They would be higher.
   c. They would be lower.
   d. It doesn't matter.

7. When monitoring the gluteus maximus and rectus femoris muscles during hip flexion and extension, how should the practitioner compare these two muscles?
   a. Compare RMS microvolts only.
   b. Compare only integral averages.
   c. Compare only normalized recordings.
   d. One cannot compare these two muscles.
8. Which filter typically eliminates or dramatically reduces any ECG artifact from SEMG recordings?
   a. 25-Hz high-pass filter
   b. 60-Hz notch filter
   c. 100- to 200-Hz band pass filter
   d. 35-Hz low-pass filter
9. During muscle fatigue, what typically happens to the median frequency of the SEMG power density?
   a. It stays constant.
   b. Its value falls.
   c. Its value rises.
   d. Its value rises in an inverse relation to SEMG amplitude.
10. Raw SEMG tracings are commonly quantified using which of the following methods?
    a. peak to peak
    b. RMS
    c. integral average
    d. raw
11. When examining the SEMG signal for interspersed rest, what is the criterion level at which rest is defined (J&J M-501 benchmark)?
    a. below 2 microvolts
    b. below 5 microvolts
    c. below 20 microvolts
    d. below 50 microvolts
12. The power spectral density curves used to examine the distribution of muscle energy across the various frequencies of the SEMG recording use which of the following methods of analysis?
    a. FFT
    b. SEMG
    c. ABC
    d. mean extrapolation

13. The energy spectrum of SEMG during work commonly resides within which of the following frequency bands?
    a. 20–300 Hz
    b. 100–200 Hz
    c. 20–1000 Hz
    d. 20–40 Hz
14. In SEMG, RMS refers to:
    a. random motor stimulation
    b. root mean square
    c. rotary motion study
    d. random motion stabilization
15. The ECG artifact is most commonly found where?
    a. on the extremities
    b. on the torso
    c. on the left aspect of the torso
    d. on the cephalic muscles
16. *Smoothing* is a term that refers to
    a. digital filtering
    b. abrading the skin for electrode placement
    c. the quality of a movement pattern during training
    d. relaxation training protocols
17. What can be said about SEMG amplitudes and force?
    a. There is a one-to-one relationship.
    b. There is a curvilinear relationship.
    c. There is no relationship.
    d. It actually doesn't make sense to focus on this relationship because the issues are far too complex.
18. The impedance at each recording electrode should be:
    a. low
    b. high
    c. low and balanced
    d. high and balanced

Electrodes and Site Selection Strategies

ELECTRODE SELECTION

Electrodes are like tiny microphones that are used to listen to the muscles. Because several types of electrodes are available on the market, practitioners should know the intended use of each and select the electrode that provides the highest quality of surface electromyography (SEMG) recording. **Figure 4–1** shows a variety of electrodes available for the practitioner.

In making the selection, practitioners should consider the size of the electrode. Electrodes with smaller detection areas (and housings) allow· closer interelectrode spacings and, therefore, offer a higher level of selectivity.[1] Small electrodes are important in recordings from the facial muscles and from some of the muscles of the upper extremities. These electrodes might be 0.5 cm in diameter and placed at an interelectrode distance of 1 cm. For larger, broad muscles, electrodes with larger surface areas are desirable and may be placed farther apart. For example, a very commonly used type of electrode provides a 1-cm diameter pellet, placed an interelectrode distance of 2 cm. This size and this spacing work for many sites. As the interelectrode spacing increases to 3 cm, larger, broader muscles may be monitored. As the interelectrode distance increases, the specificity of the recording decreases and recordings become more "regional." A 2-cm spacing on the upper

trapezius, for example, provides a very specific recording for that muscle. In contrast, the wide trapezius placement provides a regional recording of the upper back. Here, the recording electrodes are placed quite far apart, with one electrode on the right and one electrode on the left aspect of the trapezius.

Some electrodes are placed in direct contact with the skin, whereas others float on a cushion of paste above the skin. *Direct contact electrodes* are small disks that are placed directly on the skin and held in place by tape. This type of electrode was the model originally used for SEMG. In the past, these electrodes were usually made of silver or gold, and a small amount of saline paste was placed between the electrode and the skin. Some practitioners soldered a lead to a silver quarter or nickel and then taped it over the muscle of interest. Today, direct contact electrodes are commonly 0.5 to 1 cm in diameter and are made of a disposable silver-impregnated plastic that is coated with a thin layer of silver chloride to help stabilize the electrical potentials of the skin. Each is held in place with a small adhesive or foam collar that is slightly larger than the pellet. The adhesive quality of collars varies greatly. Some are diaphoretic (allowing perspiration through). One should consider the adhesion properties of the collar or electrode when choosing the appropriate electrode for the site of interest. For example,

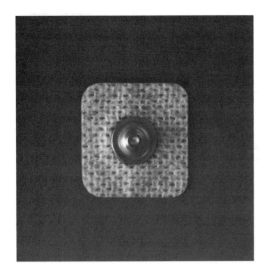
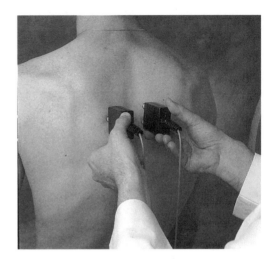

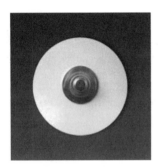
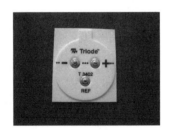
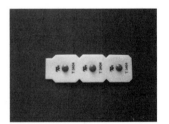

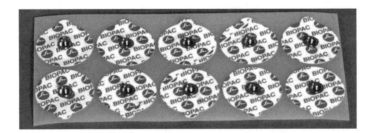

Figure 4–1 Types of SEMG electrodes.

Source: (Top left) Courtesy of Vermed, Inc.; (top right) Reproduced with permission of Myotronics, Inc.; (center left) Courtesy of Vermed, Inc.; (center center) Courtesy of Thought Technology Ltd.; (center right) Courtesy of Thought Technology Ltd.; (bottom) Courtesy of BIOPAC Systems, Inc.

electrodes placed on the low back need to adhere very well to the skin because the area is subject to extreme skin distortions and stretching during dynamic movements. However, when recording focuses on the facial muscles, some patients cannot tolerate an extremely adhesive pad. Hydrogel electrodes (discussed later in this section) provide a very gentle adhesive to be used on patients with sensitive skin.

Direct contact electrodes are ideal for quiet SEMG recordings (i.e., relaxation-based therapies). Because they reside directly on the skin, they are more subject to movement artifact (see Chapter 3) and, therefore, are not recommended for recording of dynamic movements. Activity of the body may create movement of the electrode itself upon the skin's surface, creating a direct current (DC) offset potential or movement artifact. Such artifacts commonly occur during vigorous movement, but may be present even during soft, quiet movements.

Floating electrodes are recommended for the recording of dynamic movements. They are created in such a way that the electrode is housed inside a cup, elevated above the skin by a millimeter or so. The cup is then filled with an electrolytic medium. An electrode paste or gel provides the bridge between the electrode and the skin. This substance potentiates the biological signal from the skin to the electrode and provides a cushion that absorbs the movement of the electrode (housing) on the skin's surface.

Floating electrodes may take more time to prepare and are usually a little more expensive than direct contact electrodes. While the electrolytic cushion reduces the movement artifact, it may not totally eliminate it. In addition, the use of pastes and gels may lead to a bridging of electrode paste between two active electrodes—even when electrodes are placed as much as 2 cm apart. One can reduce the probability of bridging by applying only a light pressure to the cup electrodes when they are applied to the skin. Firm pressure, however, may accidentally force the paste in one cell over to the adjoining cell. When such bridging occurs, the impedance at the electrode site is radically reduced or short-circuited. The biological energy seen by the SEMG amplifiers is significantly reduced, yielding a digital reading that is atypically low for the site and that does not change in a predictable way as a function of vigorous muscle contraction. If the practitioner is monitoring multiple sites, the SEMG readings for the site with bridging will likely appear quite low in comparison to the other sites. It is necessary to remove the bridged electrode, abrade the skin

again, and replace the electrode before a high-quality recording may be obtained. Some patients may be allergic or sensitive to the electrode paste or gel. Patients with such sensitivities should be offered hydrogel electrodes.

Hydrogel electrodes were initially developed for providing electrical stimulation to the skin (i.e., transcutaneous electrical nerve stimulation [TENS]) and have since been used to record biological potentials. They commonly consist of a silver chloride disk electrode covered with a dry, sticky layer of gel as large as the usual adhesive collar. Sometimes the electrode consists of a foil with a tab. Hydrogel has a water and acidity content that is similar to the skin and, therefore, does not adversely affect the skin. Although this type of electrode allows the electrical potentials from the muscles to flow into the amplifiers, it has a higher impedance than the direct contact electrode or floating electrode; consequently, it may be a bit noisier. In addition, the adhesion to the skin is lighter, allowing for easy removal of the electrode. Hydrogel electrodes may be moved from one electrode site to another, although this practice is not recommended. In a sense, these electrodes are replaceable. The lightness of the adhesion also means that the electrode may come loose when perspiration occurs or during movements that place a strain on the lead attached to the electrode. To ensure good adhesion, hydrogel electrodes typically have a large surface area. They are probably best used for relaxation or other forms of quiet training and are the ideal solution for patients with sensitive skin.

Electrodes for recording from the perineum (pelvic floor) have also been developed. These *vaginal and rectal electrodes* may have the dumbbell shape seen in **Figure 4-2**. Two or three electrodes are located on the middle part of the electrode. They are inserted into the rectum or vaginal barrel and allow recording from the perianal muscles or the muscles of the pelvic floor. They are somewhat intrusive and, therefore, may not be appropriate for children. In addition, sterilization of the electrode may be an issue. Therefore, it is wise to use a single-user type of electrode, so that the patient can clean and keep the sensor for repeated uses, but the same sensor is not used on multiple patients.

Ribbon electrodes are relatively new and consist of a silver ink electrode array and lead wires printed onto a thin sheet of Mylar and then covered by a thin foam pad with "cells" that define the electrode size and allow for electrode paste or gel. Such an electrode is shown in **Figure 4-3**. These electrodes are ideal for recording

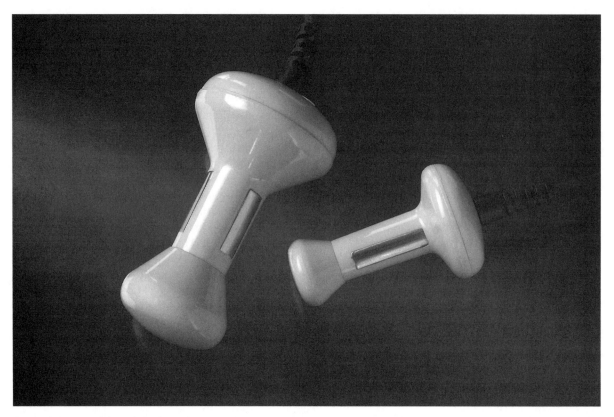

Figure 4–2 Vaginal recording electrode.
Source: Courtesy of SRS Medical.

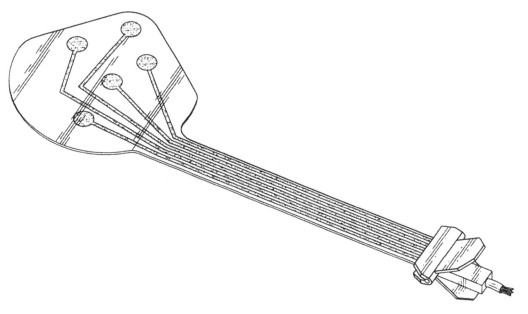

Figure 4–3 Ribbon electrode designed for specific monitoring of frontalis and corrugator muscles of the face.
Source: Courtesy of Patient Comfort.

from predetermined sets of muscles, such as those on the face. They are currently being used to monitor the facial displays of emotion from the muscle activity of the frontalis and corrugator, or the zygomaticus and orbicularis oculi during surgical procedures.[2] In addition, the flat pad allows for recordings when the patient is in a face-down position. This kind of recording would be impossible with pellet types of electrodes. Ribbon electrodes will certainly be extended to other applications in the future.

ELECTRODE LEADS AND CABLES

The lead wires transmit the SEMG signals to the SEMG amplifiers. Leads should be shielded and kept as short as possible. Otherwise, the electrode leads may act as antennae and pick up 60-Hz noise from the walls, fluorescent lighting, computers, monitors, or radio signals from a nearby transmitting tower. The longer the leads, the greater the probability of this phenomenon. Short leads (18 inches or so) not only minimize the antenna effect, but also reduce the sway of wire, which can introduce movement artifact. When a wire is moved through a magnetic field (in this case, the earth's magnetic field), a current is induced into the wire. This small current is then amplified and displayed as if it were coming from the muscles. Therefore, elimination of any unnecessary wire sway is highly desirable.

Movement of the electrode leads may be reduced by taping them to the skin or the clothing. This also provides strain relief, so that the wires do not pull on the electrodes and cause a secondary movement artifact. If electrode leads are not shielded, the leads from the two recording electrodes should be in a tightly twisted pair. Usually, the two tightly twisted wires are placed within the same plastic sheath. If a separate lead wire is provided for each electrode, the wires should be twisted or braided together with the ground lead such that they approximate the tightly twisted pair concept. Otherwise, when two lead wires run in parallel, any external noise tends to affect both wires equally and simultaneously; the external noise would be eliminated by the common mode rejection of the amplifiers.

Lead wire noise problems have also been addressed by the use of *active electrodes*. Using surface mount technology, SEMG manufacturers have developed small plastic housings that place the preamplifier directly at the electrode site. The snaps on the electrodes plug directly into the preamplifier, which eliminates head wire noise. The major benefit of the active electrode is noise reduc-

tion from wire sway and 60-cycle energy. In applications where this type of noise is an issue, an active electrode should be considered.

The disadvantage of active electrodes is that they have a fixed interelectrode distance. This parameter may be altered, however, by the use of short stem leads to allow for different interelectrode distances. If the electrodes are snapped directly into the plastic housing of the active electrode, one should remember that the plastic housing is a flat surface that works best when placed on another flat surface. Unfortunately, there are few truly flat surfaces on the human body. This mismatch may lead to poor electrode contact and faulty recordings. Practitioners should always verify their signals and electrode connections carefully when using this type of arrangement. Finally, active electrodes are slightly heavier than typical electrode housings and, therefore, may require a stronger adhesive to maintain adequate contact with the skin.

Researchers hope that, in the future, sophisticated telemetry systems will virtually eliminate the need for lead wires. With this technology, a tiny transmitting device would be located within the active electrode, which would use a radio frequency to transmit the muscle's energy to a receiving unit that would store the data, process the signal, and display it on a video screen for analysis. Unfortunately, today's telemetry systems are quite expensive and tend to introduce some unwanted noise into the signal transmission. They are primarily used in recording athletic events.

SITE PREPARATION

The electrode–skin interface is a delicate matter. It is important to keep the impedance of the skin as low and balanced as possible. Although some equipment manufacturers claim that electrode site preparation requires little attention because of the high input impedance or special characteristics of their SEMG amplifiers, these claims have not been justified. No matter how high the input impedance of the amplifier, the impedance at the electrode site could be higher. For example, in the case of a patient with skin that is dry or scaly, coated with oil-based makeup, or covered with a deep layer of hair, the impedance of the electrode at the skin could be infinite (i.e., it could produce a faulty connection). Site preparation is strongly recommended as part of all clinical protocols.

To prepare the skin, use an alcohol-soaked pad and rub the electrode site with approximately six vigorous strokes. The pad should contain some rag content so that it is a little rough. Some electrode preparation pads actually contain a small amount of pumice to facilitate abrasion. Avoid cotton balls and tissues for this purpose: They simply do not do the intended job of removing the oils and top layer of dead or hornified skin so that the biological potentials can easily reach the recording electrodes. When the task is done well, a slight rubor is commonly seen.

Site preparation sometimes includes the application of a small amount of electrode paste or gel directly onto the recording site: Take a cotton swab, dip it into the electrode paste, apply it to the skin, and then spin it lightly at the location where the electrode will be placed. Whether the practitioner preapplies electrode paste to the skin, applies it directly to the electrode, or uses pregelled electrodes, the electrolytic medium penetrates the sweat glands and provides a link to the potentials residing below the skin. This greatly facilitates the transfer of the motor unit action potentials.

In situations where the instrument manufacturer provides dry electrodes for the active electrodes, these electrodes eventually become moistened by perspiration of the skin. When the dry electrodes are applied to the skin, the skin eventually opens up its pores and exudes sweat in the body's natural attempt to shed the foreign object. Thus, the body supplies its own electrolytic medium. However, this process may be somewhat unpredictable and take several minutes. Cram and Rommen[3] have compared the impedance characteristics of several types of site preparation. As can be seen in **Figure 4–4**, the impedance improves rapidly for site preparations that include electrolytic media. Only in the case of the dry electrode does impedance take a long time. During this accommodation period, the impedance of the electrode site falls, along with the SEMG amplitude reported by the instrument. Changes in impedance affect the SEMG amplitudes as well. The amplitudes drift downward over time, and impedance improves.

Skin temperature is another factor that may noticeably affect the impedance of the site and, therefore, the SEMG recordings. Skin temperature may fluctuate as a function of room temperature, but it is more likely affected by vigorous exercise. As skin temperature increases, the impedance reduces; such fluctuations can also alter the SEMG recordings. This is particularly true if the initial impedance was poor.

STRATEGIES FOR ELECTRODE PLACEMENT

Because the electrodes are the listening devices for picking up SEMG activity, knowing where to place the

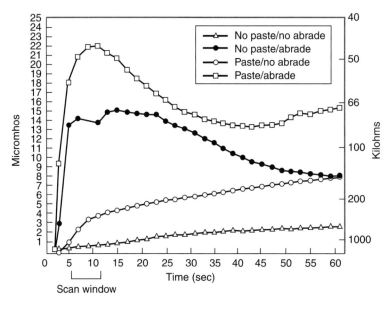

Figure 4–4 Impedance as a function of the type of electrode site preparation.

Source: Reprinted with permission from J. R. Cram and D. Rommen, Skin Preparation and Validity of EMG Scanning Procedure, *Biofeedback and Self Regulation*, Vol. 14, No. 4, pp. 75–82, © 1989, Plenum Publishing.

electrodes is a very important part of the process. Although only a small amount of information is available on this topic, Fridlund and Cacioppo[4] have highlighted six elements that can improve the fidelity of SEMG recordings:

1. Select the appropriate proximity of a proposed site to the underlying muscle mass, keeping the minimum amount of tissue between the electrodes and the muscle fibers themselves.
2. Select the appropriate position of the electrodes relative to the muscle fibers. Whenever possible, the electrodes should be placed parallel to the fibers to maximize sensitivity and selectivity (see **Figure 4–5**). Perpendicular placements tend to lead to greater common mode rejection and less selectivity.
3. Avoid straddling the motor end plate region. If this is done, the amplitudes observed are typically lower owing to differential amplification. Placing electrodes a little off the center of the muscle is better positioning.
4. Choose sites that are easy to locate (sites that have good anatomical landmarks to facilitate reliable placement of electrodes during subsequent recording sessions).
5. Choose sites that do not unduly obstruct vision or movement. Avoid areas that present problems owing to skin folds, bony obstruction, and other factors.
6. Minimize cross-talk from proximal deep or superficial muscles by selecting the best electrode size and interelectrode spacing.

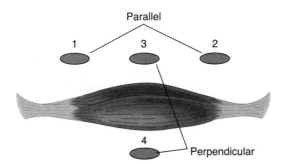

Figure 4–5 Relationship of muscle fibers to electrode placement.

Source: Copyright © J. R. Cram, *Clinical EMG for Surface Recordings: Volume 2*, Clinical Resources, Inc.

The practitioner must also decide which muscles are of clinical interest. One strategy for making this decision is the educated guess. Here the practitioner considers which muscle or muscles might be associated with the clinical phenomenon being studied or treated. The practitioner then places the electrodes over those muscle sites to test his or her clinical assumptions. This is a good model, because it encourages the practitioner to learn about muscle synergy patterns and to begin to see the movement and postural and emotional patterns as part of a larger whole.

A common but naive strategy is to place electrodes only over the area that hurts or is dysfunctional. For example, the practitioner might study only the upper trapezius muscle in someone with neck or shoulder pain. Although this may be a reasonable place to start, such a narrow focus on SEMG recordings for solitary muscles places artificial limits on the information that is obtained. The shortcoming of this strategy becomes clear when one considers the possibility that pain may be referred from a more distal site.

An alternative strategy is to use validated clinical protocols for SEMG recordings for specific disorders. For the patient with upper quarter pain, protocols have been developed that explore asymmetries and synergies of not only the upper trapezius but also the lower trapezius, and perhaps the serratus anterior.[5] Such protocols are designed to provide the practitioner with a limited, but very practical, approach to understanding the roles that muscles play in a given dysfunction. Protocols often work well, but when they fail, the practitioner must give further thought.

An extension of the protocol strategy is to develop variations based on clinical reasoning, knowledge of anatomy, and pathokinesiology. For the patient with shoulder pain, for example, the practitioner may want to consider also monitoring the deltoids, the infraspinatus, or the pectoralis. Finally, the practitioner should be open to the possibility that the disorder may be due to postural or emotional components or have its source in fascia, bone, or blood vessel. Given the complexity of the problem, the practitioner should have a strategy of going from one level of assessment to another, until all of the possible contributing factors have been examined.

In considering the strategy for assessing the postural component of dysfunction, it helpful to incorporate the sampling technique called *muscle scanning*.[6] Instead of studying just one or two sites while the patient is sitting and standing, muscle scanning allows the right and left aspects of multiple muscle groups to be studied in both the sitting and standing positions quickly using a hand-held scanner. The handheld scanner provides a chassis for two (or three) direct contact electrodes. These recording electrodes are held in place over a muscle by hand with a light pressure. For more information, see Chapter 6. The values that are obtained are then either compared to a normative reference group or are normalized and compared within the individual to determine which muscles are relatively hyperactive versus hypoactive. Right and left asymmetries may be considered within the context of various vertebral segments. Weight shifting or antalgic postures are commonly observed. Imbalances in the upper back can better be understood when imbalances in the lower back are also included. Once these relationships have been determined, the clinician can attach electrodes to gain a better understanding of how these relationships affect movement.

Strategies for studying or identifying the emotional aspect of the neuromuscular system should be considered as well. It is common for practitioners to place widely spaced electrodes on the frontal muscle, expose the patient to stressful events, and record the patient's reactions. Although such a recording procedure allows the practitioner to measure some of the major negative emotional states seen on the human face (e.g., anger, fear, and sadness), it does not provide information concerning specific emotional activation at the injured site or its homologous counterpart. One may broaden the search for an emotional component by placing a set of electrodes on the right and left aspects of the area of reported pain. Flor, Turk, and Birbaumer, for example, have demonstrated exquisite specificity of emotional reactions in the erector spinae muscles of patients with low-back pain, with little or no involvement of the facial muscles.[7]

Strategies associated with general relaxation are commonly used to treat the emotional component of dysfunction. Electrode placement for general relaxation typically involves widely spaced electrodes that cross the midline. Rather than monitoring and treating one muscle group, it is better for the practitioner to monitor and treat muscular regions. Placement of widely spaced electrodes on the frontal region increases the probability that the practitioner will see any emotional events on the patient's face. Widely spaced electrodes on the trapezius group allow the practitioner to see any activations of the neck and upper back. Wrist-to-wrist electrode placements allow the practitioner to see clearly any holding patterns or activations in the upper extremities, upper back, and chest. The ankle-to-ankle leads do the same for the lower extremities, buttocks, low back, and abdomen. In dynamic relaxation protocols, such as the ones developed by Ettare,[8] the right and left aspects of general regions are considered. For example, the right and left trapezius placement strategy would allow the practitioner to monitor the right and left aspects for the region of the upper back. Treatment would be directed at teaching the patient how to quiet the muscles quickly following their activation.

Strategies of electrode placement associated with specific muscle monitoring typically involve closely spaced electrodes that are placed parallel to muscle fibers or in areas with the least cross-talk. The electrodes are most commonly placed directly over or slightly lateral to the belly of the muscle. The electrode placement strategy for specifically monitoring the upper fibers of the trapezius, for example, is to place the recording electrode on the ridge of the shoulder, slightly lateral to the center of the muscle belly, and with the electrodes running in the direction of the fibers. In considering placement of electrodes for muscles that are partially covered by another muscle or a muscle that has very close proximity to neighboring muscles, it is sometimes possible to place recording electrodes on a distal portion of the muscle to avoid or minimize cross-talk. Recordings from the flexor digitorum in the forearm are a good example of this strategy. Although this placement is not directly over the belly of the flexor digitorum muscle, it does detect enough of the action potentials from the distal portion of its muscle fibers to reflect finger (as opposed to wrist) movement. Specific placements of electrodes may be used to assess patterns of muscle recruitment associated with movement. They are commonly used to treat the patient by teaching the patient to activate ("uptrain") a specific muscle to improve the muscular effort. They may also be used to "downtrain" a specific muscle—to teach the patient specifically to turn off the recruitment of a muscle following its use.

Chapters 5 and 6 explore in great detail the placement of electrodes for both static and dynamic procedures. These chapters contain specific recommendations about placement sites, along with examples of what one would expect to see given a particular electrode placement.

REFERENCES

1. Loeb GE, Gans C. *Electromyography for Experimentalists.* Chicago, IL: University of Chicago Press; 1986.
2. Bennett H, Kornhauser S. Assessment of general anesthesia by facial muscle electromyography (FACE). *Am J Electromed.* 1995;6:94–97.
3. Cram JR, Rommen DR. Skin preparation and validity of EMG scanning procedure. *Biofeedback Self Regul.* 1989;14 (4):75–82.
4. Fridlund AJ, Cacioppo JT. Guidelines for human electromyographic research. *Psychophysiol.* 1986;23:567–598.
5. Taylor W. Dynamic EMG biofeedback in assessment and treatment using a neuromuscular reeducation model. In: Cram JR, ed. *Clinical EMG for Surface Recordings, II.* Nevada City, CA: Clinical Resources; 1990:175–196.
6. Cram JR. EMG muscle scanning and diagnostic manual for surface recordings. In: Cram JR, ed. *Clinical EMG for Surface Recordings, II.* Nevada City, CA: Clinical Resources; 1990:1–142.
7. Flor H, Turk D, Birbaumer N. Assessment of stress-related psychophysiological reactions in chronic back pain patients. *J Consult Clin Psychol.* 1985;53(3):354–364.
8. Ettare D, Ettare R. Muscle learning therapy: A treatment protocol. In: Cram JR, ed. *Clinical EMG for Surface Recordings, II.* Nevada City, CA: Clinical Resources; 1990:197–234.

CHAPTER QUESTIONS

1. Which type of electrode is ideal for dynamic movement studies?
   a. direct contact electrode
   b. cup or floating electrode
   c. dry electrode
   d. tri-electrode
2. When bridging of electrode paste between two electrodes occurs, what effect does it have on the resulting SEMG amplitudes?
   a. It quickens the response time of the SEMG signal.
   b. It artificially increases the SEMG levels.
   c. It artificially decreases the SEMG levels.
   d. It sends the amplitude to 0.
3. Which electrode is ideal for patients who are allergic to either the paste or the adhesive collar?
   a. direct contact electrode
   b. cup/floating electrode
   c. hydrogel electrode
   d. percutaneous fine-wire electrode
4. Which of the following represent problems or artifacts that may be introduced into the SEMG signal by the electrode leads?
   a. 60-Hz noise (the antenna effect)
   b. movement artifact
   c. radio frequency interference
   d. all of the above
5. Strain relief refers to:
   a. removing the weight of the electrode leads from the electrodes themselves
   b. the effect of placing the muscle on stretch
   c. the effect on the electrode when the patient moves through the range of motion
   d. the effect of taking the muscle off of stretch
6. Site preparation for electrode placement:
   a. is always recommended
   b. is needed only with low-input impedance amplifiers
   c. is needed only with high-input impedance amplifiers
   d. is not needed

7. Poor electrode contact usually has what effect on the SEMG recording?
   a. It artificially decreases the SEMG amplitudes.
   b. It artificially increases the SEMG amplitudes.
   c. It reduces the response time of the SEMG to changes in muscle function.
   d. It changes values only in instruments with high input impedances.
8. When placing the SEMG electrodes for dynamic SEMG procedures, the practitioner should consider:
   a. symmetry of recording electrode placement
   b. agonists and antagonists (myotatic units)
   c. the anterior compartment
   d. the posterior compartment
   e. all of the above
9. When conducting assessments for the postural component of muscle dysfunction, which of the following procedures yields the most complete picture?
   a. muscle scanning
   b. dynamic SEMG protocols
   c. frontal SEMG recordings
   d. palpation examination
10. When assessing for the emotional component of dysfunction, the practitioner should:
    a. place the electrodes on the facial muscles (wide-spaced frontal)
    b. place the electrodes on the site of injury or pain
    c. place the electrodes over the zygomaticus
    d. both a and b
11. When conducting a general relaxation training session, it is extremely useful to:
    a. use widely spaced electrodes
    b. place the recording electrodes across the midline
    c. use closely spaced electrodes
    d. place the electrodes so that they run parallel to the muscle fibers
    e. both a and b

12. When placing SEMG electrodes for dynamic protocols, the practitioner should:
    a. place the electrodes over the belly of the muscle fibers of interest
    b. place the electrodes over the compartment of the muscle of interest
    c. place the electrodes such that they avoid cross-talk from other muscles
    d. all of the above

General Assessment Considerations

In the healing arts, it is commonly believed that treatment should naturally flow from the practitioner's diagnostic impressions. For surface electromyography (SEMG), this diagnosis is not the same type of *medical* diagnosis that is seen with intramuscular EMG studies; these intramuscular, needle studies have to do with structure and tissue damage. With SEMG, the practitioner makes a *functional* or clinical diagnosis; instead of diagnosing tissue damage, the practitioner considers the use or misuse of muscular energy by the central nervous system. George Whatmore, one of the pioneers of SEMG, referred to this misuse of muscular energy as *dysponesis*, or the bad use of energy.[1]

As in formal diagnosis, a strong functional diagnosis requires the practitioner to "correctly" interpret the information collected during assessment, basing the SEMG treatment protocol upon this interpretation. To that end, this chapter focuses on the interpretation of SEMG information and strategies for using SEMG to correct the observed anomaly.

FACTORS THAT AFFECT INTERPRETATION

The process of forming a clinical diagnosis begins with understanding some of the possible moderating variables that could affect the SEMG recording. This is particularly true if the practitioner is using a "standardized" assessment protocol (i.e., a protocol with a clear set of rules to allow replication). Although standardized protocols provide the practitioner with a basis to compare one patient with another and a means of communicating findings to colleagues, they fail to honor the uniqueness of the individual patient. Moderating variables provide some guidelines through which the practitioner begins to build on this individuality, adding depth and meaning to the interpretation. The practitioner must consider many moderating variables, several of which are explored next.

Anatomical and Physiological Considerations

Whenever practitioners apply surface electrodes over muscle, it is very important to palpate the site and possibly have the patient do a resisted isometric contraction of the muscle ("manual muscle test") to verify that the electrode is positioned over the muscle of interest. Only then can the practitioner ascertain that the map or atlas corresponds to the particular patient. Two practitioners have argued that morphological characteristics of the human body (muscle mass, muscle length, source of SEMG, and adipose tissue) vary so widely among individuals as to preclude the use of standardized electrode sites, let alone any associated normative values.[2,3] All practitioners, of course, recognize that people come in a variety of shapes and sizes, as do their muscles. So, rather than summarily dismissing the notion of any standardized electrode placement sites, recording procedures, and associated reference data, the practitioner must adjust the electrode placement, the clinical procedures, and the interpretation of the normative values based on the unique presentation of the patient's anatomy. Nevertheless, the establishment of standardized electrode placement sites and clinical protocols helps practitioners to communicate with colleagues concerning assessment findings and treatments.

In the assessment and treatment of tension myalgias for the upper quarter, for example, placement of electrodes on the upper trapezius muscle is quite common. In a recent review of the literature on this topic, Mathiassen, Winkel, and Hagg[4] argue strongly for standardization of research and clinical procedures to facilitate the understanding of findings across labs and clinics. One of the standardization issues concerns electrode placement over the trapezius. For many years, clinicians and researchers have used a placement described by Zipp,[5] in which the electrodes are placed at 50% of the distance between the seventh cervical vertebra (C-7) and the acromion. However, more recent research by Veiersted has clearly demonstrated that a slight lateral shift from the middle position is preferable.[6] This placement provides a stronger and more reliable signal. Clinicians are strongly encouraged to learn from the experience of others and to use this new standardized placement for trapezius (it is clearly delineated in the electrode atlas in Part III).

Consider SEMG recordings obtained during static versus dynamic assessment procedures. The recordings obtained during the static phase of assessment are generally less problematic than recordings obtained during dynamic assessment procedures. During dynamic studies, the muscles change their resting length and move differentially in relationship to the skin. As a consequence, the SEMG electrodes do not stay over the "belly" of the muscle during the entire course of the movement. Consider the placement of the electrodes 2 cm apart, parallel to the spine over the belly of the erector spinae at the L-3 (third lumbar vertebra) level, with the patient in the neutral standing posture. As the patient engages in forward flexion, the distance between the recording electrodes widens as the skin stretches to accommodate the lengthening of the back. In fact, practitioners always have to use strategies to stop the recording electrodes from "popping" or coming loose during this movement. During extension, back to midline, these electrodes return to their original interelectrode distance. Then, if the patient is asked to extend backward, the electrodes come closer together as the muscle shortens. Throughout this process, movement systematically alters the interelectrode distance and, therefore, the recording field.

Consider another example—the placement of the electrodes over the belly of the sternocleidomastoid (SCM) during axial rotation of the head. During rotation of the head, the SCM radically changes its resting length by 50%, and the recording electrodes drift either ahead of or behind the belly of the muscle, depending on the direction of the head turn. As the electrodes move from their intended location directly above the SCM, it is difficult to determine from which muscle(s) the electrode is recording data (digastric? scalene?). The electrodes probably continue to record primarily from the SCM due to volume conduction, unless one of the surrounding muscle groups (such as the scalene) is also dysfunctional and fires briskly as a function of axial rotation. Donaldson has made this observation as well, using multisite recordings around the circumference of the neck (personal communication).

DeLuca suggests one possible solution to this dilemma.[7, 8] In his studies of SEMG, DeLuca uses a sustained isometric contraction (activation without a change in muscle length). He goes so far as to state that, because of this electrode movement phenomenon, SEMG recordings observed during dynamic movement are meaningless. This is, of course, an extreme position to take. What is important to note here is that some dynamically related changes in length–tension relationships make the SEMG–force relationships variable or even unknown. Such considerations do not enter into SEMG activity during the static phase of the assessment.

Considering all of the possible contributing and contaminating factors associated with dynamic SEMG recordings, it is remarkable that we see any consistency in the SEMG recordings at all. But the truth is that both dynamic and static SEMG recordings provide reliable,[9,10] predictive,[11–13] and descriptive[14,15] information that is valuable for researchers and practitioners alike.

Adipose Tissue

Adipose tissue is well known for its insulating and attenuating effects on the SEMG signal. For this reason, it is important for the practitioner to remember that the dispersion of adipose tissue differs across individuals, within individuals, and between the two sexes. For example, females tend to carry more of this tissue in their upper chest and thighs, whereas males tend to carry more adipose tissue in the abdominal region. Because of the problems with adipose tissue dispersion, ideally the practitioner should measure and record the thickness of the adipose tissue directly at the electrode site, rather than relying on some global measure of percentage of body fat from impedance measurements. In a small, unpublished pilot study of 16 subjects, Cram conducted skin-fold measurements on six sites prior to making SEMG recordings; he observed the correlation between adipose tissue thickness and SEMG levels to be approximately 0.5 in the quiet resting state, and 0.25 during moderate levels of contraction. Adipose tissue, then, seems to bear more directly on resting or static SEMG measurements than on measurements that involve recruitment or activation of the muscle. This relationship arises because resting tone is commonly associated with low SEMG activity, which is more readily absorbed by the insulating effects of the fat. In the active muscle, higher amplitudes of SEMG activity prevail. The high amplitude allows more of the energy to pass through the fatty tissue.

Thus, information about adipose tissue helps clinicians and researchers interpret and report the SEMG data, particularly when those data are gathered while muscles are in the resting state. Until further research is conducted, however, it is difficult to provide the electromyographer with a precise correction factor for the effects of adipose tissue on the integrated levels of SEMG. Unfortunately, one rarely sees any information concerning adipose tissue in the scientific literature or clinical reports on SEMG. Nonetheless, the practitioner would be well advised to observe and record such information. This practice would allow the SEMG interpretations to be globally scaled upward or downward. Given the current state of this knowledge, when clinicians conduct SEMG assessments on the torso and upper extremities, it is recommended that they use Donoghue's[16] four-site method of skin caliper measurement—in which the thickness of the upper arm (above biceps and triceps), upper back (just below the scapula), and lower back (just above the iliac crest) is sampled and compared to normative data for percentage of body fat. The percentage of body fat would then provide the basis for the scaling of the interpretation. Finally, clinicians should note that use of a single-subject or within-patient design for SEMG assessment does not eliminate all of the problems associated with adipose tissue. As we have all noticed in the mirror, there is an uneven distribution of adipose tissue, even within the single subject.

Therefore, when interpreting the amplitudes associated with SEMG information, it is wise to consider the presence and positioning of the patient's adipose tissue. Obese individuals tend to have much lower amplitudes than thin individuals. Within the individual, assessment of symmetry would not necessarily be affected by adipose tissue levels. Comparisons of amplitudes at various body parts (i.e., upper back versus lower back) may be affected. Practitioners should remember that static values seem to be affected more by the presence of adipose tissue than recordings of dynamic procedures.

Position, Posture, and Dynamic Movement

Position, posture, and dynamic movement constitute another set of related variables that moderate the level of muscle energy reaching the electrode. During the static evaluation, the patient is typically studied in a neutral posture of standing or sitting unsupported. Here, the muscles are working against gravity, and any disturbance in the muscular activation patterns is considered to be associated with a disturbance in postural homeostasis.[17] Such a postural disturbance may be due to one or several factors: pain (antalgic postures); postural habits (slouching); anatomical features (e.g., leg-length discrepancy, scoliosis); neurological impairment (e.g., due to cardiovascular accident, spinal cord injury, herniated disk); or emotional arousal (e.g., bracing, acting "uptight"). It is not enough for the practitioner to note a disturbed activation pattern during a static assessment and let it go at that. Slight postural adjustments of the upper extremity or torso, for example, affect the resting tone in the erector spinae muscle group.[18] The practitioner must incorporate information gained from the clinical interview, physical examination, and visual observation of posture/movement to place the SEMG reading into perspective.

For the static evaluation, practitioners should use caution in the verbal instructions given to the subject regarding posture. Matheson et al.,[19] for example, observed a significant sex difference in the midback region when his subjects were instructed to "sit up straight." The power of this language caused the female subjects to vest significantly more energy in the midthoracic spine, bringing them into a more upright posture similar to what their mothers had presumably taught them to do. It is strongly recommended that the practitioner/scientist use neutral words, such as "sit comfortably." In addition, it is recommended that the practitioner/scientist have the person sit on an adjustable chair or backless stool, with the chair height set so that the patient's knees are flexed at 90 degrees. When the patient is standing, the arms should be allowed to hang comfortably at the sides.

In addition, it is important to recognize that different muscle groups have different resting tones (SEMG levels), and that the resting tone may vary as a function of posture. Some practitioners, such as Headley,[2] have advocated the use of a general criterion value for all sites. For example, the practitioner might use the "rule of 5," which holds that any SEMG value that is greater than 5 microvolts root mean square (RMS) is considered abnormal. Unfortunately, this approach is somewhat simplistic and can lead a practitioner to draw erroneous conclusions. A better solution to this problem is to use normative data collected for the various muscle sites while the patient is in various positions. Such a normative database for static recordings may be found in Chapter 6. Using such a reference group for comparison purposes, the resting tone of a patient with low-back pain was recorded using the muscle scanning procedure for two neutral postures (see **Table 5–1**). The patient appears to put on a "muscular corset" as he moves from sitting to standing; this transformation is seen in the dramatic increase in activation in the low-back area during standing. In addition, note the suprasegmental organization of the paraspinal muscles, with the neck muscles activating along with low-back muscles during standing. Normative comparisons for the various sites can assist practitioners in their initial understanding of relationships between muscle groups and neutral postures.

Some practitioners have proposed conducting the static scanning procedure while at the end range of motion (ROM). Chiropractors usually perform this step to complement an end ROM study conducted as part of the clinical exam.[20,21] To date, one study by Leach, Owens, and Geisen has provided information concerning a static assessment at full forward flexion of the low back, in an attempt to assess the flexion relaxation response.[22] These authors found that end ROM values of several low-back sites during forward flexion differed between normal subjects and patients with low-back pain. Three major problems arise when using the static procedure for end ROM studies, however:

- Electrode movement artifact due to the handheld sensors
- Potential accommodation of the SEMG amplitudes due to stretch receptor adaptation associated with the time necessary to conduct multiple samples
- Disturbances in patients' neuromuscular activation patterns associated with low-back pain when left in a flexed posture for short periods

It would seem more natural and more appropriate to use a dynamic recording procedure to study SEMG during a ROM. These dynamic procedures allow the practitioner to examine the pattern and timing of recruitment of SEMG, along with recovery from the perturbation of the movement.

Position and posture are also important issues for dynamic SEMG protocols. Practitioners who are trained in manual muscle testing procedures are familiar with the issues pertaining to assessment of recruitment patterns in muscles. The essence of these principles is that, by correctly positioning the limbs or torso, the practitioner may inhibit or potentiate attempts to isolate a given muscle group. For more information on manual muscle testing procedures, see Kendall, Kendall, and McCreary's book.[23]

Middaugh, Kee, and Nicholson describe a common example of how posture and position may affect dynamic evaluation and treatment.[24] These authors approach the assessment of upper quarter pain primarily through the monitoring of the cervical paraspinal and upper trapezius muscle groups. They pay careful attention to the position of the head and the arms, noting the forward head and arm positions for augmentation of

Table 5–1 Scan Summary Demonstrating a Strong Postural Component for a Patient with Low-Back Pain

Muscle Site	Sitting		Standing	
	Left	Right	Left	Right
C-2 paraspinal	5.6*	3.6	9.2**	7.6*
C-4 paraspinal	5.2*	3.5	7.2*	6.1 *
C-6 paraspinal	4.9*	4.5	5.5*	6.2*
Trapezius	4.9	4.2	4.7	5.0
T-2 paraspinal	2.1	2.5	4.3	5.7
T-4 paraspinal	3.4	2.5	4.9	5.0
T-6 paraspinal	3.6	3.0	4.8	5.7
T-8 paraspinal	3.3	3.0	9.1	9.2
T-10 paraspinal	3.2	3.2	7.2	8.8
L-1 paraspinal	3.4	3.4	9.9	15.6
L-3 paraspinal	7.5*	9.3*	15.8***	26.6***
L-5 paraspinal	5.6	5.3	9.1*	10.2**

*1 SD above the mean.
**2 SD above the mean.
***3 SD above the mean.
Note: A J&J M-501 with a 25- to 1000-Hz filter was used.

the resting tone of these sites. They study simple movements such as shoulder elevation, abduction, and forward flexion for their pattern of recruitment and cessation of recruitment following a request to terminate the movement. They note that recruitment patterns are inefficient when the posture is poor, becoming more efficient once the "correct" posture has been obtained. The corrected posture entails placing the elbows closer to the side of the torso and moving the head into a more neutral position. When working with a patient, the therapist may need to stretch and strengthen certain muscles to allow the patient to retract the head back over the shoulders.

Dynamic recruitment patterns may change as a function of slight alterations of limb position. Several examples of this are presented in the electrode atlas in Part III. For example, recruitment of biceps during elbow flexion changes when the hand is pronated rather than supinated (see Figure 17–33D). Recruitment of the infraspinatus during abduction differs when the arm is medially or laterally rotated (see Figure 17–24B).

In summary, both static and dynamic SEMG recordings may be affected significantly by posture, position, and movement. The astute practitioner must understand these relationships and use them in assessment and treatment protocols. It is important to note these issues in the documentation.

Volume Conduction

Another factor that affects the SEMG is volume conduction. *Volume conduction* (or far-field potentials) refers to the source of the SEMG signal residing at some distance from the surface EMG sensors. Years ago, Basmajian[25] discussed cautions regarding volume conduction. He cautioned that the frontal (wide) electrode placement is nonspecific and may record activity from muscles as far away as the first rib. Although far-field potentials from the ancillary muscles of respiration (i.e., scalene) have been noted in widely spaced electrodes at the frontal site, it is much more common to see volume conduction at this site from the corrugator, temporalis, or masseter muscles. The point is that recordings from a single set of electrodes placed over a particular muscle group may lead the practitioner to draw an erroneous conclusion about that muscle. It is helpful for the practitioner to know which sites are more easily contaminated by volume conduction or crosstalk, and which sites lend themselves to cleaner specific recordings. Although volume conduction and cross-talk are typically more problematic for dynamic recordings

than static SEMG recordings, static recordings are not completely immune to this phenomenon.

The purpose of a muscle scanning technique is to encourage the practitioner to consider the muscular system as a whole rather than drawing conclusions based on one set of electrodes. The muscle scanning technique emphasizes sampling from a variety of muscle sets, looking to identify active or inhibited sites. Such sampling is helpful in searching for the problem areas, particularly if one is not sure where to begin. For example, consider a patient who is clenching his or her jaw (activation of the masseter and temporalis). If the practitioner conducts a single-site recording at the frontalis, he or she might conclude that the patient had elevated resting tone at that site. Such a conclusion would be misleading. In contrast, by conducting multisite recording from the facial musculature, the practitioner would be able to observe that the SEMG activation from the masseter and temporalis is volume conducted, elevating the amplitudes observed at the frontalis sites as well (see **Table 5–2**). From the multisite recording, the practitioner would observe that the highest level of microvolt activity is seen at the masseter site. Such a "within-patient" pattern analysis of the multiple sites suggests that the practitioner consider volume-conducted activity from the masseteric activation. As Iacona[3] notes, such a single-subject or within-patient analysis is an essential part of correctly interpreting a static evaluation. Relying solely upon a normative database comparison in this case would lead one to conclude that the masseter, temporalis, frontalis, and SCM sites were all significantly elevated. The practitioner must sort out these volume-conduction issues.

Table 5–2 Scan Summary on Person Who Is Clenching the Teeth Intentionally

Muscle Site	Sitting	
	Left	Right
Frontalis	22.0*	24.2*
Temporalis	35.2*	41.1*
Masseter	57.2*	65.2*
SCM	12.1*	14.6*
Trapezius	2.6	2.0
T-2 paraspinal	2.3	2.1

*Severe elevations.

Note: A J&J M-501 with a 25- to 1000-Hz filter was used.

It is also important for evaluation of dynamic procedures to contemplate volume-conducted activity and place electrodes accordingly. The same type of examination of the facial muscles can be done with multiple-site dynamic SEMG recordings. Figure 17–1B demonstrates volume conduction to the frontal leads during a clench. Some sites are more vulnerable to volume conduction than others. For example, Perry, Easterday, and Antonelli have reported that only 36% of the SEMG activity recorded at the soleus site is attributable to the soleus muscle; the rest is volume conducted from the gastrocnemius and related muscles.[26] Considerable cross-talk can also occur in the muscles of the forearm. The electrode atlas (Part III) orients practitioners to the possibility of cross-talk and to those muscles that may contribute to this phenomenon.

Problems with volume conduction are also paramount when attempting to record from a "deep" muscle—that is, a muscle that resides underneath another muscle. With surface electrodes, how does one know whether the recording comes from the more superficial muscle or the deeper muscle group? This question becomes even more difficult to answer when both the superficial and deep muscles are synergists, performing slightly different functions, yet being activated by the same movement. The supraspinatus versus middle trapezius muscles, and the quadratus lumborum versus latissimus dorsi (or abdominal oblique) are two such examples. For this reason, the electrode atlas focuses on monitoring these deeper muscles by their location or site rather than by the muscle itself. For example, these two electrode placements would be called suprascapular/supraspinatus and lateral low-back/quadratus, respectively.

While it would be nice to think that SEMG recordings at multiple sites are totally independent, they are not. Just as some of the Minnesota Multiphasic Personality Inventory (MMPI) scales share some of the same stimulus items, source EMG may find its way to sensors at some distance. With SEMG (unlike intramuscular needle or fine-wire recordings), practitioners must learn to think in terms of populations of motor units, muscle synergies, and muscle dyssynergies. The system is tied together, into myotatic units.[27] Muscle scanning and multisite dynamic SEMG recording allow one to see the "bigger picture." Normative data or benchmark values for each site provide the background for beginning the interpretation, with a single-subject/within patient analysis of the pattern of activation and inhibition as a complementary step. Focusing on both types of comparisons helps the practitioner to reach sound conclusions.

Age and Gender

Age and sex variables may play substantial roles in physiological functioning and should be considered in SEMG recordings. Indeed, Wolf, Bassmajian, Russe, and Kutner[28] and Brown[29] have noted that for dynamic procedures, the level of SEMG recruitment decreases with age. This is probably the result of a loss of muscle bulk due to inactivity that comes with age. However, for SEMG recordings of static procedures, these differences disappear. Three studies have examined SEMG activity in the static, neutral posture across ages and between sexes.[11, 23, 28] All three studies note a lack of correlation between age and SEMG levels at rest. Sex differences, likewise, show too much random variation under static conditions to provide a meaningful distinction between sexes for resting tone.

SURFACE ELECTROMYOGRAPHY AND CLINICAL SYNDROMES

From a clinical perspective, the aberrant SEMG patterns that relate to myogenic etiologies for pain may arise from different types of psychophysiological and musculoskeletal dysfunctions. Following is a partial list of clinical syndromes for which a dynamic SEMG assessment may be used:

- Simple postural dysfunction
- Emotional dysfunction
- Learned guarding or bracing
- Peripheral weakness or deconditioning
- Acute, reflexive spasm or inhibition
- Learned inhibition
- Direct compensation for joint hypermobility or hypomobility
- Chronic faulty motor program

An introduction to a scheme for syndrome recognition and treatment planning, developed in large part by Kasman,[30] is presented in this section. Note that the presentation given here has been simplified, and that a more detailed exploration of these principles can be found in *Clinical Applications in Surface Electromyography* by Kasman, Cram, and Wolfe.[31] Also note that clinical syndromes presented in this framework are not mutually exclusive; that is, patients may exhibit qualities of one or more syndromes. The procedures alluded to in this framework are intended as a starting point in the practitioner's evaluation. These guidelines should be modified and tailored to the individual patient. In some cases, a team approach to patient care is required to complete the assessment.

To determine which syndromes are relevant for a given patient, the practitioner should begin by asking some of the following questions:

1. What are the significant findings from the history, intake, and clinical examination? Although the issues to consider are as varied as the patients themselves, it is helpful to consider some of following elements: trauma, vocation, medical history, type of pain description, pain-related movements, temporal aspects of pain, respiratory distress, cognitive dysfunction, visual/balance dysfunctions, headache, incontinence, paresthesia, weakness, medications, substance abuse, major life stressors, affect, coping mechanisms, and impaired activities of daily living.

2. Which specific aberrant SEMG patterns are observed? Consider amplitude, timing, and muscle groups involved.

3. Under which conditions are the aberrant patterns displayed? Consider activity/work-related aspects, posturally related aspects, and emotional overtones.

4. Under which conditions are the aberrant patterns not displayed? When are they normal? Consider environmental, emotional, postural, and movement aspects.

5. How do the answers to questions 1 through 4 come together? What is the bigger picture?

Some simplified descriptions for the clinical syndromes listed previously are provided in the remainder of this section. One case example is given for each syndrome to provide an illustration of each of the concepts presented. Treatment considerations for these different syndromes is presented in Chapter 9.

Simple Postural Dysfunction

Aberrant motor activity can be a direct function of posture. Take a case example of a patient with headache and tension myalgia of the upper quarter and neck associated with keyboard entry work. Postural examination shows that the patient sits with the head forward and with the arms extended slightly while typing. Surface EMG recordings show hyperactivity primarily in the cervical paraspinal and upper trapezius. These SEMG levels greatly improve when the patient achieves "correct" postural alignment.

Emotional Dysfunction

Heightened muscle activity may be due to maladaptive coping with stressful situations or may be a conditioned response to a traumatic event (post-traumatic stress disorder). Consider the patient who comes to the practitioner four weeks after a motor vehicle accident in which she sustained a flexion extension injury to her neck and shoulder region. Traditional medical and physical therapies have not produced long-term gains. A stress-profiling procedure is done, in which the offending muscle (wide trapezius) site and a muscle that indicates general emotions (wide frontalis) site are monitored as the patient recounts the details associated with the accident. Large emotional recruitment patterns are noted during the patient's discussion of the accident scene. Appropriate treatment of the post-traumatic stress disorder should precede or be done concurrently with the physical therapy.

Learned Guarding or Bracing

Heightened muscle activity is a learned (emotional) response to pain that occurs upon movement or postural loading. Responses are performed in an attempt to avoid pain and the possibility of further injury. In some cases, the syndrome may involve complex behavioral dysfunction that includes responses performed to declare pain and disability.

Consider an example of a patient with litigation pending, following a trauma to the left shoulder area associated with a fall two years ago. This patient commonly clutches at the neck and shoulder region, and periodically attends a session while applying her own cold pack on the area. Diffuse activation of the upper quarter and neck is observed on the muscle scan during quiet sitting and standing, and electrodes attached to the right and left upper and lower trapezius bear out this observation. Simple abduction indicates that the upper trapezius muscles on both the right and left sides have peak amplitudes that are four to seven times greater than those of the lower trapezius muscles. The right upper trapezius has a peak amplitude that is twice that of the injured left side. Anticipated and small movements of the left arm or shoulder tend to fire the right upper trapezius. With attention and SEMG feedback training, this muscle activation improves during the session, but the patient is slow to transfer gains from session to session and from the office to home. The patient responds well to relaxation-based therapies. Pain management is a key consideration in treating this individual.

Peripheral Weakness or Deconditioning

This syndrome refers to patients who have become impaired due to simple muscle disuse. This deconditioning may be caused by immobilization after injury or surgery, or it may be the cumulative effect of poor motor habits and decreased activity. The condition may include atrophic loss of muscle cross-sectional area, inefficient vascularization, and compromised biochemical and physiological function. Symptoms may include a gradual decrease in peak torque, power deficits (i.e., inability to sustain force through ROM arcs), and impaired fatigue resistance.

Consider the case of a patient who has had his knee immobilized and weight bearing restricted for 6 weeks after sustaining a leg fracture. The quadriceps has undergone disuse atrophy during the period of immobilization. Range of motion, strength, endurance, and functional mobility are impaired during the rehabilitation period. If the patient is cleared for active strengthening of the knee and is examined with SEMG, the recorded activity will likely differ between the involved and uninvolved lower extremities. Maximal effort SEMG activity will probably be decreased on the involved side, although submaximal contractions may show increased activity, presumably reflecting decreased neuromuscular efficiency. The asymmetrical SEMG activity will be associated with obvious findings of weakness and deconditioning on physical examination.

Acute, Reflexive Spasm/Inhibition

Elevated or inhibited (depressed) muscle tension presumably occurs via reflex mechanism induced by pain and/or effusion. Consider the example of a patient with a bulging or herniated disk with pain in the left aspect of the low back, radiating down into the left hip and leg. She has decreased range of motion of the torso and poor sitting tolerance. The patient might present with a flexed and laterally shifted trunk posture, and visibly and palpably elevated lumbar paraspinal tone. Pain is on the same side as the bulging disk. The patient may show discrete activations of the erector spinae muscle on the ipsilateral side of reported pain. Occasionally, this activation pattern is more diffuse to both sides of the low back, and it extends clearly into the midback region as well. Pain is increased with sitting (supported or not), and the SEMG activation level also increases. Any movements, active or passive, of the lower extremity lead to an activation of the left erector spinae muscles.

An example of acute, reflexive inhibition might be seen in a patient with a recent history of trauma and physical examination findings of swelling, tenderness, and inability to tolerate vigorous manual muscle testing of the lower extremity. Surface EMG monitoring would show a discrete focal drop in SEMG amplitude recorded from the quadriceps during a painful portion of the knee ROM arc. The focal drop in SEMG activity in this case would be a consequence of neurophysiologic inhibition. Similar scenarios involving spasm and inhibition could result from the cumulative effects of subtle, recurrent trauma to a joint.

Learned Inhibition/Weakness

Learned inhibition/weakness is a rare syndrome, but one worth considering. Here the patient unconsciously learns to inhibit motor activity so as to avoid pain. This syndrome is similar to the protective guarding syndrome discussed earlier, but with inhibition rather than spasm. Consider, for example, an otherwise healthy patient who sustains recurrent strains of the hip adductor muscles while playing racquetball. The pain becomes severe and exacerbated whenever the adductor muscles vigorously contract during functional activities. To evade the contraction-induced pain, the patient learns to reduce firing of the adductors while performing stressful physical activities. Over a period of time, the altered patterns become unconsciously incorporated into the patient's selection of motor programs.

The adductor SEMG amplitude of this patient appears symmetrical on the uninvolved side during walking and low-level activities. However, activity appears to be markedly decreased and impaired during higher-velocity and loading conditions such as sustained unilateral stance, lunging, or formal manual muscle testing. When the patient is subjected to an unanticipated postural perturbation, the adductors recruit to a level that exceeds their voluntary activation. Thus, the muscles are recruited with postural reactions to help prevent a fall. Inconsistent activation patterns might also be observed with novel tasks for which motor programming schema have not been learned, especially if simultaneous cognitive distractions are present.

Direct Compensation for Joint Hypermobility or Hypomobility

Aberrant SEMG activity may occur as a consequence of chronic joint hypermobility or hypomobility. The neuromuscular system compensates for this by attempting to stabilize lax joint structures, by affecting movement against joint stiffness, or by subserving linked compensatory movements over kinetic chains. Although SEMG activity is aberrant, the primary problem is a biomechanical articular fault (joint dysfunction). The articular fault causes a compensatory motor control pattern, which may spontaneously resolve upon improvement in joint mechanics. Chronic joint dysfunction may lead to motor control problems that themselves contribute to deterioration of the kinetic segment and persist even after joint mobility improves. The distinction between these causes is made because if aberrant motor activity is believed to be directly compensatory to articular dysfunction, then biofeedback is not a first choice of treatment. The joint dysfunction should be addressed and then SEMG activity should be reassessed.

As an example, suppose a patient with jaw pain is found on physical examination to display hypomobility at the left temporomandibular joint (TMJ). There is a deviation of the midline of the jaw during opening and closing, and a palpable difference between the motions of the left and right mandibular condyles. As opening is initiated (or closing completed), the condyles are felt to spin in place. The condyles are then felt to translate forward as opening continues. This rolling/gliding relationship is necessary for normal jaw range of motion and is expected to be symmetrical at the left and right TMJs. In this example, SEMG activity shows greater recruitment at the right masseter during jaw opening/closing range of motion. The right mandibular condyle translates a greater distance along the articular surface of the zygomatic process, and the right masseter is activated to a greater degree to subserve the greater range of movement than the right TMJ. The fundamental problem, however, is not that the right masseter SEMG activity is greater than that of the left masseter, but rather that the left joint has less mobility than the right joint. Surface EMG spontaneously becomes symmetrical once the left TMJ is mobilized with manual techniques or exercises.

Chronic Faulty Motor Programs

With chronic faulty motor control, it is assumed that the central nervous system learns to cope with pain, muscle weakness, joint instabilities, trigger points, myofascial extensibility issues, and other problems. As a result, a learned disruption of the normal agonist–antagonist–synergist relationships occurs. The assessment (and treatment) of this broad syndrome requires SEMG monitoring along with assessment of coincident joint segment dysfunction, soft-tissue dysfunction, and behavioral analysis.

Consider a patient with chronic cervical paraspinal and suprascapular pain following lifting activities at work. Motion takes place throughout the shoulder girdle to elevate the arm forward. This includes upward rotation of the scapula, achieved by the coordinated actions of the upper trapezius, the lower trapezius, the lower fibers of the serratus anterior, and numerous other muscles with direct and indirect stabilizing roles. A motor program is a planned set of commands from the central nervous system that serves to coordinate the actions of muscles so that a specific goal is achieved—in this case, shoulder flexion. If an inefficient motor program is selected, then one muscle might contract with excessive or reduced tension relative to its synergist, resulting in abnormal loading patterns of both myofascial and articular tissue. In this patient, the SEMG activity of the upper trapezius is increased on the involved side, whereas the activity of the lower trapezius or lower serratus anterior is decreased, each relative to the uninvolved side. In addition, the latter two muscles are slower to increase their activity on the involved side through an equivalent left/right ROM arc. These findings are associated with passive tightness of the upper trapezius and maximal manual muscle test weakness of the lower trapezius or serratus anterior. With close visual inspection, visual differences in the pattern of the scapular displacement between the two sides can be discerned. Physical and emotional stress tends to increase the aberrant patterns. The patient has a poor ability to recognize tension and to manipulate the SEMG signals on the involved side.

ASSESSMENT/TREATMENT LINK: AN UPPER QUARTER EXAMPLE

The clinical diagnosis should lead practitioners to a treatment plan of some sort. And, as practitioners treat their patients, it is not uncommon to assess the patient's progress continually, and to move from one treatment strategy to the next, based on the successful acquisition of neuromuscular skills. Taylor has developed a good protocol-driven approach for the upper quarter, in which assessment and treatment are intimately linked.[32] For a more in-depth examination of this protocol, refer to Taylor's chapter in *Clinical EMG for Surface Recordings, II*.[32] While the upper quarter is much more complicated than is depicted in this protocol,

Taylor takes the approach advocated by Janda,[33] in which upper quarter dysfunctions are best described as an imbalance between the postural and phasic muscles. He then provides a good model for assessing and treating this type of disorder. Further exploration of Taylor's approach to treatment is presented in Chapter 9.

Phase 1: Postural Muscle Relaxation

Relaxation of the postural tone is the first step in treatment (see **Figure 5–1**). Because posture is the foundation upon which movement rests, paying attention to the resting tone is essential to achieving successful treatment outcomes. The bilateral placement refers to independently monitoring the right and left aspects of the upper trapezius using a narrow placement (see the electrode atlas). Resting tone is tested in two postures—hands in the lap and arms hanging at the sides. If elevated levels are noted, the practitioner should begin by making general postural adjustments. For example, simply asking the patient to lower the shoulders may cause the activation pattern to disappear. If not, a relaxation-based treatment protocol is indicated. Second, the resting tone is checked out following movement. (This process is described in more detail in Chapter 8.) If the muscle does not return to a good resting baseline following movement, the practitioner should begin by teaching the patient how to rest the muscle completely following a given movement. These movements might include abduction to 90 degrees, flexion of the arms, or a shoulder shrug.

Once a good resting tone is present, the practitioner can proceed to Phase 2.

Phase 1: Postural Muscle Relaxation

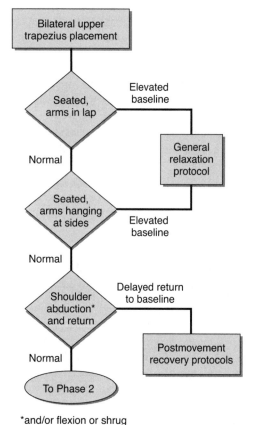

Figure 5–1 Phase 1: Postural muscle relaxation assessment and treatment linkage.

Source: Copyright © 1990, J. R. Cram, *Clinical EMG for Surface Recordings*, Clinical Resources, Inc.

Phase 2: Postural Muscle Stretching

The site for assessment may stay with the trapezius or it may focus on the scalene muscles. Muscle shortness may be a substantial contributor to problems in this region. In addition, the problem may be linked to respiration. The practitioner should examine the recording for large activation patterns that follow the breath, or ask the patient to take a deep inspiration and look for symmetrical recruitment patterns here. For initial treatment, Taylor suggests a stretching protocol similar to that suggested by Travell and Simons[27] for this site. He recommends lateral bending of the head, a passive stretch, and a protocol in which the patient is asked to breathe into the stretch and then relax into the stretch (relax-in-stretch). If the patient shows increased SEMG activity with the stretch, the goal is to teach the patient to reduce this activity while on stretch (see **Figure 5–2**).

Once the patient's muscle is at a better resting length, the practitioner can continue to Phase 3.

Phase 3: Isolation of Phasic Muscles

The practitioner typically begins this phase after observing that when the patient abducts the arms, the upper trapezius clearly dominates over the lower trapezius (with normal functioning, there is a better balance between the two muscles). This imbalance is thought to reflect inhibited lower trapezius activity, rather than overactive upper trapezius activity. (This issue is discussed in greater detail in Chapter 8.) The electrodes are placed on both the right and left aspects of the upper

Phase 2: Postural Muscle Stretching

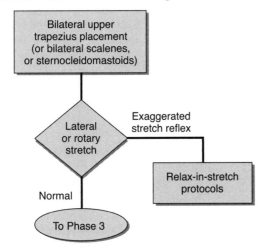

Figure 5–2 Phase 2: Postural muscle stretching assessment and treatment linkage.

Source: Copyright © 1990, J. R. Cram, *Clinical EMG for Surface Recordings*, Clinical Resources, Inc.

and lower trapezius. The patient is asked to engage in an activity that would recruit the lower trapezius. If poor recruitment patterns are noted, then isolation training is initiated (see **Figure 5–3**). The goal here is to be able to

Phase 3: Isolation of Phasic Muscles*

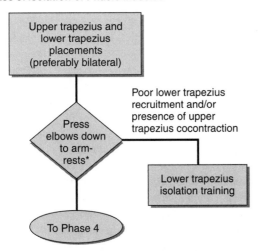

*See Lewit[34] for other isolation exercises.

Figure 5–3 Phase 3: Isolation of phasic muscles assessment and treatment linkage.

Source: Copyright © 1990, J. R. Cram, *Clinical EMG for Surface Recordings*, Clinical Resources, Inc.

activate the lower trapezius, without cocontractions from the upper trapezius or contralateral lower trapezius. Such training is described in Chapter 9.

Once the patient can isolate and contract the lower trapezius, the practitioner can move to Phase 4.

Phase 4: Postural/Phasic Muscle Balance

The purpose of this phase is to bring other muscles into play and to seek proper synergy patterns among them (see **Figure 5–4**). Again, the upper and lower trapezius are monitored. The patient does a simple abduction to

Phase 4: Postural/Phasic Muscle Balance

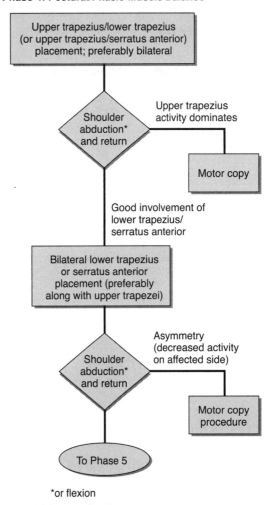

*or flexion

Figure 5–4 Phase 4: Postural/phasic muscle balance assessment and treatment linkage.

Source: Copyright © 1990, J. R. Cram, *Clinical EMG for Surface Recordings*, Clinical Resources, Inc.

90 degrees. Two levels of assessment are considered: (1) the relationship between upper and lower trapezius and (2) the relationship between contralateral muscle groups. If the upper trapezius continues to dominate, the practitioner should have the patient use the skill developed in Phase 3 to learn how to recruit the lower trapezius as part of the movement. Templates of the desired recruitment pattern are very useful and may assist the patient in acquiring the proper timing of the new response pattern. This practice is termed "motor copy," and Wolf, LeCraw, and Barton[35] have demonstrated that it accelerates learning of motor skills. Once the upper and lower trapezius can work in proper synergy, the practitioner should work on any right and left asymmetrical recruitment patterns.

After the patient has attained the proper synergy patterns, it is time to move to Phase 5.

Phase 5: Stereotyped Movement Patterns

In this phase, electrodes are usually placed on the upper and lower trapezius, although, the serratus anterior may be substituted for the lower trapezius if the task at hand suggests this new placement. The goal of this phase is to transfer the skills learned in one posture to other postures and to more complex movement patterns. A very strong focus on activities of daily living is encouraged. If excessive upper trapezius activity returns, more work is needed to promote generalization. In fact, it is better not to assume that the generalization of motor skills will occur. The training of the neuromuscular system is typically very specific, and generalization should be built into treatment procedures (see **Figure 5–5**).

CONCLUSION

Muscle dysfunction cannot be divided into disciplinary boundaries. The well-rounded practitioner must be alert to the many roles that muscles play and the ways in which muscles are affected by their external and internal environments. To be unaware of the postural aspects of muscle is to ignore the effects of gravity. To be unaware of the psychophysiological aspects of muscle is to deny the reality of emotions. To be unaware of the movement aspects of muscle is to ignore life. The rich and varied life experiences of patients must be considered and incorporated into practitioners' assessments. Along with activity or activation of the muscles, practitioners should consider the role of rest on both a macro level and a micro level. To ignore the muscle as an organ system tied to bones is to forget the physical reality of that with which we work. Practitioners should determine when function gives way to structure and should attend to the repair of the structure before working on restoring function.

Each practitioner needs to recognize fully the limits of his or her own knowledge. It is probably impossible to be knowledgeable about *all* aspects of muscle energy and function, although the practitioner should attempt to do so. Realistically, sometimes the best that can be hoped for is an awareness of one's own limits, along with knowledge that someone outside the practitioner's immediate discipline might have something additional to offer to the patient. In the best of all worlds, the patient will be treated within a truly interdisciplinary setting where all of the various aspects of muscle function can be integrated into a comprehensive and complete treatment plan. Notably, psychological or behavioral issues sometimes need to be resolved before physical issues can be addressed. A patient with a high level of stress or with major behavioral issues relating to pain will probably need to have these issues resolved before the physical treatments will be effective. Likewise, patients in whom a physical condition (e.g., joint mobility issues) makes a

Phase 5: Stereotyped Movement Patterns

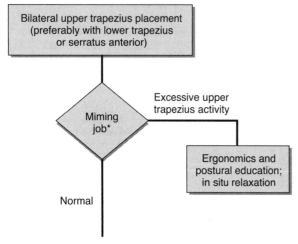

*and other tasks, e.g., driving, typing, shaving, hair care

Figure 5–5 Phase 5: Stereotyped movement patterns assessment and treatment linkage.

Source: Copyright © 1990, J. R. Cram, *Clinical EMG for Surface Recordings*, Clinical Resources, Inc.

major contribution to dysfunction will probably need to have this issue resolved before SEMG feedback for functional gains will be effective. A practitioner who knows his or her own discipline but is also aware of the other areas of concern can more effectively treat the patient through cross-referral when appropriate.

REFERENCES

1. Whatmore G, Kohli D. *The Physiopathology and Treatment of Functional Disorders.* New York, NY: Grune & Stratton; 1974.
2. Headley B. *Muscle Scanning.* Boulder, CO: IPR; 1990.
3. Iacona C. Muscle scanning: Caveat emptor. *Biofeedback Self Regul.* 1991;16:227–241.
4. Mathiassen SE, Winkel J, Hagg GM. Normalization of surface EMG amplitude from the upper trapezius muscle in ergonomic studies: a review. *J Electromyogr Kinesiol.* 1995;5:197–226.
5. Zipp P. Recommendations for the standardization of lead positions in surface electromyography. *Eur J Appl Physiol.* 1982;50:41–54.
6. Veiersted KB. The reproducability of test contractions for calibration of electromyographic measurements. *Eur J Appl Physiol.* 1991;62:91–98.
7. DeLuca C. Myoelectric manifestations of localized muscular fatigue in humans. *CRC Crit Rev Biomed Eng.* 1984;11:251.
8. DeLuca C. Keynote presentation. Presented at the Applied Psychophysiology and Biofeedback Conference, March 1992, Colorado Springs, CO.
9. Ahern DK, Follick MJ, Council JR, Laser-Wolston N. Reliability of lumbar paravertebral EMG assessment in chronic low back pain. *Arch Phys Med Rehab.* 1986;76:762–765.
10. Cram JR, Lloyd J, Cahn T. The reliability of EMG muscle scanning. *Int J Psychosom.* 1990;37:68–72.
11. Cram JR, Steger JC. Muscle scanning and the diagnosis of chronic pain. *Biofeedback Self Regul.* 1983;8:229–241.
12. Klein AB, Snyder Mackler L, Roy S, DeLuca C. Comparison of spinal mobility and isometric trunk extensors forces with electromyographic spectral analysis in identifying low back pain. *Phys Ther.* 1991;71:445–453.
13. Triano J, Schultz AB. Correlation of objective measurement of trunk motion and muscle function with low back disability ratings. *Spine.* 1987;12:561–565.
14. Dolce JJ, Raczynski JM. Neuromuscular activity and electromyography in painful backs: psychological and biomechanical models in assessment and treatment. *Psychol Bull.* 1985;97:502–520.
15. Robinson ME, Cassisi JE, O'Connor PD, MacMillan M. Lumbar iEMG during isotonic exercise: chronic low back pain patients vs controls. *J Spinal Disord.* 1992;5:1.
16. Donoghue W. *How to Measure Your Percent Bodyfat.* Plymouth, MN: Creative Health Products; 1990.
17. Cram JR. EMG muscle scanning and diagnostic manual for surface recordings. In: Cram JR, ed. *Clinical EMG for Surface Recordings, II.* Nevada City, CA: Clinical Resources; 1990:1–142.
18. Wolf L, Segal R, Wolf S, Nieberg R. Quantitative analysis of surface and percutaneous electromyographic activity and lumbar erector spinae of normal young women. *Spine.* 1991;16:155–161.
19. Matheson D, Toben TP, De Lacruz DE. EMG scanning: normative data. *J Psychopathology Behav Assess.* 1988;10:9–20.
20. Berman FS, Marcarian D. The Berman technique: a proposed standard protocol for chiropractic EMG scanning. *Am Chiropractor.* November 1990:34–40.
21. Kent C, Hyde R. Potential applications for EMG in chiropractic practice. *Digest Chiropractic Econ.* 1987;9:20–25.
22. Leach RA, Owens EF, Giesen IM. Correlates of myoelectric asymmetry detected in low back pain patients using hand held post style surface electromyography. *J Manip Phys Ther.* 1993;16:140–149.
23. Kendall FP, Kendall E, McCreary BA. *Muscles, Testing and Function.* 3rd ed. Baltimore, MD: Williams & Wilkins; 1983.
24. Middaugh SJ, Kee WG, Nicholson JA. Muscle overuse and posture as factors in the development and maintenance of chronic musculoskeletal pain. In: Grzesiak RC, Ciccone DS, eds. *Psychological Vulnerability to Chronic Pain.* New York, NY: Springer; 1994:55–89.
25. Basmajian N. Fact versus myth in EMG biofeedback. *Biofeedback Self Regul.* 1976;4:369–371.
26. Perry J, Easterday CS, Antonelli DJ. Surface versus intramuscular electrodes for electromyography of superficial and deep muscles. *Phys Ther.* 1981;61:7–15.
27. Travell J, Simons D. *Myofascial Pain and Dysfunction: A Trigger Point Manual, I and II.* Baltimore, MD: Williams & Wilkins; 1983.
28. Wolf S, Basmajian J, Russe C, Kutner M. Normative data on low back mobility and activity levels. *Am J Phys Med.* 1979;58:217–229.
29. Brown WF. *The Physiological and Technical Basis of Electromyography.* Boston, MA: Butterworth; 1984.
30. Kasman GS. *Surface EMG in Physical Therapy: Applications in Chronic Musculoskeletal Pain.* Seattle, WA: Movements Systems; 1995.
31. Kasman G, Cram JR, Wolf S. *Clinical Applications in Surface Electromyography.* Gaithersburg, MD: Aspen; 1997.
32. Taylor W. Dynamic EMG biofeedback in assessment and treatment using a neuromuscular reeducation model. In: Cram JR, ed. *Clinical EMG for Surface Recordings, II.* Nevada City, CA: Clinical Resources; 1990:175–196.
33. Janda J. Postural and phasic muscle in the pathogenesis of low back pain. Presented at the Tenth Congress of International Society Rehabilitation, 1969, Dublin, Ireland.

34. Lewit K. *Manipulative Therapy in Rehabilitation of the Locomotor System.* Boston, MA: Butterworth Heinemann; 1991.

35. Wolf S, LeCraw D, Barton L. Comparison of motor copy and targeted biofeedback training techniques for restitution of upper extremity function among patients with neurologic disorders. *Phys Ther.* 1988;69:719–735.

CHAPTER QUESTIONS

1. Surface EMG can be used:
   a. to diagnose nerve damage
   b. to diagnose herniated disk
   c. as a "clinical" diagnosis only
   d. all of the above
2. How does adipose tissue (the fat layer) affect SEMG recordings?
   a. It makes them invalid.
   b. It reduces the SEMG amplitude.
   c. It increases the SEMG amplitude.
   d. It has a stronger effect on dynamic recordings than on static recordings.
3. During the static evaluation, which approach should one take toward controlling the posture of the patient?
   a. standardize the posture by asking the patient to "sit or stand up straight"
   b. retain the patient's natural posture by asking him or her to sit or stand comfortably
   c. ask the patient to go to the end range of motion
   d. none of the above
4. Surface EMG recordings appear to change as a function of age. In general, what statement can be made concerning this finding?
   a. Dynamic SEMG amplitudes decrease over the years (decades).
   b. Dynamic SEMG amplitudes increase over the decades.
   c. Static SEMG amplitudes increase over the decades.
   d. both a and c

5. Issues regarding volume-conducted SEMG are best addressed using the following:
   a. single-site SEMG recordings
   b. multiple-site SEMG recordings
   c. an Ohm meter
   d. a volume conductor
6. Some muscle sites are more affected by volume conduction than others. Which of the following muscle sites has the lowest probability of being affected by volume conduction?
   a. frontalis
   b. upper trapezius
   c. quadratus lumborum
   d. supraspinatus
7. Which of the following is not one of the clinical syndromes described in the chapter?
   a. simple postural dysfunction
   b. weakness or deconditioning
   c. acute reflex spasm or inhibition
   d. bruxism

Static Assessment and Clinical Protocol

STATIC ASSESSMENT

The static evaluation is used to assess the "tonic" or resting state of the muscle. It provides an objective assessment of this resting tone, which correlates exceptionally well with any hypertrophied muscle mass noted during a palpation exam. To this extent, the static evaluation provides an objective measurement of chronically hyperactive muscles. In the more acute phase, these hyperactive muscles could be described as *muscle spasms*. Muscle spasms are similar to chronically hyperactive muscles, in that both are involuntary increases in alpha motor activity. However, unlike chronically hyperactive muscles, muscle spasms cannot be voluntarily released, they prevent lengthening of the muscle involved, and they are due to a painful stimulus impinging on the lower motor neuron.[1] Chronic hyperactive muscle activity may have lost its nociceptive origin and is functionally defined as excessive muscle effort that is outside the patient's conscious awareness.

Resting tone is an attribute that normally resides outside the general awareness of the patient. When we execute our conscious volition, we use primarily our alpha motor system (our large extrafusal fibers), with a secondary emphasis on gamma motor activity (the posture in which we do the movement). The resting tone is the foundation upon which volitional movement rests. It is the basis for posture. Thus, when the resting tone of a muscle is observed to be above normal and expected levels, chronic hyperactive muscle activity or muscle spasm is identified. Usually, this is a low-grade activity, and not the obvious level of spasm noted in a "cramp."

Reliance on palpation alone can lead the practitioner to draw erroneous conclusions about muscle activity. Perhaps this is why some practitioners find that the term *spasm* has limited clinical use. When the practitioner palpates the muscle, it may feel hard to the touch. If the muscle is also electrically active, it is called a hyperactive muscle. In contrast, if the muscle feels hard and is electrically silent, it is in a physiologically shortened resting length. Usually this status is brought about because of the lack of use or complete range of motion for the muscle, which adaptively shortens its resting length to fit its range of use. Thus, a hard, silent muscle will be treated differently than a hard, active one. With the former condition, the practitioner might begin with heat and gentle stretches to begin the process of lengthening the muscle, and then proceed with retraining it. With the latter condition, the practitioner would examine the agonist/antagonist/synergist relationships in the context of pain to try to determine what drives the muscle into chronic hyperactivity.

In painful conditions, it is not unusual for the patient to adopt an *antalgic posture*—a postural shift to avoid pain. This action reflects the patient's unconscious movement or a suprasegmental reflexive movement away from a painful sensation. When placed into an avoidant learning paradigm, the negative reinforcement (pain) leads the patient to learn the antalgic posture. This postural shift may become one of the signs of a painful condition and a perpetuating factor associated with the painful condition. Therefore, the muscle scanning procedure for assessing the static component of muscle is a tool for assessing hyperactive muscle and antalgic postures.

In addition, when evaluating antalgic postures, it is advantageous to assess the right and left aspects of axial muscles in both the sitting and standing postures. It is difficult to fully describe a postural shift if the practitioner monitors only one muscle site, such as the trapezius or the erector spinae muscles at the third lumbar vertebra (L-3). The practitioner could obtain a stronger description by monitoring both sites or, better yet, by looking at the activation patterns for the right and left aspects of multiple sites along the spine.

NORMATIVE DATA

In understanding muscle function, it is useful to have a sense of what the "normal" surface electromyography (SEMG) amplitudes are for a given muscle. The atlas in Part III of this book provides a "benchmark" approach for certain muscles, but only under static load conditions. These situations represent an approximate level associated with a given resting posture and are listed as a guide for interpretation. No norms are provided for dynamic procedures because of the complexity of the issues. The use of *normalized values* is recommended for dynamic procedures.

With any normative group comparisons, one should always be knowledgeable about how the testing instrument is intended to be used, how the test was constructed, on which populations it has been normed, how the standardized procedures were administered and scored, and what the guidelines for the interpretation of the test results are. The guidelines for the clinical administration of the muscle scanning procedure along with specific interpretive information for specific sites are found at the end of this chapter.

Chapter 5 discussed factors that can confound the normative data. The practitioner should weigh these factors and moderate the interpretation of the SEMG data accordingly. For example, with some obese or exceptionally lean individuals, these factors may negate the validity of the normative data. Consider the use of normative data in psychometric/personality testing. Reading level may play a significant role in the validity of psychometric testing of personality using a paper-and-pencil instrument such as the Minnesota Multiphasic Personality Inventory (MMPI). If the patient's reading ability is below that of the test construction or if the patient is significantly impaired due to the effects of a therapeutic drug, the results of the personality assessment will be invalid. Ideally, clinical examination in conjunction with pattern recognition of the test scores will help the provider to determine the validity of the test. Although such moderating factors can invalidate the use of test norms on an individual basis, such factors do not negate the potential clinical utility of standardized testing in general.

The population upon which the norms for a given test are based is very important. Standards may be developed for a variety of populations: "normal" subjects, different patient populations, vocational groups, and so forth. In addition, normative databases may vary in size, affecting our ability to generalize from them. The larger the sample population, the greater our ability to generalize. In the normative database presented for the muscle scanning procedure, the comparison group was the "normals."

But what is meant by *normal*? Does this mean "really healthy," or is it just the average for the population? Attempts to describe *normal* have proved problematic, so knowing the description of the reference population is very important. The normative data presented in **Table 6–1** and **Table 6–2** are based on a study by Cram and Engstrom,[2] in which *normal* was defined as not having had a pain-related problem requiring a physician's visit for at least two years. Thus, *normal* in this case was defined as "the absence of the symptoms." To create this sample, 104 subjects were drawn from a subset of the students attending adult education classes at the University of California at Irvine. One could argue that this normative population is limited in both size and diversity.[3] One might ask, for example, are the muscles of students the same as the muscles of truck drivers, car mechanics, or carpenters? To answer such a question, one would need to study a sample of "normal" individuals from each of these vocations and compare that database to the database for students. More research in

Table 6–1 Normative Data Based on the J&J M-501 (100- to 200-Hz Filter)

Muscle Site	Sitting				Standing			
	Left		Right		Left		Right	
	Mean	SD	Mean	SD	Mean	SD	Mean	SD
Frontal	2.0	2.1	1.8	1.9	2.0	2.0	2.1	2.0
Anterior temporalis	2.4	2.0	2.4	2.2	2.5	2.1	2.1	2.0
Sternocleidomastoid	1.3	1.2	1.3	1.9	1.3	1.7	1.6	1.6
C-2 paraspinal	1.9	1.9	1.9	1.9	1.8	1.8	1.8	1.8
C-4 paraspinal	1.9	1.2	1.9	1.1	1.8	2.0	1.8	1.9
C-6 paraspinal	2.0	2.0	2.0	2.0	2.5	2.5	2.5	2.5
Trapezius	2.2	2.5	2.3	2.8	3.1	2.7	3.3	2.9
T-2 paraspinal	2.4	2.1	2.2	1.7	2.7	2.7	3.1	3.0
T-4 paraspinal	2.3	2.3	2.3	2.3	2.3	2.3	2.3	2.3
T-6 paraspinal	2.6	2.9	2.5	2.6	2.2	2.9	2.3	3.0
T-8 paraspinal	2.4	2.4	2.4	2.4	2.7	2.7	2.7	2.7
T-10 paraspinal	2.4	2.9	2.1	2.8	2.9	3.1	3.2	3.1
L-1 paraspinal	2.0	2.0	2.0	2.0	3.1	3.1	3.1	3.1
L-3 paraspinal	2.1	2.7	1.8	2.6	3.3	3.6	3.3	3.4
L-5 paraspinal	2.0	2.0	2.0	2.0	3.1	3.1	3.1	3.1

Note: Mild = mean + 1 SD; moderate = mean + 2 SD; severe = mean + 3 SD.

Table 6–2 Normative Data Based on the J&J M-501 (25- to 1000-Hz Filter)

Muscle Site	Sitting				Standing			
	Left		Right		Left		Right	
	Mean	SD	Mean	SD	Mean	SD	Mean	SD
Frontal	2.8	2.9	2.5	2.7	2.8	2.8	2.9	2.8
Anterior temporalis	3.6	2.8	3.4	3.0	3.5	2.9	2.9	2.8
Sternocleidomastoid	1.8	1.7	1.8	2.7	1.8	2.4	2.2	2.2
C-2 paraspinal	2.7	2.7	2.7	2.7	2.5	2.5	2.5	2.5
C-4 paraspinal	2.7	1.7	2.7	1.5	2.5	2.8	2.5	2.7
C-6 paraspinal	2.8	2.8	2.8	2.8	3.5	3.5	3.5	3.5
Trapezius	3.0	3.5	3.2	3.9	4.3	3.8	4.6	4.0
T-2 paraspinal	3.4	2.9	3.0	2.4	3.8	3.7	4.3	4.2
T-4 paraspinal	3.2	3.2	3.2	3.2	3.2	3.2	3.2	3.2
T-6 paraspinal	3.6	4.0	3.5	3.6	3.0	4.0	3.2	4.2
T-8 paraspinal	3.4	3.4	3.4	3.4	3.8	3.8	3.8	3.8
T-10 paraspinal	3.4	4.0	2.9	3.6	4.0	4.3	4.8	4.3
L-1 paraspinal	2.8	2.8	2.8	2.8	4.3	4.3	4.3	4.3
L-3 paraspinal	2.9	3.8	2.5	3.6	4.6	5.0	4.6	4.4
L-5 paraspinal	2.8	2.8	2.8	2.8	4.3	4.3	4.3	4.3

Note: Mild = mean + 1 SD; moderate = mean + 2 SD; severe = mean + 3 SD.

this area is obviously needed. One might predict that a particular vocational population would differ from students to the extent that the group systematically developed or used some muscle more than other populations as a function of the work. Finally, the larger the sample and the wider the base of the sampling technique, the more confidence we have in generalizing the database to the population as a whole. For the normative database described in this section, the number of people studied is more than adequate to establish population statistics. However, the practitioner who uses this database should be aware of the limitations noted above.

Table 6–1 presents the mean SEMG value and standard deviation (SD) for a variety of cephalic and paraspinal muscle sites. Table 6–2 represents a mathematical extension of the narrow filter data to a wider filter. Here, a factor of 1.41 was used to provide the practitioner with an additional set of values to help interpret recordings from wider filters. Using the conversion factors presented in Table 3–1, the practitioner may convert the data in Table 6–1 to equivalents for his or her own particular SEMG instrument.

WITHIN-PATIENT ANALYSIS

An alternative method of analysis for muscle scanning data is the "within-patient" analysis suggested by Iacona.[3] In this type of assessment, the SEMG values for all of the sampled muscle sites in a given posture are analyzed for their central tendencies (i.e., the mean and standard deviation are calculated). Then, each of these sites is placed in relationship to the central tendency for that particular patient and in that particular posture by comparing its value to that of the mean plus the standard deviation. This practice allows for a statistical description of both hyper- and hypoactive patterns for the particular patient. The hypoactive sites or patterns are only statistically visible when using the within-patient analysis method. That is, when using population statistics, the standard deviation at a given site is usually only slightly smaller than the mean. Thus, a standard deviation of 1.0 below the mean normally lies within the noise level of the SEMG instrument and, therefore, is meaningless. The within-patient analysis provides a basis for observing both hyper- and hypoactive sites by normalizing each site to the average of all sites for the particular patient. Thus, the highs and the lows become more visible.

Table 6–3 and Table 6–4 show group norm data and within-patient data for a patient with neck pain and

Table 6–3 Scan Summary Using Group Norm Data (J&J M-501, 25- to 1000-Hz Filter)

Muscle Site	Sitting		Standing	
	Left	Right	Left	Right
Frontalis	2.2	2.5	2.5	2.5
Anterior temporalis	2.4	2.6	2.7	2.5
Masseter	2.0	2.1	2.3	2.2
Sternocleidomastoid	1.9	1.8	1.7	1.8
C-4	1.1	6.3*	0.8	8.3**
Trapezius	2.6	2.6	2.7	3.0
T-2	2.1	2.0	2.0	2.3

*Mild activation.
**Moderate activation.[2]

Table 6–4 Scan Summary Using Within-Patient Analysis (J&J M-501, 25- to 1000-Hz Filter)

Muscle Site	Sitting		Standing	
	Left	Right	Left	Right
Frontalis	2.2	2.5	2.5	2.5
Anterior temporalis	2.4	2.6	2.7	2.5
Masseter	2.0	2.1	2.3	2.2
Sternocleidomastoid	1.9	1.8	1.7	1.8
C-4	1.1†	6.3***	0.8†	8.3***
Trapezius	2.6	2.6	2.7	3.0
T-2	2.1	2.0	2.0	2.3

***Severe activation.
†Mild inhibition.

headache. The hyperactive pattern at the C-4 paraspinal site noted by the group norm comparison also has a significant hypoactive pattern on the contralateral side, as shown by the within-patient analysis. Such findings may indicate a disturbance of the gamma motor system for that myotatic unit.

Within-patient analysis is most efficiently done with computer programs that calculate the mean SEMG value and standard deviation for the sitting posture and the standing posture. These programs then mark the data fields, as in the examples described in this section, with some sort of notation. The legend below the data explains the notation. Where the practitioner wants to do a "thumbnail" of a within-patient analysis on a field of data, the practitioner calculates the mean for the sitting posture. In the example in Table 6–4, the mean is 2.45. The standard deviation is likely to be approximately one-half of the mean. We estimate it to be 1.2. Thus, the practitioner would add and subtract 1.2 from 2.45 to find the first standard deviation levels: 1.2 for hypoactive and 3.6 for hyperactive. From the field of data in Table 6–4, only one value fits the hypoactive level—left C-4, with a value of 1.1. The only value to fit the hyperactive level is found at right C-4, with a value of 6.3. To estimate two standard deviations, add an additional 1.2 to 3.6 (the total is 4.8); to estimate three standard deviations, add yet another 1.2 (the total is 6.0). The right C-4 value of 6.3 is greater than 6.0; therefore, it is at least three standard deviations away from the mean and qualifies as being "severely elevated."

In addition, within-patient analysis is highly desirable for individuals with "unique" morphologies. This technique is particularly appropriate for patients who have an extremely thin or thick layer of adipose tissue. **Table 6–5** shows muscle scan findings in an individual who is extremely thin. Many of the microvolt readings are moderately high due to the lack of adipose tissue to impede the conduction of the muscle action potentials, and the group norms comparison identifies many elevated or activated sites. When the same data are submitted to a within-patient analysis (**Table 6–6**), only a few sites show activation. The

within-patient activation pattern corresponds to the clinical examination through palpation (i.e., the hyperactive sites associated with hypertrophied muscle mass). **Table 6–7** shows scan findings for an individual who is obese. All of the microvolt readings are very low and appear to be within the normal range due to

Table 6–6 Within-Patient Analysis of an Extremely Thin Patient (J&J M-501, 25- to 1000-Hz Filter)

Muscle Site	Sitting Left	Right	Standing Left	Right
Capitis	3.0	3.5	6.4	6.2
C-4	8.2	5.2	8.6	2.1
C-6	9.0	7.0	1.1	6.2
Trapezius	52.4***	15.4	47.8***	19.7*
T-2	5.1	5.7	12.3	7.6
T-4	4.8	4.8	3.8	5.4
T-6	5.0	6.5	3.1	4.1
T-8	10.7	17.2	4.2	7.8
T-10	11.2	18.7	1.8	16.1
L-1	2.6	3.8	2.1	9.3
L-3	1.8	2.6	3.7	6.6
L-5	1.8	2.7	4.2	2.7

*Mild activation.
***Severe activation.

Table 6–5 Group Norm Analysis of an Extremely Thin Patient (J&J M-501, 25- to 1000-Hz Filter)

Muscle Site	Sitting Left	Right	Standing Left	Right
Capitis	3.0	3.5	6.4*	6.2*
C-4	8.2***	5.2*	8.6**	2.1
C-6	9.0**	7.0*	1.1	6.2
Trapezius	52.4***	15.4***	47.8***	19.7***
T-2	5.1	5.7*	12.3**	7.6
T-4	4.8	4.8	3.8	5.4
T-6	5.0	6.5	3.1	4.1
T-8	10.7**	17.2***	4.2	7.8*
T-10	11.2*	18.7***	1.8	16.1**
L-1	2.6	3.8	2.1	9.3*
L-3	1.8	2.6	3.7	6.6
L-5	1.8	2.7	4.2	2.7

*Mild activation.[2]
**Moderate activation.[2]
***Severe activation.[2]

Table 6–7 Group Norm Analysis of an Obese Individual (J&J M-501, 25- to 1000-Hz Filter)

Muscle Site	Sitting Left	Right	Standing Left	Right
Capitis	3.1	2.8	4.2	1.9
C-4	1.6	1.7	1.2	1.4
C-6	1.8	1.4	1.6	1.8
Trapezius	1.7	1.7	1.9	1.6
T-2	2.8	2.8	1.9	2.4
T-4	3.0	2.8	1.9	2.4
T-6	3.3	3.7	2.7	3.0
T-8	1.9	1.8	3.0	2.3
T-10	2.2	2.5	3.4	1.7
L-1	1.8	1.7	3.2	1.3
L-3	2.6	2.9	2.1	1.7
L-5	1.6	2.3	1.6	6.7

Note: No sites were determined to be outside the "normal limits."[2]

the absorption of the muscle action potentials by the adipose tissue. However, when the same data are submitted for a within-patient analysis (**Table 6–8**), a more meaningful activation pattern emerges from the data.

Clinicians should be aware that all of the information regarding group norms and within-patient analysis presented here would also apply to data recorded during dynamic evaluations. Both static and dynamic SEMG information must conform to the same laws of physiology and statistics. The normalization of SEMG data (as discussed in Chapter 3) provides the within-patient analysis perspective for SEMG recordings during dynamic procedures.

It is recommended that practitioners always use within-patient analysis on patients whose morphology is outside of the norm (i.e., thin and obese patients). The within-patient analysis also provides a basis for examining the muscles for hypoactive sites, which is impossible using group norms. The group norms are useful in determining when the patient's activation patterns are outside the data set of an external reference group. Their use is particularly helpful if the analysis is required for litigation.

Table 6–8 Within-Patient Analysis of an Obese Individual (J&J M-501, 25- to 1000-Hz Filter)

Muscle Site	Sitting		Standing	
	Left	Right	Left	Right
Capitis	3.1*	2.8	4.2*	1.9
C-4	1.6†	1.7	1.2†	1.4
C-6	1.8	1.4†	1.6	1.8
Trapezius	1.7	1.7	1.9	1.6
T-2	2.8	2.8	1.9	2.4
T-4	3.0*	2.8	1.9	2.4
T-6	3.3*	3.7**	2.7	3.0
T-8	1.9	1.8	3.0	2.3
T-10	2.2	2.5	3.4	1.7
L-1	1.8	1.7	3.2	1.3
L-3	2.6	2.9	2.1	1.7
L-5	1.6†	2.3	1.6	6.7***

*Mild activation.
**Moderate activation.
***Severe activation.
†Mild inhibition.

SENSITIVITY AND SPECIFICITY

The issues of sensitivity and specificity in SEMG research are complicated owing to the complex nature of the relationship of SEMG to pain. Some of the classic reviews of the literature of headache[4] and back pain[5] have found that the relationship between the location of pain and SEMG values has a concordance rate of approximately 33%. Even so, it would be unwarranted, naive, and premature to conclude that SEMG lacks sensitivity in pain assessments. Obviously, the involvement of the central nervous system in pain is more complex than a simple one-to-one relationship. For example, the response to pain via muscle may bring about a protective guarding pattern in which the painful side is "spared," while the contralateral homologous muscle group becomes activated and is overused. In this case, it is the contralateral side that would be active, not the ipsilateral side, and the one-to-one correspondence of SEMG to pain would appear to break down.

A second factor in the complicated relationship between SEMG and pain entails the spatial dislocation of pain associated with trigger points. Here the source of the painful sensation (the trigger point) may lie at some distance from the perceived location of pain.[6] When a muscle harbors a trigger point, its effect on muscle activity may not be clearly seen until the muscle is recruited during dynamic movement.[7] This phenomenon is explained in more detail in Chapter 8. Suffice it to say that when the practitioner considers protective guarding and trigger points, the relationship between pain and SEMG comes into a clearer focus.

Cram and Steger[8] originally studied the sensitivity and specificity of the static evaluation technique. They compared the SEMG data on two groups of patients—those with headache and those with low-back pain. The researchers collected SEMG data from the right and left aspects of 10 muscle sites, both in the sitting and standing postures. They found that patients with headache tended to show activation patterns in the cephalic and related muscles, while patients with low-back pain tended to show asymmetries in the paraspinal (low-back and neck) muscles. A later study by Cram and Engstrom[2] compared 104 normal subjects to 200 patients with chronic pain. This study established that the muscle scanning technique separated patients with pain from the normal population. The authors suggested that these differences occurred at a number of muscle sites, and that posture played a significant role in some muscles but not others. Scanning of the low-back muscles (L-3 and T-10), for example, more clearly separated normal patients from patients with low-back pain during the standing posture. It was primarily the left aspect of the back that afforded this distinction. The trapezius muscles showed a much larger activation pattern upon standing, as well. These results were later replicated by Kessler, Cram, and Traue[9] in a well-controlled study with a well-defined group of patients with low-back pain matched with controls for age and sex.

RELIABILITY

The reliability of a procedure is a key to its use. Tests for the reliability of the muscle scanning procedure have been conducted on two occasions with two distinct populations in different locations. In an initial and preliminary assessment of the reliability of the scanning technique,[10] a 5-minute test–retest study was conducted on a small sample of 16 patients. Here, the test–retest correlation was found to be 0.92. Later, Cram, Lloyd, and Cahn[11] studied the reliability of the scanning technique; they studied 102 patients at three points during the day. The patients had come into a multidisciplinary clinic and were scanned upon their arrival. Next, they saw either the physician or the psychologist, and then were scanned around midday. The patients were then seen by the second provider and scanned for the final time toward the end of the day. In this study, the test–retest reliability scores had a mean correlation of 0.64, indicating that the various samples of the SEMG data accounted for 64% of the variance. This figure is within the range of acceptable values for psychological tests in general,[12] and it is more than adequate for this type of physiological recording. The difference in correlations between the first and second evaluations and the first and third evaluations was not significant.

This study established the stability of the nature of the findings from muscle scanning across the course of one day. Further study of the stability of findings from muscle scannings across days, weeks, or months would be desirable. Information regarding longer-term reliability for single-site recordings using attached electrodes suggests that the longer the interval between test and retest, the lower the correlation coefficients[13] (see Chapter 8).

STABILITY OF THE SIGNAL

Because the scanning procedure entails holding the electrode over the patient's muscle site by hand and sampling from the site for relatively short periods of time, information regarding the stability of the SEMG signal during the actual data collection phase of the procedure would be of great use. When one initially places the scanning electrode onto the skin, there is an "electrical explosion" at the skin electrode interface. Soon the impedances begin to settle in, and the electrical noise of this event begins to settle out. In some instruments (e.g., J&J M-57 or M-501), this settling time is approximately 4 to 8 seconds, after which the signal becomes fairly stable. In other instruments that use an "active electrode" (e.g., Thought Technology's Smart Sensor), this settling time is two to three times longer. If one watches the integrated SEMG amplitudes (i.e., bar graphs on stand-alone instruments or curves on the computer screen) during the scanning procedure, one can see the initial large drop in the signal amplitude associated with this settling time. After that, the signal has significantly less variability.

One study[14] examined the stability issue and found that the SEMG signal obtained with the handheld scanning tool is more than adequate. **Figure 6–1A** illustrates the nature of this stability. The researchers suggested that a 10–second integration time yields slightly greater stability than 2 seconds, but the differences are relatively small and any integration between 2 and 10 seconds should adequately represent the signal. **Figure 6–1B** demonstrates that by 4 to 6 seconds, the signal has significantly less variability.

Because the SEMG signal varies somewhat once the settling has occurred, some practitioners wonder when they should collect the sample of data. In general, if the practitioner takes the sample just a few seconds after the SEMG has settled down, that sample would be the most representative. In the Thompson, Rolland, and Offord[14] study described earlier, data collection was initiated at this point, and a 10–second epoch was averaged. However, if practitioners wait too long—looking for an extremely flat and stable signal before taking a sample—they will miss the mark. Some variability in the SEMG signal ($\pm 10\%$) should always be expected. In general, practitioners simply strive to minimize that variability.

Cram and Kall have introduced an alternative algorithm into the data collection schema for muscle

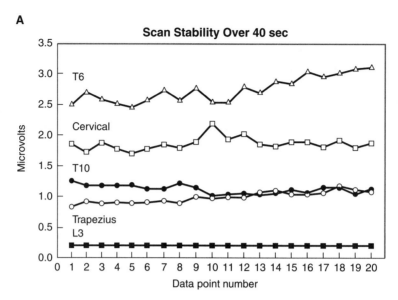

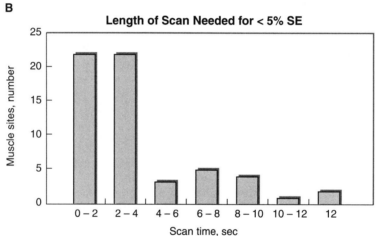

Figure 6–1 (A) Stability of SEMG signal at different sites for one subject. (B) Muscle sites grouped by length of time to achieve < 5% standard error.

Source: Reprinted with permission from J. M. Thompson, E .P. Rolland, and K. P. Offord, EMG Muscle Scanning: Stability of Hand Held Surface Electrodes, *Biofeedback and Self-Regulation*, Vol. 14, No. 1, pp. 51–61, © 1989, Plenum Publishing.

scanning software.[15] Some computerized scanning systems have deemed this the "autocollect" feature. It assesses the amount of variance around the sliding average; when this variance becomes small enough, a 2–second sample is collected.

INTERPRETATION OF STATIC FINDINGS

The interpretation of scanning information is best guided by comparison of the patient data to the reference database created by Cram and Engstrom.[2] This recommendation should be replaced with the within-patient analysis when the patient is extremely thin (< 15% body fat) or extremely obese (> 50% body fat), or when the activation pattern seen with group norm comparison does not coincide with the palpation exam. As Callet has stated, "Know what is normal, then you can discriminate what is abnormal."[16] The patient's SEMG information should be examined for its level of activation or inhibition, its degree of asymmetry, and the extent to which it is altered with postural change (see **Exhibit 6–1**). Once the SEMG information is col-

Exhibit 6–1 Keys to Clinical Interpretation of Static Surface Electromyography Data

- *Site of activation/inhibition:* Greater than two standard deviations higher (activation) when compared to the population norms or two standard deviations lower (inhibition) for within-patient normalization
- *Degree of symmetry:* 40% asymmetry between right and left sides[17]
- *Impact of posture:* Greater than two standard deviations difference between two postures
- *Comparison to clinical examination:* Sites of activation should correspond to palpation exam for hypertrophied sites

Table 6–10 Headache of Cervical or Trapezius Origin

Muscle Site	Sitting		Standing	
	Left	Right	Left	Right
Frontalis	3.1	3.0	3.2	3.0
Temporalis	2.8	3.2	3.0	3.3
Masseter	0.9	0.8	0.9	0.9
Sternocleidomastoid	0.6	0.5	0.6	0.6
Cervical	7.7	2.7	5.6	3.3
Trapezius	10.7*	3.0	14.0*	8.0
T-2 paraspinals	4.9	3.8	5.6	4.2
T-6 paraspinals	5.5	4.7	5.2	4.3

*Outside the normal and expected levels.[2]

lected, it is compared to information from the clinical examination.

HEADACHE EXAMPLE

Muscle scanning can play an important role in the examination of the headache patient, because it allows the practitioner to suspend the one-to-one model of pain sensation to causation. Consider the data from two patients with headache (**Table 6–9** and **Table 6–10**). Both patients present with identical dull, bifrontal headaches that are worse in the afternoon. Examination of the first patient (Table 6–9) suggests a myogenic headache associated with an activation pattern in the frontal region. With such a patient, the attached SEMG electrodes might be placed on the frontal region using the wide frontalis placement from the atlas. Further evaluation using stress profiling could be explored at this site. The examination of the second pa-

tient (Table 6–10), however, is more complex. It suggests referred headache pain associated with activation patterns in the cervical and trapezius region. This patient also exhibits asymmetry, along with a mild postural disturbance. Together, these findings suggest a potential biomechanical contribution to the patient's headache disorder. The practitioner might conduct further evaluation with at least two sets of attached electrodes, using the wide cervical trapezius placement listed in the atlas. Further recordings might consider the impact of stress, posture (sitting versus standing), and dynamic movement.

The scan data should always be compared with the clinical examination of the patient. The second patient, for example, was found to have a restricted range of motion in the cervical region, along with trigger points in the left trapezius muscle group that projected pain to the temporal region. This case is an excellent example of the spatial dislocation of pain, where the pain is experienced at a different site than the site of origin.

Thus, the muscle scanning procedure adds one more dimension of data to the clinical findings. Of course, it does not replace a thorough clinical exam. In addition, the muscle scan findings suggest treatment options. With the first patient, the practitioner might consider a relaxation training procedure, aided with biofeedback from the frontal EMG site. The second patient, in contrast, might initially be approached with a stretch-to-relax protocol[18] or post-isometric relaxation protocols[19] assisted by SEMG feedback. Either protocol might be followed by dynamic movement retraining suggested by Donaldson, Skubick, and Donaldson.[20] In addition, the practitioner might consider the more traditional treatments for the identified trigger point.

Table 6–9 Headache of Frontal Origin

Muscle Site	Sitting		Standing	
	Left	Right	Left	Right
Frontalis	7.3*	9.2*	8.2*	9.4*
Temporalis	6.0*	6.4*	6.1*	6.8*
Masseter	1.8	1.6	1.6	1.8
Sternocleidomastoid	1.0	1.1	1.1	1.1
Cervical	1.9	1.6	2.2	2.3
Trapezius	0.8	0.9	0.7	0.9
T-2 paraspinals	1.9	1.8	1.9	1.9

*Outside the normal and expected levels.[2]

LOW-BACK PAIN EXAMPLE

Back pain is another disorder that can be evaluated with the muscle scanning procedure, because the movements of the back muscles are orchestrated so that the muscles work together.[21] The multiple-site approach of scanning matches the multijointed, suprasegmental nature of the back muscles. But which sites should the practitioner monitor? Is the upper back involved in a patient with low-back pain? One would not know for sure without assessing multiple sites. The muscle scanning procedure provides a quick and reliable basis for deciding where to place attached electrodes for further study. This section highlights three scanning studies conducted on patients with low-back pain. The first study (**Table 6–11**) shows an example of protective guarding, the second patient (**Table 6–12** and **Table 6–13**) shows an instability in the pelvis that is posturally mediated, and the third patient (**Table 6–14**) provides an example of splinting in response to a neurological event.

The first study (Table 6–11) involves an individual with a primary complaint of low-back pain, with no objective findings on traditional tests (physical exam, plain films, magnetic resonance imaging, needle EMG). He was injured 5 months ago, when he strained his back muscles while lifting and turning. Unfortunately, traditional conservative care has not led to a diminution of his pain. The EMG scan data show high levels of EMG activation only in the erector spinae group at L-3 and T-10. This activation appears to worsen upon standing, as if the patient puts on a neuromuscular corset as he goes from the sitting to the

Table 6–11 Low-Back Pain: Protective Guarding

Muscle Site	Sitting		Standing	
	Left	Right	Left	Right
Frontalis	3.5	3.8	1.2	1.3
Temporalis	3.5	3.5	4.6	3.6
Masseter	1.3	1.5	1.5	1.6
Sternocleidomastoid	1.2	1.5	0.8	0.9
Cervical	1.6	1.7	1.9	1.9
Trapezius	2.2	2.3	3.0	2.5
T-2 paraspinals	1.5	1.5	1.3	1.1
T-6 paraspinals	3.7	3.5	4.7	4.4
T-10 paraspinals	9.6*	19.2*	44.8*	59.2*
L-3 paraspinals	2.2	11.2*	19.2*	30.4*
Abdominal	1.3	1.5	1.6	1.8

*Values are outside the normal and expected levels.[2]

Table 6–12 Low-Back Pain: Postural Shift Shows Instability in the Pelvis, Group Norms Analysis

Muscle Site	Sitting		Standing	
	Left	Right	Left	Right
Capitis	2.4	2.5	1.9	1.6
C-4 paraspinals	4.8*	4.5*	3.5	3.7
C-6 paraspinals	3.3	4.2	5.3	4.5
Trapezius	5.4	3.2	4.3	8.5
T-2 paraspinals	4.8	4.6	5.5	11.4*
T-4 paraspinals	8.2*	3.9	5.5	10.9**
T-6 paraspinals	5.5	4.8	5.0	4.7
T-8 paraspinals	6.4	5.7	5.7	4.0
T-10 paraspinals	3.7	7.6*	8.6*	8.3
L-1 paraspinals	2.9	10.1**	7.6	9.6*
L-3 paraspinals	2.6	6.7*	10.0*	7.2
L-5 paraspinals	2.3	5.1	12.9**	7.1

*Mild activation.[2]
**Moderate activation.[2]

Table 6–13 Low-Back Pain: Postural Shift Shows Instability in the Pelvis, Within-Patient Analysis

Muscle Site	Sitting		Standing	
	Left	Right	Left	Right
Capitis	2.4†	2.5†	1.9†	1.6†
C-4 paraspinals	4.8	4.5	3.5†	3.7
C-6 paraspinals	3.3	4.2	5.3	4.5
Trapezius	5.4	3.2	4.3	8.5
T-2 paraspinals	4.8	4.6	5.5	11.4*
T-4 paraspinals	8.2*	3.9	5.5	10.9*
T-6 paraspinals	5.5	4.8	5.0	4.7
T-8 paraspinals	6.4	5.7	5.7	4.0
T-10 paraspinals	3.7	7.6*	8.6*	8.3
L-1 paraspinals	2.9	10.1**	7.6	9.6*
L-3 paraspinals	2.6†	6.7	10.0*	7.2
L-5 paraspinals	2.3†	5.1	12.9**	7.1

*Mild activation.
**Moderate activation.
†Hypoactivation.

standing posture. This type of postural change commonly indicates the presence of *protective guarding*, a learned muscle activation pattern used to avoid pain. In addition, there is a striking asymmetry, with the right side more active than the left side. In cases such as this one, a hemipelvis or leg-length discrepancy may have been dis-

Table 6–14 Low-Back Pain with Herniated Disk

Muscle Site	Sitting		Standing	
	Left	Right	Left	Right
Cervical	1.2	1.5	1.5	1.7
Trapezius	2.2	3.3	3.2	3.5
T-1 paraspinals	1.2	1.3	1.2	1.2
T-6 paraspinals	3.7	3.8	5.2	5.4
T-10 paraspinals	10.3*	17.1*	4.4	5.9
L-3 paraspinals	10.4*	15.2*	4.2	5.1
Abdominal	1.3	1.5	1.6	1.8

*Outside the normal and expected limits.[2]

covered during the physical exam. However, if the pain complaint is on the opposite side of the activation pattern, the asymmetry usually represents a protective guarding mechanism in which the patient consciously or habitually shifts his or her weight away from the pain. It is far more common for the activation to be on the side opposite the pain rather than on the ipsilateral side.

The findings of this scan suggest that further SEMG assessment using attached electrodes should be conducted. Because the upper back does not appear to be involved, a multiple-electrode array in the low-back area would be indicated. (This approach is reviewed in greater detail later in the chapter.) It also suggests that biofeedback treatment should be directed toward the low-back musculature. For example, the patient might strengthen the abdominal muscles, while using SEMG feedback to learn how to use this musculature in a more biomechanically efficient fashion (i.e., anterior pelvic tilt) while standing. The equality of weight distribution, using a weight scale under each foot, would be useful feedback.

The second patient with low-back pain is a 35-year-old male who received a traumatic blow to his midback region while working in the logging industry. The muscle scan whose results are shown in Tables 6–12 and Table 6–13 was conducted using the 25- to 1000-Hz filter. Both the group norms and the within-patient analysis are presented because of the patient's moderate level of obesity. The results of both analyses are similar. The major difference is that the within-patient analysis identifies the cervical musculature and left low-back sites while sitting as hypoactive. Otherwise, the symmetry patterns shift from left to right as the patient changes from the sitting posture to the standing posture. Note how the activation patterns in the low back shift from

the right low back to the left low back, while the upper back shows a compensatory shift from the left upper back to the right upper back as the patient changes from the sitting to the standing posture. Such a shift in the activation pattern strongly suggests a hemipelvis. This finding was verified during the clinical examination and was treated through joint mobilization techniques. In addition, external support with cushions or orthoses could be used to normalize the nature of this imbalance.

The third patient with low-back pain presents during a recurrent flare-up of a long-standing pain problem. The patient reports that the pain is very severe and radiates down into his right buttocks. Radiographic studies indicate a bulging disk at L-3 and L-4. The EMG scan data shown in Table 6–14 indicate activation patterns at the L-3 and T-10 sites, with the sitting posture evoking the higher level of activation. This type of finding—an activation pattern in the T-10 to L-5 region that is stronger when sitting than when standing—has been observed in a series of 12 patients with bulging or herniated disks (Cram and Dike, unpublished). The additional pressure on the disk from sitting appears to create a larger bulge and thus places pressure on the nerve, creating a nocioceptive environment that evokes an acute muscular splinting pattern around the injured nerve to help minimize further damage. Such reflexively based splinting patterns are suggested when the pain complaint is on the ipsilateral side of the activation. In this particular case, a mild asymmetry is noted on the ipsilateral side of the patient's pain. If such an SEMG scan pattern is observed in a patient without radiographic studies, radiographic studies should be considered. One should never diagnose a herniated disk or neuropathy from SEMG data alone. For this patient, EMG biofeedback therapy might best be used within the context of McKenzie-type therapies.

Through the systematic sampling of multiple muscle sites in these two neutral postures, the SEMG scanning procedure provides a framework for identifying sites of activation. Scanning of multiple sites may also identify contributions missed by a more limited study. The major weakness of this technique is that it offers only a "snapshot" of the potential contribution of the muscles in pain-related disorders. The dynamic EMG evaluation is needed to assess the impact of pain on movement.

To summarize, the muscle scanning technique may elucidate the following interpretive elements:

- Identification of which muscle groups have been affected
- Identification of antalgic (painful) postures

- Identification of protective guarding
- Identification of splinting
- Identification of mechanical postural components

THE CLINICAL PROCEDURE ASSOCIATED WITH THE STATIC ASSESSMENT

Although a static assessment can be done with attached electrodes moved about during rest conditions, it is somewhat slow and involves a fair amount of supplies. A muscle scanning tool has been developed to make this procedure fast and reliable. A new tool to do static assessments first appeared in the 1970s as a picture in *Muscles Alive* (third edition) by John Basmajian.[22] In this picture, a specially engineered device with "post-style" direct contact electrodes was shown assessing the zygomaticus muscle; the electrodes were held in place by hand, rather than being attached with adhesives. While Basmajian had seen the wisdom of being able to sample and assess specific muscles quickly using these post-style electrodes, this technology essentially went unnoticed and undeveloped until its reintroduction in a commercialized form simultaneously by J&J Enterprises and Davicon (circa 1980).

This section reviews the technical aspects of the static assessment procedure using a muscle scanning tool. It describes the sites for electrode placement, discusses interpretation of findings for each site, and briefly highlights some of the pitfalls associated with the technique.

Although the general principles of muscle scanning are quite simple, one must adhere to the principles outlined here or the SEMG study will be significantly flawed, providing a false view of the neuromuscular system.

1. It is important to keep the impedance (resistance) at the recording site as low as possible. One must abrade the site to be scanned, so that it is free of oils and the dead or horny layer of skin.
2. If the scanning electrodes allow this practice, the practitioner should coat the scanning electrodes lightly with electrode paste or cream prior to placing them onto the site. This step will add ions to the electrode skin interface, thereby lowering the impedance while potentiating the biological signal.
3. The practitioner should hold the sensors in place with a light pressure and avoid pressing too firmly. Too much pressure might push the patient off the center of gravity, creating an artificial recruitment pattern. Some practitioners have asked whether excess pressure might place the muscle on stretch. Cram has attempted to test this hypothesis on many occasions and in many ways, but has not found excess pressure to be a source of artifact.
4. Because scanning electrodes are not held in place with adhesive tape, the electrodes must be held motionless by hand for a period of 6 to 20 seconds. It takes the signal 4 to 8 seconds to stabilize from the electrical explosion that occurs when the scanning electrodes initially make contact with the skin. In addition, going much beyond 30 seconds does nothing but add potential movement artifact into the signal. Intentional or accidental movement or sliding of the scanning electrode must be avoided, because it generates an offset potential that artificially elevates the levels of energy seen on the instrument.

A Step-by-Step Description of the Clinical Procedure

The clinical procedure described here has evolved over 10 years of refinement. Many different strategies have been tried over the years, but the following procedure yields notably reliable results.

Step 1

Identify the muscle group of interest. Think about the origin and insertion of the muscles and the direction of the muscle fibers. Visually or tactually locate the belly of the muscle.

Step 2

Abrade and clean the scan site with a rough alcohol swab. The practitioner might think of the phrase "rub to rubor." Do not use cotton balls. Let the site air-dry. Clean all of the sites that will be scanned (see **Figure 6–2**). The reference electrode simply needs to be on the patient's body.

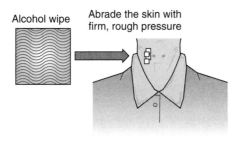

Figure 6–2 Abrade the placement site with a rough alcohol swab.

Source: Copyright © 1992, J. R. Cram, *SIS 3000 Manual*, Clinical Resources, Inc.

Step 3

Ask the patient to sit or stand comfortably. Do not otherwise verbally or physically prompt the patient's posture. Make visual observations of the "natural" posture.

Step 4

If appropriate, run a bead of electrode paste or cream on a tissue. Dip the scanning electrodes in the bead and lightly coat them with this paste. Avoid ending up with globs of paste on the electrodes (see **Figure 6–3**).

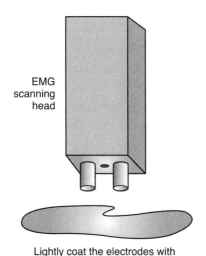

Lightly coat the electrodes with electrolyte paste or cream.

Figure 6–3 Dip the scanning electrodes into a bead of electrode paste.

Source: Copyright © 1992, J. R. Cram, *SIS 3000 Manual*, Clinical Resources, Inc.

Step 5

For recording from specific muscle groups, place the scanning electrodes so that they run parallel to the muscle fibers of the muscle of interest. When comparing data to the normative data presented in Tables 6–1 and 6–2, be certain to use the electrode placement guide used in the normative study. Once the electrodes are on the skin, hold them motionless with a light pressure (see **Figure 6–4**).

Step 6

Observe the EMG recording. Allow it to settle from its initial contact artifact. This process usually takes 4 to 20 seconds, depending on the SEMG instrument. The signal is considered stable when it is ±10% in its fluctuations and is free of artifacts (swallowing, movement) and noise (60 Hz). The level of heart rate artifact, if present, should be noted.

Step 7

When the stability of the SEMG signal seems satisfactory, record that EMG value as the best representative sample of SEMG activity for that site. The total scanning procedure for a given site commonly takes about 10 to 30 seconds.

Step 8

If a site shows values in the "severe" range (see the normative database), verify that this value results from

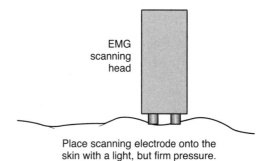

Place scanning electrode onto the skin with a light, but firm pressure.

Figure 6–4 Place the scanning electrodes on the skin and hold in place with a light, but firm, pressure.

Source: Copyright © 1992, J. R. Cram, *SIS 3000 Manual*, Clinical Resources, Inc.

SEMG signals rather than from noise of some type. If the values are excessively low, consider the possibility of bridging of electrode paste. In either event, clean the site again and rescan it to see if it remains stable in its level.

Step 9

Study the right and left aspects of each muscle site. If the SEMG system has dual-channel scanning capacity that allows the practitioner to monitor the right and left sides simultaneously, use it. If postural muscles are monitored, conduct the scan in both the sitting and standing postures.

Potential Problems and Pitfalls of the Procedure

Five problems are commonly encountered during the scanning procedure: exceptionally low values, exceptionally high values, variable EMG values, obesity, and physical appliances.

Exceptionally low SEMG readings (in the noise range for the SEMG amplifier) occur when there is a bridging of paste between the two active electrodes. If the procedure is done while the skin is still moist from the alcohol abrade, the patient's natural salts may join the moisture of the alcohol to form an electron bridge. Exceptionally low values should always be suspect. Clean the site again, let it dry, and scan it a second time.

Exceptionally high SEMG values are defined as being higher than 25 to 40 microvolts on most SEMG instruments. Surface EMG values seldom go above these amplitudes, except in posturally active muscles or muscles in "spasm." High readings may also be attributable to 60-cycle noise entering the amplifiers. This problem is commonly associated with poor contact of the electrode with the skin. If the skin has not been adequately abraded, and or if natural oils or oils from makeup have not been removed, 60-cycle noise can easily invade the signal. This problem is often associated with scanning at the hairline. Here, the practitioner may adequately abrade the skin in the cervical region, but not into the hairline, or the practitioner may use adequate electrode paste for the skin but not enough to penetrate through the hair. If there is a radical difference in the level of impedance between the two recording electrodes, the differential amplifier is defeated and becomes very vulnerable to 60-cycle noise. Practitioners are discouraged from scanning up into the hairline to reduce the

probability of impedance. Listening to the raw SEMG for the muscle action potentials (rather than the hum of the 60–cycle noise) can increase the practitioner's confidence in the validity of a high EMG reading. If the raw SEMG is not available, check the skin preparation and adequacy of electrode paste and rescan the site.

Excessive variability of the SEMG values is a third potential problem. Sometimes the practitioner places the scanning electrodes onto the skin and the SEMG values do not appear to stabilize enough. Because no consistent value is generated, it is difficult to tell which sample is the best representation of the true SEMG value. Most of the time, this problem occurs when a practitioner who is new to scanning stays on the site too long. Typically, the signal drops rapidly and then stabilizes for some 10 to 20 seconds, after which the level of variability increases. This variability likely has to do with the effects of holding the scanner in place by hand. In essence, the patient begins to sway, as he or she subtly presses back against the pressure of the scanning electrode. The practitioner should stay on the site for as little time as possible. As soon as the signal has stabilized, record that value.

A second source of variability has to do with respiration artifact. Some individuals (especially smokers and patients with chronic obstructive pulmonary disease) tend to use their ancillary muscles instead of their diaphragms for respiration. Surface EMG readings of the muscles of the upper trapezius and the dorsal region seem to be most affected by this type of artifact. When it is observed, one can readily note the correlation between the variability of the SEMG reading and the patient's respiration cycle. In such a case, the correct SEMG value to record would be the one associated with the pause between expiration and inspiration.

Obesity can also produce flawed readings. Because adipose tissue is an effective insulator, it attenuates or reduces the amount of SEMG signal reaching the skin's surface, which causes the SEMG levels on an obese individual to be much lower than normal. One should exercise extreme caution in the interpretation of scan values taken from an obese individual. When comparing an individual patient's data to the data for a normative population (see Tables 6–1 and 6–2), there is a high probability of a false negative finding.

Physical appliances (such as dentures, glasses, shoes, and lifts) are the final factor that can confound the scanning procedure. Although physical appliances may introduce an alteration in muscle activity, they may also provide powerful diagnostic clues about the etiology of pain and dysfunction. Recordings from the temporalis muscle group provide a good example of this phenomenon. Cram has noticed that patients who wear dentures have a higher probability of bracing with these muscles; where this bracing is clearly seen, the patient is having problems with loose-fitting dentures and is using the temporalis muscles to hold the dentures in place. He has also noted problems with frontalis and cervical muscles in patients who are having difficulties with glasses (usually bifocals); this problem may come from frowning, squinting, or tilting the head excessively to see through the correct area of the lens. In addition, shoes and lifts may introduce another level of variance in the SEMG values. It is up to the practitioner to inquire and make astute observations to allow for these factors in the interpretive framework.

NORMATIVE DATA COMPARISON CONSIDERATIONS

To develop the normative data provided in this book, the initial clinical protocol entailed the scanning of the right and left aspects of 11 muscle groups, first in the sitting posture and then in the standing posture. This protocol was later extended to additional muscle groups. The normative data collected on 104 normal subjects are presented in Tables 6–1 and 6–2. For practitioners to compare the EMG values collected on an individual patient to the normative data, it is essential to follow the procedure and protocol described in this section. The filter selection, skin preparation, patient instructions, posture, and electrode placement must be exactly the same as those used in the collection of the normative data. The step-by-step procedure outlined in the previous section should be followed closely. Following is a description of the instructions given to patients regarding their posture.

- *Sitting posture:* The therapist asks the patient to sit on an adjustable, backless stool or to sit sideways on a chair so that there is no support given to the back. The sitting surface should be parallel to the ground and lightly padded. It is even better if the height of the sitting surface can be altered to accommodate the leg length of the patient. If the height is fixed, the therapist will need to use devices such as pillows or boxes to create a 90–degree angle at the knee and to allow the patient's feet to rest comfortably on a surface. The patient is asked to place his or her hands in the lap, and to "sit in a comfortable fashion." Phrases such as "sit up straight" are avoided. The patient is requested not to try to help the therapist by altering posture. For example, if the patient leans the head forward to help with scanning the cervical paraspinals, the therapist gently redirects the patient to sit comfortably. No further instruction concerning posture is given. The objective is for the patient to take on as natural a sitting posture as possible.

- *Standing posture:* The therapist asks the patient to "stand comfortably" in an unsupported fashion with hands at the sides. Again, the patient is requested not to alter his or her posture to help make the scan easier. If the patient does so, the therapist redirects the patient to stand comfortably. No further instruction about posture is given. The goal is for the patient to take on the natural/habitual posture for standing.

LOCATIONS OF SCAN SITES AND INTERPRETATION FOR EACH SITE

As the placement for each site is presented in this section, consider the anatomical markers described to aid in the placement. Examine the graphic depiction for the original 11 scan sites shown in **Figure 6–5**, along with the additional extended scan sites shown in **Figure 6–6**. An interpretive framework for the recordings of each site is given. The practitioner should remember that the site labels refer most clearly to the location of the scanning electrodes rather than to the muscles from which the recordings are actually recorded. Further information on the location and interpretation of each of these sites can be found in the electrode atlas in Part III.

The practitioner should be aware that the muscle scanning procedure is most appropriately used in assessing postural muscles and emotional tone. In the sites described next, phasic muscles are also included; they are flagged with an asterisk (*). Use of the scanning protocol to assess these muscles should be limited to evaluation of the resting state and exploration of possible emotional contributions. Practitioners should not attempt to use muscle scanning to assess these phasic muscles during dynamic movement. They may use scanning to study isometric contractions, but only with extreme caution.

A

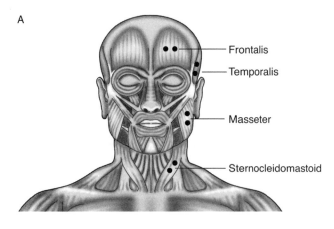

- Frontalis
- Temporalis
- Masseter
- Sternocleidomastoid

B

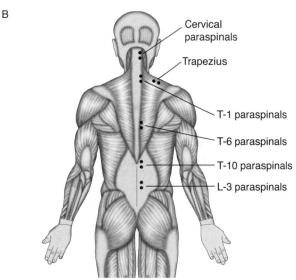

- Cervical paraspinals
- Trapezius
- T-1 paraspinals
- T-6 paraspinals
- T-10 paraspinals
- L-3 paraspinals

Figure 6–5 The original scan sites (A) for the face and (B) for the back. Abdominal site is not shown.

Source: Copyright © 1992, J. R. Cram, *The Cram Scan Manual,* Clinical Resources, Inc.

Low Frontalis

Placement

The scan electrodes are placed parallel to the eyebrow, and approximately $1/2$ inch above it. The space between the two electrodes is centered over the iris of the eye. This configuration of the recording electrodes runs perpendicular to the muscle fibers of the frontalis muscle. This nonspecific placement records from a small region on the forehead—including the frontalis, corrugator, orbicularis oculi, and temporalis muscles.

Interpretation

The primary function of this muscle or region is the nonverbal display of emotions. The emotions of anger, fear, sadness, and surprise activate this region. Movements here may also be associated with intense concentration or squinting of the eyes. Elevations in this region may represent an emotional contribution to the presenting problem. It has been suggested that elevations on the left aspect may be seen in patients who are prone to cardiac problems.

Anterior Temporalis

Placement

The scan electrodes are placed in a vertical direction. The lowest of the recording electrodes is placed across from the notch of the eye socket, approximately $1/2$ inch laterally. The electrodes run parallel to the muscle fibers of the anterior temporalis.

Interpretation

The temporalis is a major muscle of mastication and stabilization of the mandible. It elevates the jaw bone. Patients who clench their teeth during times of stress may show elevations at this site. Asymmetrical patterns (right versus left) may suggest involvement of the temporomandibular joint (TMJ), which can contribute to headache conditions. The practitioner might consider inquiring about symptoms of TMJ dysfunction, which typically include clenching, grinding, bruxing, splinting, making popping sounds, and feeling the jaw lock up.

Patients who wear dentures may show excessive activation in this muscle group. They appear to use the temporalis muscle to stabilize loose-fitting dentures. Noted elevations in this muscle group should be followed by an inquiry about the use of dentures.

Masseter

Placement

The practitioner can easily palpate the masseter muscle by placing his or her fingers on the patient's jaw and asking the patient to clench the teeth. The goal of electrode placement for the masseter muscle is to place the scanning electrodes over the belly of the muscle, with the electrodes running parallel to the muscle fibers. To do so, the practitioner should draw an imaginary line from the corner of the jaw to the cheek bone and place the

FRONT

BACK

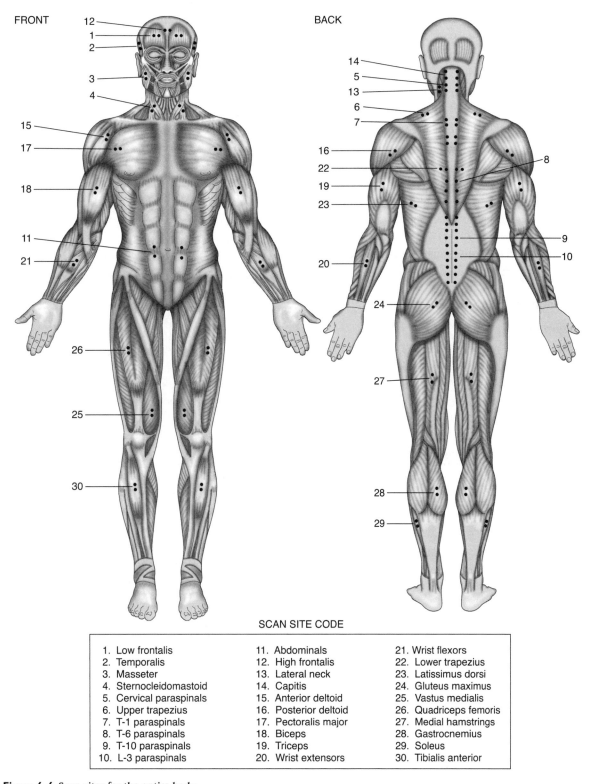

SCAN SITE CODE

1. Low frontalis	11. Abdominals	21. Wrist flexors
2. Temporalis	12. High frontalis	22. Lower trapezius
3. Masseter	13. Lateral neck	23. Latissimus dorsi
4. Sternocleidomastoid	14. Capitis	24. Gluteus maximus
5. Cervical paraspinals	15. Anterior deltoid	25. Vastus medialis
6. Upper trapezius	16. Posterior deltoid	26. Quadriceps femoris
7. T-1 paraspinals	17. Pectoralis major	27. Medial hamstrings
8. T-6 paraspinals	18. Biceps	28. Gastrocnemius
9. T-10 paraspinals	19. Triceps	29. Soleus
10. L-3 paraspinals	20. Wrist extensors	30. Tibialis anterior

Figure 6–6 Scan sites for the entire body.

Source: Modified from Copyright © 1992, J. R. Cram, *SIS 3000 Manual*, Clinical Resources, Inc.

scanning electrodes along this line over the belly of the muscle. Scanning of this site on men with beards is impossible and should not be attempted.

Interpretation

The masseter muscle is the major muscle of mastication. The vectors of force form concentric pressure on the teeth and allow chewing. When a person is not chewing, swallowing, or talking, this muscle should be quiet. Elevations or asymmetries in this muscle are commonly associated with dental problems (such as TMJ dysfunction, myofacial pain, bruxing) and may suggest an etiology for headache. In addition, such an examination could be of interest to dentists who want to determine the appropriate splint fabrication for patients with temporomandibular joint dysfunction.

Sternocleidomastoid (SCM)

Placement

This muscle runs from the back corner of the skull (mastoid process) to the collarbone (clavicle). If the practitioner asks the patient to rotate the head to the right and elevate the head slightly, the belly of the SCM on the left may be easily seen. The scanning electrodes are placed parallel to the muscle fibers of the SCM and halfway between the mastoid process and the clavicle. The head is in the midline position during the scanning.

Interpretation

The major function of this muscle is the rotation of the head: The SCM on the side that is opposite the direction of the head turn is active. The SCM also plays a minor role in respiration. Rhythmic SEMG oscillations that follow the patient's respiration pattern may suggest excessive use of the ancillary muscles of respiration. Asymmetrical patterns are clearly seen in torticollis (an abnormal twisting of the neck) and may be observed in patients with acceleration injuries to the neck. The activity in this muscle is typically quite low.

Cervical Paraspinal Muscles (C-4)

Placement

To assess the cervical paraspinal muscles, the scan electrodes are placed parallel to and approximately $1/4$ to $1/2$ inch from the spine over the belly of the muscle. If the

electrodes are placed too far laterally, slightly off the belly of the muscle, the EMG values will be significantly lower. The upper scanning electrode should be below the hairline, approximately in the vertical center of the neck. (This differs from the capitis or C-2 placement, where the upper scanning electrode may reach into the hairline.) In conducting a scan of this site, it is important to notice whether the patient attempts to help the practitioner by leaning the head slightly forward. This error is common, because so many people have been trained by the barber or hair stylist to help in this way. If the patient does lean forward, the practitioner should simply say that it is not necessary to help in this way and should instruct the patient to return to a comfortable sitting or standing posture, facing forward.

Interpretation

Many layers of muscles are present in this region; the scanning electrodes collect data from the upper fibers of the trapezius, the splenius capitis, the splenius cervicis, and the semispinalis cervicis. These muscles are primarily involved in the support and rotation of the head. With unilateral activations of these muscles, rotation or lateral flexion of the head may occur; with bilateral activation, extension of the head may occur. In patients with poor posture, where the head is held in front of its center of gravity, these muscles are required to provide chronic muscular support for the 15-pound weight of the head. In such cases, these muscles may become fatigued, and 100- to 200-Hz filter recordings may not adequately represent the nature of musclar dysfunction. In another common variation, the cervical muscles may appear to have very low EMG values, especially in comparison to trapezius T-1 or T-6. When this occurs, the patient's posture may be such that he or she has "unloaded" the cervical muscles, transferring the work to these lower muscles. This pattern of activity is an inappropriate muscle synergy. Even though the cervical muscles show low EMG values, activations in related muscle groups make these values suspect. If evaluating this region, the practitioner should consider pattern analysis comparing one site to other sites.

The cervical muscles have been indicated in headaches located in the occipital and frontal regions. There may be a concordance in activation between the frontalis muscle and the cervical paraspinal muscles. Such a concordance may indicate an emotional overlay in the patient, suggesting that stress plays a major role in conditions such as headache, for example.

Upper Trapezius

Placement

The scanning electrodes are placed so that they run parallel to the muscle fibers of the upper trapezius. Their direction follows the ridge of the shoulder. They are placed approximately 1 inch from this ridge, toward the back. The electrodes are located approximately halfway between the spine and the lateral edge of the acromion, just lateral to the belly of the muscle. The belly of the muscle may easily be determined by palpation.

Interpretation

The primary function of the upper trapezius has to do with stabilization or movement of the shoulder. It is also used in lateral bending or rotating of the head. In addition, the shoulder region is considered a strong emotional display system. Patients may elevate their shoulders when they feel threatened or are anxious and uptight. When EMG activation or asymmetries are noted on the trapezius recording, one or both shoulders are probably elevated.

The upper trapezius muscle is strongly affected by posture. In other words, its static level of discharge may be radically different during standing compared to sitting. The position of the arms in relationship to the torso may be a major factor influencing this muscle's activation. In addition, there appears to be a left-sided dominance in this region, with the left aspect generally more active than the right aspect. Some have argued that this imbalance is associated with "handedness." Others have suggested that it is associated with heart rate artifact. Because this left-sided dominance is more predictably seen during standing than during sitting, it is difficult to imagine how it might be associated with heart rate artifact.

When using the normative database as a reference, the relative activity of the trapezius should always be compared to the activity of other muscles, particularly those of the lower and midback. Compensatory shifts may be seen in some cases, when a left-sided asymmetry at the L-3 level is associated with a right-sided asymmetry at the trapezius. In addition, the trapezius may be overly active as a result of too much inhibition of the dorsal (T-8 and T-10) muscle groups. Elevations in trapezius SEMG activity may be associated with temporal headache or neck, upper back, and shoulder pain.

T-1 and T-2 Paraspinal Muscles

Placement

The scanning electrodes are placed in this region so that they run parallel to the spine and approximately 3 cm out from the vertebral ridge. The landmark for this placement is the C-7/T-1 prominence, which clearly stands out in most adults. To find it, the practitioner should follow the spinal processes in the cervical region down into the upper back until reaching the most prominent spinal process in the upper back; the chances are good that this is the C-7/T-1 prominence. The uppermost scanning electrode is placed across from this prominence.

Interpretation

Multiple muscles are located at this recording site. Indeed, the trapezius (upper/middle fibers), longissimus, semispinalis, splenius capitis, and multifidus muscle groups may all contribute to the SEMG recordings. The primary use of these muscles is the stabilization and support of the head and neck; this site appears to be a major stress point for postural support.

Elevations at this site commonly are in concordance with elevations in the trapezius muscle group. High SEMG levels of these muscles when the cervical muscles show very low SEMG values suggest that these muscles may be doing some of the work of the cervical muscles. Elevations and asymmetries at this site may be noted in patients who complain of headache or neck or upper back pain.

T-6 Paraspinal Muscles

Placement

The scanning electrodes are placed in the T-6 area so that they run parallel to the spine and are approximately 3 cm out from the vertebral ridge. The vertical level of placement is approximately between the shoulder blades (scapulae). If the spinal processes can be clearly seen or palpated on the patient, the practitioner can count down six vertebrae from T-1 to find the location. If the bottom scanning electrode is below the bottom edge of the scapula, it is too low. The bottom edge of the scapula may be easily palpated.

Interpretation

Many layers of muscles are present at this site, such that contributions from trapezius (inferior fibers), rhomboids, longissimus, semispinalis, and multifidus muscles may all affect the SEMG readings. These muscles have two functions: (1) to stabilize or move the thoracic spine and (2) to stabilize or move the scapula. In the free-sitting posture (no back support), these muscles may be very active. The T-6 area is one of the few sites where higher levels of activation are expected during free sitting than during free standing. Pain in the midback or neck is commonly associated with elevations or asymmetries at this site.

T-10 Paraspinal Muscles

Placement

The scanning electrodes are placed in the T-10 area so that they run parallel to the spine, approximately 3 cm out from the vertebral ridge. The vertical placement along the spine may be counted down from T-1 if the spinal processes are prominent. The practitioner can palpate for the ribs, placing the scanning electrodes slightly above where the rib cage disappears. Another method is to take approximately one-half the distance between the L-3 placement and the bottom of the scapula.

Interpretation

Many layers of muscles are found at this site. The primary contributors to SEMG recordings appear to be the longissimus and multifidus muscles, although there is a possibility of contributions from latissimus dorsi and serratus posterior as well. The primary function of these muscles is postural support and stabilization of the spine. Because lateral bending is possible in this region of the back, this site may reflect this action. The muscles in the T-10 area play a role in rotation of the back. Protective guarding and splinting patterns or asymmetries are commonly observed in this region in patients with back pain. This phenomenon appears to be augmented in patients who have had surgery (particularly fusions) on the lower back. Posture strongly affects this site, and elevations or asymmetries may not be observed until the patient has assumed the standing posture.

Data gathered from this region seem to correlate most highly with the total amount of muscular energy observed in a scan. If "key muscles" were to be selected that were indicative of general muscle tension, the paraspinal muscles in the T-10 area would be the choice.

L-3 Paraspinal Muscles

Placement

For the L-3 paraspinal muscles, the scanning electrodes are placed so that they run parallel to the spine and approximately 3 cm out from the vertebral ridge. The iliac crest (top of the pelvic girdle) is used as the landmark to guide the placement. The practitioner should palpate for the iliac crest. Once it is found, the practitioner should draw an imaginary horizontal line across the back toward the spine, placing the lower scanning electrodes at this level.

Interpretation

There are many layers of muscles at this site, although the muscles thought to contribute most heavily to the SEMG recording are the iliocostalis lumborum and multifidus. The major function of these muscles is postural support—the stabilization of the trunk during standing. In addition, these muscles are extensors of the lower back; they come into action with an eccentric contraction during forward bending (flexion) and in concentric fashion during the return to the upright position. Protective guarding/splinting may be seen at the L-3 site in some patients with chronic low-back pain. The site is strongly affected by posture, and the SEMG recordings may radically shift as the patient goes from sitting to standing. During quiet standing, only minimal muscle activity in the low-back region is needed as long as the patient remains over his or her center of gravity. If one shifts slightly off the center of gravity (by leaning forward a little), these muscles come into play.

It is important for the practitioner to note whether surgery has been conducted in this region. If so, the surgeon may have removed or denervated some of the muscles or in some way altered the neuromuscular structure. Needle EMG may be done to assess for denervation. Although the effect of denervation on SEMG potentials has not been adequately studied, practitioners should exercise caution in their interpretation of data in a region where surgery has been conducted.

Abdominal Muscles

Placement

To assess the abdominal muscles, the scanning electrodes are placed approximately 3 cm to the left or right of the umbilicus (belly button). The scanning electrodes are placed on opposite sides of the umbilicus. The direction of the electrodes is vertical, and they run parallel to the muscle fibers of the rectus abdominis.

Interpretation

These muscles play a role in the stabilization, elevation, and rotation of the pelvis. They are commonly underdeveloped as a result of lack of use, and they may be covered with a thick layer of fat. If this is true, readings may be lower due to the attenuation of the signals by the adipose tissue. Asymmetries may be noted in patients with low-back pain, but this is very uncommon. Elevations may be noted in patients with pain of abdominal origin.

High Frontalis

Placement

To record data for the high frontalis, the scanning electrodes are placed in the center of the forehead, 1 to $1^1/_2$ inches above the eyebrows, just below the hairline.

Interpretation

This placement provides a general recording from the frontalis muscle group. The advantage of this placement is that it separates out the potential cross-talk from the corrugator muscle group, providing a cleaner sample of frontalis muscle activity.

Lateral Neck/Scalene

Placement

The scanning electrodes are placed in the hollow on the side of the neck, which is formed by the sternocleidomastoid anterior to it, the upper trapezius posterior to it, and the collarbone below it. The electrodes run parallel to the scalene muscle.

Interpretation

The scalene muscle is well known for its stabilizing influence on the neck. It plays an active role in lateral bending and is an ancillary muscle of respiration. Practitioners should observe the SEMG signal for spontaneous signs of respiration. Large excursions are considered pathognomonic. Abnormalities at this site could play a role in thoracic outlet syndromes.

Capitis Site

Placement

The muscles just below the base of the cranium are scanned to assess the capitis site. Because these muscles are in the hairline, the practitioner must pay particular attention to site preparation. The hair must be parted, a very vigorous alcohol abrade must be done, and an ample amount of electrode paste must be applied. If the hair is too thick or coarse, it may not be possible to scan this site. The scanning electrodes are placed parallel to the spine, just lateral to the spinal process over the muscle belly.

Interpretation

High SEMG values at this site should be interpreted with extreme caution, because elevations may be due to poor impedance values. If high SEMG values are recorded, the practitioner should examine the site after the electrodes are removed to see how well the electrode paste penetrated the hair. The practitioner should then scan the site a second time to see if the same values are obtained. Exceptionally low values indicate electrode paste bridging.

The capitis site is an extensor of the head when both sides are activated and is a synergist in lateral flexion and rotation when activated unilaterally. Therefore, head position should be noted whenever this site is monitored.

Anterior Deltoid*

Placement

For this assessment, the scanning electrodes are placed so that they run parallel to the muscle fibers in the anterior deltoid group. The scanning electrodes are placed on the anterior medial surface of the upper arm, just below the shoulder joint. The upper scanning electrode is placed approximately 3 cm below the clavicle bone, with the lower electrode going laterally at approximately a 25-degree angle from vertical, so as to follow the muscle fibers.

Interpretation

This muscle group plays a role in the flexion, horizontal adduction, and medial rotation of the humerus or upper arm.

Posterior Deltoid*

Placement

With the posterior deltoid, the scanning electrodes are placed so that they run parallel to the muscle fibers. When the patient's arms hang to the side, the scanning electrodes are placed on the posterior lateral surface of the upper arm, just lateral to the shoulder joint. The upper scanning electrode is placed 3 to 5 cm below the spine of the scapula, with the lower electrode going laterally at approximately a 25–degree angle from vertical to follow the orientation of the muscle fibers.

Interpretation

The posterior deltoid group provides extension, horizontal abduction, and lateral rotation of the humerus or upper arm. Low SEMG recordings are often noted with multidirectional shoulder instability and chronic anterior subluxation or dislocation of the shoulder.

Pectoralis Major*

Placement

To assess the pectoralis major, the scanning electrodes are placed so that they run parallel to the middle fibers of this rather large and flat muscle group. The electrodes are placed below the clavicle and above the breast and nipple, with the scanning electrodes running almost parallel to the ground.

Interpretation

The primary function of this muscle group is the adduction and medial rotation of the humerus or upper arm. Activation patterns have also been noted in post-myocardial infarction patients who continue to have a fear of a future myocardial infarction.

Biceps*

Placement

With the patient's arms hanging to the sides, the scanning electrodes are placed on the anterior surface of the humerus in a vertical plane, so that the scanning electrodes run parallel to the biceps muscle fibers. They are placed over the muscle belly, approximately two-thirds of the distance between the shoulder and the elbow.

Interpretation

The primary function of this muscle is the flexion of the elbow and supination of the forearm.

Triceps*

Placement

To assess the triceps, the scanning electrodes are placed on the posterior lateral surface of the upper arm, with the

patient's arms hanging to the sides in a standing posture. The scanning electrodes are placed over the belly of the muscle, approximately half the distance between the shoulder and the elbow. The electrodes are oriented in a vertical plane so as to follow the fibers of the muscle.

Interpretation

The primary function of this muscle is to extend the elbow.

Wrist Extensors*

Placement

To assess the wrist extensors, the scanning electrodes are placed on the middle of the dorsal forearm about 6 cm down from the elbow. Asking the patient to engage in a wrist extension will help clarify the muscle belly. The scanning electrodes are placed over the muscle belly in a vertical plane so that they follow the muscle fibers. This site may be scanned with the patient in either a standing or sitting posture. In the standing posture, the patient's arms should hang naturally at the sides. During sitting, the patient should rest the arms on the lap or some other surface.

Interpretation

This muscle group causes an extension of the wrist and fingers. It may be indicated in lateral epicondylitis or arm pain in general (such as from carpal tunnel syndrome). Elevations at this site in patients with pain conditions away from the arm may indicate an overall emotional arousal problem that involves the neuromuscular system. Elevations are also noted with lack of adequate scapular stabilization.

Wrist Flexors*

Placement

To assess the wrist flexors, the electrodes are placed on the anterior surface of the forearm, approximately 6 cm from the elbow. The muscle belly is easily identified by having the patient flex the wrist. The electrodes are placed over the muscle belly in a vertical direction (while the patient is standing), such that the scanning electrodes follow the muscle fibers.

Interpretation

The primary function of this muscle group is to flex the wrist and fingers. EMG elevations may be noted in medial epicondylitis or carpal tunnel syndrome. Elevations are also noted with lack of adequate scapular stabilization.

Gluteus Maximus*

Placement

To assess the gluteus maximus, the scanning electrodes are placed in the center of the posterior surface of the buttock. The scanning electrodes are oriented laterally at approximately a 25-degree angle off vertical, so that the electrodes follow the direction of the muscle fibers.

Interpretation

This very powerful muscle is used primarily in rising from sitting, going up stairs, and running. Its primary function is the forceful extension of the hip and lateral rotation of the extended hip.

Vastus Medialis and Vastus Lateralis*

Placement

For the vastus medialis, the scanning electrodes are placed on the medial aspect of the thigh, at approximately a 55-degree angle, immediately above the patella. For the vastus lateralis, the scanning electrodes are placed on the lateral surface of the lower third of the thigh, approximately 6 cm above the kneecap. The scanning electrodes are oriented laterally at approximately a 20-degree angle from vertical, so as to run parallel to the muscle fibers.

Interpretation

These large, strong muscles stabilize the knee. In patients presenting for evaluation of total knee replacement, significant reductions in SEMG recruitment are noted in these muscles and the other quadriceps muscle groups. Asymmetries between the lateral and medial aspects have been noted in patients with patella femoral pain.

Rectus Femoris*

Placement

For the rectus femoris, the scanning electrodes are placed on the medial anterior surface of the thigh, approximately half the distance between the hip and the knee. The scanning electrodes are placed in a vertical plane from the ground so that the electrodes follow the muscle fibers.

Interpretation

The primary function of this very strong muscle is the extension of the knee and an assistive role in the flexion of the hip. This muscle helps to bring the leg forward during walking.

Hamstring*

Placement

To assess the hamstring, the scanning electrodes are placed on the medial posterior aspect of the thigh, about half the distance between the hip and the knee. The electrodes are placed in a vertical plane relative to the ground so that they run parallel to the muscle fibers.

Interpretation

These muscles primarily extend the hip and flex or rotate the knees.

Gastrocnemius*

Placement

For the gastrocnemius, the scanning electrodes are placed medially, on the upper half of the posterior aspect of the calf. There are two rather large muscle bellies. Palpate the muscle to identify the muscle belly. Place the scanning electrodes in a vertical plane relative to the ground so that they run parallel to the muscle fibers.

Interpretation

These muscles assist in the flexion of the knee and play a major role in plantar flexion (pointing of the toe).

Soleus

Placement

To assess the soleus, the scanning electrodes are placed on the lateral, posterior side of the lower leg. Because this muscle lies underneath the gastrocnemius, the practitioner must attempt to monitor it from the lateral or outside portion of the lower third of the calf, where the width of the gastrocnemius begins to narrow. The electrodes are oriented in a near vertical plane relative to the ground, with the electrodes running parallel to the muscle fibers.

Interpretation

This muscle is a very strong plantar flexor. It is actually the only muscle a person needs to stand in an erect posture (all other muscles should remain quiet while the person hangs on the ligaments). The practitioner should expect to see SEMG activity when the patient is standing.

Tibialis Anterior

Placement

To assess the tibialis anterior, the electrodes are placed about a third of the distance from the knee to the ankle, lateral to the tibia on the anterior surface of the lower leg. The electrodes are oriented in a vertical plane relative to the ground, so that they follow the muscle fibers.

Interpretation

The primary action of this muscle is the dorsiflexion of the ankle and inversion of the foot. This muscle lifts the foot during swing through as part of normal gait. Paralysis may cause "foot drop." Patients with poor foot control (i.e., excessive pronation) use this muscle excessively in an attempt to control the foot or ankle, which may contribute to the development of shin splints.

Digastric/Suprahyoid

Placement

To assess the digastric/suprahyoid, the scanning electrodes are placed under the chin, so that they run in an anterior/posterior direction, approximately $1/2$ inch to the left or right of the middle of the chin, following the muscle fibers of the digastric muscle. The patient must not raise the head to help the practitioner with this placement. The practitioner should ask the patient to sit comfortably and should provide no specific instructions regarding the position of the mandible. Men with beards cannot be scanned at this site.

Interpretation

This muscle is part of a group of muscles called the suprahyoids. Their primary function is to elevate the hyoid bone during swallowing when the mandible is stable, or to open the jaw when the hyoid is stable. It is an important muscle to assess in patients with temporomandibular joint problems.

Posterior Temporalis

Placement

To assess the posterior temporalis, the scanning electrodes are placed slightly above the ear, toward its pos-

terior flap. The electrodes are oriented downward at approximately a 45-degree angle relative to the ground. Electrodes should be clearly above the mastoid process and below the hairline.

Interpretation

This muscle, like the anterior temporalis, plays a role in elevating and stabilizing the mandible. Because of its more posterior location, the vector of force also includes the retraction of the jaw. The posterior temporalis muscles are important to consider in patients with temporomandibular joint dysfunction.

Paraspinal Muscles (C-2, C-6, T-2, T-4, T-8, L-1, L-5)

Placement

The scanning electrodes for these paraspinal muscles are placed so that they run parallel to the spine, approximately 2 to 3 cm out from the vertebral ridge over the belly of the paraspinal muscle. These muscles may be visually seen in some individuals but may need to be palpated in others. The vertical placement for each site is as follows:

- C-6 placement: For the cervical region, it is probably best to start at the bottom and move upward. The electrode placements go from easy to more difficult. The C-6 electrodes are placed so that the lowest scanning electrode is directly across from the C7/T-1 prominence.
- C-2 placement: This is a very important, yet very difficult site to scan. The potential problems lie with the hairline. The most accurate method for vertical placement is to count up five vertebrae from the C-7 prominence and place the middle of the scanning electrode opposite this spinous process. Alternatively, place the lower electrode for the C-2 scan at the spot where the upper scanning electrode was for the C-4 scan. The residue left behind should help guide this placement, but the practitioner should avoid problems with bridging of the electrode paste.
  - Placing electrodes at the hairline can be problematic. Make certain that the abrade for the site is rough and adequate, particularly around the hairline. If the patient's hairline is too low, so that the upper scanning electrode clearly reaches into a thick patch of hair, it will push scanning technology to its limits. If the scanning electrode that reaches into the

hairline does not make a good, clean contact with the skin (scalp), the poor contact will artificially drive up the SEMG readings as a result of interference with the differential amplifier. When this situation occurs, the practitioner must decide if a high reading is real SEMG or just instrument noise.

○ As an alternative means of monitoring the area, the practitioner can place the electrodes at an oblique angle, just below the mastoid process, rather than up into the hairline. This arrangement might better reflect the activity of the group of muscles that cross the atlas/axis joint. Practitioners who use this concept should give it a different label to differentiate it from the C-2 configuration.

- T-4 placement: To locate this site, simply count down four vertebrae from the C-7/T-1 prominence and place the space between the active electrodes directly across from the vertebral prominence.

- T-8 placement: It is typically very easy to count down from the C-7/T-1 prominence, placing the space between the active electrodes directly across from the vertebral prominence. The location of this site is approximately where a woman's bra strap would run.

- L-1 placement: To locate this site, count down 13 vertebrae from the C-7/T-1 prominence. Another method is to use the iliac crest to determine the L-3 vertebra (see the L-3 placement in the original scan site descriptions), and count up two vertebrae from that point.

- L-5 placement: To locate this site, count down 17 vertebrae from the C-7/T-1 prominence or two vertebrae down from the L-3 vertebra determined using the iliac crest method described previously. This site is typically below the belt line.

Interpretation

When monitoring from the paraspinal muscles, there are many layers of muscles to consider: The longissimus, spinalis, semispinalis, and multifidus may all contribute to the signal. All of these muscles play a substantial role in stabilization of the spine. In addition, when both the right and left aspects are activated, extension of the spine occurs. Unilateral contractions of one side lead to either rotation or lateral bending of the spine.

Some chiropractors believe that an asymmetry in SEMG at one level indicates a rotated or subluxated vertebra at that level. This may or may not be true. An unpublished pilot study on 25 chiropractic patient records for SEMG (neutral posture) and radiographic findings (using the Gonsted method) indicated that the relationship between asymmetry in SEMG and vertebra rotation/subluxation varied from level to level. The strongest relationships were found at sites of the greatest spinal instability: the axis and L-5 levels. At the axis, 21 of 25 patients showed abnormal radiographic findings. Of the 23 patients who were scanned at this site, 9 (39%) showed significant SEMG asymmetries. Of those with SEMG asymmetries, 6 (67%) had concomitant radiographic evidence. At L-5, 18 of the 25 patients showed radiographic evidence. Of the 22 patients who were scanned at this site, only 6 (27%) had clinically significant asymmetries. Of those with asymmetries, 5 (83%) had concomitant X-ray findings. At the T-1 paraspinals, only 4 abnormal X-ray findings were identified for the 25 patients. Of the 14 patients scanned at that site, only 4 (29%) had clinically significant SEMG asymmetries. Of those 4, only 1 (25%) had a concomitant X-ray finding. At a similar site, T-7, 4 patients had abnormal X rays; of the 14 patients receiving an SEMG scan at this site, only 2 (14%) were asymmetrical. Both of these patients (100%) had abnormal radiographic findings.

From this brief study, it may be concluded that it is too simplistic to say that an SEMG asymmetry at a given level indicates a rotated or subluxated vertebral body. X-ray evidence of rotation is not always associated with asymmetrical SEMG activity. In addition, when clinically significant asymmetries of SEMG activity are noted, they are not always associated with radiographic evidence of rotation. In conjunction with rotation, practitioners should consider other diagnostic concepts such as scoliosis, pain displays of splinting/guarding, functional problems, hypermobile and hypomobile segments, and emotional displays.

REFERENCES

1. Stedman TL. *Stedman's Medical Dictionary.* 25th ed. Baltimore, MD: Williams & Wilkins; 1990.
2. Cram JR, Engstrom D. Patterns of neuromuscular activity in pain and non-pain patients. *Clin Biofeedback Health.* 1986;9:106–116.
3. Iacona C. Muscle scanning: caveat emptor. *Biofeedback Self Regul.* 1991;16:227–241.
4. Haynes S. Muscle-contraction headache: psychophysiological perspective in etiology and treatment. In: Haynes S, Gannorn W, eds. *Psychosomatic Disorders: A*

Psychophysiological Approach to Etiology and Treatment. Westport, CT: Greenwood Press; 1981.

5. Dolce JJ, Raczynski JM. Neuromuscular activity and electromyography in painful backs: psychological and biomechanical models in assessment and treatment. *Psychol Bull.* 1985;97:502–520.

6. Travell J, Simons D. *Myofascial Pain and Dysfunction: A Trigger Point Manual, I and II.* Baltimore, MD: Williams & Wilkins; 1983.

7. Donaldson S, Skubick D, Clasby B, Cram J. The evaluation of trigger-point activity using dynamic EMG techniques. *Am J Pain Manage.* 1994;4:118–122.

8. Cram JR, Steger JC. Muscle scanning and the diagnosis of chronic pain. *Biofeedback Self Regul.* 1983;8:229–241.

9. Kessler M, Cram JR, Traue H. EMG muscle scanning in pain patients and controls: a replication and extension. *Am J Pain Manage.* 1993;3:20–28.

10. Cram JR. *Clinical EMG for Surface Recordings, I.* Poulsbo, WA: J&J Engineering; 1986.

11. Cram JR, Lloyd J, Cahn T. The reliability of EMG muscle scanning. *Int J Psychosom.* 1990;37:68–72.

12. Kaplan RH, Saccyzzo DP. *Psychological Testing: Principles, Applications and Issues.* Monterey, CA: Brooks/Cole; 1989.

13. Ahern DK, Follick MJ, Cocurcil JR, Laser-Wolston N. Reliability of lumbar paravertebral EMG assessment in chronic low back pain. *Arch Phys Med Rehab.* 1986;76:762–765.

14. Thompson JM, Rolland EP, Offord KP. EMG muscle scanning: stability of hand held surface electrodes. *Biofeedback Self Regul.* 1989;14:55–61.

15. Cram JR, Kall R. *The CAM Scan Software.* Nevada City, CA: Clinical Resources; 1990.

16. Callet R. *Soft Tissue Injury and Disability.* Philadelphia, PA: FA Davis; 1977.

17. Donaldson S, Donaldson M. Multi-channel EMG assessment and treatment techniques. In: Cram JR, ed. *Clinical EMG for Surface Recordings, II.* Nevada City, CA: Clinical Resources; 1990:143–174.

18. Cram JR. Diagnostic frameworks for surface EMG. *Biofeedback Self Regul.* 1988;13:123–137.

19. Lewit K. *Manipulative Therapy in Rehabilitation of the Locomotor System.* Boston, MA: Butterworth Heinemann; 1991.

20. Donaldson S, Skubick D, Donaldson M. *Electromyography, Trigger Points and Myofascial Syndromes.* Calgary, Alberta: Behavioral Health Consultants; 1991.

21. Hollingshead WH. *Functional Anatomy of the Limbs and Back.* Philadelphia, PA: WB Saunders; 1976.

22. Basmajian N. *Muscles Alive.* 3rd ed. Baltimore, MD: Williams & Wilkins; 1974.

CHAPTER QUESTIONS

1. The muscle scanning procedure requires:
   a. a scanning head
   b. abrading the site
   c. electrode paste
   d. holding the electrodes motionless
   e. all of the above

2. Typically, one must stay on the site for how long before it becomes stable?
   a. 2 seconds
   b. 10 to 20 seconds
   c. 2 minutes
   d. 5 minutes

3. Which of the following is *not* one of the pitfalls of muscle scanning?
   a. bridging of electrode paste (values too low)
   b. excessive resistance (values too high)
   c. excessive variability (too long at the site)
   d. excessive movement during range of motion

4. Which of the following is *not* one of the general clinical concepts associated with muscle scanning?
   a. site of activation/inhibition
   b. level of symmetry
   c. impact of posture
   d. degree of reciprocal inhibition

5. During muscle scanning, which approach should be used in positioning the patient's posture?
   a. Place the patient in the ideal posture.
   b. Allow the patient to assume his or her natural posture.
   c. Ask the patient to sit or stand up straight.
   d. Always study the end range of motion of a posture.

6. The muscle scanning assessment of the static component of the neuromuscular system provides information about which of the following?
   a. hyperactive muscles
   b. antalgic postures
   c. trigger points
   d. both a and b

7. During a muscle scan, an antalgic posture (protective guarding) is noted when:
   a. the activation is greater during standing than during sitting
   b. the activation is on the ipsilateral side of the pain
   c. the activation is on the contralateral side of the pain
   d. both a and c

8. During a muscle scan, muscle splinting is noted when:
   a. the activation is greater during sitting than during standing
   b. the activation is on the ipsilateral side of the pain
   c. the activation is on the contralateral side of the pain
   d. the activation is greater during standing than during sitting
   e. both a and b

Emotional Assessment and Clinical Protocol

MUSCLES AND EMOTIONAL DISPLAY

Along with posture and movement, another key attribute of muscles is emotional display. In fact, one can conceptualize emotional display as muscle activation patterns that are but one step removed from intentional movement (e-motion). When muscle activation associated with emotions occurs, more energy is sent into the neuromuscular system, taking up the "slack" in the system and increasing the tonic or resting level. This emotional bracing or increased tonus may also affect the quality of movement.[1,2]

Professional athletes certainly know how emotional arousal can unintentionally alter levels of exertion and change the timing associated with coordinated movement. In addition, it is not uncommon for a patient to react to stressful events in a stereotypical fashion. "Individual response stereotypy"[3] is the tendency for an individual to respond to a variety of stressors with a similar physiologic response. This tendency was first noted in the early 1960s, when some individuals were always observed to respond to a stressful event by, say, speeding up their heart rates or tensing their shoulder muscles. Within the neuromuscular system, emotional arousal and associated stereotypy have been studied for the facial muscles,[4] the postural muscles,[5] and the muscle spindle.[6]

The procedure used to study the emotional reactivity of the body is called *stress profiling*. Throughout the history of psychophysiology, researchers have looked for the psychophysiological correlates to emotions.[7-9] Researchers hoped that this technique would help them to determine the individual's emotional state without having to rely upon the patient's self-report. As investigations have moved into applied clinical research, the questions have been directed more at how to identify individuals who are at risk for a particular disorder. Haynes, for example, has considered this question, looking at both the reactivity and recovery of the individual's physiology to a stressor.[10] This chapter reviews the procedures used in stress profiling. For a more complete description of stress profiling in assessment of psychological and medical disorders, refer to *Biofeedback: A Practitioner's Guide*, edited by Mark Schwartz.[11]

THE FACIAL MUSCLES

One form of emotional display is found on the human face, creating the movements of the skin that are recognizable around the world.[4] Muscle scanning of the cephalic muscles may reveal some of the rudimentary aspects of these facial displays. In addition, the wide frontalis placement presented in the atlas in Part III provides an excellent barometer of negative emotional displays. Such emotional displays are most prominently seen on the upper face or forehead. For this reason, the wide frontalis placement is commonly used in stress profiling. **Figure 7–1** shows surface electromyography (SEMG) activation in the frontalis muscles in patients with headache during a simple stressor such as "serial sevens" (i.e., counting backward from 1000 by sevens).

Normative data have been collected on healthy subjects of different ages. In the reference base reported in **Table 7–1**, the resting and stress values are presented for the facial and shoulder muscles and for two autonomic nervous system (ANS) indicators. It is very common to monitor sympathetic activation along with the central nervous system (CNS) patterns of the neuromuscular system. The SEMG recordings for this normative sample were conducted using an Autogen 1700 with a

100- to 200-Hz band pass filter and wide placements on the frontalis and upper trapezius sites. When Beaton, Egan, and Mitchell studied 46 healthy adults from 18 to 75 years of age,[12,13] they found no significant differences as a function of age, although they studied the data across three age spans.

THE TRUNK MUSCLES

The impact of emotions on the neuromuscular system may also be seen in the postural muscles. Simple visual observation of depressed patients often reveals their stooped shoulders, while anxious patients may have their shoulders markedly elevated. Whatmore[2,14] has verified this phenomenon using SEMG recordings. The SEMG activation of the trunk muscles may take on a general form, affecting all muscles and generally taking up the slack in the system as a whole—a phenomenon that Whatmore referred to as *bracing*. In addition, the trunk muscles may show a high level of specificity.

Figure 7–2 shows the SEMG recordings of the right and left trapezius muscle groups using the cervical trapezius placement from the electrode atlas for a patient who injured the right upper quarter during a fall down some stairs. This patient presented with headache and right upper quarter pain. Only the right cervical trapezius lead initially responded to the stressor, followed by a very poor recovery pattern (return to baseline).

The effects of stress can result in emotional displays from the neuromuscular system that involve the muscles of the face and shoulders. Some suggest that these muscles have phylogenetically evolved from the gills of the fish and are "hard wired" for emotional displays.[15] The emotional nature of the gills of the fish, for example, is well represented in the threat displays of Siamese fighting fish. When threatened, these fish instinctively enlarge their gills to appear much larger than they really

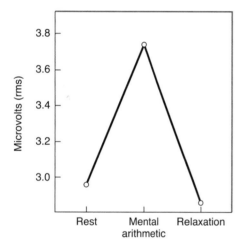

Figure 7–1 Surface EMG response of frontalis muscles during stress profiling.

Source: J. R. Cram, EMG Biofeedback and the Treatment of Tension Headaches: A Systematic Analysis of Treatment Components, *Behavior Therapy*, Vol. 11, pp. 699–710, Copyright © 1980 by the Association for Advancement of Behavior Therapy. Reprinted by permission of the publisher.

Table 7–1 Surface Electromyography and Autonomic Nervous System Values During Stress Profiling Procedure

Physiological Measure	Rest		Stressor (Serial Sevens)	
	Mean	Standard Deviation	Mean	Standard Deviation
Wide frontalis SEMG (µv)	2.58	0.63	3.2	0.86
Wide trapezius SEMG (µv)	3.30	0.69	3.75	0.51
Hand temperature (°F)	83.95	0.28	83.4	0.32
Skin conductance (mOhm)	9.05	0.41	12.0	0.78

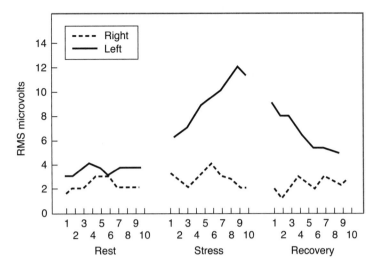

Figure 7–2 Stress profiling response in right and left trapezius of a patient with injury to the right trapezius.
Source: Reprinted with permission from J. R. Cram, Surface EMG Recordings and Pain Related Disorders: A Diagnostic Framework, *Biofeedback and Self Regulation*, Vol. 13, p. 127, © 1988, Plenum Publishing.

are, so as to frighten off the intruder. When this theory is extended to the human species, it suggests that the head and neck muscles have a genetic predisposition for reacting to stressful events with activation patterns. Anatomists[16,17] have studied the facial muscles extensively, finding that these muscles have direct anatomical connections to the lower centers of the brain (i.e., the facial nerves of the pontine nucleus). Given this strong connection to the reptilian brain, they have concluded that the facial muscles could be considered an autonomic organ.

Flor, Turk, and Birbaumer also demonstrated the specific effects of emotions on the muscles of the low back.[18] They studied the right and left aspects of the erector spinae muscles in a group of patients with low-back pain, a group of patients with general pain (i.e., pain other than in the low back), and a group of healthy control subjects. Each group was presented with various types of stressors. The findings clearly showed that only the patients with low-back pain demonstrated an emotional response (activation pattern) in the left erector spinae muscles, and only during stressors relevant to the patient's condition. In other words, while the serial sevens subtraction task evoked an activation response, the task of describing their pain and its effects on these patients' lifestyles evoked the largest response. This study strongly suggests the need to study the relationship of personally relevant stressors to painful states.

RELATIONSHIP OF EMOTIONAL AROUSAL TO MUSCLE ACTIVATION

The effects of stress may be observed throughout the neuromuscular system.[5] On rare occasions, emotional activation may affect the entire neuromuscular system. More typically, it is reflected in patterns of activation of specific muscles. These muscles are usually involved in the patient's symptom complex. For example, if the patient reports a painful neck, the muscles of the neck or upper back have a higher probability of being activated during a stress profiling procedure than those of the lower legs.

How does stress find its way into the muscles? The more traditional formulations suggest that emotional stress facilitates a shift in the balance of the hypothalamic system toward an ergotropic (and sympathetic) dominance. This, in turn, activates the limbic/autonomic circuits mentioned earlier and increases the efferent outflow to the muscles.[19] In their recent study, McNutty, Gevertz, Berkoff, and Hubbard suggested a more specific mechanism by which stress finds its way into the neuromuscular system: autonomic innervation of the muscle spindle.[6] In this study, the researchers demonstrated that stressful events increased activation of fine wires placed in tissue thought to be muscle spindles. The intrafusal muscle fibers are known to be innervated by[19] and stimulated to contract[17] via the sympathetic nervous system. Hubbard and Berkoff[20] have demonstrated that activity from the tissue into which McNutty and colleagues inserted their fine wires was not blocked by agents that block acetylcholine, yet was blocked by sympathetic blocking agents. Thus, ANS activation through the muscle spindle may play a role in pain-related disorders. Such a mechanism may affect the general resting tone of the extrafusal muscle fibers from the muscle group of origin, as well as increase the muscles' responsivity to stressful events. Alternatively, as Hubbard and Berkoff have argued, excessive activation of the muscle spindle itself may provide a pathway for nociception, thereby playing a role in the perpetuation of painful states.

RELIABILITY OF STRESS PROFILING

How consistent are these individual response stereotypes to stressful events? Three studies have attempted to answer this question. In their study, Walters, Williamson, Bernard, Blouin, and Faulstich[21] demonstrated that approximately half of the patients continued for 2 weeks with the same stereotypic response patterns (they continued to respond to a variety of stressors in the same way, such as increased frontal activity). The other half of the subjects fell more into some form of "stimulus stereotypy." This result indicates that the patients tended to respond physiologically to slightly different stressors in slightly different ways. For example, during the first assessment, they might have responded with increased frontal activity to mental stressors, while at 2 weeks they might have responded to a loud noise with increased trapezius activity.

In a second study, Arena and Hobbs[22] found approximately the same percentage of response stereotypy (42%), with 20% of the remaining subjects showing stimulus specificity. The intraclass correlation coefficient for the wide frontal placement was 0.87, with observations taken on four occasions distributed across 4 weeks. This suggests a strong level of persistence in the type of response pattern.

The third study, by Voas,[23] sampled from a broad set of muscle groups (including lower leg muscles, forearm muscles, trapezius, masseter, and frontalis) under three conditions (rest/relaxation, mental arithmetic, and stress/frustration) over the course of 9 days. His findings demonstrate that one cannot generalize the findings from one site to another, or from one condition to another. For example, Voas found the lower leg muscles to have the lowest level of reliability across all conditions (0.15 to 0.48). The forearm muscles showed the greatest

reliability during the active tasks (0.59 to 0.93), with lower levels of reliability during quiet activities (0.17 to 0.46). Trapezius and masseter muscles showed the greatest consistency during mental arithmetic (0.69 to 0.87), with much lower correlations during the other tasks (0.23 to 0.39). Only the wide frontal placement showed consistently high test–retest correlations across all tasks (0.80 to 0.91). This study suggests that the concepts of stimulus specificity are found in the trapezius and arm muscle groups, with response stereotypy occurring in the wide frontal placement.

THE STRESS PROFILING PROTOCOL

In conducting a stress profile, the first thing the practitioner must consider is which muscle sites to monitor. One general rule of thumb is to monitor SEMG activity at the site of the pain complaint. Two-thirds of the time, the resting muscle tone at the site of pain may look normal,[10] but the possibility of referred pain patterns[24] may still exist. The neuromuscular component at the painful site may not be ruled out until one has observed the effects of perturbation on the muscle(s) being monitored. Thus, the practitioner should not draw any conclusions regarding a myogenic component of pain based on resting tone alone. Instead, he or she would be wise to see how the painful site reacts to a mental stressor before reaching conclusions. If the site reacts easily to the stressor or has a poor rebound or recovery, this factor may potentially explain the myogenic origin of the patient's pain. In addition, the practitioner may want to select and study muscle sites away from the reported site of pain. The selection of these sites could be based on the findings of the muscle scan study or on knowledge about which muscle sites could harbor potential trigger points that could refer to the area of described pain.

Next, the practitioner should select a "stressor" to be used to create the perturbation of the emotional system. One standard stressor is the mental arithmetic task termed "serial sevens," in which the patient is asked to count backward from 1000 by sevens. In other words, the patient is to take the number 1000 and subtract 7, take that number (993) and subtract 7 from it, take that number (986) and subtract 7 from it, and so forth. The patient is instructed to do this calculation aloud, and as quickly and accurately as possible. The astute practitioner encourages the patient to stay on task and go quickly, while tracking the patient's responses and pointing out any errors. For some patients, this task is an excellent stressor. In such cases, the practitioner can observe the results from the perspective of the physiological response in the SEMG or ANS channels. For other patients, this task is too difficult and they simply give up. The practitioner must monitor the mental arithmetic process of the patient to capture the timing of this event. For still other patients, the task may be too easy and they will not react to it. If the task is too easy, one might consider administering another test such as the Pace Serial Arithmetic Test (PSAT), a serial arithmetic task that all subjects will eventually find stressful and fail to complete successfully.

If the task is too hard, the practitioner may want to explore other potential stressors. An alternative standardized stressor might include the introduction of a sudden sound that startles the patient. Here the practitioner might stand outside the patient's view and suddenly slam a book down on a hard surface. The unexpected noise acts as the stressor. Other options include playing the patient an audiotape that presents a series of environmentally stressful sounds (e.g., phones ringing, cars honking, dogs barking, babies crying).[25] Or, as Flor and colleagues[18] did, the practitioner might make the stressor relevant to the patient by asking the patient to describe the pain or the impact of the pain on his or her life.

Once the practitioner has selected the muscle sites to monitor and the appropriate stressor for the patient, the practitioner should follow some sort of standardized single-subject protocol. Typically, such a procedure uses an A-B-A type of design. Here, the practitioner runs a baseline SEMG reading (condition A), introduces a stressor (condition B), and completes the assessment with a recovery phase, commonly termed the postbaseline recording (return to condition A). In practice, most practitioners usually conclude the stress profile with a combination of return to baseline while the patient is encouraged to engage in some form of relaxation. Thus, the patient's relaxation skills are tested "under fire." The design of such a protocol is presented in **Exhibit 7–1**.

PATTERNS OF ACTIVATION AND RECOVERY

The psychophysiological assessment protocol is examined for three elements: (1) initial resting baseline levels, (2) level of response to the stressor, and (3) ability of the emotional component of the muscular system to recover to resting baseline (prebaseline) levels.

Baseline Levels

An assessment for some of the resting baseline values may be roughly determined by comparing the resting values for the site of placement to the electrode atlas benchmark values or those presented in the group norms listed earlier in this chapter. If elevations in the resting levels are noted, they could influence the ability of the system to react to the stressor. This effect is attributable to the "law of initial value,"[26] which states that physiological systems operate within certain limits or boundaries. If the person is near the ceiling of a given system, that system has less room for "reactivity" than when the prestimulus levels are toward the bottom end of the range.

Level of Response to the Stressor

Next, the practitioner examines the patient's level of response to the stressor. If multiple sites are monitored, the practitioner examines the SEMG signals to learn which sites react first and which sites react with the strongest SEMG activation. There is approximately a 50/50 chance of seeing a significant physiological reaction to a stressor. In a meta-analysis of a variety of stressors on diverse populations of subjects, Haynes[10] found that 45% of the studies showed nonsignificant reactivity to a stressor. To increase the probability of finding significant clinical results, the practitioner should study more than one portion of the neuromuscular system, study sites of painful complaint as well as sites away from the pain (i.e., trigger points for referred pain), or use personally relevant stressors.

Exhibit 7–1 Typical Design of a Stress Profile

Baseline (A)	Stressor (B)	Recovery/Relaxation (A)
2–4 minutes (or until stable)	3–5 minutes (or until there is some sort of physiological response)	5–10 minutes minimum (or until there is recovery)

To determine reactivity to a stressor, the practitioner would want to see if the activation pattern during stress exceeds the natural variations in the resting tone for a given site. Many computerized physiological monitoring systems generate information on a patient regarding the mean level of SEMG activity for the site as well as the variability of the signal. Taking the mean level of the prebaseline activity and adding the standard deviation to it will indicate whether the stressor had a mild effect on the muscle site that exceeds the ambient variations of its resting tone. The practitioner should note that it is normal for the neuromuscular system to react to emotional stress with increased activation. In fact, the success of the stress profiling protocol depends on this outcome; it is the validity check that indicates whether the neuromuscular system is actually stressed. What is abnormal, however, is for one aspect of the system to react more strongly than another aspect. A headache patient with dull bifrontal headache, for example, may be within "normal" SEMG limits for the cephalic and neck muscles at rest, but react more strongly with the frontal musculature during a stressful event.

The certainty of this type of conclusion is enhanced by examining the means and standard deviations for each muscle group during the stressful event. Taking the mean and both adding and subtracting the standard deviation to this mean will provide an average range of operation for the SEMG channel that is used. If the means for either of the muscles fall *within* the range of the other muscle, then the conclusion about one muscle reacting more than the other would be weakened. If the mean of one muscle falls *outside* the range of the other muscle, then the conclusion is strengthened and clinically significant. If the standard deviation is doubled before it is added or subtracted to the mean and the mean is still outside the range of the other muscle, then this finding suggests a "moderate" reactivity; in this case, the conclusion is not only clinically significant but also statistically significant. In either event, when one muscle group reacts to a greater extent than another muscle group, this finding must be considered in the etiology of pain. This conclusion is strengthened even further when hyperreactivity is coupled with poor recovery to prebaseline levels.

Recovery to Prebaseline Levels

Finally, the pattern of stress profiling is examined for the level of recovery. Here, one would expect the recovery pattern to return to the prebaseline levels. When the recovery phase remains one standard deviation above the initial baseline level, it is considered mildly elevated; when it remains two standard deviations above baseline level, it is considered moderately elevated. Lack of recovery is important because it can change the biochemistry of the muscle. For example, 10% to 50% of maximum voluntary isometric contraction (MVIC) is known to reduce the blood flow to a muscle significantly.[27,28] Prolonged reduction of blood flow leads to the buildup of lactic acid, which stimulates the chemoreceptors in the muscle that signal pain. Ischemia also leads to an increase in the release of bradykinins, prostaglandins, and serotonin,[29] which brings about an increased sensitization of pain reception at a local level. If the reactive muscle group is activated frequently, with activation followed by only a partial recovery, each reactivity cycle could lead to a gradual buildup of lactic acid over the course of the day; this could result in a dull, bilateral headache that is felt toward the latter part of the day.

Table 7–2 provides an example of these comparisons. In this table, the mean SEMG level of both muscles is within the range of the other muscle during the prebaseline phase. During the stressor, muscle A shows a mild reaction. When the mean SEMG level of muscle A during stress is compared to the range of its own prebaseline phase, the stress mean is greater than the first standard deviation for the prebaseline period. For muscle B, the stress mean is greater than the second standard deviation of the prebaseline period, suggesting a moderate level of reactivity. In addition, the mean for the reactivity of muscle B is outside the range of the second standard deviation for the reactivity of muscle A, strongly supporting the notion that muscle B reacted more strongly to the stressor than did muscle A. Finally, muscle A recovered quickly from the stressor, and the recovery mean for muscle A is within the range of the prebaseline values for muscle A. Muscle B, by comparison, did not recover well; the mean for the recovery phase for muscle B is greater than the range of the second standard deviation for the prebaseline phase. In addition, the recovery mean for muscle B is outside the second standard deviation range for the recovery phase of muscle A. This finding provides substantial evidence that the recovery patterns of muscles A and B are different.

The lack of recovery to prebaseline levels reflects a dysregulation of the homeostasis of the body. In a normal muscle system, a return to baseline is expected. Because muscle reactivity potentially leads to a change in

Table 7–2 Surface Electromyography Data Obtained from Two Muscle Sites During a Stress Profiling Procedure in Which There Is a Differential Reaction to Stress and Recovery

Condition	Muscle A				Muscle B			
	Mean	SD	Number of SDs	Range	Mean	SD	Number of SDs	Range
Prebaseline	2.3	1.7	1	0.6–3.0	2.5	1.5	1	1.0–4.0
			2	0.0–5.7			2	0.0–5.5
Stressor*	4.1	2.5	1	1.6–6.6	12.3	5.2	1	7.1–17.5
			2	0.0–9.1			2	2.1–13.4
Recovery*	2.5	1.8	1	0.7–4.3	7.3	2.3	1	5.0–9.6
			2	0.0–6.1			2	2.7–11.9

SD = standard deviation.
*Indicates difference between muscle A and muscle B or between the various conditions within a given muscle.

the pH balance of the tissue (and accumulation of lactic acid), delayed recovery to prestress levels increases the probability of this metabolic imbalance.

How long should it normally take to recover from a stressor? Arena and Hobbs[22] suggest that 6 minutes is adequate for the facial muscle reactivity but inadequate for hand temperature. The 10-minute time frame suggested in Exhibit 7–1 is usually more than adequate for both the central nervous system and autonomic nervous system components. To define the recovery process better, one might measure the length of time it takes for the muscle activity to return to within 5% of its prebaseline levels following the cessation of the stressful event.

REFERENCES

1. Jacobson E. Electrophysiology of mental activities. *Am J Psychol.* 1932;44:77–94.
2. Whatmore G, Kohli D. *The Physiopathology and Treatment of Functional Disorders.* New York, NY: Grune & Stratton; 1974.
3. Engel BT. Stimulus response and individual-response stereotypy. *Arch Gen Psychiatry.* 1960;2:305–313.
4. Ekman P, Friesen WV. *Unmasking the Human Face.* Englewood Cliffs, NJ: Prentice-Hall; 1972.
5. Goldstein B. Electromyography: A measure of skeletal muscle response. In: Greenfield S, Sternbach R, eds. *Handbook of Psychophysiology.* New York, NY: Holt, Rinehart & Winston; 1972.
6. McNutty W, Gevertz R, Berkoff G, Hubbard D. Needle electromyographic evaluation of a trigger point response to a psychological stressor. *Psychophysiology.* 1994;31:313–316.
7. Lacey J, Lacey B. Verification and extension of the principle of autonomic response-stereotype. *Am J Psychol.* 1958;71:50–73.
8. Lader MH, Mathews AM. A physiological model of phobic anxiety and desensitization. *Behav Res Ther.* 1968;6:411–421.
9. Malmo RB, Shagass C. Physiologic studies of reaction to stress in anxiety and early schizophrenia. *Psychosom Med.* 1949;11:9–24.
10. Haynes S. Muscle-contraction headache: psychophysiological perspective in etiology and treatment. In: Haynes S, Gannorn W, eds. *Psychosomatic Disorders: A Psychophysiological Approach to Etiology and Treatment.* Westport, CT: Greenwood Press; 1981.
11. Schwartz M, ed. *Biofeedback: A Practitioner's Guide.* New York, NY: Guilford; 1987.
12. Beaton R, Egan K, Mitchell P. Frontalis and trapezius electromyographic activity in healthy non-patients and in clinical headache samples. *Am J Clin Biofeedback.* 1984;7:3–12.
13. Egan KJ, Beaton R, Mitchell P. Autonomic indicators in healthy non-patients and in clinical headache samples. *Am J Clin Biofeedback.* 1984;7:31–41.
14. Whatmore G, Ellis R. Some neurophysiologic aspects of depressed states. *Arch Gen Psychiatry.* 1959;1:70.
15. Skubick D, Clasby R, Donaldson CCS, Marshall W. Carpal tunnel syndrome as an expression of muscular dysfunction in the neck. *J Occup Rehab.* 1993;3:31–43.
16. Horst GJ, Copray JCVM, Lein RSB, Van Willgren JD. Projections from the rostral parvicellular reticular formation to pontine and medullary nuclei in the rat: involvement in autonomic regulation and orofacial motor control. *Neuroscience.* 1991;40:735–758.
17. Paloheimo M. Quantitative surface electromyography (qEMG): applications in anesthesiology and critical care. *Acta.* 1990;93(suppl):34.
18. Flor H, Turk D, Birbaumer N. Assessment of stress-related psychophysiological reactions in chronic back pain patients. *J Consult Clinic Psychol.* 1985;53(3):359.

19. Santini M, Ibata Y. The fine structure of thin unmyelinated axons within muscle spindles. *Brain Res.* 1971;33:289–302.
20. Hubbard D, Berkoff G. Myofascial trigger points show spontaneous needle EMG activity. *Spine.* 1993;18:1803–1807.
21. Walters WF, Williamson DA, Bernard BA, Blouin DC, Faulstich ME. Test-retest reliability of psychophysiological assessment. *Behav Res Ther.* 1987;25:213–221.
22. Arena JG, Hobbs SH. Temporal stability of psychophysiological response profiles: analysis of individual response stereotypy and stimulus response specificity. In: *Proceedings of the 23rd Annual Meeting of the Association for Applied Psychophysiology and Biofeedback.* Colorado Springs, CO; 1992.
23. Voas RH. *Generalization and Consistency of Muscle Tension Levels.* Dissertation. Reviewed in Goldstein IB. Electromyography: a measure of skeletal muscle response. In: Greenfield S, Sternbach R, eds. *Handbook of Psychophysiology.* New York, NY: Holt, Rinehart & Winston; 1972.
24. Travell J, Simons D. *Myofascial Pain and Dysfunction: A Trigger Point Manual, I and II.* Baltimore, MD: Williams & Wilkins; 1983.
25. Thomas A. *The Psycho-Physical Assessment.* Nevada City, CA: Clinical Resources; 1993.
26. Wilder J. The law of initial value in neurology and psychiatry. *J Nerv Ment Dis.* 1957;125:73–76.
27. Bonde-Peterson F, Mork AL, Nielson E. Local muscle blood flow and sustained contraction of human arm and back muscles. *Eur J Appl Physiol.* 1975;34:43–50.
28. Mortimer JT, Kerstein MD, Magnusson R, Petersen H. Muscle blood flow in the human biceps as a function of developed muscle force. *Arch Surg.* 1971;103:376–377.
29. Robard S. Pain in contracting muscles. In: Crue BL, ed. *Pain Research and Treatment.* New York, NY: Academic Press; 1975.

CHAPTER QUESTIONS

1. When a patient responds to a variety of stressful events in the same physiological way (e.g., always increasing muscle tension in the forehead), this is called:
a. response stereotypy
b. stimulus response specificity
c. stress profiling
d. stress profile response specificity
2. The law of initial values states that when the prestimulus level of physiological activity is near the ceiling level for that system, the magnitude of the stress response will be:
a. larger than normal
b. limited because of the lack of room to respond
c. smaller than normal
d. enhanced as a result of the ceiling effect
3. Negative emotions are found primarily on the:
a. upper face
b. neck
c. back
d. legs
4. Stress responses can find their way into:
a. the face
b. the muscle spindle
c. an injured area
d. all of the above
5. The term *serial sevens* refers to:
a. adding by sevens
b. multiplying by sevens
c. subtracting from 1000 by sevens
d. none of the above
6. In stress profiling, one would interpret:
a. initial baseline data
b. level of reactivity
c. recovery data
d. all of the above

Dynamic Assessment

DYNAMIC EVALUATION OF THE NEUROMUSCULAR SYSTEM

The dynamic evaluation of the neuromuscular system is a much broader, more generic, and older procedure than the static evaluation or stress profiling techniques. It has been used in kinesiologic studies for decades. One of the oldest clinical studies of pain that used surface electromyography (SEMG) as its primary descriptive tool was conducted by Price, Clare, and Ewerhardt[1] in the 1940s. Floyd and Silver[2] provided a nice base of information about the back during the 1950s. In addition, Basmajian and DeLuca's book, *Muscles Alive*,[3] served as a foundation of SEMG work and stimulated broad interest in electromyography.

The use of dynamic SEMG in the clinical assessment of various syndromes entails examining how the muscular energy is used to support the body against gravity, how it is used to do work through movement, and how often it rests. Practitioners want to examine the muscles not only to determine disordered movement patterns, but also to note how these movements are affected by prior baseline levels and how the movements might disturb the ability to return to resting levels. In dynamic assessment procedures, muscles are monitored using attached electrodes that "float" above the skin. Information about exact placement of electrodes to monitor a specific mus-

cle group is found in this book's electrode atlas (Part III). The specific sets of muscles to monitor are primarily determined by the nature of the patient's complaint. The static assessment may provide clues about where the disturbances in resting tone might lie. In dynamic assessment, usually four to eight channels of SEMG are monitored to allow the practitioner to study the right and left aspects of two opposing muscle groups. For example, in patients with neck problems, the sternocleidomastoid and cervical paraspinals might be examined during flexion, extension, rotation, and lateral bending of the neck. The practitioner should ask the patient to go through the desired movements several times and in verbally guided and paced fashion. In this way, the SEMG tracings of the movement can be easily examined for the quality of the movement.

The electrode atlas in Part III provides some templates of SEMG recordings from a variety of muscles and movements. Practitioners can compare these templates to their patients' movements. The SEMG record can be examined for some key elements. For instance, issues pertaining to the amplitude of SEMG activation are extremely important, as are issues pertaining to timing and rest. Kasman[4] has developed two figures that describe these issues. **Figure 8–1** depicts the issues pertaining to amplitude, and **Figure 8–2** presents the issues

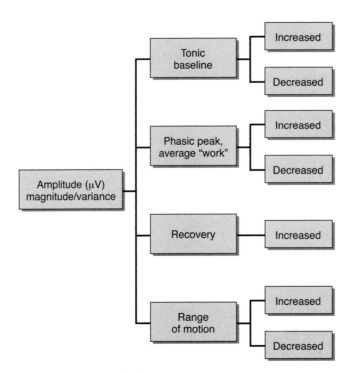

Figure 8–1 Aberrant SEMG activity: Issues in amplitude.

Source: Reprinted with permission from G. Kasman, *Surface EMG in Physical Therapy: Applications in Chronic Musculoskeletal Pain*, © 1995, Movements Systems.

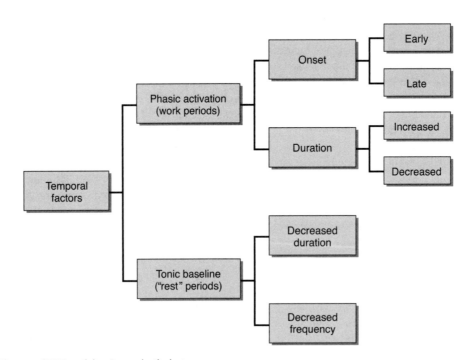

Figure 8–2 Aberrant SEMG activity: Issues in timing.

Source: Reprinted with permission from G. Kasman, *Surface EMG in Physical Therapy: Applications in Chronic Musculoskeletal Pain*, © 1995, Movements Systems.

pertaining to timing. These features are briefly reviewed in the sections that follow.

THE "TONIC BASELINE" AMPLITUDE

The levels of muscular energy present prior to and following a movement can be markers for dysfunction. Figure 8–1 identifies two "tonic baseline" components: tonic baseline and recovery. In the absence of voluntary movement, abnormal muscle tone (an elevated or depressed tonic level) reflects a dysregulation in posture and/or emotional tone. In a neutral posture—one where the body alignment is at its theoretical ideal—the weight of the body should stack on the bones and hang on the ligaments with little muscular involvement. Elevations in the tonic baseline state may result from increased emotional tone or postural disturbances, as described in previous chapters. Usually, elevated resting tone must be treated in some way before disordered movement can be addressed. If one describes the elevated resting baseline as the "noise" in the neuromuscular system, then it is best to reduce that noise before trying to refine timing issues.

RECOVERY OF BASELINE LEVELS FOLLOWING MOVEMENT

When surface electrodes are attached, the practitioner can assess the patient for the effects of movement on postural resting tone. This effect is termed *recovery*. The patient is asked to engage in a movement (e.g., abduction of the shoulder), followed by a return to the neutral position. As in stress profiling, it is important to establish a stable resting baseline prior to a movement. The practitioner should then introduce the movement and examine how well the muscles return to the prebaseline level following the movement. The movement can be regarded as a mechanical stressor on the postural system, and the practitioner assesses how well the postural network recovers following this movement/stressor. Ettare and Ettare[5] have created a therapeutic protocol based on their work in training individuals to recover successfully following various movements and in a variety of postures.

When a muscle fails to recover to prebaseline levels following movement, the condition is termed *postmovement irritability*. What is the mechanism associated with the lack of recovery? One explanation is that irritable muscles harbor a trigger point that disturbs the resting tone. Hubbard and Berkoff[6] have presented some very interesting data that suggest the trigger point may

reside within the muscle spindle. According to their theory, the trigger point may be a muscle spindle in "spasm"; this is the palpable "pea-like" tissue noted in a trigger point examination. When a muscle spindle is disturbed, it sends out impulses to the spinal cord and reflexively activates the motor unit from which it is housed. This activation could create the taut band, along with more general activation of the muscle as a whole and increased resting tone. The individual who exhibits a poor recovery following movement is rarely consciously aware that the muscle is still active.

As an example, observe the recruitment pattern shown in **Figure 8–3**. Failure to recover following movement is noted by comparing the thickness of the postcontraction and precontraction tracings. In the postcontraction tracing, note the frequent "solitary" excursions that rise above and fall below the common width of the tracing. It looks as if the tracing needs a "haircut," because it has so many straggly ends. These "long hairs" probably represent a disturbance in the muscle spindle and, therefore, the potential presence of a trigger point within the muscle. When the muscle is examined and treated for trigger points, the appropriate resting tone returns. In addition, it may be necessary to train the patient regarding how to terminate a movement pattern appropriately. It is helpful to eliminate this postmovement irritability before attempting to retrain and refine dynamic movements. Think of this postmovement irritability as a source of noise within the system that hinders the acquisition of refined motor skills.

ASSESSMENT OF TRIGGER POINTS

Considerable research on the topic of trigger points has been conducted. In particular, the exemplary research by Fishbain, Goldberg, Meagher, Steel, and Rosomoff documents the important role of trigger points in pain-related work.[7] Among the 283 consecutive admissions to a comprehensive pain center that these authors studied, a primary organic diagnosis of myofascial pain syndrome was assigned to 85% of the cases. In a related study of 164 patients with chronic neck pain and headaches,[8] 55% of the cases had a primary diagnosis of myofascial pain. Given its prevalence, it is wise for a practitioner working with muscles to become familiar with myofascial pain. The most comprehensive text on this topic may be found in a two-volume set by Travell and Simons.[9] For an update on the area, the recent review by Simons is recommended.[10]

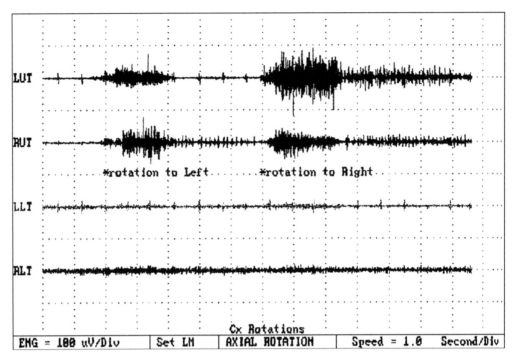

Figure 8–3 Abnormal raw SEMG tracing of upper and lower trapezius during head rotation. Note postmovement irritability, along with "long hairs" suggestive of trigger point.

Source: Copyright © Clinical Resources, Inc.

Assessment and treatment of trigger points should help to normalize muscle function. In fact, it may be impossible to retrain a disordered movement pattern using SEMG feedback without first eliminating trigger points within the muscle. The anatomical foundation of trigger points is still being explored, but the diagnostic criteria have become clearer. The clinical features associated with the presence of a trigger point are outlined in **Table 8–1**.

Treatment of trigger points is achieved either through ischemic pressure applied directly to the trigger point, dry needling of the trigger point, or application of a coolant spray during stretching of the affected muscle. For further information on this topic, consult the books by Travell and Simons.[9]

RANGE OF MOTION

During dynamic movement, the practitioner should visually examine the movement for the range of motion (ROM). Differences in the symmetry of the movement pattern could help to explain patterns of symmetry or asymmetry of SEMG recruitment. Assessment of ROM

may also provide valuable information regarding mechanical impediments to SEMG retraining. It may be necessary to institute manual therapies prior to undertaking dynamic SEMG training for such training to be effective.

ISSUES PERTAINING TO THE WORK PEAK

Symmetry of Recruitment

Along with the range of motion, the practitioner should concurrently examine the recruitment pattern for its amplitude, paying particular attention to the amplitude of the maximum recruitment or peak(s). In many cases, the practitioner should monitor the right and left aspects of homologous muscle groups and inspect for the level of symmetry of the peak contractions. The following rule should apply: *During symmetrical movements, such as forward flexion of the trunk, expect to see a symmetrical recruitment pattern from homologous muscle pairs.*

Donaldson and Donaldson[11] have described lack of symmetry at the peak of movement in cervical and

Table 8–1 Clinical Features Associated with the Presence of a Trigger Point

Clinical Concept	Description
History	The patient has a history of spontaneous localized pain associated with acute overload or chronic overuse of the muscle. The pattern of described pain provides valuable clues about the location of the potential trigger point.
Palpable band	A cord-like band of fibers is palpable. The band assists in locating the tender points.
Spot tenderness	A very tender and very small spot is found in the band. Sensitivity of the band is directly related to the amount of pressure applied.
Jump sign	Pressure on the spot of tenderness causes the patient to react physically to the pain with a spontaneous exclamation or movement.
Pain recognition	Pressure on the spot induces at least some of the pain of which the patient complains, and the patient recognizes it as his or her pain.
Twitch response	The local twitch response is a transient contraction of the fibers of the taut band associated with a trigger point. It can be elicited by vigorous snapping palpation of the taut band. This criterion is possible only in sufficiently superficial and accessible muscles.
Elicited referred pain and tenderness	The trigger point refers pain in a pattern that is characteristic for that muscle. Often, this pain is not local; some 85% of the pain is referred to some distant site. Adequacy of the amount of pressure may determine whether referred pain patterns are discovered.
Restricted range of motion	Full-stretch range of motion of the affected muscle is restricted by pain. This restriction is relieved by the release of the taut band through the inactivation of the trigger point.
Muscle weakness	Clinically, the patient is unable to develop normal strength on static muscle testing as compared to an unimpaired homologous muscle group. Surface EMG findings show greater peak amplitudes on the affected side during repeated movements.

lumbar flexion studies as commonly associated with injury or pain. These authors collected data on both healthy subjects and patients who experienced pain during forward flexion of the neck and trunk, and determined that a 20% difference in peak values is within the normal range. Differences exceeding that level are less common and should be considered abnormal. As a result of the natural variation in these normalized percentage asymmetry scores, differences greater than 20% should be of interest, and differences of 40% or greater should be considered *clinically significant*—the average level of asymmetry for the pain population was slightly greater than 40% in Donaldson and Donaldson's study.

Donaldson and Donaldson also introduced the concept of the hypoactive site.[11] In their symmetry model, the side that evidenced the least recruitment would be labeled as *hypoactive*. Similarly, the site with the most activity would be considered *hyperactive*. Note that "hyperactive" and "hypoactive" are merely relative terms; they do not refer to a referential database, and these authors did not use a statistical basis to obtain these labels. In fact, the so-called hypoactive site is usually in the same range of peak amplitudes as those seen in healthy subjects. It is the *asymmetry* that is considered the red flag.

In addition, Donaldson and Donaldson reported that the hypoactive site is commonly the injured one. Using flexion extension injury to the cervical region associated with motor vehicle accidents as an example, these authors suggest that the hypoactive site is likely to be the side to have experienced the hyperextension injury. This injury is thought to alter the sensitivity of the muscle spindle. These authors argue that the injured site falls into a "disuse" pattern secondary to pain; following the injury, protective guarding does not allow the muscle spindle to come back "online." As a consequence, the hyperactive side takes over the workload for the protected side and becomes overused. This overuse pattern often results in the development of a trigger point in the overused muscle. In one study of recruitment patterns of the upper trapezius and cervical paraspinals during forward flexion and reextension of the head, Donaldson, Skubick, Clasby, and Cram[12] demonstrated increased activation during the reextension phase of the movement pattern in muscles that harbor a trigger point.

Cocontractions

Issues concerning peak work values may also be observed during asymmetrical movements, such as rotation or side bending. The following rule applies: *During an asymmetrical movement, such as rotation, the recruitment pattern from homologous muscles should be asymmetrical.* In the rotation of the head, for example, one would expect the sternocleidomastoid to become activated so that primarily the left sternocleidomastoid is active during the right rotation, while primarily the right sternocleidomastoid is active during left rotation. Abnormal findings are noted when this synergy pattern breaks down and a coactivation of the right and left aspects of a muscle group occurs during an asymmetrical movement. This coactivation is called a *cocontraction.* Here, the prime mover is not allowed to do its work efficiently because of excessive activation of the opposing or antagonistic muscle group.

Tracings from normal and abnormal recruitment patterns may be seen in **Figure 8–4** and **Figure 8–5.** In assessing any movement pattern, the practitioner should be alert to the patient's active ROM. Asymmetrical recruit-ment is commonly accompanied by an asymmetrical ROM. When an asymmetrical ROM is observed, further investigation of the recruitment patterns is suggested. For example, the clinician could ask the patient to do the movement so that it has symmetry in ROM at the smaller end of the ROM; the practitioner would observe this movement to see whether a separation of muscle function occurs or whether the cocontraction persists. While respecting the patient's comfort zone, the practitioner should have the patient increase the ROM in a symmetrical fashion; the practitioner would then observe at what point the excessive activation kicks in.

ISSUES PERTAINING TO TEMPORAL FACTORS
Flexion/Extension

Temporal factors have to do with timing. Does the recruitment pattern come on too soon or too late? Does it last too long, or is it too brief? A good clinical example of timing issues is the study of forward flexion and return to midline of the trunk. **Figure 8–6** shows a normal recruitment pattern for the erector spinae site at the third

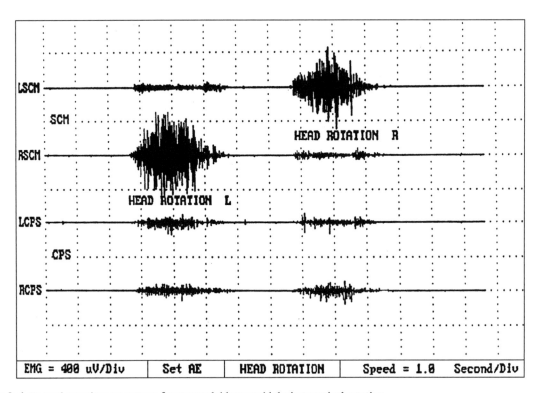

Figure 8–4 Normal recruitment pattern for sternocleidomastoid during cervical rotation.

Source: Copyright © Clinical Resources, Inc.

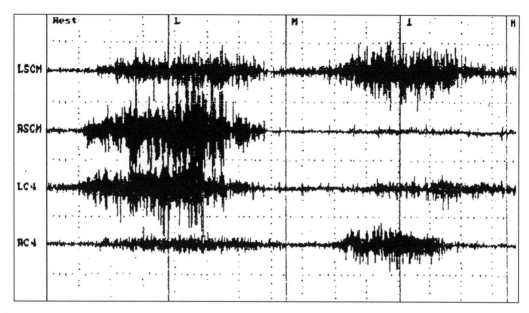

Figure 8–5 Abnormal recruitment pattern for sternocleidomastoid during cervical rotation. Note cocontraction during the right rotation (right portion of EMG).

Source: Copyright © Clinical Resources, Inc.

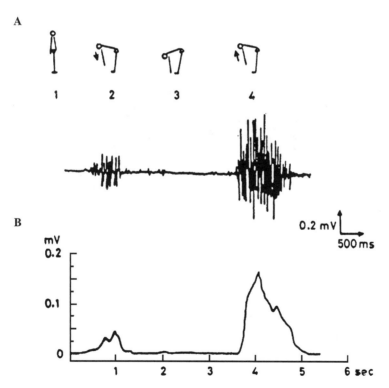

Figure 8–6 Normal flexion and reextension pattern at L-3 for the trunk. (A) Tracing reflects a fine-wire recording from the erector spinae; (B) tracing reflects an RMS (root mean square) display from concurrent surface electrodes.

Source: Reprinted with permission from T. Sihvonen, J. Partanin, H. Osmo, and S. Soimakalio, Electric Behavior of Low Back Muscles During Lumbar Pelvic Rhythm in Low Back Pain Patients and Healthy Controls, *Archives of Physical Medicine and Rehabilitation*, Vol. 72, pp. 1080–1087, © 1991, WB Saunders Company.

lumbar vertebra (L-3), while **Figure 8–7** shows an abnormal one. Here, timing is as important as amplitude. The normal recruitment pattern for this movement should show recruitment during both the eccentric and concentric phases, but a greater level of recruitment should be notable during the concentric phase of the work (return to midline). In addition, during the last 45 degrees of flexion and hang, one should observe a flexion–relaxation response of the erector spinae muscles. The abnormal recruitment pattern in Figure 8–7 shows a lack of the flexion–relaxation response during the hang phase of trunk flexion.

Agonist/Antagonist/Synergy Issues

Evaluation of timing issues is complex and usually requires examination of multiple muscles under various conditions. Surface EMG relationships may change as a function of isometric versus concentric versus eccentric phases of work, or over repeated loadings or movements. In a complex system, the practitioner should examine agonist/antagonist reciprocation versus cocontractions to determine if the movement has agonist/synergist balance. The practitioner should assess whether a muscle recruits at the right time or whether it comes on early or late; whether, once it is recruited, its duration is appropriate for the task; whether the work period is too long or too short; whether the muscle gets a chance to rest between repetitions; whether those rest periods occur often enough; and whether they are long enough.

The following paragraph provides a simple example of the timing issues the practitioner will confront. For an examination of these issues in greater depth, see the electrode atlas section (Part III) and *Clinical Applications in Surface Electromyography* by Kasman, Cram, and Wolf.[13]

In the stabilization of the shoulder during abduction, Will Taylor[14, 15] has argued that the lower trapezius is the major stabilizer during this movement. **Figure 8–8**

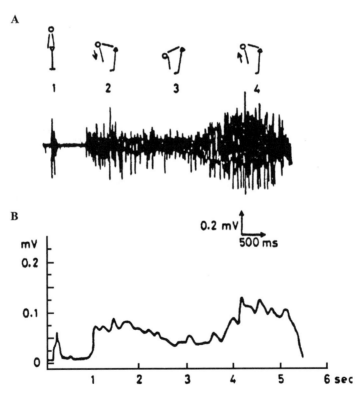

Figure 8–7 Abnormal flexion and reextension pattern at L-3 for the trunk. (A) Tracing reflects a fine-wire recording from the erector spinae; (B) tracing reflects an RMS (root mean square) display from concurrent surface electrodes.

Source: Reprinted with permission from T Sihvonen, J Partanin, H Osmo, and S, Soimakalio, Electric Behavior of Low Back Muscles During Lumbar Pelvic Rhythm in Low Back Pain Patients and Healthy Controls, *Archives of Physical Medicine and Rehabilitation*, Vol. 72, pp. 1080–1087, © 1991, WB Saunders Company.

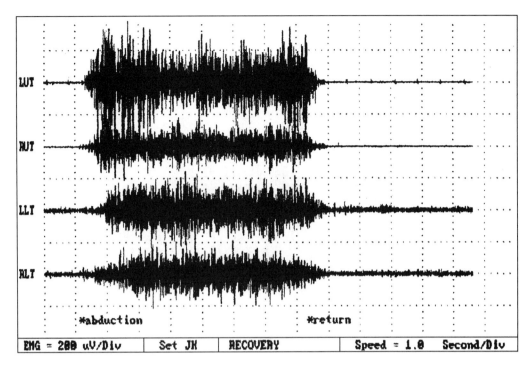

Figure 8–8 The "nearly normal" relationship of upper and lower trapezius during abduction to 90 degrees. It is mildly abnormal with an asymmetry in left upper trapezius to right upper trapezius, with the left upper trapezius being hyperactive.

Source: Copyright © Clinical Resources, Inc.

demonstrates a fairly typical synergy pattern: There is a relative balance between the upper and lower trapezius, with the lower trapezius showing a slightly larger burst pattern. According to Taylor, the general rule is that the ratio between the upper and lower trapezius (upper trapezius/lower trapezius) should be less than 1:0. **Figure 8–9** shows an exaggeration of lower trapezius dominance; the lower trapezius muscle groups show a strong burst of activity, while the upper trapezius site remains relatively quiet. In the normal body, however, such synergy is rarely seen and would probably disturb the glenohumeral rhythm of the shoulder. **Figure 8–10** demonstrates a recruitment pattern where the upper trapezius dominates over the lower trapezius during this movement. The tracing is grossly abnormal. Here, the weight of the arms would be transferred to the neck instead of being borne on the thorax.

The examination of the movement and stabilization of the shoulder and arm as depicted here is greatly simplified. A more comprehensive study of shoulder movement and stabilization would require that one consider more than simply the relationship of the upper and lower trapezius, and that one study more movement

patterns than abduction. With more channels of SEMG available, the practitioner could consider other muscle groups such as serratus anterior; supraspinatus/upper trapezius; infraspinatus; anterior, posterior, and middle deltoids; and the clavicular aspect of pectoralis. Recruitment patterns associated with abduction, flexion, scaption (abduction halfway between the frontal and sagittal planes), shoulder elevation, internal rotation, external rotation, and real and varied life activities could be examined. Amplitude and timing issues will vary, depending on which muscle groups are monitored and under which movement conditions. The electrode atlas (Part III) provides information about what some of the synergy patterns would look like.

THE ISSUE OF REST

As a result of the current level of computerized technology readily available to the practitioner, timing issues pertaining to recruitment are easier to examine than timing issues pertaining to rest. Yet, for the neuromuscular tissue to remain healthy, it needs to rest from time to time. Sustained contractions of moderate intensity

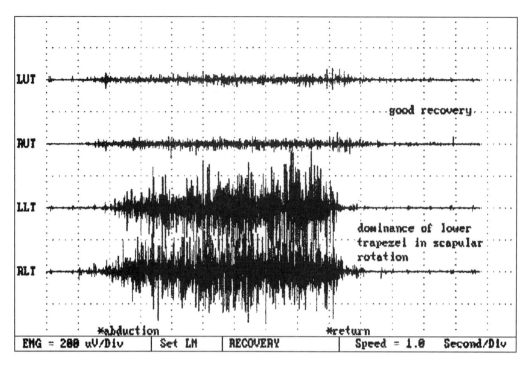

Figure 8–9 An abnormal relationship in which the lower trapezius overrecruits in relation to the upper trapezius during abduction to 90 degrees.

Source: Courtesy of Will Taylor, Portland, Oregon.

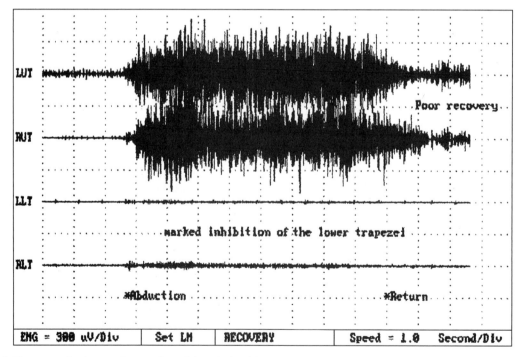

Figure 8–10 A "grossly abnormal" recording of the relationship between the upper and lower trapezius muscles during abduction to 90 degrees, in which the upper trapezius dominates over the lower trapezius.

Source: Copyright © Clinical Resources, Inc.

(i.e., 50% of maximum voluntary contraction) for relatively short periods of time (a minute or two) will lead to muscle fatigue and eventually to a failure point. The physiology of this phenomenon is discussed in Chapter 2, and the electrophysiology is discussed in Chapter 3. During real and varied life activities, there is usually a rhythm to work. On a macro level, the human body is limited by the basic rest–activity cycle (BRAC)[16] of approximately 90 minutes of work. This period should then be followed by a 20-minute rest period. In a normal, healthy body that is allowed to self-regulate, this 2-hour rhythm is reflected as natural fluctuations in such things as the neuroendocrine system, arousal levels, and attentional processes. Human cortisol levels fluctuate, as do body temperatures, brain rhythms, and mentation. Unfortunately, many of us have lost touch with these natural body rhythms and attempt to stay aroused or active or to remain productive.

Scandinavian researchers[17,18] have been studying micromomentary rest or "EMG gaps" that occur during the work cycle. Visually, Taylor[14] has presented this concept as shown in **Figure 8–11**. In his depiction, he has superimposed four 1.5-minute tracings of the right upper trapezius while the patient undergoes four separate conditions:

- The first tracing is taken while the patient is at rest (arms in the lap), with the baseline resting levels appearing quite low.
- The second tracing is taken while the patient undergoes stress profiling. Here, there is a slight increase in the SEMG levels.
- The third tracing shows SEMG activity while the patient is typing. Here, there are periodic and momentary drops in the SEMG activity below 5 microvolts throughout the tracing. These brief drops are the "EMG gaps."

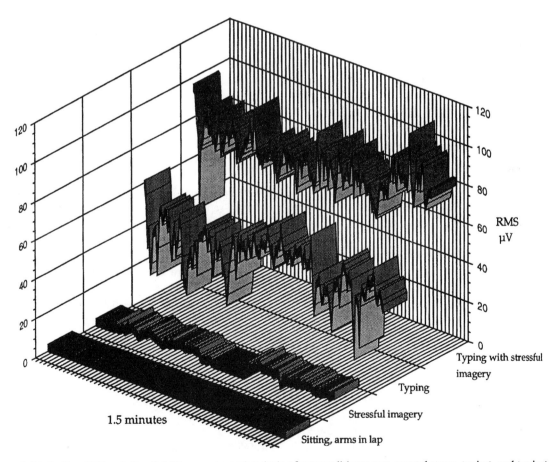

Figure 8–11 Surface EMG activity of right upper trapezius during four conditions: rest, mental stress, typing, and typing while under stress. The micromomentary rest phenomenon may be observed during a typing task. These brief periods of rest are represented by momentary drops in the SEMG activity.

Source: Courtesy of Will Taylor, Portland, Oregon.

- The fourth tracing is taken while the person is typing while simultaneously undergoing a stressful event. A comparison of this tracing to the third tracing indicates that not only does the level of SEMG activity rise, but the EMG gaps also disappear. This places the patient in a form of "double jeopardy": The patient has increased metabolic demands due to increased levels of activation, but the mechanism for profusion of the muscular tissue—rhythmic and interspersed rest—is missing. The buildup of retained metabolites (lactic acid) is very likely.

Another method for examining the SEMG record for interspersed rest is the *probability amplitude distribution* discussed in Chapter 3. Briefly, the occurrence of discrete amplitude "bins" of the SEMG are plotted for a given unit of time. In **Figure 8-12**, the probability amplitude distribution for a patient with right-sided neck and headache pain is displayed. The distribution curve represents a 20-minute period of typing. Note that the recording of the left upper trapezius (LUTr) shows a clear bimodal distribution with a work peak in the 9 to 10 microvolt range and a nice, strong rest peak in the 2 to 3 microvolt range. This distribution looks "normal." The amplitudes of work are relatively quiet, and there is ample rest. The recording of the right upper trapezius (RUTr), however, shows a work peak in the 22 microvolt range and a much smaller rest peak (50% smaller) in the 2 to 3 microvolt range. Although the work amplitude is strikingly higher in the affected right upper trapezius compared to the left upper trapezius, the smaller levels of rest may account for the tension myalgia observed in the right side of this patient's neck.

The second example provides a much clearer picture of the phenomenon, as presented in **Figure 8-13**. Here a 20-minute recording from the right and left upper trapezius muscles during typing is taken on a patient with left-sided carpal tunnel syndrome. Note that the recording of the left upper trapezius takes the form of a unimodal distribution with a work peak around 11 to 12 microvolts, with no distinct rest peak. The recording of the right upper trapezius shows a work peak in the 6 to 10 microvolt range, with a very solid rest peak in the 3 to 4 microvolt range. Here, because the work peaks are nearly the same, the primary difference is in the presence or absence of a rest peak.

RELIABILITY OF DYNAMIC SURFACE ELECTROMYOGRAPHY ASSESSMENTS

The reliability of SEMG recordings is a complicated issue. An excellent discussion of the issues and potential solutions is presented in a recent article by Knutson, Soderberg, Ballantyne, and Clarke.[19] The issues are complicated by the type of contraction studied (isometric versus open chain), level of contraction (10% versus 80% maximum voluntary contraction), type of statistic utilized (Pearson, internal consistency coefficient, or co-efficients of variation), same versus multiple days, and other factors. Major questions include how consistent these recordings should be as one performs the same movement several times on the same occasion, and from one occasion to another. Donaldson has studied the reliability of the peak amplitude during forward flexion of the neck over five repetitions (personal communication). The correlations between the first movement peak and the other four movement peaks was relatively low (< 0.40). However, the correlation between the second to fifth movement peaks was very high (> 0.90). This finding suggests that the first movement pattern of an assessment is an unreliable measure that should always be thrown out, whereas the third repetition represents a reliable estimate of the recruitment pattern for the patient.

Knutson et al.[19] reviewed nine studies that assessed the reliability of SEMG recordings within the same day on a variety of muscles and found the Pearson correlations to be between 0.77 and 0.98. Mathiassen, Winkel, and Hagg[20] reported coefficients of variation (CV) to be in the range of 6% to 14% for a series of studies on upper fibers of the trapezius conducted on the same day. The within-day reliability values were quite respectable. Knutson et al.[19] reviewed five studies that assessed reliability across days and found Pearson correlations as high as 0.92 and as low as 0.32. Mathiassen et al. reported a CV of 23% to 25% in upper trapezius recordings across days.[20] Thus, variability of findings increases as time between recordings increases.

Ahern, Follick, Cocurcil, and Laser-Wolston[21] have investigated the reliability of SEMG over an extended period of time using dynamic assessment procedures. In this study, the researchers found initially high test–retest correlations on day 1. As they reassessed a small sample of individuals at longer and longer time intervals, however, the test–retest correlations fell off substantially. This finding may be restricted to SEMG

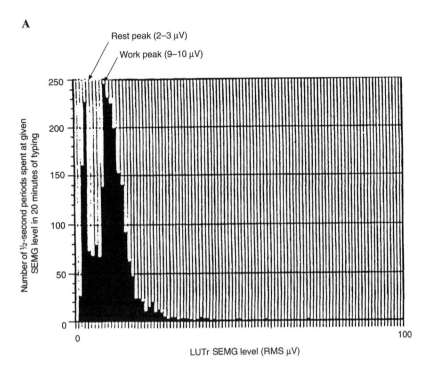

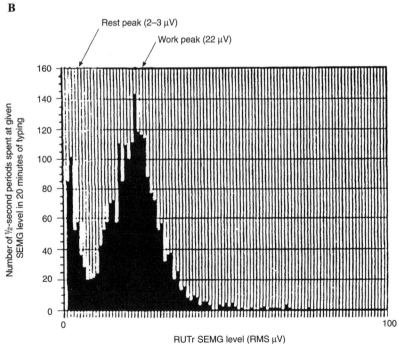

Figure 8–12 Probability amplitude distribution for (**A**) left and (**B**) right upper trapezius during a typing task for a patient with chronic neck and headache pain primarily on the right side. Note change of scale for LUTr and RUTr.

Source: Courtesy of Will Taylor, Portland, Oregon.

A

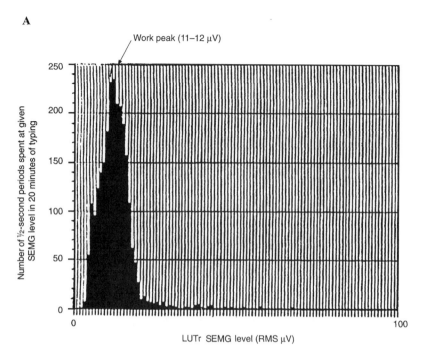

B

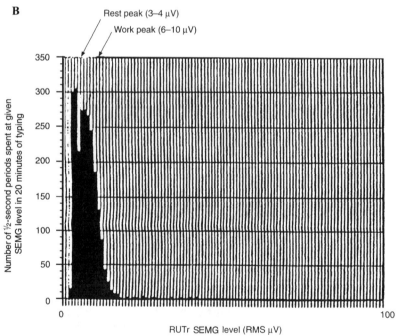

Figure 8–13 Probability amplitude distribution for the left (**A**) and right (**B**) upper trapezius during 20 minutes of typing for a patient with left-sided carpal tunnel syndrome. Note absence of rest peak on the left upper trapezius.

Source: Courtesy of Will Taylor, Portland, Oregon.

patterns observed in the population studied—"normal" backs. Also, perhaps this finding is a signature of health: One could argue that because the neuromuscular system is a fluid and dynamic one, high test–retest correlations for days, months, or years would be found only in pathological populations. Patients with chronic back pain, for example, might show higher test–retest scores over time because of their pathology. In this sense, one might want to consider SEMG as a "state" rather than a "trait" measure, changing in response to the task and the environment. Highly consistent and persistent bracing or postural patterns of activation or habitual movement patterns might indicate an emerging or expressed pathology.

ASSESSMENT OF THE PELVIC FLOOR

Surface EMG recordings may assist the practitioner in the assessment and treatment of urinary and fecal incontinence, as well as pelvic floor pain such as vulvodynia and vulvar vestibulitis. The scope of these problems is immense: An estimated 80% of the geriatric population is incontinent,[22] and 15% of all women suffer from some sort of pelvic pain disorder.[23] (See Chapter 13.)

The same assessment protocol is used for all of these conditions. Consistent with the functions of the pelvic floor musculature (sexual, sphincteric, and supportive), and so as to look at recruitment and endurance, three types of contractions are studied using different durations[24] (see **Figure 8–14**). Six attributes of SEMG are examined (see **Table 8–2**). Once the electrodes are in place and the patient is comfortable in a reclining position, the practitioner records a resting level for 3 to 5 minutes and checks the level of resting tone. It should be low and with good stability. Next, in each of six 5-second periods, the patient is asked to create a strong, brief contraction (called a "flick") in

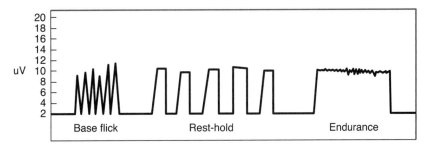

Figure 8–14 Normal patterns of SEMG recruitment observed during assessment of the pelvic floor.

Source: Reprinted with permission from J. Corocos, S. Drew, and L. West, Urinary and Fecal Incontinence, *Electromyography: Applications in Physical Therapy*, © 1992, Thought Technology.

Table 8–2 Surface Electromyography Attributes/Criteria for Comparisons of Normal Subjects (Nonmorbid) and Patients with Vulvar Vestibulitis

SEMG Attribute	Criterion* (SEMG Value)	Nonmorbid Subjects (N = 55)	Vestibulitis Patients (N = 32)
1. Resting baseline (supine posture)	> 2.0 µv (RMS)	18%	71%
2. Contraction amplitude (averaged over 6 occasions)	< 17.5 µv (RMS)	13%	65%
3. Postcontraction resting baseline variability (6 occasions)	> 0.2 µv (RMS)	21%	93%
4. Recruitment time	> 0.2 second	1%	3%
5. Derecruitment time	> 0.2 second	6%	86%
6. Mean spectral frequency during contraction (6 occasions)	> 115 Hz	12%	69%

*Based on Flexiplus SEMG and intravaginal sensors. All values represent the criterion cutoff used in determining the percentage of correct classification.

Source: Copyright © Marek Jantos, PhD.

the middle of the epoch. The practitioner examines these SEMG recordings for latency of recruitment, amplitude, and fatigue. This phase is followed by a rest period of approximately 15 seconds. Next, a series of ten 10-second periods is studied in which the patient alternates between resting and contracting. The patient is asked to make a full contraction and hold it for 10 seconds, and then to stop the contraction and rest for 10 seconds. This recording is examined for the ease of recruitment and derecruitment, the amplitude of contraction, and the presence of any fatigue. It is followed by a 10-second rest period. Finally, the patient is asked to contract fully and hold for as long as possible over a 60-second period. The practitioner examines this SEMG recording for amplitude and the rate of fatigue. This recording is followed by monitoring of a resting baseline, which the practitioner examines for its amplitude and stability.

A normal recruitment pattern for a 10-second hold can be seen in **Figure 8–15**. Initially, the resting tone is low, and there is a crisp recruitment to a high amplitude. At the cessation of the 10-second hold, the SEMG level falls off rapidly and returns to a low resting tone level. In **Figure 8–16**, an abnormal recruitment pattern is evident. Here, the patient exhibits an elevated and unstable resting baseline. When the patient is

asked to contract completely for 10 seconds, low amplitude/poor recruitment is seen, followed by fatigue (indicated by declining amplitude over time). Upon cessation of the recruitment, the release is not crisp, but slow. Finally, postbaseline levels remain elevated and variable.

Table 8–2 lists the criteria for examining attributes of SEMG recordings from the pelvic floor.[25] These recordings are based upon Flexiplus SEMG instrumentation (see Table 3–1 for benchmark equivalence). Comparison of the hit rate for 55 "nonmorbid" subjects (no pain, no incontinence) to 32 vulvar vestibulitis patients is presented in Table 8–2. The percentages of these two cohorts meeting the diagnostic criteria are given as well. Some of the SEMG attributes distinguish the two groups better than others. The level of variability seems to be the most sensitive indicator, suggesting that the pelvic muscles are quite "noisy" in that population. Inability to cease the contraction, which suggests irritability in the neuromuscular system, is also a key indicator of a problem. Contractile amplitudes and resting baselines also separate the two groups.

The assessment criteria also suggest potential biofeedback treatment opportunities, which are discussed in Chapter 9.

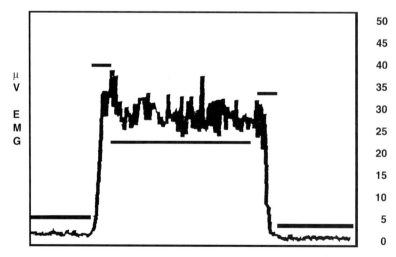

Figure 8–15 A normal recruitment pattern recorded from the pelvic floor using an intravaginal recording electrode.
Source: Copyright © Marek Jantos, PhD.

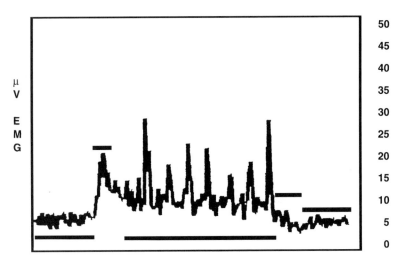

Figure 8–16 An abnormal recruitment pattern recorded from a patient with vulvar vestibulitis.

Source: Copyright © Marek Jantos, PhD.

REFERENCES

1. Price JP, Clare MH, Ewerhardt RH. Studies in low backache with persistent spasm. *Arch Phys Med.* 1948; 29:703–709.
2. Floyd WF, Silver P. The function of the erector spinae muscles in certain movements and postures in man. *J Physiol.* 1955;129:184–203.
3. Basmajian JV, DeLuca C. *Muscles Alive.* 5th ed. Baltimore, MD: Williams & Wilkins; 1985.
4. Kasman GS. *Surface EMG in Physical Therapy: Applications in Chronic Musculoskeletal Pain.* Seattle, WA: Movements Systems; 1995.
5. Ettare D, Ettare R. Muscle learning therapy: a treatment protocol. In: Cram JR, ed. *Clinical EMG for Surface Recordings, II.* Nevada City, CA: Clinical Resources; 1990: 197–234.
6. Hubbard D, Berkoff G. Myofascial trigger points show spontaneous needle EMG activity. *Spine.* 1993;18: 1803–1807.
7. Fishbain DA, Goldberg M, Meagher BR, Steel R, Rosomoff H. Male and female chronic pain patients categorized by DSM-II psychiatric diagnostic criteria. *Pain.* 1986;26 181–197.
8. Fricton JF, Kroening R, Haley D, Siegert R. Myofascial pain syndrome of the head and neck: a critical review of clinical characteristics of 164 patients. *Oral Surg.* 1985; 60:615–623.
9. Travell J, Simons D. *Myofascial Pain and Dysfunction: A Trigger Point Manual, I and II.* Baltimore, MD: Williams & Wilkins; 1983.
10. Simons D. Clinical and etiological update of myofascial pain from trigger points. *J Musculoskeletal Pain.* 1996;4: 97–125.
11. Donaldson S, Donaldson M. Multi-channel EMG assessment and treatment techniques. In: Cram JR, ed.

Clinical EMG for Surface Recordings, II. Nevada City, CA: Clinical Resources; 1990:143–173.
12. Donaldson S, Skubick D, Clasby B, Cram J. The evaluation of trigger-point activity using dynamic EMG techniques. *Am J Pain Manage.* 1994;4:118–122.
13. Kasman G, Cram J, Wolf S. *Clinical Applications in Surface Electromyography.* Gaithersburg, MD: Aspen; 1997.
14. Taylor W. *Patterns of SEMG.* Presented at meeting of the Surface EMG Society of North America; 1993; Boston, MA.
15. Taylor W. Dynamic EMG biofeedback in assessment and treatment using a neuromuscular reeducation model. In: Cram JR, ed. *Clinical EMG for Surface Recordings, II.* Nevada City, CA: Clinical Resources; 1990:175–196.
16. Shannahoff-Khalsa D. Lateralized rhythms of the central and autonomic nervous system. *Int J Psychophysiol.* 1991; 11:225–251.
17. Veiersted KB, Westgaard RH, Andersen P. Electromyographic evaluation of muscular work pattern as a predictor of trapezius myalgia. *Scan J Work Environ Health.* 1993;19:284–290.
18. Veiersted KB, Westgaard RH. Work related risk factors for trapezius myalgia. *Int Arch Occup Environ Health.* 1990; 62:31–41.
19. Knutson LM, Soderberg GL, Ballantyne BT, Clarke WR. A study of various normalization procedures for within-day electromyographic data. *J Electromyogr Kinesiol.* 1994; 1:47–59.
20. Mathiassen SE, Winkel J, Hagg GM. Normalization of surface EMG amplitude from the upper trapezius muscle in ergonomic studies: a review. *J Electromyogr Kinesiol.* 1995;5:197–226.

21. Ahern DK, Follick MJ, Cocurcil JR, Laser-Wolston N. Reliability of lumbar paravertebral EMG assessment in chronic low back pain. *Arch Phys Med Rehab.* 1986;76: 762–765.
22. Portnoi VA. Urinary incontinence in the elderly. *Am Fam Physician.* 1981;23:151–154.
23. Goetsch MF. Vulvar vestibulitis: Prevalence and historic feature in a general gynecologic practice population. *Am J Obstet Gynecol.* 1991;164:1609.
24. Glazer HI, Rodke G, Swencionis C, Hertz R, Young A. Treatment of vulvar vestibulitis syndrome with electromyographic biofeedback of pelvic floor musculature. *J Reprod Med.* 1995;40:283–290.
25. White G, Jantos M, Glazer H. Towards establishing the diagnosis of vulvar vestibulitis. *J Reprod Med.* 1997;42: 157–160.

CHAPTER QUESTIONS

1. Resting baseline of muscle tone is primarily affected by:
   a. posture
   b. emotional tone
   c. kinematics
   d. both a and b
2. When a muscle fails to return to baseline following a movement, it is called:
   a. dysfunctional
   b. irritable
   c. hypoactive
   d. hyperactive
3. During a symmetrical movement, one would expect to see:
   a. an asymmetrical activation pattern
   b. a symmetrical activation pattern
   c. a symmetrical activation pattern for homologous muscle groups
   d. an asymmetrical activation pattern for homologous muscle groups
4. During an asymmetrical movement, one would expect to see:
   a. an asymmetrical activation pattern
   b. a symmetrical activation pattern
   c. a symmetrical activation pattern for homologous muscle groups
   d. an asymmetrical activation pattern for homologous muscle groups
5. Symmetrical movement is to asymmetrical recruitment as asymmetrical movement is to:
   a. irritability
   b. cocontraction
   c. flexion–relaxation
   d. synergy
6. The probability amplitude distribution of SEMG should be:
   a. bimodal
   b. unimodal
   c. curvilinear
   d. multiphasic
7. In assessing vulvodynia, which SEMG attribute best separates normal subjects from patient populations?
   a. amplitude of contractions
   b. resting baseline amplitudes
   c. resting baseline variance
   d. spectral frequency
8. A "flick" consists of a short, brisk contraction. For which disorder is it commonly used as a diagnostic indicator?
   a. upper quarter pain
   b. incontinence
   c. vulvodynia
   d. both b and c
9. In incontinence assessments, fatigue is noted by:
   a. an increase in amplitude
   b. a decrease in amplitude
   c. an increase in blood flow
   d. an increase in urine flow
10. How much asymmetry is considered to be within the normal range?
    a. 5%
    b. 10%
    c. 20%
    d. 50%
11. The erector spinae muscles are expected to _____ during full-trunk flexion.
    a. cocontract
    b. turn off
    c. recruit
    d. become hypoactive
12. During abduction of the arms to 90 degrees, what should be the ratio of SEMG activity for the upper and lower trapezius muscles?
    a. approximately 1 to 1
    b. 2 to 1
    c. 1 to 2
    d. none of the above
13. Which of the following is not a sign of a trigger point?
    a. jump sign
    b. taut band
    c. muscle weakness
    d. referred pain
    e. all of the above

Treatment Considerations and Protocols

AN OVERVIEW OF TREATMENT

Once the clinical assessment has been completed, the formation of treatment plans and the setting of goals are the next order of business. Whenever possible, the practitioner should place the patient's particular dysregulation pattern into the context of its emotional, postural, and movement components. Once all three elements are considered, a treatment plan is developed. If the practitioner proceeds through all three elements of treatment, it is recommended to start with relaxation, then initiate postural treatment, and finally incorporate movement. The area of interest and expertise of the practitioner and the nature of the patient's dysfunction will determine the extent to which each element is emphasized. **Exhibit 9–1** provides a partial list for the scope and sequence associated with surface electromyography (SEMG) treatments.

Treatment using SEMG falls within an educational model. In the most general sense, biofeedback entails providing patients with information concerning their physiology—in this case, muscle activity. In the world of physical medicine, this process is called *neuromuscular reeducation*. The SEMG feedback is used to teach the patient how to normalize his or her muscle function. The approaches described in this section are suggestions for how to optimize the learning experience. Two cases are considered: (1) dysfunction of the upper and lower trapezius and (2) dysfunction of the cervical muscles.

Exhibit 9–1 A Partial List of Scope and Sequence for Treating the Neuromuscular System Using SEMG Feedback

1. Reduce excessive resting tone.
   - Possible relaxation strategies to lower emotional tone
     —Progressive relaxation
     —Autogenic therapy
     —Guided imagery
     —Breath work
   - Possible dynamic relaxation strategies to fine-tune the movement system
     —Muscle learning therapy
     —Recovery training
     —Feldenkrais Method
2. Make postural corrections.
   - Cuing and SEMG feedback
     —Physical prompting
     —SEMG training
   - Stretching
     —SEMG guided stretches
3. Develop recruitment and timing synergies.
   - Isolation training
   - Discrimination training
   - Coordinated recruitment/synergy training
4. Promote generalization through activities of daily living.

Relaxation

If a patient's dysfunction has emotional, postural, and movement components, the practitioner should begin with quieting or relaxation therapies. Although relaxation work is not a necessary ingredient of all successful SEMG therapy protocols, it is advisable to teach patients how to become quiet before attempting to teach them how to self-regulate the neuromuscular–musculoskeletal system. By *downtraining* the neuromuscular system, one reduces the "noise" in the system. This step is taken before initiating a dynamic, uptraining phase; it allows the patient to begin the reeducation process with a quiet nervous system, which enables the patient to better attend to the proprioception associated with the SEMG feedback signal and facilitates the learning process.

Another potential source of noise in the learning process is behavioral or socioemotional issues (i.e., significant pain displays). If these issues are clearly present, the practitioner should address them before moving on to more physical components of SEMG treatments. Dynamic relaxation should also be considered. Micromomentary rest periods can be learned or at least encouraged. The practice of longer rest periods, in which the patient returns the muscle to a low level of activity following its use, is a form of dynamic relaxation and may be a key to successful treatment.

Posture

Postural aspects of dysfunction should be considered next. These factors may have a significant relationship with the emotional or movement components of dysfunction, and it may be impossible to separate out posture as a separate component. Movement, for example, cannot occur without posture. Postural correction will not be retained if it is strongly linked to emotional elements, because the emotional display tends to dominate over volitional control of posture in the long run. If movement patterns are based on a faulty posture, they seldom have the correct agonist/antagonist/synergist relationships. Correcting the limitations placed on a movement by faulty postures greatly enhances any movement-oriented exercise.

Movement

The movement component of dysfunction is superimposed on the emotional and postural components. Provided that the muscle and connective tissues have not been altered, the fluidity of movement depends on the presence of well-regulated emotional tone along with proper postural alignment. Movement is directed by many aspects of our being; it cascades down through the complex neural network described in Chapter 2. The idea for the movement originates in the frontal lobes, the prefrontal cortex sets the general plan for the movement, the motor cortex tunes the finer aspects of the movement, and the cerebellum integrates the movement with the other senses, sets the postural tone through its control of the collateral gamma motor activity, and provides the final link in the actual execution of the movement. Segmental and suprasegmental reflex arcs from the muscle spindle, Golgi tendon organs, Ruffini endings, and free nerve endings impinge on the descending information at a spinal tract level, bringing about the output for the final common pathway—the lower motor neuron.

Disease in any aspect of this very complex system alters this recruitment pattern and the resultant movement. The job of the practitioner is to understand and tease apart this puzzle, to determine which part of the system has gone awry, and to work with those aspects of the problem that can be corrected. This effort may involve joint mobilization, stretching exercises, isolation training for specific muscle groups, integrating the solitary muscle into correct agonist/antagonist/synergist relationships with other muscles, and finally shaping the movement pattern to fit the patient's lifestyle.

Generalization of Training

It simply is not enough to teach the patient to relax in one posture or to move through one plane of motion. Cram and Freeman[1] have demonstrated that SEMG relaxation-based feedback to the frontal muscles does not spontaneously generalize to the neck or the shoulder, nor does it generalize from the reclining posture to the standing posture. In addition, posturally based SEMG feedback to the upper back while standing does not generalize to the seated posture. These authors found the same to be true for the erector spinae muscle group. In other words, you reap what you sow. When practitioners conduct SEMG training in one posture, there is no guarantee that this training will spontaneously generalize to another posture. This lack of generalization applies to quieting the neuromuscular system as well as to learning how to activate it and coordinate it. Therefore, the practitioner must employ strategies that enable patients to generalize their newly acquired motor skills to new settings. For this reason, practitioners should encourage patients to demonstrate their SEMG abilities during activities of daily living.

Relaxation Strategies

The muscular system typically accounts for 50% of an individual's body weight, and it consumes a major amount of a person's metabolic resources. Thus, it is reasonable to assume that the muscles could reflect or influence other aspects of the body system.

The fine art of relaxation has been passed down through the ages. Even the ancient yogis embedded relaxation into their yoga posture rituals, recognizing its role in learning to control one's life.[2] During the early 1900s, Edmund Jacobson became well known for his use of general relaxation in the treatment of a variety of functional or "psychosomatic" disorders.[3] At the same time that Jacobson was introducing his treatment in the United States, a German named Wolfgang Luthe[4,5] developed a series of autogenic phrases or formulae that patients could be taught as a means to treat a variety of psychosomatic disorders. Unfortunately, these relaxation techniques were replaced by Valium during the 1950s as the cultural model shifted to "better living through chemistry."

During the 1960s, Wolpe[6] reintroduced Jacobson's technique to American psychology in an abbreviated form known as *progressive relaxation*. This technique was used as the relaxation component for a psychological procedure called systematic desensitization. A little later, George Whatmore, a student of Jacobson, published *The Physiopathology and Treatment of Functional Disorders*.[7] In this work, Whatmore detailed his adaptation of Jacobson's techniques in which he used SEMG instrumentation as part of the relaxation-based training.

During the 1970s, relaxation protocols flourished with the publication of hundreds of relaxation-based, guided-imagery tapes. One of the most prolific producers of these tapes was psychiatrist Emmett Miller.[8] Some fine-tuning of these imagery tapes for medical uses has also occurred. For example, Hank Bennett,[9] using language very specific to the human body, produced an audiotape entitled *Preparation for Surgery*, the use of which has been shown to reduce blood loss during surgery, reduce the need for narcotic analgesia following surgery, and reduce the number of days of required hospitalization significantly.

Progressive Relaxation Training

Relaxation training is a verbally mediated event in which the practitioner helps the patient change his or her physiology through the use of actions. For Jacobson, the preferred model was one of tensing and releasing various muscle groups. That is, the therapist instructs the patient about how to tense and release muscles in isolation, with an emphasis upon downtraining.

A typical beginning session works on the upper extremity. The patient is instructed to progress up the forearm, one arm at a time, through the following muscles:

1. *Wrist extensors:* "Lift the wrist up, tensing the muscle responsible for this up here on your upper arm until you can feel the tension in that muscle. Then let go of that tension quickly. Let your wrist drop, and feel the tension leave your arm. Relax that muscle completely for the next minute."
2. *Wrist flexors:* "Next, push your wrist down. Tense the muscles, making that movement happen until you can feel them on the bottom of your arm. Then suddenly let go of that tension. Feel the tension leave the muscle, letting the arm relax as completely as it can for the next minute."
3. *Biceps:* "Next, bend your arm up at the elbow, tensing the muscle of your upper arm until you can clearly feel the tension in that muscle. Then suddenly let it go. Feel the tension leave your upper arm as you let it relax as completely as you possibly can for the next minute."
4. *Triceps:* "Next, let your arm go straight, tensing the muscle responsible for the movement so that you can feel the tension on the back of your upper arm. Then let it go quickly, feeling the tension leave that muscle as you relax to the best of your ability for the next minute."

Figure 9–1 and **Figure 9–2** show the effects of progressive relaxation over a course of sessions. In Figure 9–1, the tensing and releasing of each specific muscle group affects other sites as well. There is an overgeneralization of the muscular effort to multiple sites, resulting from the patient's moving the extremity in an effort to feel and sense a particular site. The patient is treated using a combination of SEMG feedback and progressive relaxation procedure. Figure 9–2 shows that by the third session, the patient demonstrates a good ability to make very specific small isometric contractions at the

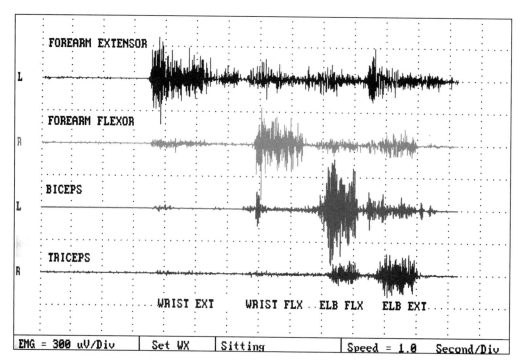

Figure 9–1 Surface EMG recordings from forearm extensors and flexors (wide placement), biceps, and triceps are shown during voluntary activation of each site. Note the lack of specificity of activation, as there is spillover of muscular effort to multiple sites.

Source: Copyright © Clinical Resources, Inc.

various sites without the excessive spillover of muscular efforts seen in Figure 9–1.

Progressive relaxation training involves several components. Initially, the patient is asked to move the joint associated with the muscle as he or she intentionally tenses the muscle to the point of tension perception. As training progresses across sessions, the practitioner encourages the patient to become more aware of tension at lower levels of activation. Toward the end of training, the patient is able to activate and sense a specific muscle group without moving the associated joint. It takes a very relaxed muscle and a fair amount of training for the patient to sense a brief burst of isometric tension in a muscle. In the 1960s, Whatmore demonstrated that SEMG instrumentation and feedback made this task much easier.[7]

Second, the practitioner must teach the patient to "let go" of tension. The preceding example suggests that practitioners teach the patient to let go quickly. Jacobson used the term "zero down" to describe what it means to let go of muscle tension quickly and com-

pletely. It is the relaxation component that has the greatest therapeutic effect. "Tense with will, relax and feel." The "relax and feel" component is at least twice as important as tensing the muscle.

Third, a long period of quiet time and relaxation follows each tension cycle. The ratio of tension to relaxation should be 1 to 5.

Fourth, opposing pairs of muscles are systematically activated. This systematic activation is intended to maintain a healthy balance in the neuronal pool of spinal segments that control these muscles. At a segmental and suprasegmental level, the output from the Golgi tendon organ and muscle spindles provides collateral excitatory or inhibitory influences on related contralateral or opposing lower motor neurons (see Chapter 2).

Finally, the practitioner progresses from one muscle group to another, working through the various kinetic chains. The second session might work on the arms and then address the muscles of the shoulder and upper back. The third session might work on the arms, the

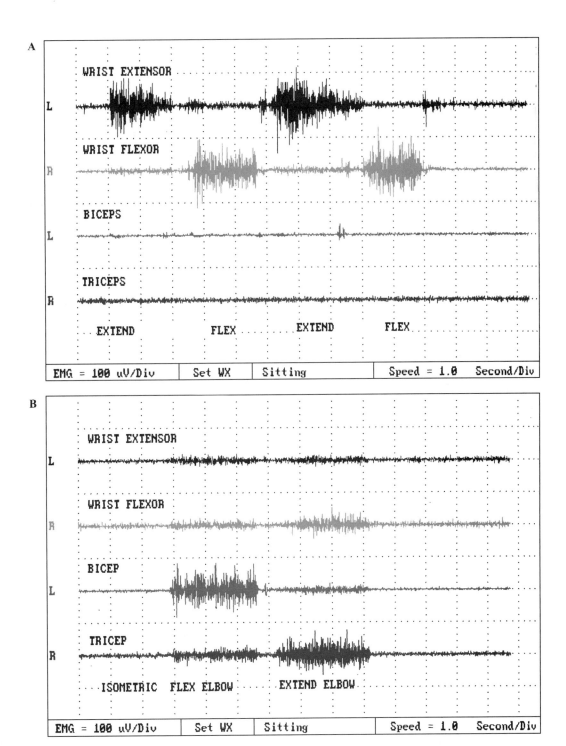

Figure 9–2 After a few sessions of SEMG feedback and progressive relaxation training, SEMG recordings from forearm extensors and flexors (wide placement), biceps, and triceps sites are shown during voluntary activation of each site. (**A**) Isolated wrist extensor and flexor activity, (**B**) isolated bicep and tricep activity.

Source: Copyright © Clinical Resources, Inc.

shoulder, and the head and neck. As the therapy progresses, patients become increasingly more adept at activating only the muscles that they intend to activate. For more elaborate and specific information on this technique, the original work of Edmund Jacobson, *You Must Relax*,[3] is highly recommended.

Briefer adaptations of Jacobson's protocols are available as well.[6] Typically, they reduce the specificity of the contraction by asking the patient to cocontract the agonist/antagonist muscles (e.g., "Make a fist and feel the tension throughout your entire forearm"). The focus is on feeling large contractions, and there is no effort to recognize the smaller "efforts." In addition, those protocols use a shorter, 15-second relaxation phase. These briefer relaxation protocols are appropriate and adequate if the patient is already fairly relaxed or has some rudimentary relaxation skills, and if the practitioner wishes to induce a lighter level of relaxation.

Autogenic Therapy

Autogenic therapy (AT) uses words and images without action. It is a form of self-hypnosis. The patient learns to use very specific self-suggestions or phrases to affect his or her physiology. AT approaches six different domains:

1. Heaviness—neuromuscular relaxation
2. Warmth—vascular dilatation
3. Slow and regular heartbeat—cardiac regulation
4. Slow and regular breath—respiratory regulation
5. Abdominal warmth—visceral relaxation
6. Cooling the forehead—cooling the brain

The structure of the therapy is very specific. It begins with setting the correct posture. The therapy can be done while the patient is lying, reclining, or sitting. In the lying posture, the head is supported by pillows, the palms are down, and the feet are slightly apart. In the reclining posture, the feet are on the ground, the arms are positioned on the armrests of the chair with the palms down, and the head is supported in some way. In the sitting posture, the feet are on the ground, the arms are in the lap (palms down), and the torso is slumped forward with the head in the fully flexed posture.

The patient is encouraged to use *passive volition*. That is, the individual is encouraged to focus on the body part in question, respond to phrases spoken by the practitioner, yet have a casual attitude about the outcome of the effort. It is more like wishing for something to happen, rather than making it happen. It is helpful for the practitioner to begin the exercises with a verification phrase, one in which the patient is asked to close his or her eyes and mentally visualize the part(s) on which he or she is going to work. Then the practitioner speaks a phrase to the patient to repeat internally. This phrase is followed by a minimum of a 30-second observation period in which the patient observes what is happening. Finally, the exercise is terminated by asking the patient to move the part(s) of interest vigorously, breathe out heavily, and open his or her eyes. This process is followed for each autogenic phrase or set of phrases, and the patient is asked to note any discharges that result from the procedure. These discharges are thoughts, feelings, or physical sensations associated with the autogenic phrase.

In summary, the autogenic phrases are spoken to the patient, and the patient thinks the phrases himself or herself, five or six times over the course of 30 to 60 seconds per phrase. During the first visit, the practitioner usually begins with one phrase and goes through the entire cycle. On subsequent visits, the practitioner adds more phrases to the patient's suggestions, making the training sessions longer and deeper. The standard autogenic phrases are as follows:

- My right (left) arm is heavy.
- My right (left) leg is heavy.
- My right (left) arm is warm.
- My right (left) leg is warm.
- Both my arms (legs) are heavy.
- Both my arms (legs) are warm.
- I am at peace.
- My heart beat is slow and regular.
- My breathing is slow and regular.
- It breathes me.
- My abdomen (solar plexus) flows warmly.
- My forehead is cool.

For a more in-depth review of autogenic training, see Luthe's *Autogenic Therapy: Autogenic Methods*, volume 1. In addition, a tremendous amount of literature is available on the physiological effects of this technique. The reader is referred to volume 4 of the *Autogenic Therapy* series for an in-depth review of the literature.[5]

The effects of this type of training appear to be quite specific. The suggestions of heaviness appear to bring about reductions in SEMG activity, suggestions of warmth bring about increased hand temperature, suggestions of slowness of the heart and breath seem to slow both systems, and suggestions of coolness of the forehead appear to lower the temperature of the upper face. If practitioners want to work on quieting down a particular organ system or part of the body, they should direct their language in very specific ways to those body parts and organs.

Guided Imagery

Guided imagery is a much broader concept than AT. It is a form of self-hypnosis, in which patients are encouraged to think, visualize, hear, feel, and/or smell their way into a relaxed and comfortable state.

Guided imagery procedures attempt to begin with a state of general relaxation. The script by Thomas[10] provided in **Exhibit 9-2** is directed toward this generic sense of relaxation. From there, many practitioners may overlay a particular therapeutic theme for the patient. For example, a tape may be specifically designed to assist the patient in drifting off to sleep.[11] The images used for sleep differ significantly from those used to cope with pain.[12]

One of the best tapes with a specific application area has been authored by Bennett[9,13,14] on preparing the patient for surgery. Like the language for AT, the language for this tape has been selected for its desired effect. For example, the surgical preparation tape uses a very specific approach to suggestions, which make the suggestions quite believable, if not literally true. It then uses language that asks the body to take the physiologically correct action to minimize the trauma of surgery. Strange as it may seem, this approach actually works: Patients tend to bleed less, use less medication following surgery, have fewer complications, and be discharged earlier.

Practitioners who want more information on which types of images seem to work with which types of disorders should refer to Barber's article on this topic.[15]

Breath Work

Respiration should be considered as part of the comprehensive view of the neuromuscular network. After all, it is the muscles that bring the air into our bodies. When breathing is done efficiently, the diaphragm is predominantly involved. When respiration becomes inefficient and disordered, it begins to overuse the ancillary muscles of respiration such as the sternocleidomastoid, scalene, or upper trapezius. This type of response may be seen in **Figure 9-3**. In the case of upper back or neck pain, it is essential to consider inappropriate breathing patterns as part of the assessment. If these are noted, training in

appropriate respiratory patterns is indicated. In addition, training of the respiratory system can be one of the avenues for teaching the patient general relaxation. Such training reduces the metabolic demands on the breath and increases the mechanical efficiency of the upper back in general.

Teaching a relaxed respiratory pattern involves teaching the patient to breathe abdominally. This goal can be achieved in several ways. The easiest, non-instrumented method involves placing a small (5-pound) sandbag or small phone book on the patient's abdomen as he or she lies in a well-supported supine posture. Next, the practitioner asks the patient to invite his or her breath down into the abdomen while pressing up against the weight of the sandbag or book. As the patient exhales, he or she then lets the weight fall. The patient is asked to let his or her body tell him or her how quickly or slowly he or she should breathe. As the patient increases the tidal volume of each breath (the amount of air breathed), it is not uncommon for the respiration rate to fall and for the patient to report feelings of relaxation. If the patient notes sensations of arousal or anxiety associated with this procedure, the practitioner might suspect a hyperventilation syndrome and the breathing disorder will need to be treated somewhat differently.[16] If all goes well with supine abdominal breathing, the practitioner should make sure that the behavior is generalized to other postures. The practitioner should observe the patient's ability to breathe abdominally in the sitting and standing postures. Further training may be needed for specific postures. Patients should be encouraged to practice the abdominal breathing in the various postures.

The practitioner may want to use SEMG to monitor the ancillary muscles of respiration during training in abdominal breathing. Electrodes attached to the scalene, sternocleidomastoid, or trapezius muscle groups would provide information concerning excessive use of these muscles. Thresholds can be set that encourage the patient to practice breathing while keeping these muscles relaxed.

Treating patients with respiratory anomalies may be quite complex. If simple training in abdominal breathing does not correct the problem or makes matters worse, the practitioner may want to consult a respiratory therapist. For further information on teaching patients how to breathe correctly, see Rama and colleagues' *The Science of Breath*[17] or Fried's *The Breath Connection*.[16]

Exhibit 9–2 Guided Imagery Script for General Relaxation

"Now relax and let all stressful memories fade away . . . for the next 20 minutes you can just relax as you listen to suggestions on how to allow yourself to be calm . . . as you begin this period of relaxation let your body get as comfortable as you can . . . if you need to adjust anything, do it now . . . be sure that you can breathe easily . . . keep your eyes gently closed . . . this is your time to forget all cares and worries . . . give yourself permission to use this time to simply be . . . to let go of tension . . . to relax . . .

"Now allow your mind to drift far, far away . . . away from your everyday life . . . away from all your anxieties, worries, and responsibilities . . . let your mind drift to a place where you can feel safe, comfortable, and tranquil . . . as this happens just passively listen to suggestions for relaxation . . . don't try to make anything happen . . . just let it happen . . . just let your muscles relax all by themselves . . . suggest to your muscles that they may take a vacation now . . . the chair will hold you . . .

"Now focus on your breathing . . . become aware of your breathing . . . let it be deep, and abdominal . . . let it be slow, and regular . . . let the air come in through your nose and go directly to your abdomen . . . feel your stomach muscles expand as you breathe in . . . let your stomach muscles relax as you breathe out . . . just let your breathing be calm . . . and take no effort at all . . . inhale and exhale . . . inhale and exhale . . . calm, and placid, and tranquil . . . with no cares or worries . . . just think about relaxing every muscle in your body . . . from the top of your head to the tips of your toes . . . just let the air breathe for you . . . as you focus your attention elsewhere . . .

"Let your attention focus on your face and head . . . let the muscles in your forehead relax . . . imagine all those tiny muscles becoming smooth and relaxed . . . let the muscles around your nose relax . . . let the muscles around your eyes relax . . . let the muscles in your jaw relax . . . let your teeth part slightly . . . let the muscles in your eyelids relax . . . allow your eyelids to find a place that is just right for them to rest comfortably . . . now let this relaxation spread into the temple area . . . allow your temples to relax . . . as your temples relax you may even be able to feel your ears letting go . . . and dropping with gravity ever so slightly . . . notice how good that feels . . . remember to keep your breathing slow, deep, and regular . . . maybe you can even feel the slight tug of gravity on your face and head . . . more and more calm . . . more and more serene with each breath you take . . . feeling your body becoming heavier and heavier . . . now let the muscles in your throat just let go entirely . . . let them relax . . . let all the muscles in your throat just let go completely and relax . . . maybe you can imagine that all the muscles from the neck up have become loose . . . and soft . . .

"Now just think about relaxing all the muscles in your shoulders . . . imagine the back of your neck and your shoulders feel all the muscles in the back of your neck and shoulders becoming very loose and very slack . . . just let all the muscles in your neck and shoulders sink deeper and deeper into the chair . . . each time you exhale you may notice the contact of your body with the surface it is on . . . feeling the surface beneath you, becoming more and more comfortable . . . let this relaxation flow down your spinal column . . . let all the muscles from the base of your head all the way down to your tailbone relax . . . let them be smooth, and soft . . . loose, and slack . . . feel the comfort of the chair as it holds you . . . let go of the tension as that wonderful feeling spreads into your chest and abdomen . . . feel all your abdominal muscles become smooth, and soft . . . loose, and slack . . . keep your breathing slow, and deep . . . let all your internal organs be soft, and comfortable . . . and now your arms . . . feel your arms let go . . . and become heavy, and soft . . . loose, and slack . . . just let your arms and hands be heavy, and warm . . .

"Let all the tension in the muscles of your entire body relax . . . and now focus on your hips and buttocks . . . let those large muscles be at ease . . . smooth, and soft . . . loose, and slack . . . let the large muscles in your thighs relax . . . and the joints of your knees . . . let the calves of your legs relax . . . going very loose and slack . . . and now your feet . . . let them relax . . . perhaps you can imagine that the joints in each and every toe relax . . . as you feel more and more calm . . .

"Now we are going to spend 10 more minutes visualizing a pleasant experience . . . just passively follow the suggestions and enjoy yourself . . . as you begin this next period of relaxation allow your body to feel comfortable . . . now let yourself focus again on your breathing . . . once again becoming aware of your breathing . . . let it be deep . . . and abdominal . . . let it be slow . . . and regular . . . feel your abdomen expand as you breathe in . . . feel your abdomen relax as you breathe out . . . just let your breathing be still . . . and make no effort at all . . . inhale and exhale . . . inhale and exhale . . . calm . . . relaxed . . . tranquil . . . no cares . . . no worries . . . just think about relaxing every muscle in your body . . . just let the air breathe for you . . . as you focus your attention elsewhere . . .

"Now I am going to 'paint' a picture with words . . . listen to the words and see the picture in your mind's eye . . . allow this 'voice picture' to be vivid and real . . . see the colors . . . taste the tastes . . . feel the feelings . . . smell the smells . . . and hear the sounds . . . as I describe the scene, let it be real for you . . . as if you were really there . . . allow your mind to roam freely . . . maybe you can discover new places I may not even describe . . . that would be okay . . . this can become your picture . . . let it develop all on its own . . .

"Now imagine you are on a wonderful vacation . . . with no cares . . . with no worries . . . with no one to be responsible to . . . completely free from your daily pressures and expectations . . .

Exhibit 9–2 *(Continued)*

"You are walking along the beach; it is mid-summer . . . it is warm and comfortable . . . it is late afternoon . . . this perfect summer day . . . the sun is a blazing golden yellow in the brilliant blue sky . . . the sun shines down and warms you . . . as you casually walk along you can feel the hard-packed sand beneath your bare feet . . . feel the warmth of the sand . . . feel the dampness of the sand . . . wiggle your toes in the sand . . . isn't it wonderful? . . . as you continue to walk you can hear the sound of the surf on the beach . . . the gentle rhythm of the waves lapping in and out . . . in and out . . . hear the distant cry of a gull as it soars through the sky . . . you look toward the sound . . . the sky is a beautiful deep blue . . . it is filled with fluffy white clouds . . . see the clouds slowly moving and changing their shapes . . . you feel overcome with a feeling of peace and tranquility . . . it is a lazy day that reminds you of many wonderful experiences from your past . . .

"You come to a small mound of pure white sand . . . you find a comfortable place to sit . . . you feel alone and still . . . now you lie back and watch the wispy clouds as they float by . . . you drift, and dream that warm summer day . . . you feel the warmth of the sand beneath you . . . you feel the warmth of the sun as it shines down on you . . . you continue to enjoy this wonderful place for what seems like hours . . . allowing your mind the freedom to wander as it wishes . . . you enjoy this stillness . . . this warmth . . . this quiet . . .

"Now you slowly sit up again . . . as you look toward the sea . . . the sun is beginning to set in the west . . . it reflects in beautiful patterns off the sea . . . colors dance and skip in all directions . . . along the horizon there is a sparkling glimmer where the sky touches the water . . . you can see a sailboat, its sails billowing in the wind . . . you can almost feel yourself on that sailboat piercing through the sea . . . there is a gentle ocean spray . . . it is cooling and refreshing . . . you are aware of the fresh smell of the salt in the spray . . . there is a light residue on your lips . . . you can taste it if you lick your lips . . . with each movement of the sun as it slowly sets you find yourself becoming more and more relaxed . . . all your senses are merging with the calm environment around you . . . you allow yourself to enjoy this wonderful time . . . with no cares . . . no worries . . . no uneasiness . . . ."

Source: Copyright © 1995, A. Thomas, *The Psychophysical Evaluation*, Clinical Resources, Inc.

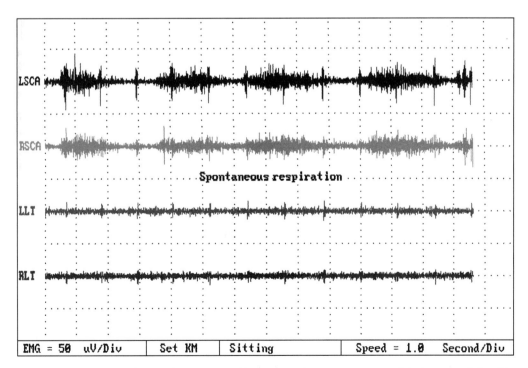

Figure 9–3 Surface EMG recordings from scalene (SCA) and lower trapezius (LT) are presented during quiet sitting. The pattern of rhythmic activation is associated with respiration and the inappropriate use of the ancillary muscles.

Source: Courtesy of Will Taylor, Portland, Oregon.

Generalization of Relaxation Training

In relaxation training, there are issues relating to the transfer of training effects from one muscle group to another, from one posture to another, and from one situation to another. Several studies have shown that relaxation-based SEMG feedback directed toward one muscle group does not necessarily generalize to other muscle groups.[1,18,19] In addition, Cram and Freeman[1] found that relaxation effects do not generalize from the sitting posture to the standing posture. Although no formal studies have been conducted on the generalization of relaxation skills from the clinic to the home or office setting, it would be safe to assume that such generalization does not happen spontaneously. It appears that the central nervous system is fine-tuned for specificity in the learning of physiological regulation. The practitioner must enhance and promote generalization rather than expect it. For example, to transfer skills from one posture to another, the practitioner should train the client in both postures. (See Chapters 11 and 12.)

DYNAMIC RELAXATION STRATEGIES

Relaxation training does not need to occur only in the quiet, recumbent posture. It is possible to teach a patient to turn off the muscular system quickly following its use or simply to move in a more relaxed and synergistic fashion. Two such therapies are described in this section: muscle learning therapy developed by Ettare and Ettare[20] and the Feldenkrais Method.[21] These are not the only such therapies to consider; other possible avenues to quiet, relaxed movement include tai chi, the Alexander Technique, and Aston-Patterning, among other techniques.

Muscle Learning Therapy

This unusual SEMG training technique has been described in detail by Ettare and Ettare.[20] Its essence and beauty lie in the emphasis on teaching the patient, from the first day, to quiet the muscles following their use. Rather than using the Jacobson technique of an isometric contraction of a specific muscle, a change of posture or a functional movement is the perturbation that precedes the practice of relaxation. Dynamic relaxation is defined here as the ability to voluntarily quiet or *derecruit* the muscles following movement.

The muscle learning therapy system is intentionally a regional one. Electrode placement recommendations are presented in the electrode atlas section of this book (Part III) and are represented by widely spaced, nonspecific recordings at the cervical trapezius (wide), cervical dorsal (wide), and dorsal lumbar (wide) muscles.

During the assessment phase, the protocol for the upper back and neck entails having the patient go from sitting, to standing, to walking, to standing, and back to sitting (see **Figure 9–4**). During training, the practitioner should have the patient go from sitting to standing; once the patient is standing, the practitioner should find ways in which the patient can quiet the upper quarter as much and as quickly as possible. Next, the patient is trained to lower the SEMG levels to a "normal" resting level (less than 2 microvolts using a J&J M-501), following the change in activity. This may entail postural changes, stretching, and intentionally learning to "let go." Finally,

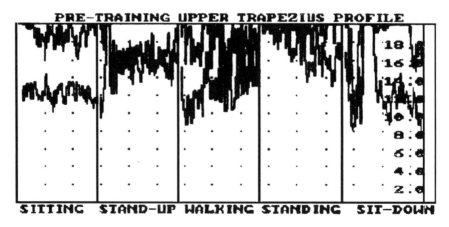

Figure 9–4 Typical pre-training guarding or hypertonic profile for upper trapezius. This represents a 20-second epoch.
Source: Copyright © 1990, J. R. Cram, *Clinical EMG for Surface Recordings: Volume 2*, Clinical Resources, Inc.

the patient is encouraged to recognize the sensations of released tension as soon as the SEMG amplitude has dropped. The goal is to transfer the awareness of tension from the biofeedback displays to proprioception. By the end of several visits of training, the sit, stand, walk, stand, sit protocol is transformed into the SEMG recordings shown in **Figure 9–5**.

Ettare and Ettare's rich protocol includes several variations on the theme of using controlled relaxation to facilitate transfer of skills. For example, there is sit–stand training, sit–stand training with reverse counting; blind sit–stand training; typing; walking; sit–walk–sit; and stand-to-lying. An excellent description of this protocol, including a 12-session description, may be found in the article by Ettare and Ettare.[20]

Recovery Training

Recovery training is a variation of the Ettare protocol, in that the goal is to teach the patient how to turn off his or her muscle after it has been intentionally activated. As noted in Chapter 8, muscles may be subject to postcontraction irritability. In this condition, the muscle continues to remain active even after the patient has intentionally ceased the activity. **Figure 9–6** illustrates a mild example of this phenomenon following the movement of abduction. There is a 2-second period in which the muscle remains active following the return of the arms to the sides of the body. In more extreme examples, the persistent activity may last for several minutes following the termination of the action.

As with the Ettare protocol, SEMG biofeedback training can be directed toward teaching the patient how to turn off the recruitment as quickly as possible following the activating event. **Figure 9–7** provides an example of how this scenario might look after just a few trials of feedback. Once the patient is able to achieve this goal with visual feedback, the practitioner should ask the patient to close his or her eyes, practicing without external feedback and tuning into proprioceptive feedback instead. Generalization to other postures may be important as well. The level of asymmetry in Figure 9–7 is large enough (approximately 40%) to be of clinical interest. Working on issues pertinent to symmetry of recruitment might be the next therapeutic task at hand.

Quieting exercises may also be conducted using isometric contractions. Here, one would want to begin with small efforts and gradually move to larger and larger efforts. The training increases the patient's awareness of the muscle of interest by teaching him or her how to turn it on and off. This training takes some of the "noise" out of the neuromuscular system.

The Feldenkrais Method

Moshe Feldenkrais developed another excellent technique to teach dynamic relaxation, which is currently taught around the world by his students. For more in-depth reading, several books are available on this topic.[21,22] Surface EMG biofeedback and Feldenkrais movement exercises complement each other. The Feldenkrais movement strategies provide a structure for instructing the patient and encouraging normalized movement patterns, while the SEMG feedback documents that these patterns are recruiting the desired muscles, at the desired amplitude, and with the

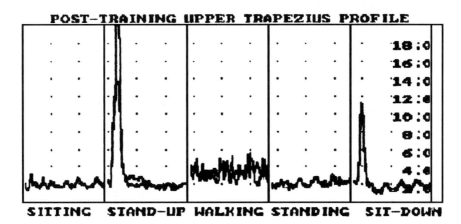

Figure 9–5 Typical post-training profile for upper trapezius using the Ettare model of treatment.

Source: Copyright © 1990, J. R. Cram, *Clinical EMG for Surface Recordings: Volume 2*, Clinical Resources, Inc.

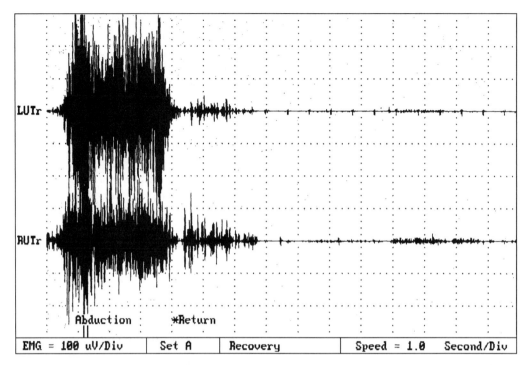

Figure 9–6 Surface EMG recording from the left and right upper trapezius during abduction of the arms to 90 degrees and return. Note the persistent activity for 2 seconds following the return of the arms to the sides.

Source: Courtesy of Will Taylor, Portland, Oregon.

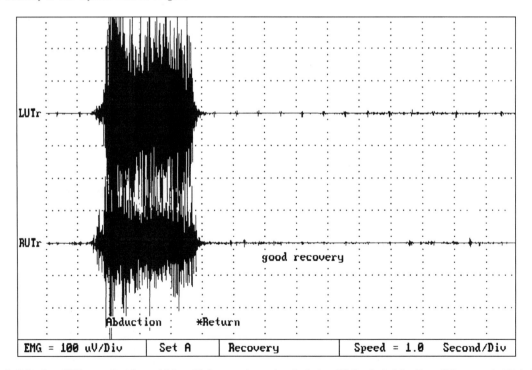

Figure 9–7 Surface EMG recording from right and left upper trapezius during and following abduction of the arms to 90 degrees. Here the patient is intentionally trying to quiet the muscles as quickly as possible following the cessation of the movement.

Source: Courtesy of Will Taylor, Portland, Oregon.

desired timing. The movement exercises are used to correct asymmetries, cocontractions, and poor timing of recruitment.

The cornerstone of this therapy entails teaching the patient to engage in gentle movement patterns that facilitate the normal recruitment of muscle. The practitioner should instruct the patient as follows:

1. Ask the patient to make small movements. The patient should do only what is comfortable and easy, without pushing himself or herself. Do not encourage the movement pattern to progress to the point of pain.

2. Encourage the patient to reduce any unnecessary movement. According to Feldenkrais, less muscular effort will bring the patient more physical benefit. His theory is that the brain can detect differences more easily when the senses are less stimulated. Slow, small, and easy movements allow the nervous system to detect any unnecessary muscular effort.

3. Encourage the patient to do each movement slowly—to take time to sense and feel what he or she is doing. By doing the movement slowly, the patient will be able to detect any unnecessary effort and strain. Feldenkrais states that once the patient becomes aware of this extra effort, the nervous system will automatically attempt to reduce it.

4. Encourage the patient not to try too hard. Learning of new movements will be enhanced if the patient forgets about competing or trying to succeed. Trying too hard is one of the ways in which the patient introduces excessive effort into the movement.

5. Allow the patient to go at his or her own rate. The rate at which the muscles and nervous system change is different for each person.

6. Make certain that the patient rests between each movement. The patient should return to the neutral position and stop there for several seconds before going on to the next movement. Also, allow the patient to stop and rest for a half minute or so every few minutes. After the patient has done an entire sequence of movements, allow the patient to rest before introducing a new movement, or even a repetition of the same movement.

There are many Feldenkrais movement patterns from which to choose. Movement exercises to add flexibility to the neck region are described in this section. The patient can do these exercises while either sitting or lying. The instructions below are given for the sitting position. The practitioner should begin by having the patient rotate the head as far as it is comfortable to the left and to the right. The patient should note how far it is that he or she turned. The exercises described next involve rotating to the left. Once the patient has done the left aspect, he or she should follow through with the right aspect.

1. Using the six pointers given earlier in this section, ask the patient to rotate the head to the left and back while keeping the eyes fixed forward. Do this two or three times.

2. Ask the patient to allow the eyes to lead the rotation as they would normally do. Do this a couple of times.

3. Ask the patient to rotate the shoulders to the right while he or she is rotating the head to the left. Do this two or three times.

4. Ask the patient to rotate the shoulders in the direction of the head turn, as he or she would normally do. Do this a couple of times.

5. Ask the patient to push the right knee forward. Have the patient observe any tension felt in the torso. Encourage the patient to find the natural rotation of the torso associated with this knee push. See if the patient can find his or her way into rotating not only the torso, but also the shoulders and head. Do this rotation two or three times.

6. Conclude by asking the patient simply to rotate the head to the left, and see if it rotates any farther than it did before the patient started Step 1.

These simple rotational patterns can bring about more normalized recruitment patterns in the sternocleidomastoid and C-4 paraspinal muscles. Such relatively simple exercises may be given to the patient as part of the home exercise program. Patient-oriented books[22] and audiotapes[23] are available commercially.

SURFACE ELECTROMYOGRAPHIC FEEDBACK AND NEUROMUSCULAR REEDUCATION

These protocols place dynamic SEMG feedback training into an active neuromuscular training paradigm. Once specific deficits are noted from the assessment, these deficits may be addressed by working with the muscle itself as well as with the central nervous system. This therapy guides the efforts of the practitioner and patient in the restoration of muscle function.

Unfortunately, the dynamic SEMG can go awry in many ways. The assessment issues of amplitude, recovery, symmetry, timing, cocontraction, agonist/antagonist/synergy, and rest are explored in Chapter 8. During treatment, it may be necessary to address any of these elements within the context of a full physical, postural, emotional, and dynamic movement perspective.

Some of the strategies associated with neuromuscular reeducation are reviewed in this section. Specific treatment approaches to the various syndromes detailed in Chapter 8 are developed in depth in *Clinical Applications in Surface Electromyography* by Kasman, Cram, and Wolf.[24] The descriptions given here are intended to introduce readers to some of the general clinical concepts associated with the use of SEMG for treatment.

Correction of Simple Postural Dysfunctions

As noted earlier, posture makes movement possible. Thus, dynamic movement patterns are frequently improved as a function of postural change. The practitioner, therefore, must consider posture and postural correction as part of any dynamically oriented work. Once a postural dysfunction is noted, it is best approached by placing the SEMG electrodes over the postural muscles of interest and assisting the patient in finding his or her way into the "correct" posture. If muscle shortness somewhere in the musculoskeletal system limits the individual's ability to attain the correct posture, stretching is necessary. If muscle weakness prevents the patient from attaining or maintaining the correct posture, strengthening exercises are in order.

Middaugh and colleagues[25] have presented a chapter on problems associated with the neck and shoulder region. Monitoring from the upper trapezius and suboccipital sites, they have demonstrated that a head-forward posture is associated with increased activation of the upper trapezius muscle group. In addition, they have demonstrated that this issue is frequently normalized when the head is placed in proper alignment above the shoulders. These authors commonly use the suboccipital muscle as a feedback site for uptraining the endurance of these muscles, so as to facilitate the normal posture of the head. Because placement of electrodes into the hairline is difficult, temporal mastoid placement (found in the

atlas in Part III) with specific reference to the cervical site location is recommended.

Once these electrodes are in place, the therapist instructs the patient how to retract the head back over the neck ("turkey tuck") while observing the SEMG recruitment pattern. A strong burst of activity should be noted during the tuck, followed by a return to prior resting tone. A 10-second recruitment followed by a 50-second rest, with five repetitions, is a good starting place and provides a basis for an easy home program to follow between visits.

Surface Electromyographic-Guided Stretching

A reeducation program might require stretching shortened muscles before they can be retrained. Stretching can be done with or without instrumentation. Clinical books on the topic have been written by Travell and Simmons,[26] McKenzie,[27] and Lewit,[28] along with a book for laypersons authored by Andersen.[29]

Practitioners who work with patients who have cervical or upper quarter pain may notice restrictions in movement in one or more planes. Such restrictions are commonly associated with exaggerated stretch reflexes during demonstration of the active and passive range of motion. These exaggerated stretch reflexes may impede progress when uptraining a normal recruitment pattern. When the practitioner uses SEMG feedback during stretching, the goal is to teach the patient to place the muscle on stretch while keeping the stretch receptor drive on the alpha motor system as low as possible (i.e., at an RMS level as low as possible). In this way, the practitioner maximizes the patient's ability to quiet the gamma motor system, allowing it to recalibrate to a lower level of activity while simultaneously lowering the stretch receptor threshold.

To use SEMG as part of a stretching program, the practitioner should place electrodes over the muscle that he or she plans to stretch. Then, the practitioner should ask the patient to place that muscle gently on stretch, moving to lengthen it. Many times, these stretches are guided by gravity; at other times, they are assisted by the patient. The patient should stay in the stretched position for at least 20 to 60 seconds. During this time, the patient should breathe into the stretch (i.e., take a deep breath) and then relax into the stretch for at least three respiration cycles. The practitioner should suggest that with each breath, the patient should relax more completely into the stretch. The SEMG feedback should guide the patient to lower the levels of SEMG activity associated with each breath into the stretch. Audio feedback is extremely helpful in this regard, because it allows the patient to hear the amplitude of the muscle activity without looking at a screen. If an audio threshold is available, the practitioner could systematically shape increasingly lower levels of SEMG activity by gradually changing the threshold to lower levels of SEMG. The goal is to be able to go to full range of motion passively, without causing SEMG activity. **Figure 9–8** shows a 30-second stretch to relax for the cervical paraspinals. Notice how they began with a mild asymmetry. By the end of the stretch, the amplitudes are much lower and more symmetrical.

SURFACE ELECTROMYOGRAPHIC FEEDBACK: DEVELOPMENT OF RECRUITMENT AND TIMING SYNERGIES

Once a recruitment pattern is noted for abnormalities in amplitude or timing and the practitioner has a sense of why the recruitment is abnormal, he or she may choose to *uptrain* the muscles for a correct recruitment pattern. Knowing what is normal is sometimes tricky; this knowledge develops from hours of clinical experience. The practitioner must also consider which muscles to monitor under which movement conditions. Although the tracings given in the electrode atlas provide a basis for such knowledge, the practitioner should remember that the atlas provides only a limited set of examples of possible recruitment patterns and is not intended to be exhaustive. Practitioners are encouraged to use their own knowledge of the neuromuscular system to explore SEMG and movement.

Isolation Training

The uptraining process is a matter of working on quality—rather than quantity—of the recruitment pattern. Uptraining typically begins by teaching the patient to isolate a particular muscle group. If the abnormal recruitment pattern features one muscle group that is literally not pulling its weight, SEMG feedback would be directed toward bringing that muscle group back online. Commonly, this disorder is observed as a cocontraction pattern during an attempted effort to activate a specific muscle. As can be seen in **Figure 9–9**, the patient is able to recruit and isolate the right lower trapezius readily, but the attempt to isolate the recruitment of the left lower trapezius is met with low levels of recruitment on the left and a cocontraction on the right.

Consider a case where the lower trapezius is severely inhibited during simple abduction of the arms to 90 degrees, while the upper trapezius overrecruits during the same movement (see Figure 9–9). The SEMG uptraining is directed toward the lower trapezius muscles. During training, the practitioner should pay attention to the posture of the rib cage and suggest that the patient lift the sternum if he or she is slouching. The patient is then asked to isolate the recruitment of only the left aspect of

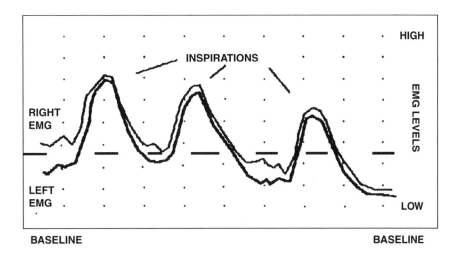

Figure 9–8 Surface EMG recordings from the right and left C-4 paraspinals as the patient breathes into the stretch.
Source: Copyright © 1990, J. R. Cram, *Clinical EMG for Surface Recordings: Volume 2*, Clinical Resources, Inc.

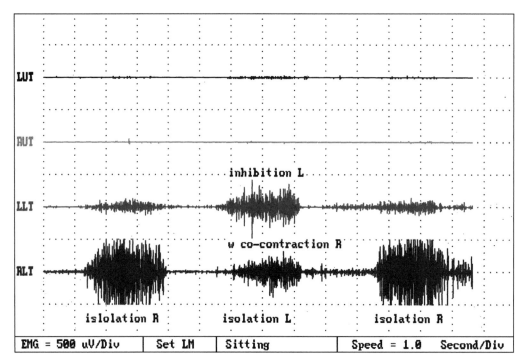

Figure 9–9 Surface EMG recordings from lower trapezius during an attempted isolated recruitment of the right and left muscles. Note the cocontraction present during the attempted recruitment of the left lower trapezius.

Source: Courtesy of Will Taylor, Portland, Oregon.

the lower trapezius. The practitioner instructs the patient on how best to attempt to recruit this muscle using isometric muscle-testing protocols. In this case, the patient is asked to press the elbow either into the palm of the therapist or the arm of the chair.

The patient must create just enough effort in the right lower trapezius to show a small burst pattern on the screen, but only for the left trapezius. There should be no overflow recruitment to the left lower trapezius or either upper trapezius muscle (see **Figure 9–10**). If the patient puts out a muscular effort for the left lower trapezius that begins to recruit other muscles, the patient is encouraged to cease the muscular effort at the time when the other muscle site(s) become active. As the patient gets better at isolating the particular muscle, he or she is asked to increase gradually and sustain the amplitude of the isolated recruitment. If at any time a spillover of recruitment to other sites occurs as the patient increases the amplitude, he or she is asked to cease the muscular effort (see **Figure 9–11**).

As a general strategy, Donaldson's 10-50-5 model (10 seconds of activation, followed by 50 seconds of rest, for 5 repetitions) of training is used.[30] As the patient improves at managing the left aspect of the lower trapezius,

he or she is asked to do the same for the right aspect. Placing a template of the desired movement up on the screen for the patient to copy with his or her own muscular efforts may accelerate acquisition of the desired recruitment pattern.[31] Sometimes this learning can be fostered by having patients do the recruitment pattern on the side where they have already learned the desired pattern, followed by the other side. The memory from the learned side can serve as the template.

Discrimination Training

Once the patient has demonstrated an ability to recruit the desired muscle while being guided by the visual or audio feedback associated with the SEMG recording, the practitioner must help the patient transfer the guidance to proprioceptive cues. The practitioner can ask the patient to close his or her eyes, conduct the isometric contraction, and then open the eyes and peek out at the results. By doing so, the patient begins to transfer the isolation skills to his or her own internal sensations. Variations on this process can also be useful in scaling. Here, the practitioner asks the patient to practice producing first 100

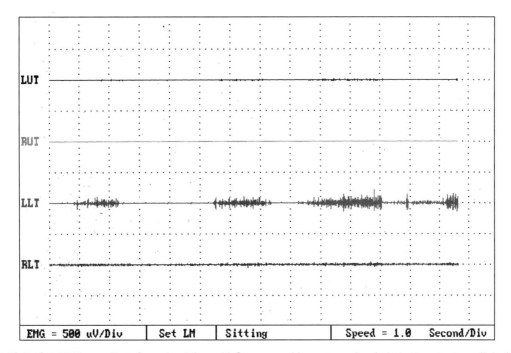

Figure 9–10 Surface EMG recordings from the right and left upper and lower trapezius during attempts at small, isolated efforts for the left lower trapezius.

Source: Courtesy of Will Taylor, Portland, Oregon.

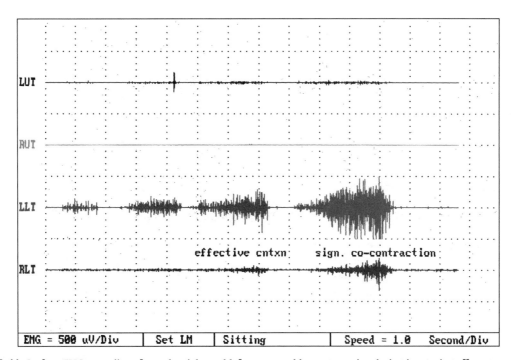

Figure 9–11 Surface EMG recordings from the right and left upper and lower trapezius during increasing efforts to recruit and isolate the left lower trapezius. Note that by the fourth attempted recruitment, the patient begins to cocontract the right trapezius along with the left.

Source: Courtesy of Will Taylor, Portland, Oregon.

microvolts of recruitment, then 50 microvolts, and finally 25 microvolts. After the patient practices, the peeking exercise is instituted again. But now, the patient relies on proprioceptive cues for whether a muscle is activated and for much recruitment. In the case of lower trapezius isolation, both the right and left aspects of the lower trapezius muscles are passed through this discrimination task.

Coordinated Recruitment

Once the lower trapezius muscles are isolated using isometric contractions, the patient is asked to engage them during the coordinated dynamic movement of abduction. Remember, the targeted SEMG goal is to recruit the lower trapezius along with the upper trapezius during abduction of the arms. Therefore, the patient is asked to initiate the abduction of the arms, with an intentional effort to engage the lower trapezius area. If the upper trapezius muscles come to grossly dominate during the movement, the abduction movement is stopped at less than 90 degrees and the arms are returned to the sides. The patient's recruitment pattern is gradually shaped across successive attempts at abduction using this technique, until there is a relatively balanced activation of the upper and lower trapezius muscles during 90 degrees of this movement. This may entail having the patient raise the rib cage with a sternal lift prior to attempting the movement, or it might simply involve suggesting that the patient activate the lower trapezius muscles prior to initiating the movement. Again, it is helpful to provide computer screen templates for the patient to copy using his or her own muscular efforts.

Functional/Daily Activities

The patient's newly acquired ability is next tested in both the sitting and standing postures. It is very important to begin the process of generalizing the newly learned recruitment pattern to varied environments and tasks. Forward flexion of the arms may be studied as well. Here, the serratus anterior is monitored along with the lower trapezius, since the serratus anterior muscle is better known for scapular stabilization during forward flexion of the arms. It is important to consider the work environment of the individual and to test for the generalization of appropriate lower trapezius activity in the various postures and activities associated with the patient's work.

AN EXAMPLE INVOLVING THE CERVICAL MUSCLES

Let's now examine a second example. In this case, a co-contraction is noted during rotation of the head to the left (see **Figure 9–12**). After some trigger-point work and stretching exercises, uptraining is initiated. Uptraining begins by teaching the patient to isolate the sternocleidomastoid muscle that shows the lowest peak amplitude. In this case, the right sternocleidomastoid underrecruits during left rotation, so the SEMG-guided uptraining is directed at that side. The easiest way to isolate the right sternocleidomastoid is to have the patient rotate the head to the left. To augment this recruitment, if necessary, a slight extension at the end of the rotation to the left can be added. Through instructed movement strategies along with SEMG feedback, the patient is taught to isolate and activate the right sternocleidomastoid. Once the patient can selectively recruit the left sternocleidomastoid, he or she is asked to activate the muscle for approximately 10 seconds, then to rest for 50 seconds; the patient does five repetitions of the movement. The patient is asked to continue with this exercise regimen three times a day at home until the next office visit. The same protocol is used during the second visit. By the third visit, the patient should be able to engage in axial rotation without a cocontraction in the recruitment pattern (see **Figure 9–13**).

Once the desired recruitment pattern is achieved, the patient attempts to generalize it. The practitioner should note whether the recruitment is symmetrical in both the sitting and standing postures, and observe what the symmetry is like during other activities of daily living such as reading, washing the dishes, or activities related to work.

SUMMARY FOR UPTRAINING

All uptraining protocols have several elements in common. First, postural and stretching considerations usually occur prior to or at the beginning of treatment. Second, uptraining begins with isolation training. Such training usually involves small, isometric contractions that attempt to avoid inappropriate recruitment of other muscles during the isolation. One may need to start with smaller movements and recruitment patterns and gradually increase the strength of the contraction. Motor copy strategies seem to accelerate the learning process. As isolation training becomes successful, the

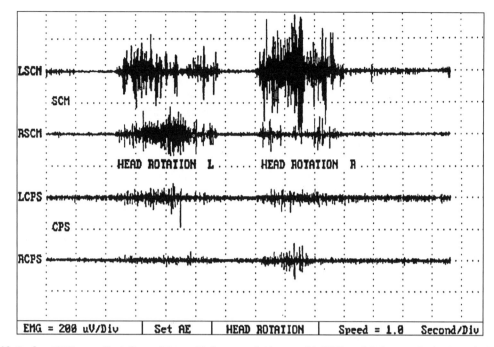

Figure 9–12 Surface EMG recordings from right and left sternocleidomastoid (SCM) and C-4 paraspinals (CPS) during rotation of the head prior to treatment. Note the cocontraction that occurs during rotation to the left.

Source: Reprinted with permission from Donaldson et al., *Electromyography, Trigger Points and Myofascial Syndromes,* © 1991, Behavioral Health Consultants.

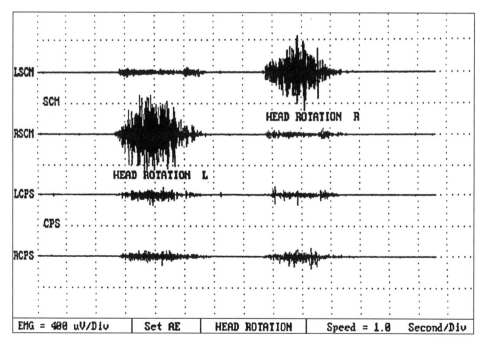

Figure 9–13 Normal SEMG recordings from right and left sternocleidomastoid (SCM) and C-4 paraspinals (CPS) during rotation of the head following three treatment sessions.

Source: Reprinted with permission from Donaldson et al., *Electromyography, Trigger Points and Myofascial Syndromes,* © 1991, Behavioral Health Consultants.

movement pattern is taken from the isometric contraction to a coordinated dynamic movement. Third, generalization is facilitated by exploring the movement during different postures and during activities of daily living.

PELVIC FLOOR CONSIDERATIONS

Weakness and noise in the pelvic floor are thought to play a substantial role in incontinence and pelvic pain. A recent report from the U.S. Department of Health and Human Services Agency for Health Care Policy and Research[32] on urinary incontinence recommends that behavioral approaches, such as biofeedback, be attempted before surgical or other invasive procedures are considered as treatment options. For an excellent review of the issue of incontinence, see an article by Tries[33]; for the premier article on the treatment of pelvic pain, see the 1995 article by Glazer, Rodke, Swencionis, Hertz, and Young.[34]

Surface EMG biofeedback procedures alone are not sufficient to treat incontinence. Diet and lifestyle must be considered, and a bowel and bladder monitoring program must be put into place. Vulvodynia cannot be approached without the appropriate concurrent medical treatment of the disorder. The cornerstone to SEMG treatment of both disorders is training in isolating, strengthening, and controlling the pelvic floor muscles. Arnold Kegel recognized this relatonship in the 1940s when he introduced the Kegel exercises. What biofeedback adds to the Kegel exercises is the specificity of training effects. With Kegel exercises, the patient may inadvertently contract other muscles (such as the abdominals, buttocks, or thighs), leading to greater levels of fatigue and inappropriate pressure on the bladder itself. Through the use of feedback and trial-and-error learning, the patient quickly learns to isolate the pelvic floor muscles. Simultaneous monitoring of the abdominal muscles (or other muscles) can help shape the appropriate use of pelvic floor muscles. With this approach, the

patient is instructed to contract the pelvic floor muscles but to stop the effort when the ancillary muscles (i.e., abdominals) recruit as well.

The methods for assessing the pelvic floor, which are discussed in Chapters 8 and 13, may now be used to treat it as well. Treatment usually begins by teaching the patient to do "flicks." The patient is instructed to engage in short, strong contractions, resting briefly between each action. These efforts continue until there are signs of fatigue (reduced amplitude) or the recruitment spills over into ancillary muscles. Once this happens, a longer rest period is given and a different contraction strategy is initiated. The patient is encouraged to practice these finely tuned flicks or Kegel exercises frequently throughout the day. They are extremely useful in helping the patient to reduce stress incontinence associated with exertional efforts.

Endurance training comes next. This is done with submaximal contractions held for increasing periods of time (e.g., a 50% maximum voluntary isometric contraction starting at 10 seconds and working up to 30 seconds and finally to 60 seconds). These endurance exercises truly strengthen the support of the pelvic floor.

Next, the cycle of recruitment and derecruitment is practiced repetitively and rapidly. The patient can even attempt 1-second flicks, making certain that the SEMG quiets down following each effort. In a variant on this approach, the practitioner instructs the patient to tense and release slowly over a 10-second period of time. The goal is to increase the patient's awareness of the pelvic floor muscles, while strengthening them and bringing the muscles more and more under the patient's control. The total SEMG feedback training time is usually about 15 minutes. Additional session time is needed to review the bowel and bladder diaries and to provide education concerning nutrition and lifestyle choices. Office visits for further training are typically carried out every 7 to 10 days, and many incontinent patients are "cured" by the third visit. Others need more time. Pelvic pain patients are typically offered approximately six SEMG feedback sessions.[34]

REFERENCES

1. Cram JR, Freeman C. Specificity in EMG biofeedback treatment of chronic pain patients. *Clin Biofeedback Health.* 1985;8:106–119.
2. Walters D. *The 14 Steps to Higher Awareness.* Nevada City, CA: Crystal Clarity; 1985.
3. Jacobson E. *You Must Relax.* New York, NY: McGraw-Hill; 1976.
4. Luthe W, Schultz JH. *Volume 1: Autogenic Methods.* In: Luthe W, ed. *Autogenic Therapy.* New York, NY: Grune & Stratton; 1969.
5. Luthe W. *Volume IV: Research and Theory.* In: Luthe W, ed. *Autogenic Therapy.* New York, NY: Grune & Stratton; 1969.
6. Wolpe J. *The Practice of Behavior Therapy.* Elmsford, NY: Pergamon Press; 1973.

7. Whatmore G. *The Physiopathology and Treatment of Functional Disorders.* New York, NY: Grune & Stratton; 1974.

8. Miller E. *Source Cassettes.* Stanford, CA: Source Cassettes; 1989.

9. Bennett H. *Preparation for Surgery* [audiotape]. Nevada City, CA: Patient Comfort Incorporated; 1995.

10. Thomas A. *The Psycho-Physical Assessment.* Nevada City, CA: Clinical Resources; 1993.

11. Barton B. *Relax to Sleep* [audiotape]. San Francisco: Crystal Clear Productions; 1994.

12. Miller E. *Changing the Channel on Pain* [audio cassette]. Stanford, CA: Source Cassettes; 1989.

13. Bennett HL, Disbrow E. Preparation for surgery and medical procedures. In: Golman D, Gurin J, ed. *Mind Body Medicine.* New York, NY: Consumer Reports Books; 1994:401–428.

14. Disbrow EA, Bennett HL, Owings JT. Effects of preoperative suggestion on postoperative gastrointestinal motility. *West J Med.* 1993;158:488–492.

15. Barber TX. Changing "unchangeable" bodily processes by (hypnotic) suggestions: a new look at hypnosis, cognitions, imagining and the mind–body problem. In: Sheikh AA, ed. *Imagination and Healing.* Amityville, NY; Baywood; 1984.

16. Fried R. *The Breath Connection.* New York, NY: Plenum; 1990.

17. Rama S, Ballentine R, Hymes A. *The Science of Breath.* Honsdale, PA: Himalayan Institute; 1990.

18. Alexander AB, Smith DD. Clinical applications of EMG biofeedback. In: Gatchel RJ, Price KR, eds. *Clinical Applications of Biofeedback: Appraisal and Status.* New York, NY: Pergamon; 1979.

19. Suarez A, Kohlenberg R, Pagano R. Is EMG activity from the frontalis site a good measure of general bodily tension in clinical populations? *Biofeedback Self Regul.* 1979;4:293–297.

20. Ettare D, Ettare R. Muscle learning therapy: a treatment protocol. In: Cram JR, ed. *Clinical EMG for Surface Recordings, II.* Nevada City, CA: Clinical Resources; 1990:197–234.

21. Feldenkrais M. *Body and Mature Behavior: A Study of Anxiety, Sex, Gravitation and Learning.* New York, NY: International University Press; 1950.

22. Zemach-Berson D, Zemach-Berson K, Reese M. *Relaxercise.* San Francisco, CA: Harper; 1990.

23. Reese M, Zemach-Berson D. *Relaxercise* [audiotape]. Berkeley, CA: Sensory Motor Learning Systems; 1986.

24. Kasman G, Cram J, Wolf S. *Clinical Applications in Surface Electromyography.* Gaithersburg, MD: Aspen; 1997.

25. Middaugh SJ, Kee WG, Nicholson JA. Muscle overuse and posture as factors in the development and maintenance of chronic musculoskeletal pain. In: Grzesiak RC, Ciccone DS, eds. *Psychological Vulnerability to Chronic Pain.* New York, NY: Springer; 1994:55–89.

26. Travell J, Simons D. *Myofascial Pain and Dysfunction: A Trigger Point Manual, I and II.* Baltimore, MD: Williams & Wilkins; 1983.

27. McKenzie R. *Treat Your Own Neck.* Low Hut, New Zealand: Spinal Publications; 1985.

28. Lewit K. *Manipulative Therapy in Rehabilitation of the Locomotor System.* Boston: Butterworth Heinemann; 1991.

29. Andersen B. *Stretching.* Bolinas, CA: Shelter Publications; 1980.

30. Donaldson S, Donaldson M. Multi-channel EMG assessment and treatment techniques. In: Cram JR, ed. *Clinical EMG for Surface Recordings, II.* Nevada City, CA: Clinical Resources; 1990:143–174.

31. Wolf S, LeCraw D, Barton L. Comparison of motor copy and targeted biofeedback training techniques for restitution of upper extremity function among patients with neurologic disorders. *Phys Ther.* 1988;69:719–735.

32. Agency for Health Care Policy and Research. *Urinary Incontinence in Adults: Clinical Practice Guidelines.* Rockville, MD: US Dept of Health and Human Services; March 1992. AHCPR pub. 92–0038.

33. Tries J. Kegel exercises enhanced by biofeedback. *J Enterosomal Ther.* 1990;17:67–76.

34. Glazer HI, Rodke G, Swencionis C, Hertz R, Young A. Treatment of vulvar vestibulitis syndrome with electromyographic biofeedback of pelvic floor musculature. *J Reprod Med.* 1995;40:283–290.

CHAPTER QUESTIONS

1. If problems are noted in more than one area of the neuromuscular system (posture, emotion, and movement), in which order should they be approached?
   a. movement, emotion, posture
   b. posture, emotion, movement
   c. emotion, posture, movement
   d. emotion, movement, posture

2. Progressive relaxation training was developed by:
   a. Jacobson
   b. Schwartz
   c. Whatmore
   d. Luthe

3. During progressive relaxation the patient is taught to:
   a. make large tension contractions followed by relaxation of the muscle

   b. make small tension contractions followed by relaxation of the muscle
   c. relax without tensing first
   d. both a and b

4. In autogenic training, which key word is associated with muscular relaxation?
   a. warmth
   b. heaviness
   c. coolness
   d. slow and regular

5. Autogenic training utilizes:
   a. passive volition
   b. active volition
   c. quiet movement
   d. guided imagery

6. Guided imagery is a form of:
   a. self-hypnosis
   b. inner child work
   c. self-actualization
   d. self-analysis

7. During breath work, which goal would the patient have for the scalene muscles?
   a. increase their participation in quiet breathing
   b. decrease their participation in quiet breathing
   c. use them to help breathe into the chest
   c. use them to help breathe into the abdomen

8. What can be said concerning the generalization of relaxation effects?
   a. They automatically transfer from one muscle to another.
   b. They automatically transfer from one posture to another.
   c. Generalization must be cultivated to other muscles, various postures, and a variety of settings.
   d. Both a and b.

9. In muscle learning therapy, the patient is taught to:
   a. turn on specific muscle groups
   b. turn off the muscle following its use
   c. use specific muscles for real and varied life activities
   d. none of the above

10. The Feldenkrais Method teaches the patient how to recruit muscles in their normal fashion. Which of the following is not one of the keys to teaching this concept?
    a. make large movements
    b. move slowly
    c. rest between movements
    d. reduce unnecessary movements

11. In treating simple postural dysfunctions, the practitioner may need to:
    a. teach correct postural alignment
    b. strengthen weakened muscle
    c. stretch shortened muscles
    d. all of the above

12. To use stretching effectively, one should go out onto stretch for a minimum of:
    a. 2 seconds
    b. 5 seconds
    c. 20 to 60 seconds
    d. It really doesn't matter how long you stretch as long as you can feel the stretch.

13. Isolation training is used to:
    a. teach the patient how to turn on a specific muscle
    b. reduce the activity of a specific muscle
    c. reduce the range of motion of a joint segment
    d. quiet the mind

14. Discrimination training refers to:
    a. being able to know which muscles are working
    b. being able to know whether a muscle has been activated
    c. being able to discern large recruitment amplitudes from small recruitment amplitudes
    d. both a and b
    e. a, b, and c

15. Donaldson's 10-50-5 rule pertains to:
    a. the number of repetitions of a recruitment sequence
    b. the amount of time spent on a series of three recruitments
    c. 10 seconds of contraction, followed by a 50-second rest, over 5 repetitions
    d. none of the above

16. Uptraining refers to:
    a. learning to stand in an upright posture
    b. learning how to uplift one's emotions
    c. learning to isolate and activate a specific muscle group
    d. learning how to lift up the arm during abduction

17. Surface EMG feedback to the pelvic floor is useful in the treatment of:
    a. urinary incontinence
    b. fecal incontinence
    c. vulvodynia
    d. all of the above
    e. both a and b

18. The SEMG assessment procedures commonly used to assess incontinence may also be used to treat incontinence.
    a. true
    b. false
    c. true for fecal incontinence only
    d. true for vulvodynia only

CHAPTER

10

Documentation

Clinical documentation is vitally important, for it allows practitioners to know what has been done. It provides a basis for analysis and the sharing of information with others, it allows for replication and comparison during future visits, and, in many cases, it provides the basis for insurance reimbursement. Documentation can be broken into basic elements, which meet the medical–legal requirements, and supplementary elements, which are essential for research purposes or would be nice to document if time permits.

BASIC DOCUMENTATION

Documentation must cover at last four main items. A few years back, these elements were referred to as SOAP: subjective, objective, assessment, and planning information.

The first layer of information represents the subjective—the self-report of the patient or the general status of the patient. The practitioner's records should reflect how treatments are affecting the patient. A practitioner who is primarily treating pain, for example, should consider having the patient rate the pain on a scale of 1 to 10 for each visit, and the practitioner should chart the patient's progress in mitigating this pain.

The second layer of information represents objective information. Surface electromyography (SEMG) provides a very powerful set of objective information to share with others. However, detailed information re-garding the clinical procedure should be given, so that a similarly trained individual could take a practitioner's notes and replicate the electrode setup and training procedure. If practitioners are using standard electrode placements, such as the ones listed in the atlas of this book, giving the muscle site name should be sufficient. If standard electrode placements are used, this convention should be documented in a policy and procedures manual for the Joint Commission on Accreditation of Healthcare Organizations, the Center for Accreditation of Rehabilitation Facilities, other accrediting agencies, and general liability coverage purposes. It is preferable to state interelectrode distance if the practitioner has the option to use more than one set of interelectrode distances. If the SEMG instrument supports more than one band pass filter, it is essential to specify which one is used. Even if the band pass filter is fixed, incorporating this specification into the report provides the basis for other electromyographers to interpret findings correctly.

Once the electrodes are in place, the record of the SEMG study should be preserved. This information can take the form of analogue tracings (strip charts/screen dumps) or digital representations of the data (e.g., mean, standard deviation). Both graphic displays and digital representations should give some indication about the form of signal processing, such as "root mean square microvolts" (μV RMS), integral average (μV/sec), or microvolts peak-to-peak (μV pp). Analog graphs should contain information

163

concerning the sensitivity of the graph (scale), along with the sweep speed. In more sophisticated reporting, a normalization procedure is commonly used. In this protocol, the type and conditions under which the reference contractions were collected must be specified.

The next layer of information refers to the practitioner's assessment of the patient's information. Clinical diagnoses (or changes in diagnosis that have occurred over the course of treatment) are helpful. Comments about what works for the person and what does not can help to remind practitioners which treatments have been tried previously. Information about obstacles to improvement is also very important. The motivational attitude of the patient may be useful in understanding compliance issues. Some patients overdo it, while others do not give maximum effort.

The last layer of information refers to the practitioner's treatment plan. Given all of the preceding information, where does the practitioner plan to go next? This information may help the related staff to provide continuity in care of the patient.

ASSESSMENT CONSIDERATIONS

Documentation associated with assessment typically includes a finer level of detail than documentation associated with treatment. As the assessment protocol unfolds, some descriptions regarding its findings might include the following considerations:

- Posture of the body/position of the limb
- Resting baseline values
- Movement peak amplitude attained
- Rate of change from baseline to peak (fast, slow, smooth, jagged)
- Recovery from movement
  —Postmovement baseline levels
  —Rate of recovery (fast, slow, "descending" notch)
- Concentric versus eccentric phase of the recruitment pattern (amplitude comparisons)
- Isometric contractions
- Comparison of one channel of activity to another*

---

*These comparisons may be made for homologous muscle groups with confidence. However, comparison between different muscle groups may be problematic because of a number of anatomical features, such as area of muscle bulk. Such comparisons should be made with caution. They are best done in muscles where the magnitude of relationships is already known—such as upper to lower trapezius or vastus medialis oblique to vastus lateralis. Normalized comparisons, of course, are preferred.

—Appropriate isolated muscle activity without cocontractions for asymmetrical movements
—Appropriate cocontraction for symmetrical movements
—Appropriate activation and timing of agonist/antagonist groups for joint stabilization
—Relative signal magnitude at peaks during range of motion
—Relative timing of recruitment/derecruitment during the eccentric and concentric phases of the movement
- Interpretation of the findings
  —Magnitude
    1. Insufficient magnitude (inhibited/hypoactive) relative to the task or in relation to other synergists
    2. Excessive magnitude (hyperactive) relative to the task or in relation to other synergists
  —Timing
    1. Delayed onset required for the movement
    2. Premature onset for the required movement
    3. Excessive duration for the particular phase of the movement
- Recommendation for further assessment or treatment

Comparisons may be made between homologous recording sites from the involved versus uninvolved sides, or between a site and the normal template for that movement at that site (if available), or integrated and digitalized information may be compared to normative data. Using the protocol developed by Donaldson and Donaldson,[1] movement patterns should be conducted for at least three repetitions to ascertain stability. Typically, the first movement pattern is tossed out because it is frequently dissimilar to the other two repetitions. The third movement is usually kept because it is the most stable.

A sample text for **Figure 10–1** might read like this:

Nancy Smith. 36 years old. Female. Dx: Upper quarter pain.

The patient presents with complaints of upper quarter pain (7 on 10-point scale), which is exacerbated with use of the left upper extremity. Recordings from upper, middle, and lower trapezius along with serratus anterior were taken during a simple shoulder elevation and release (see Scan 8). Initial baselines were observed to be within normal limits. Shoulder elevations show fairly equal

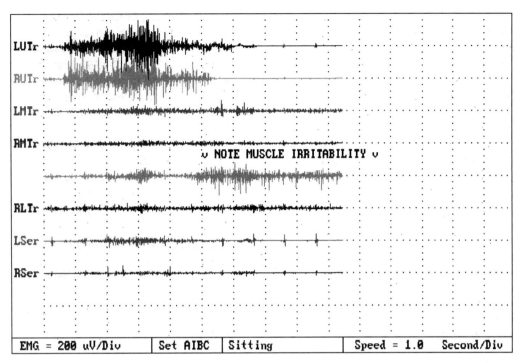

Figure 10–1 Surface EMG recording from upper trapezius, middle trapezius, lower trapezius, and serratus anterior during shoulder elevation. Note the muscle irritability that emerges following the shoulder elevation.

Source: Copyright © Clinical Resources, Inc.

symmetry, with some slowness to derecruit at the cessation of the movement, more on the left than the right. Left recruitment greater than right for lower trapezius and serratus anterior during shoulder elevation. Left lower trapezius shows spontaneous recruitment and irritability postmovement. Irritability suggests possible trigger point involvement. Assess and treat potential trigger point at next visit. Work on recovery training of SEMG.

A sample text for assessing abduction of the arms, while monitoring upper and lower trapezius, might read something like this:

Nancy Smith. 36 years old. Female. Dx: Headache and neck pain.

The patient presents with headache (4 on 10-point scale) and neck pain (5 on 10-point scale). Recordings from upper and lower trapezius were taken during abduction of the arms to 90 degrees. Resting baselines were low and symmetrical, around 2 to 3 μV RMS. Peak values were symmetrical but showed upper trapezius muscles to be 2× that of lower trapezius (20 μV versus 10 μV). Lower

trapezius muscles appear to be hypoactive or inhibited, placing additional mechanical loads on the neck. Headache probably secondary to neck-related problems. Upper quarter SEMG training protocol indicated.

Some cases are more complicated. The case presented next would be greatly enhanced if the physical exam preceded the SEMG finding and if examination results were integrated into the interpretations and recommendations.

Nancy Jones. 37 years old. Female. Dx: Left upper quarter pain.

The patient presents with upper quarter pain, primarily on the left (8 on 10-point scale). Pain made worse with upper extremity work. Palpation exam indicates active trigger points at T-1. Head, neck, and shoulder posture fairly normal. Manual muscle testing indicates normal strength in cervical and upper trapezius muscles. Recordings from upper and lower trapezius were recorded during abduction and forward flexion of the arms to 90 degrees. Resting baselines show the right upper trapezius as mildly elevated (7.2 μV RMS), with all others within normal limits. During forward flexion, synergy pattern is within normal limits. During abduction, however, right upper trapezius is nearly 2× more active (45 μV RMS peak) compared to the left upper trapezius (25 RMS μV peak). Both lower trapezius muscles were inhibited, with the left lower being more severely inhibited (2.5 μV RMS peak) than the right lower trapezius (12.5 μV RMS peak). During unilateral abduction, the right upper recruits for both left and right movements. This suggests a protective guarding pattern noted on the right, along with dyssynergy between upper and lower trapezius muscles, especially on the left. Left lower trapezius inhibited/hypoactive. Recommend neuromuscular retraining for shoulder muscles, with particular emphasis on uptraining the left lower trapezius.

TREATMENT CONSIDERATIONS

When SEMG is used as part of a biofeedback or neuromuscular reeducation program, it is very important to document the sites of electrode placement, thereby enabling replication of this placement during future visits. This is particularly true if the practitioner wants to compare the same sites over sessions. For consistent electrode placement, the practitioner should consider use of some of the following elements: standard electrode sites (see Part III), reference of anatomical landmarks, anatomical templates, or indelible marker.

Uptraining Considerations

Because the goal of uptraining is to maximize muscle output, the practitioner should note the highest microvolt level attainable without feedback. Then the practitioner should document the highest level of microvolt output observed during feedback. Sometimes as a variation, the average peak value for a training session is reported. If a threshold is used to provide an incentive for increasing the peak contraction, record either this threshold or the percentage of time the patient reached and exceeded the threshold. Because the initial resting length of muscle or the posture associated with training can enhance or inhibit one's ability to recruit a muscle, these parameters should be noted. If resting values are an issue, the effects of uptraining on resting values should be noted during a postbaseline period.

Following is an example of a brief chart note:

Nancy Jones

Visit 2. Patient reports pain levels are about the same. Uptraining/isolation training of lower trapezius conducted using standard upper and lower trapezius electrode placements and the wide (25–1000 Hz) filter during the seated posture. Initial resting levels (RMS (V) were RUTr = 7.9, LUTr = 2.5; RLTr = 1.3; LLTr = 1.5. Initial isometric peak contraction of RLTr = 9.2; LLTr = 2.6. Discrimination with eyes closed utilized. Ending isometric peak contraction RLTr = 14.7; LLTr = 7.9. Resting baseline at end of session for RUTr = 3.3. Intervention appears to bring a better balance to muscle synergies. Patient instructed to practice lower trapezius recruitment using 10-50-5 rule, three times a day. Continue isolation training on next visit.

Relaxation or Downtraining Considerations

The goal of downtraining is to minimize the SEMG output using relaxation protocols (i.e., progressive relaxation, autogenics) or quiet movements (i.e., Ettare protocol, Feldenkrais Method). Baseline levels should be recorded, along with the lowest level of SEMG activity achieved during the session. Because the ability to downtrain is acquired in a particular posture, one must attempt to generalize it to other postures through training in these alternative postures. Thus, the posture in which the training is conducted should be noted. Again, a threshold may be used to provide an incentive during training for lowering the SEMG levels. This threshold is usually lowered across time to help shape the desired behavior. If this feature is used, the threshold level should be recorded along with the percentage of time the patient spends below that threshold.

A sample progress note is presented here:

Randy Greene

Visit 3. Patient reports that the headache is slightly improved (4 on 10-point scale). Has practiced relaxation at home 3 times since last visit. R and L wide cervical trapezius placement used. Relaxation-based therapy offered using autogenics heavy/warm to arms. Initial baseline R = 17, L = 12. Postbaseline R = 7.3, L = 5.3. Nice in-session response to autogenic therapy. Home-training exercises given with handout. Plan: Check on transfer of initial baseline, deepen relaxation abilities.

DOCUMENTATION AS AN OUTCOME MEASURE

Surface EMG may be used as an outcome measure for other treatment modalities. With this approach, SEMG baselines are collected in relevant postures and/or during functional movement patterns, prior to and following the alternative therapies (e.g., mobilization). Such recordings may help to document the therapeutic effects of the alternative therapy and provide a basis for continuing or discontinuing a particular therapy.

RELATIONSHIP OF SURFACE ELECTROMYOGRAPHY TO OTHER MEASURES

Surface EMG information should be related to other forms of clinical information, such as pain, manual muscle testing, range of motion, isolated joint control, and other indexes of function. If the patient is taking medications that might interact with the treatment, these should be noted. These medications include, but are not limited to, muscle relaxants, tranquilizers, some analgesics, central nervous system depressants, and antispasticity agents.

COMPREHENSIVE LIST OF ELEMENTS TO DOCUMENT

This secton provides a comprehensive list of the potential variables that could potentially affect SEMG recordings. Depending on the setting, some variables may be more important to document than others. Attributes that are worthwhile to consider for medical–legal reasons are followed by *L*. Attributes that are considered germane to research protocols or procedures involving SEMG are followed by *R*. The research recommendations are adapted from those recommended by the International Society for Electromyography and Kinesthesiology.[2] Attributes that are considered essential for the clinical record are followed by *C*.

Recording Parameters

1. Target muscle (and use of anatomical markers if relevant) (*C, L, R*)
2. Recording electrode location, distance for anatomical markings, use of electrode locator templates or indelible markings for intersession reliability (*C, L, R*)
3. Electrode type, diameter, manufacturer, type of paste or gel used if relevant (*L, R*)
4. Interelectrode distance and orientation to muscle fibers (*C, L, R*)
5. Ground electrode placement location (*R*)
6. Instrumentation specifications: band pass filter range (*C*), site of preamplification (active electrode), notch filter, type of signal display (raw versus processed), integration times (time constants), common mode rejection ratio, input impedance, signal-to-noise ratio, time constant, type of signal processing (i.e., RMS), and sampling rate for computerized systems (*L, R*)

Patient/Task Considerations

1. Subjective impressions associated with the clinical evaluations and procedures (*C, L*)
2. Informed consent for procedure and goals of training (*C, L, R*)
3. Associated physical exam findings (*C, L*)
4. Patient positioning and movement: task, trunk/limb support, open versus closed kinetic chain, control of single versus multiple joints, movement plane (*C, L, R*)
5. Type of contraction: isometric, eccentric, concentric (*C, L, R*)
6. Joint angle (*R*)
7. Contraction intensity, load, and velocity (*R*)
8. Work: rest times, number of repetitions, exercise sets, task duration (*R*)
9. Relaxation strategy (*C, R*)
10. Threshold levels (*C, R*)

Surface Electromyography Characterization and Interpretation

1. Verification that SEMG placement records from the muscle of interest (*L, R*).
2. Verification that the clinician/scientist has attempted to document or eliminate cross-talk from neighboring muscles (*L, R*).
3. Baseline amplitude, maximum, minimum, standard deviation (*C, L, R*).
4. Peak magnitude or symmetry during a movement (*C, L, R*).

5. Average amplitude during a defined phase of cyclic movement (*C, L, R*).

6. Normalization methods (*C*) are becoming more common and are essential when the practitioner/scientist wants to compare SEMG levels across muscle groups. They are essential when one wants to quantify SEMG under dynamic conditions. They are just as important for the clinician as for the researcher. In fact, many journals do not allow authors to present dynamic SEMG data unless they are normalized. When a normalization procedure is used, it must be accompanied by a description of the conditions under which the maximum value was collected (i.e., joint angle, intensity, positioning). Several types of normalization are described in Chapter 3 and are briefly summarized here. Types a and b are the most common, but types c through f are also very practical (*L, R*).

   a. *Maximum voluntary isometric contraction.* Here the patient exerts the maximum muscular effort under isometric conditions. All SEMG values are calculated as a percentage of that value:

   (SEMG activity ÷ maximum SEMG activity) × 100
   This is highly reliable, but compliance and motivation of patients with pain to exert a maximal effort is potentially problematic.

   b. *Submaximal voluntary isometric contraction.* Here the patient is asked to exert a force against a dynamometer to a specified level. The SEMG level is then used to express all other values as a percentage of this level:

   (SEMG activity ÷ submaximal SEMG activity) × 100
   This is a more realistic benchmark for pain-related disorders.

   c. Surface EMG is defined as a *percentage of the peak magnitude* recorded during a defined dynamic movement.

   d. Surface EMG is defined as a *percentage of the average magnitude* recorded during a defined dynamic movement.

   e. Surface EMG values averaged over a defined movement sequence are expressed as a *percentage of the average* during another reference movement.

   f. Surface EMG values from homologous muscles are expressed as *a left–right percent difference*:

   (Larger side – smaller side ÷ larger side) × 100
   This may be done for resting tones or from peak contraction data. The peak conversion is commonly used in the work of Donaldson.[1]

7. *Frequency spectral analysis* has been used to monitor muscle fatigue. The initial frequency, the slope of the frequency during the exertive task, and the rate of recovery to the initial frequency are commonly measured (*R*).

ISSUES PERTAINING TO THIRD-PARTY REIMBURSEMENT

Surface EMG is generally considered to be a reimbursable procedure—simply one of the tools that the practitioner uses in his or her field. The secret to qualifying for third-party reimbursement is to use the existing codes for one's profession. For the physical medicine practitioner, the 97 series CPT code (the American Medical Association's *Current Procedural Terminology* code) is suggested. Some practitioners routinely use neuromuscular reeducation in conjunction with kinetic exercises. For mental health practitioners, the 98 series CPT code is suggested for "behavior therapy," interactive medical psychotherapy, or psychophysiologic therapy including biofeedback. Both physical medicine and psychology providers might consider using the 90901 CPT code for biofeedback. Unfortunately, this code remains somewhat controversial, even 20 years after its emergence.

Fortunately or unfortunately, depending on one's point of view, there are no specific CPT codes that pertain to the diagnostic use of SEMG. Because of this ambiguity, there was a period during which many providers used the neurological section of the CPT code, billing the SEMG procedure as if it were the functional equivalent to a needle EMG study, and charging a similar amount. Eventually, third-party carriers had these studies reviewed by their experts, all of whom were familiar with needle EMG procedures but knew very little about SEMG procedures. These reviewers stated, correctly, that SEMG procedures were not valid to study neurological conditions, and reimbursement for SEMG procedures was denied. Because of this confusion, many third-party payers began to issue guidelines to deny reimbursement for all SEMG procedures.

The clamor regarding this blurring of SEMG and needle EMG procedures led to responses from several professional organizations. In 1992, the Surface EMG Society of North America (SESNA) organized a multidisciplinary panel to produce a position paper, "Responsible Use of SEMG."[3] After studying the issues, it stated that SEMG procedures were valid for static and dynamic studies for musculoskeletal conditions, but for only 4 weeks following onset of injury.

In 1992, a commission of 35 chiropractic physicians produced what is known as the Mercy Conference Guidelines.[4] It rated static assessment procedures as "experimental," while describing dynamic procedures as "promising." To some, these guidelines appeared to be a political move to stop the abuse of submissions for static assessments.

In 1996, the American Association of Electrodiagnostic Medicine (AAEM) produced a position paper stating that there are no indications for the use of SEMG in the diagnosis and treatment of disorder of nerve or muscle.[5] The AAEM position is correct: Surface EMG is not intended to study muscle and nerve disease; this is to be done with needle EMG recordings. But what AAEM is missing is the utility of SEMG for clinical or functional diagnoses, which is where SEMG proves most valuable. Needle EMG studies for this purpose are considered to be overly invasive and a poor representative of gross and fine motor activities. In fact, when a needle EMG assessment is performed and the patient is asked to make a significant contraction, the term used for this phenomenon is *interference pattern*. Volume-conducted activity from surrounding motor units inevitably interferes with the needle electromyographer's ability to see the single motor unit—the primary area of interest. As Sihvonen, Partanin, Osmo, and Soimakalio have noted,[6] SEMG recording better describes the flexion–relaxation phenomenon in the low-back muscles than simultaneous needle EMG recordings. The needle EMG is designed to record from very specific muscle fibers and truly misses the larger picture that SEMG can see. The only case in which needle EMG performs better than SEMG in dynamic movement assessments is when the muscle of interest lies beneath other muscles. In this situation, the needle EMG could come closer to eliminating the volume conduction and cross-talk so commonly noted in SEMG. However, the needle recordings are also subject to volume-conducted activity or far-field potentials. So the political debate among the various professional groups goes on.

Providers who wish to educate the insurance industry concerning the sensitivity, specificity, and clinical efficacy of SEMG should consider all of the references for the assessment and treatment chapters. A list of the most relevant ones appears in the Suggested Readings section at the end of this chapter. An asterisk (*) appears next to the most critical readings.

REFERENCES

1. Donaldson S, Donaldson M. Multi-channel EMG assessment and treatment techniques. In: Cram JR, ed. *Clinical EMG for Surface Recordings, II.* Nevada City, CA: Clinical Resources; 1990:143–174.
2. International Society for Electromyography and Kinesthesiology. Standards for reporting EMG data. *J Electromyogr Kinesiol.* 1996;6(1):III.
3. Surface EMG Society of North America. SESNA position paper: responsible use of SEMG. *SEMG Potentials,* Summer 1992.
4. Haldeman S, Chapman-Smith D, Petersen D. *Guidelines for Chiropractic Quality Assurance and Practice Parameters:*

Proceedings of the Mercy Center Consensus Conference. Gaithersburg, MD: Aspen; 1992.
5. Haig AJ, Gelblum JB, Rechtein JJ, Gitter AJ. Technology assessment: the use of surface EMG in the diagnosis and treatment of nerve and muscle disorders. *Muscle Nerve.* 1996;19:392–395.
6. Sihvonen T, Partanin J, Osmo H, Soimakalio P. Electric behavior of low back muscles during lumbar pelvic rhythm in low back pain patients and healthy controls. *Arch Phys Med Rehab.* 1991;72:1080–1087.

SUGGESTED READINGS

Agency for Health Care Policy and Research. *Urinary Incontinence in Adults: Clinical Practice Guidelines.* Rockville, MD: Agency for Health Care Policy and Research; March 1992. U.S. Department of Health and Human Services publication AHCPR 92-0038.

*Arena JG, Sherman R, Bruno G, Young T. Temporal stability of paraspinal electromyographic recordings in low back pain and non-pain patients. *Int J Psychophysiol.* 1990;9:31–37.
Basmajian JV, DeLuca C. *Muscles Alive.* 5th ed. Baltimore, MD: Williams & Wilkins; 1985.

Bittman B, Cram JR. Surface EMG: An electrophysiological alternative in pain management. In: Weiner RS, ed. *Innovations in Pain Management: A Practical Guide for Clinicians.* St. Petersburg, FL: Deutsche Press, 1993.

*Cram JR, Engstrom D. Patterns of neuromuscular activity in pain and non-pain patients. *Clin Biofeedback Health.* 1986;9:106–116.

*Cram JR, Steger JC. Muscle scanning and the diagnosis of chronic pain. *Biofeedback Self Regul.* 1983;8:229–241.

Dolce JJ, Raczynski JM. Neuromuscular activity and electromyography in painful backs: psychological and biomechanical models in assessment and treatment. *Psychol Bull.* 1985;97:502–520.

Fishbain DA, Goldberg M, Meagher BR, Steel R, Rosomoff H. Male and female chronic pain patients categorized by DSM-II psychiatric diagnostic criteria. *Pain.* 1986;26:181–197.

*Glazer HI, Rodke G, Swencionis C, Hertz R, Young A. Treatment of vulvar vestibulitis syndrome with electromyographic biofeedback of pelvic floor musculature. *J Reprod Med.* 1995;40:283–290.

*Kessler M, Cram JR, Traue H. EMG muscle scanning in pain patients and controls: a replication and extension. *Am J Pain Manage.* 1993;3:20–28.

*Klein AB, Snyder-Mackler L, Roy S, DeLuca C. Comparison of spinal mobility and isometric trunk extensor forces with electromyographic spectral analysis in identifying low back pain. *Phys Ther.* 1991;71(6):445–453.

Leach RA, Owens EF, Giesen JM. Correlates of myoelectric asymmetry detected in low back pain patient using hand held post style surface electromyography. *J Manipulative Physiol Ther.* 1993;16:140–149.

Mathiassen SE, Winkel J, Hagg GM. Normalization of surface EMG amplitude from the upper trapezius muscle in ergonomic studies: a review. *J Electromyogr Kinesiol.* 1995;5:197–226.

*Middaugh SJ, Kee WG, Nicholson JA. Muscle overuse and posture as factors in the development and maintenance of chronic musculoskeletal pain. In: Grzesiak RC, Ciccone DS, eds. *Psychological Vulnerability to Chronic Pain.* New York, NY: Springer; 1994:55–89.

Peper E, Wilson V, Taylor W, et al. Repetitive strain injury. *Phys Ther Products.* September 1994:17–22.

Price JP, Clare MH, Ewerhardt RH. Studies in low backache with persistent spasm. *Arch Phys Med.* 1948;29:703–709.

Robinson ME, Cassisi JE, O'Connor PD, MacMillan M. Lumbar iEMG during isotonic exercise: chronic low back pain patients vs controls. *J Spinal Disord.* 1992;5:1.

*Roy SH, DeLuca CJ, Casavant DA. Lumbar muscle fatigue and chronic back pain. *Spine.* 1989;14:992–1001.

*Roy SH, DeLuca CJ, Snyder-Mackler L, et al. Fatigue, recovery and low back pain in elite rowers. *Med Sci Sports Exerc.* 1990;22:463–469.

Sherman R, Arena J. Biofeedback for assessment and treatment of low back pain. In: Basmajian JV, Wolf S, eds. *Rational Manual Therapies.* Baltimore, MD: Williams & Wilkins; 1994:177–197.

Skubick D, Clasby R, Donaldson CCS, Marshall W. Carpal tunnel syndrome as an expression of muscular dysfunction in the neck. *J Occup Rehab.* 1993;3:31–43.

Soderberg GL, ed. *Selected Topics in Surface Electromyography for Use in the Occupational Setting: Expert Perspective.* Washington DC: National Institute for Occupational Safety and Health; 1992. U.S. Department of Health and Human Services publication NIOSH 91-100.

*Triano J, Schultz AB. Correlation of objective measurement of trunk motion and muscle function with low back disability ratings. *Spine.* 1987;12:561–565.

Veiersted KB, Westgaard RH. Work related risk factors for trapezius myalgia. *Int Arch Occup Environ Health.* 1990;62:31–41.

*Veiersted KB, Westgaard RH, Andersen P. Electromyographic evaluation of muscular work pattern as a predictor of trapezius myalgia. *Scand J Work Environ Health.* 1993;19:284–290.

Wolf S, Basmajian J. Assessment of paraspinal electromyographic activity in normal subjects and chronic back pain patients using a muscle biofeedback device. In: Asmussen E, Jorgensen K, eds. *International Series on Biomechanics; VI-B.* Baltimore, MD: University Press; 1978.

Wolf S, Basmajian J, Russe C, Kutner M. Normative data on low back mobility and activity levels. *Am J Phys Med.* 1979;58:217–229.

Wolf S, LeCraw D, Barton L. Comparison of motor copy and targeted biofeedback training techniques for restitution of upper extremity function among patients with neurologic disorders. *Phys Ther.* 1988;69:719–735.

*Wolf S, Nacht M, Kelly J. EMG feedback training during dynamic movement for low back pain patients. *Behav Ther.* 1982;13:395–406.

CHAPTER QUESTIONS

1. Chart notes should include at least four basic elements. They are:
   a. name, age, Social Security number, and marital status
   b. subjective, objective, assessment, and planning information
   c. age, diagnosis, objective findings, and plan
   d. resting microvolt levels, peak microvolt levels, recovery microvolt levels, and synergy pattern

2. How does the saying "Can't see the forest for the trees" relate to electrodiagnosis?
   a. describes SEMG recordings
   b. describes needle EMG recordings
   c. none of the above

3. In functional kinesiology, needle EMG recordings are useful when:
   a. the practitioner wants to record activity from a deep muscle
   b. the practitioner wants a definitive quantification of gross motor activity
   c. both a and b
   d. none of the above

4. Surface EMG assessment procedures should be billed out as a neurological procedure.
   a. True
   b. False

Surface Electromyography: Past, Present, and Future

The History of Muscle Dysfunction and Surface Electromyography

Jeffrey R. Cram and Maya Durie

Humans have had to deal with sore muscles since the beginning of time. Initially, muscle assessments and treatments were conducted by hand; during the last century, the use of electronic instruments came into play.

To put muscle function and the clinical use of surface electromyography (SEMG) into a perspective of history, it seems prudent to utilize a broad nomothetic net, or conceptual framework. In *Clinical Applications for Surface Electromyography*, Kasman, Cram, and Wolf[1] consider chronic muscle dysfunction from a fourfold perspective: histologic (tissue-related issues); psychologic (psychophysiology and emotions), sensorimotor (movement), and mechanical dysfunction (e.g., cumulative trauma, posture). In this chapter we provide a brief historical overview related to each of these four areas. This will provide a deep background for the emergence of the clinical use of SEMG, including information on the history of body work, psychophysiology, rehabilitation, and electricity and SEMG instrumentation.

TISSUE-RELATED ISSUES

We begin with issues pertaining to the tissues of the body. The muscle, as an organ system, contains many sensory mechanisms. The muscle spindles tell the nervous system about the instantaneous length and force of contraction of segments of muscle tissue. The Golgi tendon organ measures the actual force that the muscle is exerting, and the Ruffini endings of the joints inform the nervous system of the relationship of angles of the bones. However, it is the free nerve ending within the muscle that senses local pain. And it is metabolic disturbances such as too much (lactic) acid or too much internal pressure due to swelling, congestion, or edema that activate the free nerve ending.

From a clinical point of view, up until the last two centuries, palpation and observations about movement and posture were the only tools available for assessing muscle-oriented pain. Through the manual sense of touch, the practitioner can learn to feel many things. Is the muscle tissue hard to the touch? Does it feel stiff? Does it have lumps, tough fibers, or overly firm areas, or is it

Reprinted with permission from Shannon and Heidi Cram, J. R. Cram, and M. Durie, and *Somatics Magazine*, which first published the article "The History of SEMG and Muscle Soreness" in 2003.

soft, supple, and relaxed? What do the fascia feel like? Is there a normal cranial–sacral rhythm? As the body moves passively through its range of motion, does it seem restricted, suggesting a shortened muscle resting length? During active movement, does it appear that the body is using the correct muscles for the movement, or is a substitution pattern evident? Is the patient afraid of movement because of pain? Has a trauma become lodged in the nervous system or even the muscle tissue itself? Can one see or feel problems with ligament laxities or joint fixations? These are just some of the examples of questions practitioners want to address, both by hand and by instrument. Thus, one could think of body work as a means to help normalize the disturbance of tissue that might foster and create muscle pain, and SEMG as an instrumented way of assessing some of these conditions.

Massage and touch therapy date back many thousands of years. The oldest known book to have been written about massage was from China in 3000 B.C. The Egyptians are credited with developing reflexology in 2500 B.C. The East Indian holistic health approach called Ayurveda dates back to around 1800 B.C. and includes massage techniques. The Greeks massaged their athletes prior to the Olympic Games in 776 B.C. Even Hypocrites, the father of Western medicine, used a massage technique, known as friction rub, to treat sprains and dislocations.

The most common massage approach in the Western world is Swedish massage. It had its origins in the early 1800s and was formulated by Per Heinrik Ling, who developed a repertoire of five basic massage strokes.[2] The two main purposes of Swedish massage are to induce the relaxation response in the body, which promotes the release of stress, and to improve both blood and lymph circulation, which helps the body remove toxins more efficiently. Athletes whose muscles become sore and stiff from physical exercise, overuse, or trauma, for example, routinely receive massage. The massage strokes help to relax the muscles, allowing more oxygen to flow, and assist in flushing lactic acid buildup that comes from exercise. In addition, Swedish massage strokes are used to break down adhesions that form around joints from injury, thereby increasing joint mobility.

Structural Integration—or, as it is more commonly called, Rolfing—was named after its creator, Ida Rolf, and first gained recognition in the 1960s.[3] This method is considered deep-tissue body work. It works to release the myofascial system, thereby reestablishing flexibility and ease of movement in the body. Rolf believed that gravity is the major force that shapes our posture and movement patterns. She postulated that gravity causes the body to slump forward and thus shorten muscles. The Rolf practitioner softens the fascial tissue so it can be realigned properly, allowing the force of gravity to flow through the natural vertical and horizontal planes of the body. The vertical plane is defined as an imaginary plumb line passing through the landmarks of the ear, shoulder joint, hip joint, knee, and ankle. The Rolfer, through a series of 10 body work sessions, works to realign all of the major body segments to achieve this proper vertical alignment. Rather than working on specific symptoms, the aim of Rolfing is to bring the whole body into alignment, in the process eliminating the cause of the symptoms. By softening the fascia, the body is freed from restrictions and can return to its natural relationship with gravity.

Another type of body work that focuses on the myofascial system is called Myofascial Release (MFR). This technique is most commonly associated with John Barnes,[4] a physical therapist who began developing it in the 1960s. This approach seeks to release distortions and tension in the fascia, thereby allowing the body to return to a more healthful balance. In its healthy, natural state, fascia, which spreads like a three-dimensional web throughout the body, is elastic and relaxed. The fascial system's purpose is to allow the body to absorb compressive forces to the body while protecting the position of the vital organs and retaining the body's normal shape. Through injury, stress, poor postural habits, and illness, the fascia may develop restrictions. For example, it can become hardened and tight, pulling muscles and bones out of alignment. This tightening effect can spread over time. The MFR practitioner believes that just removing restrictions in the muscles will not bring lasting results because constrictions in the fascial system will cause the muscle tension to return. The MFR technique uses long, sustained pressure along the fascial planes for at least 3–5 minutes to elongate and stretch the fascia, returning it to a gelatinous consistency. As the softening is felt, the practitioner moves the tissue in the direction of ease until the next barrier/restriction to this ease of movement is felt. This softening allows more freedom of movement and removes the pressure on nerves and restrictions to the blood supply created by the fascial hardening.

The history of muscle pain syndromes has been presented several times[5–7] and will not be repeated here. Suffice it to say that the notion of muscle-oriented pain grew out of the clinical concept of rheumatism. By the mid-1800s, writings were beginning to appear describing "tender points," or localized areas of pain within the muscle. It was not until the early part of the last century that the term "referred pain" found its way into the medical literature.[8] A little later, a physician by the name of Gutstein[9] is credited as having introduced the observation of tender spots associated with a "jump sign." A decade later, Kelly[10] described "nodules" associated with these tender points along with patterns of referred pain. By this time, the concept of a functional, reflex component to trigger points was beginning to emerge. In 1942, Janet Travell and her colleagues wrote their first paper on trigger points.[11] By 1976, Travell had authored or co-authored 38 papers on these tender/trigger points, and summarized her theory that trigger points depended on a feedback mechanism between the trigger point and the central nervous system.[12] The prevalence of the problem of trigger points was highlighted by Sola in 1955, who found that 60% of the population had latent, or inactive, trigger points. More recently, Fishbain et al.[13] noted that 85% of the patients in pain clinics had active trigger points.

Janet Travell and her colleague David Simons are probably best known for their work in this area. Their book *Myofascial Pain and Dysfunction: A Trigger Point Manual*[14] is a very scholarly work that provided the basic foundation of understanding the mechanisms behind trigger points, along with the body maps for knowing where to palpate for trigger points and diagrams of their pain distributions. The trigger point, when palpated, feels like a small pea or area of congestion, with an associated "taut band" located within the muscle. When the taut band is stimulated, it twitches; when the trigger point is pressed upon, it provides several possible responses, including the jump sign and referred pain distribution to distant locations. Trigger points may be treated or cleared by needling them with or without an anesthetic. Alternatively, they may be treated with ischemic pressure techniques used in massage therapy. In essence, trigger points within the muscle are a sign of muscle-based pain, and are associated with a disturbance in the neuromuscular system and myoelectric potentials within the muscle.

From an electrophysiological perspective, needle EMG studies of trigger points[15,16] have shown a high level of spontaneous electrical activity (SEA) at the locations of the trigger points. Hong and Simons,[17] after reviewing the research on this topic, concluded that myofascial trigger points are related to integrative mechanisms in the spinal cord that respond to sensitized nerve fibers associated with SEA and extrafusal end-plate noise activity. Another point of view is voiced by Hubbard and Berkoff,[18] who argue that the SEA emanates from the intrafusal fibers of the muscle spindle. They observed that the SEA was found only in the trigger point zone, and not a few millimeters away in adjacent extrafusal muscle tissue. The location of the SEA is very specific, and has now been termed the "nidus" of the active trigger point. In addition, Hubbard[19] clearly demonstrated that the SEA was diminished or blocked by a beta adrenergic (sympathetic) blocker (phentolamine), and not by an alpha motor blocker (curare). McNulty et al.[20] demonstrated that the SEA activity at the trigger point increased during a stress induction, while the EMG activity in the adjacent extrafusal muscle tissue did not. Earlier research on muscle spindles by Passatore et al.[21] had clearly demonstrated autonomic innervation of the muscle spindle, thereby illuminating one of the mechanisms for contraction of the intrafusal muscle fibers.

The question of whether trigger point activity can be seen using SEMG recording techniques has yet to be answered. Simons and Dexter[22] noted that the SEA seen with needle electrodes could not be observed using surface recording techniques. Donaldson et al.,[23] in contrast, found muscles containing trigger points, when studied using the dynamic SEMG procedure of flexion/extension, to be more active than previously supposed. Symptomatic muscles showed a higher peak amplitude during movement compared to asymptomatic muscles. Cram and Kasman[24] have also noted that muscles that contain trigger points tend to have a poor recovery following movement (termed postmovement irritability). Lastly, Donaldson (personal communication) has stated that SEMG biofeedback retraining techniques will be impeded if initiated before the trigger point is eradicated from the muscle. Thus, body work should precede SEMG retraining when trigger points are present.

THE PSYCHOLOGIC AND EMOTIONAL LEVEL

As Cacioppo et al.[25] state, "The skeletomotor system is the final common pathway through which humans interact with and modify their environment." This statement has very broad implications for SEMG. The emergence of psychophysiology at the turn of the last century held forth the promise of being able to study complex human behaviors such as thoughts and emotions by monitoring human physiology. Among all of the physiological systems available for study, the neuromuscular or skeletomotor system, owing to its the specificity and sophistication, provided a very strong basis for studying the nonverbal language of emotions.

While Duchenne[26] is best known for the original studies of the dynamics and functions of intact skeletal muscles, it was Charles Darwin[27] who announced a rather complex theory of overt emotional behaviors in both animals and humans. Most of his visual observations were limited to emotional displays on the face along with postural gestures. A few years later, William James[28] introduced the ideomotor theory of emotions, which placed the proprioception of facial muscle activity at the forefront of the emotional experience. Using crude measuring instruments, attempts were made at quantifying the micro-momentary displays of emotions seen on the human face. But it was not until Edmund Jacobson[29-32] conducted a series of experiments using biological amplifiers while displaying the signal on the cathode ray tube to monitor the facial muscles of his subjects that the concept truly took hold. Using this new technology, clear and convincing evidence was brought forth to show that SEMG responses were evoked by imaginal tasks (visualizations), and that these responses were very minute and highly localized. This understanding was confirmed a few years later by R. C. Davis,[33] a major researcher in psychophysiology and SEMG.

Facial displays of emotions were given additional value when Ekman et al.[34] demonstrated an almost universal quality to the recognition of emotions across cultures. Ekman and Friesen[35] provided a very powerful guide to understanding facial action patterns in their book *Unmasking the Face*. During the 1970s, detailed investigations of SEMG activity of the human face were attempted. For example, Rusalova et al.[36] used method actors and normal subjects to study the intentional display of emotions. When asked to show four emotions (anger, fear, joy, and sadness), the method actors showed consistent patterns of facial SEMG for all four emotions, while the untrained subjects were able to clearly display only joy and sadness. Gary Schwartz and his colleagues[37,38] were able to show that facial SEMG allowed the practitioner to observe "covert" emotional responses to imaginal tasks of various emotions. Interestingly, their study demonstrates one of the primary goals of psychophysiology: to see patterns of emotional responsiveness that could not be seen through usual sensory channels of information (such as seeing the emotions on the face).

Over the years, numerous studies have examined patterns of SEMG in psychiatric populations. For an excellent review of these, see the works by Thompson[39] and Goldstein.[40] As early as 1941, Reusch et al.[41] had observed that patients who reported feeling fidgety, uncomfortable, or tense showed elevations in resting forearm SEMG. Malmo et al.[42] observed the startle response in extremely anxious patients and noted a poor recovery in forearm SEMG, compared to controls. Later, Malmo et al.[43] demonstrated that psychotic and neurotic patients showed higher levels of SEMG in the forearm flexors and neck muscles, compared to controls. Of course, the history of SEMG is replete with contradictory findings. This difficulty could be seen as early as 1956, when Martin[44] failed to replicate Malmo's findings.

George Whatmore, a student of Edmund Jacobson, studied the arousal patterns of SEMG in various disorders. Whatmore and Ellis[45] found higher levels of SEMG in the forehead, jaw, forearm, and leg muscles in patients with schizophrenia as compared to normal subjects. Interestingly enough, the same type of elevated SEMG was noted in severely depressed individuals.[46] These tension levels were observed to decrease as a function of treatment of the depression, and to return prior to relapse.

Whatmore went on to study and treat a variety of disorders using SEMG measurement techniques, culminating in the book *The Physiopathology and Treatment of Functional Disorders*.[47] Here, he and Kohli present a thesis that all psychosomatic disorders are due to dysfunctional muscular efforts that they term "dysponesis," or bad muscle energy. The authors distinguish four types of muscular efforts: bracing, performing, representation, and attention. When one puts too much muscular effort into any one of these four types of efforts, physiological symptoms are thought to develop due to imbalances in the nervous system. According to Whatmore, treatment of these disorders is best conducted by teaching the patient how to reduce these dysponetic efforts. To do so, he embellished Jacobson's progressive relaxation technique[48] in 1952, by adding an analog audio tone (or feedback) driven by the SEMG signal.[47] In some ways, Whatmore should be considered to have created the first SEMG biofeedback instrument and, therefore, is the unrecognized father of SEMG biofeedback.

Eventually the "key muscle" hypothesis emerged,[49] in which the frontalis or forearm musculature was thought to be a strong indicator of overall muscle tension. Unfortunately, several studies have reported low correlations between the frontal or forearm site to other sites.[50,51] Interestingly, Cahn and Cram[52] found the T-10 paraspinals to correlate strongly (0.76) with the overall resting muscle activity of 24 sites. Perhaps the mid-back is the best indicator of general tension levels. However, the vast majority of the SEMG literature supports a model of specificity of the neuromuscular system rather than a generalized arousal model.

Clinically, several treatment techniques have been developed to treat the emotional layer of muscular disturbance. The technique of progressive relaxation was introduced by Edmund Jacobson in 1934.[53] Jacobson's thesis was that nearly all muscular and functional disorders (e.g., irritable bowel syndrome) were attributable to a dysregulation of the nervous system and that all could be treated with his technique. In some ways, his therapy was replaced with Valium when the pharmaceutical revolution took place in the 1950s.

Jacobson developed a set of exercises in which the patient was instructed in how to systematically tense and release the major muscle groups of the body. The patient would initially be taught to tense the muscles to the extent that they would vibrate with intense effort, and then "zero down" and let go of the muscle contraction or tension as completely as possible. As time went on, the patient was to learn how to let go of small, even minute levels of tension. This was the key to Jacobson's success. He focused on 16 muscle sets: forearm (wrist flexors and extensors), upper arm (biceps and triceps), lower leg (foot flexors and extensors), upper leg (quadriceps and hamstrings), abdomen and back extensors, chest and scapular retractors, shoulders and neck, forehead, eyes, lips, and jaw. Such tensing and releasing behaviors remain popular components of current SEMG biofeedback work.

Autogenic training, a more cognitive approach, was developed in Germany in the 1950s by Wolfgang Luthe.[54] His intense interest in the phenomenon of hypnosis and the effects it could have on the human body led him and his colleagues to begin researching the effects of words on physical functioning. Using physiological monitoring devices, they tested more than 1000 phrases. From this research, a series of key phrases or "formulae" were discovered to consistently evoke physiological responses. The key word for the neuromuscular system was "heavy," and the phrase consisted of four variations of "my right arm is heavy" for the different limbs. The autogenic (self-cleansing) phrases may be used to induce emotional and general physiological relaxation: "I am completely calm," "My right arm is heavy," "My right arm is warm," "My heartbeat is slow and regular," "My breathing is slow and regular," "My abdomen flows warmly," and "My forehead is cool."

A number of body work therapies have been created to work with the emotions. The Rosen Method was developed in the mid-1900s by Marion Rosen,[55] a physical therapist who believes that old, forgotten emotions and memories are stored in the body and that these are the source of the holding patterns that cause pain and dysfunction. The Rosen Method consists of gentle touch. With the fingertips, pressure is applied to areas of tension in the muscles. The pressure is applied slowly and seeks to meet the level at which the resistance, or muscle tension, is felt. The practitioner uses one hand to work with the muscle tension, while the other hand remains still to detect changes in the tissue or in the movement of the breath. These changes typically indicate that some emotional release has occurred.

Rosen believes that as we become socialized, we develop patterns of holding and restriction to be socially appropriate. We tighten our muscles to inhibit the expression of emotions and physical motions of defense, such as hitting, kicking, or pushing away. These inhibited emotions and motions are stored in the body, limiting our freedom of expression and movement. Restriction of breathing is a key way in which we learn to inhibit our emotions. For this reason, freeing up the tightness in the diaphragm is a major focus in the Rosen work. As muscle tension and holding patterns from past injury and trauma are released, the individual is freer to respond more authentically to the present moment.

SENSORY MOTOR ASPECTS: MOVEMENT-ORIENTED APPROACHES AND REHABILITATION

As surface EMG emerged in the 1940s, studies on dynamic movement began. Inman and his colleagues,[56] for example, conducted a widely accepted SEMG study that was able to measure the muscle activity associated with movements of the shoulder. This interest in dynamic movement quickly spread to the clinical arena. By the early 1950s, Floyd and Silver[57] had presented an exceptionally strong study of SEMG and the erector spinae muscles. They clearly demonstrated that as the person goes through forward flexion of the trunk, the back muscles shut off as the trunk goes out onto ligament support. Thirty years later, Wolf and colleagues[58,59] utilized SEMG biofeedback techniques in the assessment and treatment of low-back pain. For a comprehensive review of the history of SEMG assessment and biofeedback treatments for low-back pain up into the early 1990s, see the chapter by Sherman and Arena in Wolf and Basmajian[60] or the earlier review article by Dolce and Raczynski.[61]

During the 1960s, biofeedback was born. Part of the impetus for its introduction was the work on single-motor-unit training of the neuromuscular system conducted by Basmajian.[62] While this type of training entailed the use of fine wire electrodes rather than surface electrodes, it clearly demonstrated that the neuromuscular system could be trained using EMG biofeedback techniques, down to its most basic element: the single motor unit. With all the excitement around his discovery, Basmajian conceived of an international forum to share information on SEMG, and in 1965, the International Society of Electrophysiological Kinesiology (ISEK) was formed. It still exists today and provides one of the only journals that specifically addresses issues pertaining to SEMG: *The Journal of Electromyography and Kinesiology*.

From a biofeedback perspective, the history of surface EMG began with Elmer Green[63] at the Menninger Clinic. Green modified the concepts behind Basmajian's single-motor-unit training paradigm and applied them to a general relaxation training paradigm. A few years later, Budzynski and Stoyva[64] began using SEMG feedback to treat muscle contraction headaches. From there, the SEMG biofeedback arena began to expand rapidly.

Clinical use of SEMG biofeedback for the treatment of more specific neuromuscular disorders also began in the 1960s. Hardyck et al.[65] were among the first to use SEMG to teach students not to subvocalize during silent reading, thereby accelerating their reading development. Booker et al.[66] demonstrated neuromuscular reeducation methods for patients with various conditions, and Johnson and Garton[67] utilized SEMG to assist in the restoration of function among hemiplegic patients. In the 1980s Brucker began working with patients who had experienced stroke and spinal cord injury, taking on cases where traditional physical therapies had given up. His work on neuromuscular reeducation has recently been published,[68] reporting success where others had failed. In addition, a meta-analysis[69] compared traditional methods of treating cardiovascular stroke to traditional methods augmented with the use of SEMG biofeedback. Across these studies, its authors found that the use of SEMG biofeedback improved the outcome of the therapy. Given these findings, it remains a source of amazement that SEMG biofeedback is not part of the standards of care for the stroke patient.

Neuromuscular applications in dentistry were introduced in the early 1970s by Bernard Jankelson.[70] Jankelson recognized that the traditional concept of "centric relation" failed to consider the status of mandibular posturing muscles. He developed procedures that used SEMG as an aid in determining a physiologically balanced occlusion and building of orthotics ("splints") for treatment of myofacial pain disorders. In addition, Cooper et al.[71] and Yamashita[72] have extensively studied the role of SEMG in the assessment, understanding, and treatment of occlusal and temporomandibular joint (TMJ) disorders. Recently, Jankelson[73] has summarized this type of clinical work. Lastly, Glaros[74] and Hudzynski and Lawrence[75] have extensively studied the role of SEMG in the psychophysiological assessment, understanding and treatment of TMJ disorders.

During the late 1980s, Donaldson and Donaldson[76] normalized his SEMG recordings by calculating the degree of symmetry of homologous muscle pairs during dynamic movement. He studied the degree of symmetrical recruitment during symmetrical and asymmetrical movement patterns in both normal subjects and patients with pain, concluding that a 20% asymmetry provided adequate sensitivity between the two groups. In addition, Donaldson popularized the concept of "cocontractions." During asymmetrical movements, asymmetrical recruitment patterns should be seen in homologous muscle pairs. When this doesn't occur, an abnormal finding is identified that potentially could be treated using SEMG biofeedback retraining techniques. More recently, Sella[77] has expanded Donaldson's concepts of monitoring homologous muscle pairs to a higher level, presenting a systematic method of testing many of the muscles of the human body for deficiencies.

Also during the 1980s, Will Taylor[78] introduced the concept of measuring synergy patterns in the upper and lower trapezius during abduction of the arm. Following the work of Karol Lewit,[79] Taylor noted that myalgias in the upper quarter were commonly associated with a "postural" muscle doing the work of its "phasic" counterpart. For example, in upper back or neck pain, the upper trapezius (a phasic muscle) commonly dominates the stabilizing muscular action associated with abduction of the arm to 90 degrees, even though it should share this workload with the lower trapezius (a postural muscle). The hyperactivity of the upper trapezius, then, is seen as being facilitated by the inhibition of the lower traps. Susan Middaugh et al.[80] have also clearly delineated the role of a hyperactive upper trapezius in headache and neck and shoulder pain. These authors came to the conclusion that almost all of the dysfunctional patterns in the upper back involve hyperactivity of upper trapezius.

The American, European, and international academic communities have provided a strong fundamental basis for understanding electromyography in general and surface electromyography in particular. Space limits the ability to acknowledge the many contributors to this field, so only a limited sample of the major contributors are mentioned here. The influence of DeLuca and his colleagues at the Neuromuscular Research Institute in Boston cannot be overlooked. Much of their work on spectral analysis and muscle fatigue[81] has shed light on both the physiology of muscle and methods of muscle measurement. Kadefors et al.[82] from Sweden and Masuda et al.[83] and Sadoyama and Miyano[84] from Japan have also contributed to our understanding of muscle fatigue. Clinically, the role of muscle fatigue in back pain was clearly delineated in a study by Roy et al.[85]

The work of the Scandinavian community on tension myalgia in the workplace is very impressive. Hagg[86] has provided a vast amount of information concerning work and the upper trapezius muscle, as have Mathaissen,[87] Hagberg,[88] Westgaard and Bjorklund,[89] and Jonsson.[90] They have clearly added to our understanding of muscle dysfunctions in the workplace. Veiersted et al.[91] and Hagg and Astrom[92] should also be recognized for their studies on the importance of rest. In addition, an excellent summary of SEMG issues related to the workplace may be found in a publication by Soderberg.[93]

European researchers have also focused strongly on the engineering and technical aspects of SEMG, and have created an organization called Surface Electromyography for the Noninvasive Assessment of Muscles (SENIAM). Through this effort, several books have been written that look at standardizing the recording methods for SEMG,[94] the state of the art for SEMG sensors and sensor placements,[95] European activities on SEMG,[96] and European applications of SEMG.[97] SENIAM has also undertaken a "concerted action"[98] to help clarify technical standards for SEMG.

Clinically, several body work techniques have been developed to work dynamically with muscle-oriented pain. The Feldenkrais Method[99] is an approach to movement reeducation. Moshe Feldenkrais believed that we learn the vast majority of our movement patterns during the first few years of life, and then repeat these compulsively to the exclusion of other possible movement patterns. He was so bold as to say that we use only 5% of our total potential movement ability.

Feldenkrais also believed in the innate movement wisdom of the body. The goal of the Feldenkrais practitioner is to assist the patient in experiencing more efficient forms of movement. Once experienced, the ease associated with this new pattern may automatically become part of the patient's movement repertoire, or may become consciously available to the patient.

Feldenkrais was a master at understanding and breaking down movement patterns into their components. As part of a Feldenkrais session, the therapist might ask the patient to begin with his or her habitual pattern. The therapist might then scramble these components, introducing chaos into the system, in an attempt to disrupt the habitual pattern. For example, normally the eyes move in the same direction as the rotation of the head. In working with neck problems, the Feldenkrais practitioner might ask the patient to move the eyes in the direction opposite to the head's rotation. In general, six elements are important when doing Feldenkrais movements: be consciously aware of each movement, move in a relaxed fashion, make the movements very small, make them slowly, never go into pain, and practice these movements through visualization only as well as through actual movement. For some nice examples of Feldenkrais exercises, consult *Relaxercize* by David Zemach-Bersin et al.[100]

The Trager Approach was developed by Milton Trager in the mid-1900s.[2,101] The underlying theory of this work is that pain and dysfunction begin and are maintained in the unconscious portion of the mind. Trager's approach seeks to communicate with the unconscious aspect of the client's mind and to reeducate the nervous system toward a more relaxed way of being. To do so, the Trager practitioner enters into a deep meditative state that Trager called a "hookup." While in this active, yet meditative state, the practitioner moves the client's body while mentally asking the client's unconscious such questions as "How should this feel? What could be softer? Lighter? Freer?" The practitioner is at the same time being aware of his or her own body, seeking to have it be as light, free, and soft as it can be. In this fashion, the practitioner's body can transmit the desired way of being to the client's body.

The Trager technique consists of gentle wiggling and jiggling of different parts of the client's body. Through this jiggling, habitual holding patterns in the nervous system are disturbed, introducing chaos into the muscular system and allowing for a healthier reorganization of the muscle energy patterns. During a Trager session, the practitioner encourages the client to become aware of changes in his or her body and to remember how this new sense of ease or lightness feels. This "recall" is believed to assist in the mind's ability to release these habitual holding patterns.

BIOMECHANICS AND THE ROLE OF POSTURE

Posture is the foundation upon which movement rides. Therefore, the history of SEMG would not be complete without some information concerning posture. Posture can be thought of as a purely biomechanical event—that is, bearing weight against gravity—or it may be thought of as a manifestation of emotions. We will look briefly at both.

Janet Price and her colleagues[102] began in the 1940s to study clinical populations of patients with back pain using SEMG. They noted that SEMG activation patterns began to migrate away from the site of original injury to other muscle sets in these individuals. This study represents the first documentation on antalgic postures or protective guarding patterns.

One of the SEMG assessment techniques provides a "big picture" of bracing and holding patterns, thereby allowing the practitioner to describe and quantify postural disturbances from a muscular point of view. The muscle scanning procedure developed by Cram[103] utilizes handheld electrodes that allow the practitioner to sample the right and left aspect of multiple muscle groups quickly. If one were to sample the paraspinal muscles at each fourth vertebral segment, for example, the postural pattern of resting tone along the spine would emerge. Using this technique, Cram and Engstrom[104] studied 104 normal individuals and compared them to more than 200 patients with chronic pain to demonstrate the clinical sensitivity of this technique in studying pain-related disorders. From this study, a normative database was developed that may be used to guide clinical interpretations of patterns or sites of muscular activation, asymmetrical activation patterns, and postural (antalgic) disturbances. Cram and Kasman[24] present a clear case study of antalgic (painful) posture. Here activations on the left erector spinae are evident as the patient's weight shifts away from a right sciatic-type pain. With the ability to see SEMG resting tone at higher vertebral sites, this case study allows one to see a compensatory bracing pattern in the right T-2 and C-4 paraspinals. It is no wonder that patients with low-back pain, as Price had noted, eventually begin to hurt in the upper back and neck as well.

The role of SEMG in the chiropractic community cannot be ignored, given that this community has adopted paraspinal muscle scanning as a method for helping to describe the neuromuscular elements of the subluxation complex.[105,106] A few studies have demonstrated the usefulness of SEMG paraspinal scanning as an outcome measure.[107] Cram[108] has encouraged the chiropractic community to expand the scope of its use of SEMG to include dynamic procedures as well.

Florence Kendall and colleagues,[109] in their most recent book, *Muscles: Testing and Function*, provide a beautiful guide to understanding and assessing the mechanical aspects of posture. The book shows stances against postural grids, and simultaneously describes postural disturbances for the involved muscles. Along with the "ideal posture," the faulty postures of kyphosis-lordosis, sway back, military type, flat back, and scoliosis are presented. Special sections on head position, shoulders and scapulae, and knees, feet, and legs are included as well.

Body-oriented psychotherapists and somatics practitioners have also focused on the role of emotions and posture in neuromuscular health. Stanley Keleman[110] has developed a model of layers and compartments in understanding how the body and muscles function as a whole in physical and emotional health. He conceptualizes the body as having three compartments or pouches located roughly in the abdomen, chest, and head. In addition, he views the body as having three distinct layers. The outer layer represents our interaction with the world and includes the nervous system and the skin. The middle layer encompasses the muscles, bones, and connective tissues. The inner layer consists of the internal organs of digestion, assimilation, respiration, and distribution. The biological and psychological integrity of the body entails adequate pumping of life-bearing fluids and biological energy through all three layers and between all three compartments.

According to Keleman, the fluidity of these compartments may become disturbed by stress and insults to the organism. He describes a startle/stress continuum that affects posture through six variations. The first three postures involve getting bigger and expanding outward. The postures evolve from a rigid cautionary stance to a threatened bracing and finally a turning, as if getting ready to run away. The next three postures involve getting smaller and shorter and becoming fixed; they represent a freezing-type response. The postures evolve through the stages of a contracted bracing, to a withdrawal and submission, and finally to a downward collapse in defeat. Over time, if the stressors are perpetuated, Keleman suggests that the density of the layers and the directions in which the pouches pulsate or flow will change. The postural muscles and postures involved can lead to one of four somatic defenses: rigid and controlled, dense and shamed, swollen and manipulative, and collapsed compliant. Each type has a variety of complex physical, social, and psychological sequelae.

Thomas Hanna,[111] who studied with Feldenkrais, has described three common reflexive postural stances. The first, called the "red light" reflex, is best represented as a withdrawal response from perceived stress or danger. Here, the facial muscles contract, the shoulders rise, the head moves forward, the elbows and knees bend, and the abdominal muscles contract, pulling the trunk forward and the chest down. This posture limits the ability to breathe and affects the heart and other internal organs. It may become habitual in individuals who live in a high state of alertness or fear.

In contrast, the "green light" reflex is considered assertive and active. This reflexive pattern opens the eyes, pulls the neck backward and the shoulders downward, hyperextends the elbows and knees, lifts the chest, and activates the lumbar muscles to hyperextend the back. When this reflex is repeatedly triggered, as it commonly is in Western society, Hanna suggests that it may be the primary culprit for the high incidence of back pain.

Both red light and green light reflexes are triggered by the individual's response to the environment. While the red light reflex brings us to a stop, the green light puts us into action. Both reflexes coexist, yet there is also a competition between the two. Over time, both postural reflexes may be seen in the same individual, a development that Hanna refers to as the "senile posture." One reflex may dominate over the other. If, for example, the red light reflex has been dominant over the course of a person's life, he or she will have a more pronounced stooped-over posture and may even develop a dowager hump.

The third reflex, known as the "trauma" reflex, develops as a result of accidents, surgery, and repetitive use. It consists of chronic muscle contraction patterns resulting in an asymmetrical posture: side bending and rotations.

Hanna has presented a very nice series of sensory motor exercises in his book *Somatics*. These floor exercises (somatics exercises) focus on becoming sensorially aware of movement, and may be used to break up dysfunctional habitual postural reflexes and patterns. Underlying the emphasis on sensory awareness is Hanna's concept of "sensory-motor amnesia." He utilizes floor exercises to bring a renewed sensory awareness to the afflicted areas and to reset the resting tonus of the muscles. The set of floor exercises includes learning to control the extensor muscles of the back, the flexor muscles of the stomach, and the muscles of the waist, as well as efforts related to rotation of the trunk, controlling of the hip joints and legs, and controlling of the muscles of the neck and shoulders. There are also exercises for improving breathing and improving walking. Practitioners using SEMG to treat various pain disorders may want to familiarize themselves with Hanna's work.

Another approach to understanding and treating posture was developed by F. Matthias Alexander[112,113] at the turn of the last century. His system emphasizes postural reeducation with a focus on the proper relationship of the head, neck, and torso. Alexander posited that most people have learned a less than optimal way of carrying themselves, thus causing pain and discomfort. He states that when the head and neck are in proper alignment with the torso, the head "floats" upward and the neck and spine are released and lengthened. The Alexander teacher provides a combination of gentle guidance by touch and verbal instruction to encourage the student's awareness of his or her postural alignment. The Alexander process includes three steps that the SEMG practitioner might want to adopt in his or her own work. The first is to assist the student in becoming consciously aware of his or her posture and movement patterns. The second is for the student to master the ability to inhibit dysfunctional and habitual patterns. The third step is to consciously break old habits and establish new and better postural and movement patterns. SEMG practitioners working on cervical problems would be wise to familiarize themselves with the tactile and verbal suggestions utilized in this technique.

ELECTRODE ATLASES

In the world of SEMG, knowing where to place the recording electrodes is essential. The SEMG electrodes are like little microphones that "listen" for the muscle action potentials (MAPs). Having these microphones in the right locations facilitates the nature of the recording. The SENIAM group has demonstrated that even slight changes in the placement of the recording electrodes may dramatically alter the amplitude and quality of the SEMG recording.[94]

The first SEMG electrode atlas was constructed by Davis.[114] Given that Davis conducted much of the original SEMG research, he provided researchers with electrode placement maps to assist in the standardization of

SEMG recordings. Nearly 30 years later, Basmajian and Blumenstein[115] wrote a small book to guide electrode placements. This manual expanded and updated the initial recommendations of Davis to include more sites relevant to rehabilitation. Cram and Kasman[24] produced an electrode atlas of 69 sites, classifying each recording site for the quality of the recording (specific, quasi-specific, and general recordings). Because SEMG recordings may be subject to issues of volume conduction from surrounding and distant muscles, "specific" recordings were felt to be relatively free of such contamination. "Quasi-specific" sites were thought to record from the muscle named, as well as volume-conducted signals from surrounding muscles. "General" recordings were considered recordings from a region rather than from specific muscles. In addition to the sites for placement, sample recording from standardized movements are presented in both raw SEMG and processed modes.

SENIAM, the European effort, has also created a very concise and well-illustrated book on standardized SEMG electrode placements for 27 muscle sites across the areas of the shoulder and neck, the back muscles, the arm and hand, the upper leg and hip, and the lower leg.[94]

A BRIEF HISTORY OF ELECTRICITY AND SEMG INSTRUMENTATION

The history of SEMG has to do with the discovery of electricity, and the ability to see through the aid of instruments phenomena that one could not see, feel, or touch with the normal senses.

The theme of the development of SEMG can be traced back to Francesco Redi[116] in the mid-1600s, whose work with the electric ray fish documented that a highly specialized muscle was the source of its energy. By 1773, Walsh had been able to clearly demonstrate that the eel's muscle tissue could generate a spark of electricity. During the 1790s, Luigi and Lucia Galvani[117] had conducted a series of studies that demonstrated that muscle contractions could be evoked by the discharge of static electricity. Concurrently, Volta[118] had developed a powerful tool that could be used to generate electricity, which, incidentally, could be used to stimulate muscle. The technique of using electricity to stimulate muscles gained wide attention during the 1800s. The documentation of the use of electrical stimulation to study muscle function was conducted by Duchenne.[26] As mentioned earlier, his work is truly the first systematic study of the dynamics and function of the intact muscle.

It was not until the early 1800s that the galvanometer, a robust tool for measuring electrical currents and therefore muscle activity, was invented. In 1838, Matteucci[119] used the galvanometer to clearly demonstrate an electrical potential between an excised frog's nerve and its damaged muscle. By 1849, Du Bois-Reymond[120] had provided the first evidence of electrical activity in human muscles during voluntary contraction. Du Bois-Reymond's classic experiment involved placing blotting cloth on each of the hands or forearms of his subject and immersing them in separate vats of saline solution, while connecting the electrodes to the galvanonmeter. He noted very minute but very consistent and predictable deflections whenever the subject flexed his hand or arm. Du Bois-Reymond thought that the magnitude was diminished by the impedance of the skin; thus he removed a portion of the skin of the subject, replaced the electrodes, and noted a dramatic increase in the magnitude of the signal during wrist flexion. (Note that the importance of good skin preparation before electrode placement has been present from the very beginning of SEMG.) By the early 1900s, Pratt[121] had demonstrated that the magnitude of the energy associated with muscle contraction was due to muscle and the recruitment of individual muscle fibers, rather than due to the size of the neural impulse. By 1922, Gasser and Erlanger[122] were able to use the newly invented cathode ray oscilloscope to show the signals from muscles, a feat that won them the Nobel Prize in 1944.

The concentric needle electrode, developed by Adrian and Bronk[123] in 1929, provided a powerful tool that is still widely used today for needle EMG studies. Vacuum tube amplifiers[124] and later solid-state differential amplifiers made it possible to obtain a better and cleaner EMG signal. By 1962, John Basmajian[125] had compiled all of the information available on electromyography into his book *Muscles Alive*. Over the years, it has been updated through five editions. In the last edition, he shared authorship of the book with DeLuca.[126]

DeLuca pioneered much of the mathematical language and models for understanding the motor unit action potential (MUAP) of the EMG.[127] This modeling was further elaborated upon by Dimitrova,[128] who provided mathematical tools for understanding the biophysics of EMG and, therefore, the information contained within the signal. Later, Lindstrom and Magnusson[129] provided the mathematical foundation for decomposing the EMG using spectral analysis. Spectral analysis was further considered in DeLuca's[81] description of muscle fatigue. Broman et al.[130] introduced a method of linear electrode arrays and double differential amplification techniques that allows the researcher to see the electrophysiological characteristics of the MUAP as it travels down the muscle fiber. Recently, Merletti et al.[131] have presented information on the use of these linear electrode arrays.

CONCLUSION

Surface EMG technology is found across many disciplines, ranging from manual therapies to psychology. Those providers who have come into SEMG work through psychology may have been unfamiliar with some of the body work approaches to treatment, and the manual therapists may be unfamiliar with the emotional aspects of SEMG.

By reviewing the history of the four domains of tissue, emotions, movement, and posture, a broad understanding of muscle soreness and SEMG can be appreciated by all disciplines involved. It is hoped that such a broad exposure will encourage providers to learn more about applications with which they are currently unfamiliar, to consider referral to other providers when necessary, or to learn how to blend new techniques into what they are doing. As one uses SEMG and body work to their fullest potential, one learns to walk the mind–body interface and to practice a body-oriented psychotherapy.

REFERENCES

1. Kasman G, Cram JR, Wolf S. *Clinical Applications in SEMG*. Gaithersburg, MD: Aspen; 1998.
2. Claire T. *Bodywork*. New York, NY: William Morrow: 1995.
3. Rolf I. *Rolfing: Re-establishing the Natural Alignment and Structural Integration of the Human Body for Vitality and Well-Being*. Rochester, VT: Healing Arts Press; 1989.
4. Barnes JF. *Myofascial Release: The Search for Excellence*. Paoli, PA: MFR Seminars; 1990.
5. Simons DG. Muscle pain syndromes: part I. *Am J Phys Med.* 1975;54:289–311.
6. Simons DG. Muscle pain syndromes: part II. *Am J Phys Med.* 1976;55:15–42.
7. Port K. Eine fur den orthopaden wichtige Gruppe des chronischen rheumatismus (Knotchenrheumatismus). *Arch Orthop Unfallchir.* 1920;17:465–506.
8. Kellgren JH. A preliminary account of referred pains arising from muscle. *Brit Med J.* 1938;1:325–327.
9. Kraft GH, Johnson EW, LaBan MM. The fibrositis syndrome. *Arch Phys Med Rehab.* 1968;9:155–162.
10. Kelly M. The nature of fibrositis: 1. The myalgic lesion and its secondary effects: a reflex theory. *Ann Rheum Dis.* 1945;5:1–7.
11. Travell J, Rinzler S, Herman M. Pain and disability of the shoulder and arm: treatment by intramuscular infiltration with procaine hydrochloride. *JAMA.* 1942;120:417–422.
12. Travell J. Myofascial trigger points: clinical view. In Bonica JJ, Albe-Fessard D, eds. *Advances in Pain Research and Therapy: Volume 1*. New York, NY: Raven Press; 1976: 919–926.
13. Fishbain DA, Goldberg M, Magher BR, Steel R, Rosomoff H. Male and female chronic pain patients categorized by DSM-II psychiatric diagnostic criteria. *Pain.* 1986;26: 181–197.
14. Travell J, Simons D. *Myofascial Pain and Dysfunction: A Trigger Point Manual*. Baltimore, MD: Williams and Wilkins; 1983.
15. Weeks VD, Travell J. *How to Give Painless Injections: AMA Scientific Exhibits*. New York, NY: Grune and Stratton; 1957:318–322.
16. Chen JT, Chen SM, Kuan TS, Chung KC, Hong CZ. Phentolamine effect on the spontaneous electrical activity of active loci in the myofascial trigger spot of rabbit. *Arch Phys Med Rehab.* 1990;79:790–794.
17. Hong CZ, Simons D. Pathophysiologic and electrophysiologic mechanisms of myofascial trigger points. *Arch Phys Med Rehab.* 1998;79:863–872.
18. Hubbard D. Chronic and recurrent muscle pain: pathophysiology and treatment, and review of pharmacologic studies. *J Musculoskel Pain.* 1996;4:123–143.
19. Hubbard D, Berkoff G. Myofascial trigger points show spontaneous needle EMG activity. *Spine.* 1993;18:1803–1807.
20. McNulty W, Gevertz R, Berkoff G, Hubbard D. Needle EMG evaluation of a trigger point response to a psychological stressor. *Psychophysiology.* 1994;31:313–316.
21. Passatore M, Grassi C, Filippi G. Sympathetically induced development of tension in jaw muscles: the possible contraction of intrafusal muscle fibers. *Pflugers Arch.* 1985;405:297–304.
22. Simons DG, Dexter JR. Comparison of local twitch responses elicited by palpation and needling of myofascial trigger points. *J Musculoskel Pain.* 1995;3:49–61.
23. Donaldson CCS, Skubick D, Clasby R, Cram JR. The evaluation of trigger point activity using dynamic EMG techniques. *Am J Pain Manage.* 1994;4(3):118–122.
24. Cram JR, Kasman G. *Introduction to Surface EMG*. Gaithersburg, MD: Aspen; 1998.
25. Cacioppo JT, Tassinary G, Fridlund AJ. The skeletomotor system. In: Cacioppo JT, Tassinary G, eds. *Principles of Psychophysiology*. New York, NY: Cambridge University Press; 1990.
26. Duchenne GB. *The Physiology of Motion: Demonstrated by Means of Electrical Stimulation in Clinical Observations and Applied to the Study of Paralysis and Deformities*. Trans., ed. E Kaplan. Philadelphia, PA: Lipincott; 1959. (Original work published 1867.)
27. Darwin C. *The Expression of Emotion in Man and Animals*. New York, NY: Appleton; 1986. (Original work published in London by Murray in 1872.)

28. James W. *The Principles of Psychology*. New York, NY: Holt; 1890.

29. Jacobson E. Voluntary relaxation of the esophagus. *Am J Phys*. 1925;72:387–394.

30. Jacobson E. Action currents from muscular contractions during conscious processes. *Science*. 1927;66:403.

31. Jacobson E. Electrical measurements of neuromuscular states during mental activities: I. Imagination of movement involving skeletal muscles. *Am J Phys*. 1930; 91:567–608.

32. Jacobson E. Electrical measurements of neuromuscular states during mental activities: V. Variation of specific muscles contracting during imagination. *Am J Phys*. 1931;96:115–121.

33. Davis RC. Patterns of muscular activity during "mental work" and their constancy. *J Exper Psych*. 1939;24: 451–465.

34. Ekman P, Sorebsib ER, Friesen WV. Pan-cultural elements in facial displays of emotion. *Science*. 1969;164:86–88.

35. Ekman P, Friesen WV. *Unmasking the Face*. Englewood Cliffs, NJ: Prentice Hall; 1975.

36. Rusalova MN, Izard CE, Simonov PV. Comparative analysis of mimical and autonomic components of man's emotional state. *Aviation, Space Environ Med*. September 1975:1132–1134.

37. Schwartz GE, Fair PL, Greenberg PS, Mandel MR, Klerman GL. Facial EMG in the assessment of emotion. *Psychophysiology*. 1974;11:237.

38. Schwartz GE, Fair PL, Salt P, Mandel MR, Klermant GL. Facial muscle patterning to affective imagery in depressed and non depressed subjects. *Science*. 1976; 192:489–491.

39. Thompson JG. *The Psychobiology of Emotions*. New York, NY: Plenum Press; 1988.

40. Goldstein IB. Electromyography: A measure of skeletal response. In: Greenfield NS, Sternbach RA, eds. *Handbook of Psychophysiology*. New York, NY: Holt, Rinehart and Winston; 1972:329–366.

41. Reusch J, Cobb S, Finesinger JE. Studies on muscular tension in the neuroses. *Trans Am Neurol Assoc*. 1941;67: 186–189.

42. Malmo RB, Shagass C, Davis FH. A physiological study of somatic symptom mechanisms in psychiatric patients. *Res Publ Assoc Nerv Mental Dis*. 1950;29:23–261.

43. Malmo RB, Shagass C, Bellanger DJ, Smith AA. Motor control in psychiatric patients under experimental stress. *J Abnormal Social Psychol*. 1951;46:539–547.

44. Martin I. Levels of muscle activity in psychiatric patients. *Acta Psychologica*. 1956;12:326–341.

45. Whatmore G, Ellis RM. Some motor aspects of schizophrenia. *Am J Psychia*. 1958;114:882–889.

46. Whatmore G, Ellis RM. Some neurophysiologic aspects of depressed states. *Arch Gen Psychiatry*. 1959;1:70.

47. Whatmore G, Kohli D. *The Physiopathology and Treatment of Functional Disorders*. New York, NY: Grune and Stratton; 1974.

48. Jacobson E. *You Must Relax*. New York, NY: McGraw-Hill; 1976. (Original work published in 1934.)

49. Alexander B, Smith DD. Clinical applications of EMG biofeedback. In: Gatcher RJ, Price KR, eds. *Clinical Applications of Biofeedback: Appraisal and Status*. New York, NY: Pergamon; 1979:112–133.

50. Suarez A, Kohlenberg RJ, Pagano RR. Is EMG activity from the frontalis site a good measure of general bodily tension in clinical populations? *Biofeedback Self Regul*. 1979;4:293.

51. Shedivy DE, Kleinman KM. Lack of correlation between frontalis EMG and either neck EMG or verbal ratings of tension. *Psychophysiology*. 1977;14:182–186.

52. Cahn T, Cram JR. Muscle scanning: support for the back. *Perceptual Motor Skills*. 1900;70:851–857.

53. Jacobson E. Electrical measurement concerning muscular contraction (tonus) and the cultivation of relaxation in man: relaxation times of individuals. *Am J Phys*. 1934;108:573–580.

54. Luthe W, ed. *Autogenic Therapy*. New York, NY: Grune and Stratton; 1969.

55. Mayland EL. *Rosen Method*. CA: Inksmith Printing, 1984.

56. Inman VT, Saunders JB, Abbot LC. Observations on the function of the shoulder joint. *J Bone Joint Surg*. 1944;26:1–30.

57. Floyd WF, Silver P. The function of the erector spinae muscles in certain movements and postures in man. *J Physiol*. 1955;129:184–203.

58. Wolf S, Basmajian JV. Assessment of paraspinal electromyographic activity in normal subjects and chronic back pain patients using a muscle biofeedback device. In: Asmussen E, Jorgensen K, eds. *International Series on Biomechanics, Vol. 6b*. Baltimore, MD: University Press; 1978.

59. Wolf S, Nacht M, Kelly J. EMG feedback training during dynamic movement for low back pain patients. *Behav Ther*. 1982;13:395–406.

60. Sherman R, Arena J. Biofeedback for assessment and treatment of low back pain. In: Basmajian JV, Wolf S, eds. *Rational Manual Therapies*. Baltimore, MD: Williams and Wilkins; 1994.

61. Dolce JJ, Raczynski JM. Neuromuscular activity and electromyography in painful backs: Psychological and biomechanical models in assessment and treatment. *Psychol Bull*. 1985;97(3):502–520.

62. Basmajian JV. Control and training of individual motor units. *Science*. 1963;141:440–441.

63. Green EE, Walters ED, Green A, Murphy G. Feedback techniques for deep relaxation. *Psychophysiology*. 1969;6:371–377.

64. Budzynski T, Stoyva J, Adler C. Feedback-induced muscle relaxation: Application to tension headache. *J Behav Experi Psychiat*. 1970:205–211.

65. Hardyck CD, Petrincovich LV, Ellsworth DW. Feedback of speech muscle activity during silent reading: rapid extension. *Science*. 1966;154:1467–1468.

66. Booker HE, Rubow RT, Coleman PJ. Simplified feedback in neuromuscular retraining: an automated approach using EMG signals. *Arch Phys Med*. 1969;50:621–625.

67. Johnson HE, Garton WH. Muscle re-education in hemiplegia by use of electromyographic device. *Arch Phys Med.* 1973; 54:320–322.
68. Brucker B, Bulaeva NV. Biofeedback effect on electro-myography responses in patients with spinal cord injury. *Arch Phys Med Rehab.* 1996;77(2):133–137.
69. Moreland JD, Thomson MA, Fuoco AR. Electromyographic biofeedback to improve lower extremity function after stroke: a meta-analysis. *Arch Phys Med Rehab.* 1998;79(2): 134–140.
70. Jankelson B. Electronic control of muscle contraction: a new clinical era in occlusion and prosthodontics. *Sci Educ Bull.* 1969;2(1):29–31.
71. Cooper BC, Cooper DL, Lucente FE. Electromyography of masticatory muscles in craniomandibular disorders. *Laryngoscope.* 1991;101(2):150–157.
72. Yamashita A. Management of TMJ syndrome with the use of myomonitoring equipment. *Hotetsu Rinsho.* 1985;spec no:234–239.
73. Jankleson R. *Neuromuscular Dental Diagnosis and Treatment.* Tukwila, WA: Myotronics; 1998.
74. Glaros AG. Awareness of physiological responding under stress and non stress conditions in TMJ disorders. *Biofeedback Self Regul.* 1996;21:261–272.
75. Hudzynski L, Lawrence BA. Myofacial pain and the temporomandibular joint. In: Cram JR, ed. *Clinical EMG for Surface Recordings, Volume 2.* Nevada City, CA: Clinical Resources; 1990.
76. Donaldson S, Donaldson M. Multi-channel EMG assessment and treatment techniques. In Cram JR, ed. *Clinical EMG for Surface Recordings: Volume 2.* Nevada City, CA: Clinical Resources; 1990.
77. Sella G. *Neuro-muscular Testing with Surface EMG.* Martins Ferry, OH: GENMED Publishing; 1995.
78. Taylor W. Dynamic EMG biofeedback in assessment and treatment using a neuromuscular re-education model. In: Cram J, ed. *Clinical EMG for Surface Recordings: Volume 2.* Nevada City, CA: Clinical Resources; 1990.
79. Lewit K. *Manipulative Therapy in Rehabilitation of the Loco-motor System.* Boston, MA: Butterworth Heinemann; 1991.
80. Middaugh SJ, Kee WG, Nicholson JA. Muscle overuse and posture as factors in the development and maintenance of chronic musculoskeletal pain. In: Grzesiak RC, Ciccone DS, eds. *Psychological Vulnerability to Chronic Pain.* New York, NY: Springer; 1994.
81. DeLuca CJ. Myoelectric manifestations of localized muscular fatigue in humans. *CRC Crit Rev Biomed Eng.* 1984;11(4):251.
82. Kadefors R, Lindstrom L, Petersen I, Ortengren R. EMG in objective evaluation of localized muscle fatigue. *Scand J Rehabil Med.* 1978;suppl.6:75–93.
83. Masuda K, Masuda T, Sadoyama T, Inaki M, Katsuta S. Changes in surface EMG parameters during static and dynamic fatiguing contractions. *J Electromyogr Kinesiol.* 1999;9(1):39–46.
84. Sadoyama T, Miyano H. Frequency analysis of surface EMG to evaluation of muscle fatigue. *Eur J Appl Physiol Occup Physiol.* 1981;47(3):239–246.
85. Roy SH, DeLuca CJ, Cassovant DA. Lumbar muscle fatigue and chronic back pain. *Spine.* 1989;14:992–1001.
86. Hagg GM. Static work load and occupational myalgia: a new explanation model. In: Anderson P, Hobart D, Danoff J, eds. *Electromyographical Kinesiology.* Amsterdam, Netherlands: Elsevier Science; 1991: 141–144.
87. Mathiassen SE, Winkel J, Hagg GM. Normalization of surface EMG amplitude from the upper trapezius muscle in ergonomic studies: a review. *J Electromyogr Kinesiol.* 1995;5:4, 197–226.
88. Hagberg M. Muscular endurance and surface EMG in isometric and dynamic exercise. *Arch Phys Med.* 1981; 60(3):111–121.
89. Westgaard RH, Bjorklund R. Generation of muscle tension additional to postural muscle load. *Ergonomics.* 1987;39: 911–923.
90. Jonsson B. Kinesiology: With special reference to electro-myographic kinesiology. *Cont Clin Neurophysiol EEG.* 1978;suppl34:417–428.
91. Veiersted KB, Westgaard RH, Andersen P. Electro-myographic evaluation of muscular work pattern as a predictor of trapezius myalgia. *Scan J Work Environ Health.* 1993;19:284–290.
92. Hagg GM, Astrom A. Load pattern and pressure pain threshold in the upper trapezius muscle and psychosocial factors in medical secretaries with and without shoulder/neck disorders. *Int Arch Occup Environ Health.* 1997;69:423–432.
93. Soderberg GL, ed. *Selected Topics in Surface Electromyography for Use in the Occupational Setting: Expert Perspective.* Washington DC: NIOSH, 1992. DHHS (NIOSH), publication no. 91-100.
94. Hermens H, Freriks B, Merletti R, Stegeman D, Joleen B, Gner R, Disselhorst-Klug C, Hagg G. *SENIAM: European Recommendations for Surface Electromyography.* Roessingh Research and Development; 1999.
95. Hermens H, Freriks B, eds. *SENIAM: The State of the Art on Sensors and Sensor Placement Procedures for SEMG.* Roessingh Research and Development; 1997.
96. Hermens H, Merletti R, Freriks B, eds. *SENIAM: European Activities on SEMG.* Roessingh Research and Development; 1996.
97. Hermens H, Hagg G, Freriks B, eds. *SENIAM: European Applications on SEMG.* Roessingh Research and Development; 1997.
98. Merletti R, Hermens H. Introduction to the special issue on the SENIAM European concerted action. *J Electromyo Kinesiol.* 2000;10:283–286.
99. Feldenkrais M. *Awareness Through Movement: Easy-to-Do Health Exercises to Improve Your Posture, Vision, Imagination, and Personal Awareness.* San Francisco, CA: Harper & Row; 1972.
100. Zemach-Berson D, Zemach-Berson K, Reese M. *Relaxercise.* San Francisco, CA: Harper; 1990.
101. Juhan D. *An Introduction to Trager Psychophysical Integration and Mentastics Movement Education.* Mill Valley, CA: Trager Institute; 1989.

102. Price JP, Clare MH, Ewerhardt RH. Studies in low back-ache with persistent spasm. *Arch Phys Med.* 1948;29:703–709.

103. Cram JR. *Clinical EMG for Surface Recordings: Volume 1.* Poulsbo, WA: J&J Engineering; 1986.

104. Cram JR, Engstrom D. Patterns of neuromuscular activity in pain and non-pain patients. *Clin Biofeedback Health.* 1986;9(2):106–116.

105. Brody S. Practical chiropractic EMG. *Dig Chiro Econ.* 1987;9:28–31.

106. Kent C, Hyde R. Potential applications for EMG in chiropractic practice. *Dig Chiro Econ.* 1987;9:20–25.

107. Myerowitz M. Scanning paraspinal surface EMG: a method for corroborating post treatment spinal and related neuromusculoskeletal symptom improvement. *J Occup Rehab.* 1994;4(3):171–179.

108. Cram JR. (1993). Muscle scanning: The 18% solution. *J Manipulative Physiol Ther.* 1993;16(4):274–277.

109. Kendall FFP, Kendall, E, McCreary BA. *Muscle Testing and Function.* 3rd ed. Baltimore, MD: Williams and Wilkins; 1993.

110. Keleman S. *Emotional Anatomy.* Berkeley, CA: Center Press; 1985.

111. Hanna T. *Somatics.* New York, NY: Addison-Wesley; 1988.

112. Alexander FM. *The Use of the Self.* Long Beach, CA: Centerline Press; 1985. (Original work published by E. P. Dutton in 1932.)

113. Maisel E, ed. *The Alexander Technique: The Essential Writings of F. Matthias Alexander.* New York, NY: Lyle Stuart; 1990.

114. Davis RC. *Manual of Surface EMG Laboratory for Psychological Studies.* Montreal, Canada: Allen Memorial Inst of Psychiatry; 1952.

115. Basmajian JV, Blumenstein R. Electrode placement in electromyographic biofeedback. In: Basmajian JV, ed. *Biofeedback: Principles and Practice for Clinicians.* Baltimore, MD: Williams and Wilkins; 1989.

116. Redi F. Esperienze intorno a diverse cose naturali e particolarmente a quelle che ci sono portate dalle Indie. Reprinted in: Giacosa P. ed., *Le Piu Belle Pagine di Francesco Redi.* Milan: 1925:105–109. (Original work published in 1617.)

117. Galvani L. De viribus electricitaatis in motu musculari. Typographia Instituti Scientiarum. Trans. RM Green. [Commentary on the effect of electricity on muscular motion.] Cambridge, MA: Elizabeth Lict; 1953. (Original work published in 1791.)

118. Volta A. Mommoria prima sull' elettricita animatle. In: *Collezione dell'Opere, Vol. 2.* Florence: G. Piatti; 1792.

119. Matteucci C. *Traites des Phenomenen Electrophysiologiques.* Paris, France; 1844.

120. Du Bois-Reymond E. *Untersuchungen ueber Thiersiche Electricitae, Volume 2, Second Part.* Berlin, Germany: Teimer-Verlag; 1983.

121. Pratt FH. The all or none principle in graded response of skeletal muscle. *Am J Physiol.* 1918;44:517–542.

122. Gasser HS, Newcomer HS. Physiological action currents in the phrenic nerve: an application of the thermionic vacuum tube to nerve physiology. *Am J Physiol.* 1921;57:1–26.

123. Adrian ED, Bonk DW. The discharge of impulses in motor nerve fibers II: the frequency of discharge in reflex and voluntary contractions. *J Physiol.* 1929;67:119–115.

124. Mathews BHC. A special purpose amplifier. *J Physiol.* (London). 1934;81:28–29.

125. Basmajian JV. *Muscles Alive.* Baltimore, MD: Williams and Wilkins; 1962.

126. Basmajian JV, DeLuca C. *Muscles Alive.* Baltimore, MD: Williams and Wilkins; 1983.

127. DeLuca CJ. Physiology and mathematics of myoelectric signals. *IEEE Trans BME.* 1979;26:313–325.

128. Dimitrova N. Model of the extracellular potential field of a single striated muscle fiber. *Electromyogr Clin Neurophysiol.* 1974;14:53–66.

129. Lindstrom L, Magnusson R. Interpretation of myoelectric power spectra: a model and its applications. *Proc IEEE.* 1977;65:653–662.

130. Broman H, Bilotta G, DeLuca CJ. A note on the noninvasive estimation of muscle fiber conduction velocity. *IEEE Trans Biomed Eng.* 1985;32:341–344.

131. Merletti R, Farina D, Gazzoni M. The linear electrode array: a tool with many applications. In: *VIV Congress of the International Society of Electrophysiology and Kinesiology*; 2002.

CHAPTER QUESTIONS

1. The muscle, as an organ system, contains many sensory mechanisms. The sensory mechanisms include:
   a. Golgi tendon organs
   b. muscle spindles
   c. Ruffini endings of the joints
   d. all of the above
2. Palpation is:
   a. used to probe the condition of the body
   b. no longer practiced
   c. a manual sense of touch used to learn many things about the body
   d. not a valid source of information
3. Approaches to body work include:
   a. Structural Integration
   b. trigger point injections
   c. Feldenkrais Method
   d. both a and c
4. Facial displays of emotions were given additional life when:
   a. Paul Ekman discovered the universal quality of emotions across cultures
   b. the cultural uniqueness of emotions was discovered
   c. SEMG was used to monitor facial displays of emotions
   d. Paul Ekman discovered the large number of facial emotional displays

5. Dysponesis refers to:
   a. "bad" muscle energy
   b. misplaced effort
   c. bracing
   d. all of the above

6. In what way are progressive relaxation and autogenic training different?
   a. One guides the person to make physiological changes.
   b. One must be guided by the practitioner.
   c. One requires muscle contraction and relaxation; the other includes other nervous systems as well.
   d. One cannot be used with SEMG training.

7. Single-motor-unit training of the neuromuscular system was:
   a. introduced by Thomas Budzenski and Johann Stoyva
   b. pioneered by John Basmajian
   c. discovered by Maurice B. Sterman
   d. developed by NASA

8. Neuromuscular reeducation:
   a. has been used with patients with various conditions
   b. is practiced only by physical therapists
   c. cannot assist in the restoration of function of patients with hemiplegia
   d. encourages the patient to decrease motor unit activity of the muscles

9. Cocontraction of muscles:
   a. refers to the work of Stuart Donaldson
   b. rarely happens to the healthy person
   c. automatically increases with age
   d. refers to the contraction of homologous pairs of muscles

10. The goal of the Feldenkrais practitioner is:
   a. to assist the patient in experiencing more efficient forms of movement
   b. to break down movement patterns
   c. to diagnose and treat physical ailments
   d. to differentiate movements

11. Body-oriented psychotherapists and somatics practitioners have focused on:
   a. memories stored in the body
   b. movement patterns
   c. emotions and cognitions
   d. the role of emotions and posture in neuromuscular health

12. Thomas Hanna described which common reflexive postural stances?
   a. the red light reflex
   b. the green light reflex
   c. the trauma reflex
   d. all of the above

13. The Alexender Technique developed by F. M. Alexander:
   a. is a system of postural reeducation with a focus on the proper relationship of the head, neck, and torso
   b. focuses on breathing patterns
   c. restores speaking ability
   d. is practiced only by actors

14. An SEMG electrode atlas:
   a. allows appropriate placement of the recording electrodes
   b. allows for consistency in electrode placements
   c. encourages communication of results
   d. all of the above

15. The origins of SEMG can be traced back to:
   a. Benjamin Franklin
   b. Francesco Redi
   c. Luigi and Lucia Galvani
   d. Plato

16. Understanding the motor unit action potential (MUAP) of the EMG:
   a. cannot be done without needle electrodes
   b. requires the understanding of biophysics
   c. was pioneered by DeLuca
   d. is not necessary for work in SEMG

Somatics and Surface Electromyography

Eleanor Criswell

"The SEMG practitioner constantly needs to remember and explore the three masters of muscle: posture, emotions, and dynamic movement."
—Jeffrey Cram[1] (p. 213)
"Somatology [somatics] sees the human person as a self-aware, self-controlling organism, an organic unity of many functions which have traditionally been thought of separately as 'bodily' and 'mental.'"
—Thomas Hanna[2] (p. 5)

Surface electromyography reflects the function of the entire body. It demonstrates the integration of mind and body or somatics. Because SEMG reflects the entire body, it is important to consider the entire mind–body system or the somatics dimension in SEMG work. SEMG work includes both SEMG monitoring and SEMG feedback. Therefore, this chapter addresses the following topics: the definition of somatics, SEMG monitoring and somatics, SEMG feedback as a somatics discipline, somatic exercises and SEMG, the elements needed for the practice of SEMG and somatics, and SEMG and somatic psychotherapy.

WHAT IS SOMATICS?

Somatics is a term coined by Thomas Hanna (**Figure 12–1**) in 1976 to label the emerging field of the mind–body disciplines. This term is based on *soma*, the Greek word meaning "the living body." Hanna further defined soma as "the body experienced from within." As the body is experienced from within, there is no mind–body separation. "It was his [Hanna's] brilliant solution for the [philosophical] mind–body problem."[3] (p. xviii)

Somatology, from the Modern Latin word *somatologia* (sixteenth century), is the name of the study of the body that later became anatomy and physiology. This distinction between anatomy and physiology separated the study of the bodily structure from the study of its functions. Hanna used the term *somatology* to label the science or study of the soma. René Decartes, the seventeenth-century French philosopher, is credited with having initiated Western culture's separation of mind and body. At this point in history, many are aware of the limitations of that separation. Hanna's definition of the soma, however, has no Cartesian mind–body split. In somatics, the soma is considered function first and structure second. According to Hanna, the soma originated with the creation of the universe (the "Big Bang") and evolved over time.[4]

Somatics focuses on the first-person perspective versus the third-person perspective. First-person perception refers to the perception of oneself; third-person perception is the perception of others and the world. SEMG monitoring provides external, third-person information. The client then uses the SEMG feedback information for

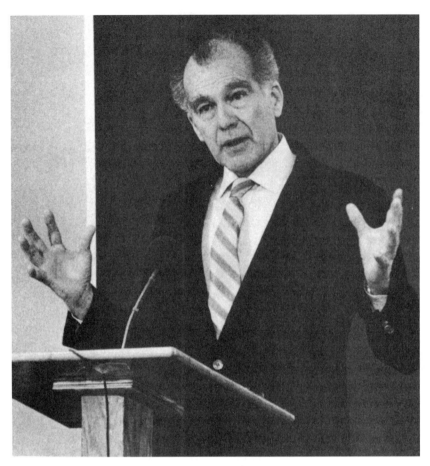

Figure 12–1 Thomas Hanna.
Source: Copyright © Joel Gordon.

first-person experiences: self-understanding and self-regulation. Somatics and SEMG feedback both involve a shift from the "reflexive, automatic physiological programs to the more voluntary control areas of the brain and behavior, involving more cortical control."[3] [(p. 34)]

History of Somatics

A number of disciplines in the field of somatics are relevant to SEMG. These disciplines are intentionally, first and foremost, somatic. Although some somatics disciplines, such as yoga, are 5000 years old, the contemporary field of somatics emerged in the 1970s. Including Eastern and Western traditions, all disciplines that feature mind–body integration are considered somatics disciplines.

Somatics can be educational or clinical. Many practitioners consider somatics disciplines educational, which means that the focus is on the client learning and making changes. Somatics is often practiced in an educational,

wellness, or fitness setting. The leader of the class is considered a teacher; the class is very student centered. Even in a private one-on-one setting, the practitioner is considered a teacher.

Somatics is also used for clinical purposes. The client with somatic issues or needs seeks out a practitioner from a particular somatics background, training, and orientation. The presenting complaint is addressed using somatics techniques. There is a problem and it is resolved through somatic methods. Somatics disciplines are used in private practices, centers, spas, clinics, and complementary medical settings.

Somatics Disciplines

The somatics disciplines bring in awareness and the psychological dimension. Changing the client's psychological state changes its effect on the client's muscle contraction levels. The human, or other animal, moves to express emotions and to satisfy needs. Somatics is not a treatment, but rather an educational process. Therefore, it requires that the client be mentally and emotionally involved in the process.

Western and Eastern cultural approaches to the mind–body disciplines have much in common. This commonality is created by working with the natural tendencies of the body and by the historical borrowing of techniques from other cultures. The somatics disciplines come from many different cultural and philosophical traditions. For example, "The highly disciplined Indian practice of hatha yoga is driven by the belief that all matter is a materialized form of the one great spirit motivating the universe."[5 (p. 65)] The word *yoga* comes from the Sanskrit word *yuj*, meaning "yoke or union." It refers to the unification or reunification of the self with the universal Self. In Western culture, the body is considered from a physiological perspective only and its function is frequently relegated to the unconscious.

Examples of Eastern somatics traditions include martial arts disciplines such as aikido, judo, karate, and so forth,[6] yoga,[7] zen, tai chi chuan, Tibetan Buddhist practices,[6,7] and many others. Western somatics traditions include the Alexander Technique,[8] Feldenkrais's Functional Integration[9] and Awareness through Movement,[10] Somatic Exercises[11] and Hanna Somatic Education,[12] Ida Rolf's Structural Integration and related methods,[13] Charlotte Selver's Sensory Awareness,[14] somatically oriented dance and athletics,[6] massage therapy,[15] body-oriented psychotherapy,[16] biofeedback training,[3] and many other disciplines. Medicine, chiropractic, physical therapy, occupational therapy, and other disciplines may be considered somatic when they integrate mind and body.[17]

Somatics disciplines have a variety of orientations. Allison[5] grouped them under the following categories: martial arts, mind–body medicine, energy work, movement therapies, yoga, meditative approaches, expressive arts therapies, and body-oriented psychotherapies. For example:

- Martial arts: aikido and tai chi chuan
- Mind–body medicine: biofeedback/neurofeedback training, autogenic training, guided imagery, hypnotherapy, interactive guided imagery, and progressive relaxation
- Energy work: qigong and reiki

- Structural work: Rolfing or Structural Integration, Hellerwork, Rosen Method
- Movement therapies: Alexander Technique, Aston-Patterning, Body-Mind Centering, Feldenkrais Method, Continuum, Gurdjieff Movements, Hanna Somatic Education, and Sensory Awareness
- Yoga: Integral Yoga, Iyengar Yoga, Kripalu Yoga, and others
- Meditative approaches: relaxation response and Transcendental Meditation
- Expressive arts therapies: Authentic Movement, Hakomi Integrative Somatics, Halprin Life/Art Process
- Body-oriented psychotherapies: Bioenergetics, Bodynamic Analysis, Focusing, gestalt therapy, Psychosynthesis, Rubenfeld Synergy Method, Somatic Experiencing, and others

Sidney Jourard, the American psychologist, believed that "all these techniques share one common feature; they entail an abrupt cessation of destructive, anesthesia-producing lifestyles, they enliven consciousness in general and somatic perception in particular."[18 (p. 6)]

Thousands of people practice somatics disciplines, and millions of people in the United States and other parts of the world practice the somatics discipline of yoga. It is the oldest and largest of the somatics disciplines. Yoga approaches include hatha, raja, jnana, karma, bhakti, and others. Hatha yoga, the path of physical discipline and postures, is particularly relevant to SEMG. Current developments in the yoga world include yoga and Yoga Therapy as part of complementary medical care. The International Association of Yoga Therapists (IAYT) is actively encouraging research into the efficacy of yoga and Yoga Therapy.

Psychophysiology of Somatics

Somatics disciplines emphasize the mind, body, or both. They also emphasize different aspects of the mind–body. Because of their unique emphases, they have different psychophysiological effects. For example, the somatics discipline of biofeedback training helps to make conscious those functions that are usually unconscious. As a consequence, previously involuntary functions come under greater voluntary control: Functions that are usually automatically controlled by the brain stem, and other subcortical areas, are controlled at the cortical level where functions can be organized more effectively for the task at hand.[3]

The somatics disciplines vary as to how they approach the integrated mind–body. Some of them focus on the neuromuscular system; others focus on the sensory system; still others encourage greater awareness and therefore involve the part of the brain that has to do with self-awareness, the prefrontal lobe. Some of them are verbal interventions; others are primarily nonverbal. Although approaching the soma uniquely, all of the somatics disciplines have an effect on the soma as a whole.

Goals and Outcomes of Somatics

The goals and outcomes of somatics include decreased pain, increased ease of movement, increased ease of activities of daily living (ADLs), and enhanced arts and sports performance. Somatics is used for both clinical purposes and personal development. It is also used to promote the actualization of potential and peak or optimal performance. It is used by people who are experiencing sensory–motor amnesia (SMA–unconsciously chronically contracted muscles) and other deficiencies as well as by people who want to learn how to move more efficiently. It is primarily an educational process. Neurological changes accompany the learning of new movements, so the research on neural plasticity is applicable here.

Indications for Somatics

Indications for somatics or mind–body disciplines can include "migraine headaches, insomnia, hypertension, asthma and other respiratory conditions, ulcers and other gastrointestinal disorders, incontinence, cardiac and vascular irregularities, muscular problems cause by strokes or accidents, arthritis, anxiety, attention and learning disorders, depression, chemical and emotional addictions, and phobias and other stress-related disorders."[5 (p. 67)] Somatics is indicated for any condition for which sensory-motor amnesia is a factor unless there are contraindications.

Contraindications for Somatics

The somatics practitioner must assess whether there is a contraindication or a situation requiring caution prior to embarking on somatic work. Hippocrates' "Do no harm" admonition is appropriate here.

Medical contraindications include the following conditions:

- Diabetes
- Lowered blood sugar level
- Cancer, including potential metastases
- Osteoporosis
- Acute injuries, such as fractures
- Blood clots
- Cardiac issues
- Hypertension
- Fibromyalgia
- Active disease processes
- Medication interactions
- Other medical conditions

Psychological contraindications include the following:

- Secondary gain—litigation (auto, workplace, and other accidents); other perceived or unconscious losses or gains
- Dissociative identity disorder (DID)
- Anxiety disorder
- Depression
- Bipolar disorder
- History of physical or psychological abuse
- Post-traumatic stress disorder
- Other psychological issues

Somatics Research

More research needs to be done regarding the efficacy of the somatics disciplines. Often, research has been conducted in the classical empirical fashion. That is, the practitioner or teacher provides the service; the client has the responses and outcomes. The practitioner and the client then assess how well the client's outcomes match the goals for the session. Many clients and students, having similar experiences, begin to confirm the validity of the practice. Some of the creators of these disciplines come from strong physiological backgrounds and clinical or experiential arenas; others come from somatics lineages, trained by originators; still others have studied and brought together their knowledge and experiences to create new disciplines. The practitioners' somas and client experiences have been significant contributors to the development of the field.

Somatics research needs to be both qualitative and quantitative in nature. SEMG, quantitative electroencephalography (QEEG), MRI, functional MRI (fMRI), and other modalities can contribute to the quantitative measures, along with use of other data-gathering devices (e.g., questionnaires, behavioral observations, rating scales). Quantitative measures represent third-person sources of information. Qualitative or phenomenological data (interviews, journal entries, and other sources) can help in understanding the first-person experience of the client and the context in which somatics is taking place. Because somatics is first-person oriented, it is necessary for the data to be triangulated to blend the different kinds of data. Double-blind studies would be a challenge for somatics: Clients need to be aware and receptive to the somatics approach, and it is difficult to disguise the activity.

Although there has been very little research on somatics per se, except occasional studies on particular disciplines, the somatics disciplines are based on thousands of studies within the whole of anatomy, physiology, and psychology. Indeed, the somatics disciplines are applications of the principles of these sciences. The field of biofeedback has demonstrated that physiological functions once thought to be automatic and not subject to voluntary control are, in fact, trainable. More research needs to be done on the psychophysiological mechanisms and efficacy of the somatics disciplines. Surface electromyography has enormous potential for further exploring the validity of the somatics disciplines and for enhancing those practices through allowing the practitioner and client to observe the changes as they happen. The more the practitioner and the client know about the psychophysiology of these practices, the more effective the practices will be.

SEMG MONITORING AND SOMATICS

Surface electromyography monitoring enables clients to refine their self-regulation skills, confirms the progress they have made, and enables them to expand their skills. It is important to pursue self-regulation practices because the effects of stress and repetitive movements begin to accumulate unless something is done to return to baseline. Without a return to baseline, this accumulation increases over time.

It is possible to use SEMG combined with somatics. When beginning as a somatics client, it may become relevant for the client to see what is happening to SEMG levels and to understand his or her capacities to change those levels. For example, clients can see the microvolt level of relevant muscles and watch themselves change the level of contraction of the muscle. Alternatively, the individual might begin as an SEMG feedback client for

whom somatics work seems necessary in preparation for SEMG feedback training or use somatics to develop his or her SEMG feedback skills.

Surface EMG allows for quantification and documentation of neuromuscular events. An important consideration in making use of SEMG data is the potential for artifacts to contaminate the recording (see Chapter 3). Other clinical information needs to be included as well. SEMG is used for patient feedback; it lets clients know the outcomes of their voluntary control of movements. Armed with the SEMG information, clients can then explore more refined patterns of motor control. Using SEMG with other therapies, the practitioner can greatly enhance the outcomes. For example, when SEMG is combined with other therapies, movement difficulties can be decreased and motor function enhanced more easily than with a single therapy. SEMG data can support the principles of the somatics disciplines, and sometimes it leads to new understandings. Much research still needs to be done regarding which techniques are effective and how they might best be applied.

SEMG in the somatics context can be used for the following purposes:

- Assessment regarding the goals of the somatics discipline (pre- and post-assessment)
- Demonstration of the mind–body connection for clients
- Feedback to the client during the techniques of the somatics discipline
- Help in generalizing the somatic results into everyday life
- Training of somatics practitioners or educators
- Research as to the mechanisms and effectiveness of the somatics discipline
- Exploring the different somatics disciplines and how SEMG might be used

Hanna Somatic Education and Surface EMG

This section will explore in greater detail one of the somatics disciplines—Hanna Somatic Education (HSE)—to demonstrate the integration of SEMG and somatics. This approach has been chosen because of its emphasis on the neuromuscular system. Hanna Somatic Education was created by Thomas Hanna, an American philosopher and somatics educator, as an outgrowth of his Functional Integration (FI) work. He first studied with Moshe Feldenkrais, the Israeli physicist and originator of

FI, in 1972. Hanna became director of the Humanistic Psychology Institute (now Saybrook University) in San Francisco and organized the first Feldenkrais professional training program in the United States in 1973, which he attended. Hanna practiced FI at the Novato Institute for Somatic Research and Training, which he cofounded in 1975.

Over the next 13 years, Hanna's work continued to evolve. While maintaining some of the features of FI, it became something quite different. When Hanna conducted the first training program for his approach in 1990, he named the approach Hanna Somatic Education.

Both FI and HSE include hands-on work and floor exercises. The difference between FI and HSE lies mainly in the hands-on or table work. In the table work, the FI practitioner/teacher moves the client to approximate origin and insertion of muscles to allow muscles to relax along with other maneuvers. With HSE, the client is the center of the process and does the main work of the session. Different areas of the brain are involved in the two approaches: FI primarily affects the sensory cortex, while HSE primarily affects the motor cortex. Thomas Hanna felt that what he had added to FI, he learned from biofeedback, especially SEMG feedback. He brought in the concepts of self-regulation and the knowledge of muscle function.

The HSE approach relies on several key concepts, including the postures (*red light*, *green light*, and *trauma* postures) discussed in Chapter 11. There is a fourth posture that Hanna called the *senile* posture, in which all of the muscles are contracted with many cocontractions present. First- versus third-person perception and sensory-motor amnesia (chronic muscle contractions and loss of awareness and control) are additional HSE key concepts.

Postural patterns affect the person's psychophysiological state. For example, postural patterns such as the red light posture discussed in Chapter 11 may interfere with respiration and cardiac function. Postural patterns, stress of the posture, emotions that accompany postures, and distress resulting from pain or restricted movement may also affect brain wave activity, increasing beta brain waves (13–30 Hz). Beta brain waves are characteristic of the alert brain. The alert brain cannot go to sleep or stay asleep easily, so contracted muscles impact negatively on sleep. Sleep deprivation, in turn, affects the general physiological state and muscle contraction levels. Many other somatic complaints also result from the habitual postural patterns. (For more information on the postural patterns observed by Thomas Hanna, see Chapter 11.)

Hanna's concept of SMA describes the tendency of humans to "forget" certain movements or ways of organizing muscles or muscle groups, leaving the muscles chronically contracted. The contraction is the result of ongoing brain stem–level motor tracts, sending impulses to the motor units and causing contractions of muscle fibers. (A motor unit is an alpha motor neuron and all the muscle fibers on which it synapses.) This increased cortical control returns the control of the muscles to the client. HSE enables the client to gain or regain greater control with increased awareness and enhanced conscious self-regulation. In HSE, the client is invited to move neuromuscular control from the brain stem–level tracts to the corticospinal tract that originates in the primary motor cortex. The corticospinal tract is the only part of the motor system that can voluntarily relax the muscles. The other four brain stem motor tracts—reticulospinal, vestibulospinal, rubrospinal, and tectospinal—are largely involved with postural reflexes and muscle tone.

In HSE, there are three protocols devoted to addressing the basic postures; specialized work with extremities follows the basic protocols as needed. Three techniques are used in HSE: *meanswhereby*, which is an adaptation of F. M. Alexander's Alexander Technique; *kinetic mirroring*, Hanna's term for the approximation of the origin and insertion of muscles used by Moshe Feldenkrais; and *pandiculation*,[12,19] the technique developed by Hanna and named after the reflexive full-body contraction or contraction of parts of the body and slow release of the contraction used by all healthy animals. In the voluntary pandiculation, the client is asked first to voluntarily contract a muscle or muscle group (concentric contraction), creating a movement against gravity or the practitioner's hand, and then to slowly return to a neutral position, decreasing the contraction(s) (eccentric contraction). All three techniques can benefit from SEMG monitoring during the activity. This technology enables the practitioner to see what is happening more clearly and the client to engage in the activity more effectively.

Hanna somatics techniques that can be done using SEMG include meanswhereby, kinetic mirroring, and pandiculation. In the meanswhereby technique, the practitioner moves the client's body through various ranges of motion. Using SEMG, the client and the practitioner are able to see and hear the SEMG changes that accompany the movement as well as monitor the pre- and post-SEMG measures. The movements provide sensory input to the brain.

The effect of kinetic mirroring occurs at the spinal cord level, subsequently informing the brain of the changes. As the practitioner brings the origin and insertion of the client's muscle closer together and the muscle shortens, gently pulling on its tendons, a message is sent to the spinal cord to decrease the motor unit firing rate. The Golgi tendon organs (structures within the tendons) create the change, which allows the muscle to relax. With SEMG, the practitioner and client can hear the changes.

Pandiculation, the technique developed by Hanna, includes a voluntary concentric contraction of a muscle or muscle group with a movement and a subsequent relaxation of the muscle(s). With the use of the SEMG, the client can see the microvolt reading for the muscle contraction increasing and decreasing. Pandiculation uses gravity as the load on the muscle; alternatively, the practitioner can provide resistance as the client moves. For example, while SEMG electrodes are attached to the shoulders (upper trapezius), the client can raise the shoulders. At the practitioner's direction, the client will slowly lower his or her shoulders, decreasing the output to the upper trapezius and levator scapulae muscles. The slow release of the contractions is the most important part of the pandicular process. The client can be asked to watch the microvolt levels decreasing on the computer graph as the muscle contractions decrease and the shoulders slowly lower. Finally, both the client and the practitioner can see the lowered resting tonus of the muscle as measured by the SEMG. The decrease in muscle contractions happens in the absence of SEMG feedback, of course, but SEMG can aid in refinement of the technique and facilitate the learning.

SEMG FEEDBACK AS A SOMATICS DISCIPLINE

Surface EMG feedback works with the brain and the peripheral nervous system, particularly the somatic nervous system. The motor system includes motor tracts that consciously and unconsciously control movement. The areas of the brain that are largely unconscious are also significant in controlling behavior. For example, Yochanan Rywerant[20] has written a valuable monograph on corollary discharge, the process that the brain uses to prepare the person for coming movements and to decrease sensory feedback from the person's own movements that might disrupt the intended movement. SEMG feedback involves learning how to shift the areas of brain control of motor functions. Learning

how to organize all of this information more effectively is the task.

SEMG feedback is a somatic practice that includes both first- and third-person perceptions. First-person perception refers to the client's personal perceptions from his or her subjective center. The client is "subject" and everything else is considered an "object." The third-person perception is the outside information about the person. It includes information about how the person behaves, the observations of the SEMG feedback practitioner, and external data recorded by the SEMG instrument.

Clients who have experienced SEMG training respond very quickly to somatic work because they are used to self-regulating their bodies on subtle and not-so-subtle levels. They are used to sending messages along their nervous systems to create activity or to inhibit activity; they are used to being aware of their bodies precisely and coordinating body sensations with the feedback signals of the SEMG feedback equipment. Conversely, people who have learned and practiced somatics respond quickly to the SEMG feedback training experience. They are used to asking their bodies to engage in the movements; they are used to sensing the effects of the movements that come from internal feedback from the muscles (neuromuscular spindles), tendons (Golgi tendon organs), joints, skin, and other position sensing mechanisms.

Somatics Assessment in the SEMG Session

A brief somatics assessment can be added to the SEMG intake. Begin by noting the presenting complaint(s) and client goals and assess the posture of the client. Have the person stand (fully clothed). Determine whether the person is tilting to one side or the other. Are the muscles of the trunk tighter on one side, resulting in a tilt to that side? Is the head tilted to that side or the opposite side? Are the arms rotated inward? How are the legs positioned? Is the person standing with legs spread apart or close together? Are the feet turned out or in?

Walk to the side of the client. If a plumb line were hung from the external meatus (the hole in the ear), would it hang to the ground through the shoulder, hip, leg, and ankles (posterior), or would it hang down in front of the person?

From the rear, run a hand down the client's spine. Is it straight, curved, or multiply curved? How are the head, shoulders, and legs as seen from the back?

Assess the client's posture from the opposite side.

Now ask the client to walk across the room. Does the postural pattern become more exaggerated in walking? Is there free movement of the arms and shoulders? Does the person walk contralaterally—that is, do his or her shoulders move in opposition to the legs (for example, the right shoulder and arm move back as the right leg comes forward) or ipsilaterally (when the same shoulder and leg move forward)?

These data are clues as to which postural pattern is extant. The clues can be used for SEMG training and for planning the somatics session or lesson. Psychological elements such as emotions/mood, self-concept, learning/modeling of family members, response to expectations from others, cultural and gender roles, and so forth, can all influence posture. In turn, SEMG training, somatics disciplines, and allied therapies can directly or indirectly address some of these issues.

Somatics Disciplines as Adjuncts to SEMG Feedback

The somatics disciplines as adjuncts can bring to SEMG feedback training an expansion of its effects throughout the person's physiological systems and lifestyle. A pure blend of somatics and SEMG includes SEMG feedback and somatics from the beginning. The client might be hooked up to the SEMG system while doing the somatic movements. This type of training requires telemetry or special cables to allow an artifact-free recording during movement. It enables the practitioner to see the subtle changes that are taking place; it also allows the client to use the information in organizing the body for the somatics movements.

James Kepner,[16] in his book *Body Process*, has discussed various levels of blending somatic practices with psychotherapy. The levels that he listed are the singular, alternating, layered, and integrated approaches. In this case, the relationship between SEMG and somatics is the focus, but the comparison is useful. In the singular approach, the two sessions are kept separate. The client might have an SEMG feedback session once during the week and a somatics session with another practitioner at another time. In the alternating approach, the client might have an SEMG feedback session one week and a somatics session the next week, each session with the same practitioner. In the layered approach, SEMG feedback and somatics take place during the same session. Finally, integration of somatics and SEMG feedback occurs during the same session at the same time. In the integrated approach, mind–body integration happens within the experience of the client and is fostered by the practitioner.

At times, SEMG and somatics are blended such that somatics practices are used with SEMG feedback to enhance the client's learning and awareness. One of the benefits of SEMG feedback is the increase in awareness and the specificity of the client's self-regulation. In somatic work, the client self-regulates mind–body states; SEMG feedback adds another level of awareness and integration to this process.

Somatics practices that are taught by the SEMG practitioner in session can be used outside of the session as home practice. At home, they can be used with SEMG monitoring and feedback or without.

Ways to Blend SEMG and Somatics

Surface electromyography can be blended with somatics in the following ways:

- SEMG as part of assessment
- SEMG feedback during session
- SEMG feedback for differential use of muscles
- SEMG in post assessment

Benefits of Blending Somatics and SEMG Feedback

Blending somatics and SEMG allows for the following benefits:

- Addressing the whole person
- Completing the protocol so that all psychophysiological systems are addressed
- Enhancing the person's ability to continue the somatics/SEMG work through home practice and self-regulation
- Enhancing assessment for SEMG and somatics disciplines
- Helping evaluate the results of somatics practices in achieving SEMG goals
- Refining the client's learning

Who Can Benefit from Somatics and SEMG?

Many clients who present with musculoskeletal complaints are candidates for somatics and SEMG. Whether the client is ultimately receptive to an approach depends on the readiness of the client to engage in the somatic practices. Many clients with postural patterns that might contribute to their presenting complaints and many clients with chronic muscle contractions, regardless of whether the condition affects the focus of SEMG training, can benefit from this type of therapy. Somatics can also be used with neurofeedback clients because muscle contractions affect brain activity. Somatics disciplines affect a variety of areas of the brain in a holistic manner.

Persons of all ages, from all walks of life, can potentially benefit from the somatics/SEMG combination. Many somatics disciplines are not attached to any belief system and blend nicely with most lifestyles; that is, they are based on pure physiological principles confirmed by much research. Although research on somatics per se is scarce, the physiological systems that are targeted in somatics have a long history of research in physiology, biology, medicine, psychology, and other fields. Somatics/SEMG combinations also work very well in complementary, integrative medicine contexts.

A Typical Somatics/SEMG Session

A typical somatics/SEMG session begins with an assessment. The assessment includes a brief visual inspection and palpation to determine the postural pattern the client is presenting during that session, a review of the progress with the presenting complaint, and goals for the session. The client is hooked up to the SEMG instrument; SEMG baseline data are recorded. Other physiologies may be measured as well. The client's life context is discussed briefly at that time. Somatic practices that the client has been doing and somatic issues that the client would like to work on during the session are discussed. The client might also talk about current stressors. If the client is reporting shoulder pain, a look at where the pain is being felt and which muscles are contributing to the pain is necessary. Postural patterns that may be contributing to the pain are observed. Based on that information, palpation, and a visual assessment of posture and movement, a protocol for the session will be selected by the practitioner.

After the assessment, which lasts approximately 15 minutes, a treatment or training plan is selected. Depending on the setting, the client is invited to lie on a low padded table or sit in a chair, and to move in certain directions to voluntarily contract the relevant muscles. Then the client will slowly move out of that position, decreasing the contraction. Movement must occur with the contraction. To simply contract muscles represents an isometric contraction (a change in muscle tonus without

a change in muscle length). Unfortunately, there is no decrease in muscle tone following an isometric contraction because of the activation of the gamma motor neurons accompanying the contraction, the subsequent excitation of the neuromuscular spindles, and the lack of inhibition of the gamma motor neurons following the contraction.

For 30 minutes, the client works through relevant muscles—contracting, moving, and slowly relaxing—along with muscles that are not being monitored by the SEMG instrument. Post-SEMG baselines are recorded and noted. At the end of the session, there is a debriefing period during which the client discusses his or her insights about the session, learns somatic exercises for home practice, and looks forward to the subsequent applications of the learning (such as generalization to everyday life or enhanced performance).

With some somatics disciplines, it is only feasible to take prebaseline and postbaseline measurements due to the active nature of the practices. In contexts such as insurance reimbursement or demonstration of clinical outcomes, pre- and post-SEMG data are invaluable.

SOMATIC EXERCISES AND SEMG

Many of the somatics disciplines include floor exercises and other exercises. Some exercises can be used adjunctively within the SEMG training session (i.e., they can be done before, during, or after the training). The somatic exercises can be done in the SEMG session or as home practice exercises. As home practice, somatic exercises may be combined with other adjunctive procedures, such as guided relaxation and visualization procedures the client is learning and making part of his or her lifestyle.

Why Do Somatic Exercises?

The somatic exercises can prepare the client for the day's activity and reduce the accumulated muscle contractions at the end of the day. Somatic exercises foster mind–body integration. The effects of somatic exercises are cumulative. The client becomes increasingly more somatically integrated over time. The client begins to actualize more potential along the lines of natural talents, rather than stopping development somewhere in life.

Somatic exercises can retard or reverse some of the negative effects of aging. The client becomes maximally effective in all aspects of life, whether it is business or family (for example, being able to play with his or her children or grandchildren). The client remains healthier, maintaining a higher level of general health. If accidents or health issues occur, the client responds to them more effectively and moves through the healing process more easily. For example, when a horse bucked its rider off recently, the rider's pelvis was fractured in several places; an external fixator was surgically installed, and the rider used somatics and SEMG feedback skills along with physical and occupational therapy to move through the healing process quickly and easily.

Clients who engage in somatic exercises report that they are happier and feel more like themselves. They become self-responsible and self-confident. Becoming their own somatic educators, clients are able to deal with most problems using their somatics and SEMG skills. If they are dealing with health issues, they bring the same self-responsibility to handling the situation effectively.

WHAT IS NEEDED FOR THE PRACTICE OF SOMATICS AND SEMG?

For clients and practitioners to practice somatics and SEMG, a knowledgeable SEMG practitioner needs to be involved who can use the equipment effectively with the appropriate electrode or sensor placements (see Chapters 4 and 17), rule out artifacts, and interpret the results. Somatics practitioners need to be trained in SEMG or to work in partnership with someone who is trained and certified by the Biofeedback Certification Institute of America (BCIA) in general biofeedback, which includes SEMG. Somatics practitioners and educators need enough knowledge about SEMG to produce useful data. In addition, the somatics practitioner needs to be trained and certified in his or her somatics discipline. Clients need information about and experience with SEMG, so that they can become desensitized to the stimulus properties of the recording process, and be able to focus on their physiological and SEMG responses.

SURFACE EMG AND SOMATIC PSYCHOTHERAPY

Surface EMG can be integrated into somatic psychotherapy or body-oriented psychotherapy. This combination can also include other biofeedback and neurofeedback modalities.

For example, elevated psychophysiological levels typically occur with stress. In this approach to SEMG/somatic psychotherapy, the client under stress is hooked up to the SEMG instrument and is able to view the computer screen; visual and/or auditory displays are available. With the patient's eyes closed, SEMG baseline measures are recorded. After the baseline is established, the client is allowed to see the SEMG baseline level. After some initial downtraining or relaxation, the talking portion of the session begins. The client may be instructed to talk about something stressful or to talk about the most important or salient topic(s) of the day. The therapist and client are both attending to the information presented by the SEMG system. Previously, the client was educated about the nature of SEMG and the ways in which it relates to arousal, alertness, stress responses, relaxation, emotions, and so forth. Clients are taught what the microvolt signal represents (i.e., the graphed quantity goes up or down, correlated with the contraction level of the muscle). The correlation between microvolt level and motor unit activity may be discussed. (The number of motor units firing—frequencies of firing of motor units or number of motor units recruited—correlates with the microvolt level of the SEMG recording.) The SEMG-knowledgeable client is able to experience the physiological changes (i.e., decreasing muscle tension) and to associate them with the corresponding graphed changes.

Both the therapist and the client may notice the SEMG changes accompanying emotions, cognitions, and images that are being experienced or discussed. The physiological changes are not positive or negative except as the client subjectively assesses them. The therapist can also bring meaning to the data by remembering the client's experiences from the past and current issues. Facial expressions and other physical indicators, such as posture, respiration rate, and movements, will be observed as well. In the session, it is possible to pause to further explore the topic while the client brings the microvolt levels down or to stop to practice a relaxation procedure to allow the client to relax.

In some cases, the purpose of the SEMG feedback is to increase SEMG levels (uptraining), such as in the case of depression or apathy. For example, a client was referred for biofeedback training for insomnia. Her baseline data as recorded via all modalities were unremarkable. The referral source felt that some psychological issues were involved, however. Because all her biofeedback modalities were relaxed, her frontalis SEMG was monitored with the goal of noticing the changes in the microvolt levels, especially her responses to various topics. Over time, the client was able to reengage with her somatic responses, decrease her insomnia, and move forward with her life. She went back to school, completed her university degree, married, and began a career. These were all things she previously felt she would never be able to do.

The SEMG/somatic psychotherapist uses all his or her knowledge to assess the situation. If appropriate, the *Diagnostic and Statistical Manual of Mental Disorders* (DSM-IV-TR) criteria are used to create a psychological diagnosis. The SEMG data complement the therapist's and client's understanding of the client's responses to issues and themes. These issues frequently relate to where the client is in his or her life development. The SEMG/somatically oriented psychotherapist is interested in the whole person—the mind/body/spirit—and the development of the client's full positive potential. The client's awareness of somatic responses in making life decisions is an important outcome.

CONCLUSION

There is a growing appreciation for the role of somatics in mind–body health. SEMG is an important somatics discipline owing to its feedback capabilities and its compatibility with the other somatics disciplines. A call for more research in somatics is now coming from several directions: Some psychotherapists are becoming aware of the body's role in psychological health and the impact of emotions on the body; some somatics practitioners and healthcare providers are becoming aware of the effect of emotions on physiological states; some SEMG practitioners are becoming aware of the ability of the psychological state of the client to affect SEMG levels. In addition, clients are becoming more interested in their mind–body health: The body is a system of systems that is characterized by feedback. For all these reasons, SEMG is a significant contributor to research relevant to the field of somatics.

Growing fields such as SEMG and somatics need to continue to explore, to deepen their understandings, and to draw from other disciplines—to be interdisciplinary. The SEMG field is very interdisciplinary; that has always been one of its charms. Together, SEMG and somatics have a bright future. Blending the two brings SEMG into the holistic field of health, healing, and wellness. What is unique about somatics is that it brings greater awareness or self-awareness into the mix. Somatics is a valuable adjunct to SEMG and SEMG has enormous riches to offer somatics.

REFERENCES

1. Cram JR, Kasman GS, Holtz J. *Introduction to Surface Electromyography.* Gaithersburg, MD: Aspen; 1998.
2. Hanna T. Three elements of somatology: preface to a holistic medicine and to a humanistic psychology. *Somatics.* 1975/1994;IX(4):4–9. [Originally published in *Main Currents in Modern Thought.* 1975;31(3):82–87.]
3. Criswell E. *Biofeedback and Somatics: Toward Personal Evolution.* Novato, CA: Freeperson Press; 1995.
4. Hanna T. *The Body of Life: Creating New Pathways for Sensory Awareness and Fluid Movement.* Rochester, VT: Healing Arts Press; 1979/1993.
5. Allison N. *The Illustrated Encyclopedia of Body–Mind Disciplines.* New York, NY: Rosen; 1999.
6. Murphy M. *The Future of the Body: Explorations into the Further Evolution of Human Nature.* Los Angeles, CA: Jeremy Tarcher; 1992.
7. Criswell E. *How Yoga Works: An Introduction to Somatic Yoga.* Novato, CA: Freeperson Press; 1989.
8. Alexander FM. *The Use of the Self: Its Conscious Direction in Relation to Diagnosis, Function and the Control of Reaction.* New York, NY: E. P. Dutton; 1932.
9. Rywerant Y. *The Feldenkrais Method: Teaching by Handling.* New Canaan, CT: Keats; 1983.
10. Feldenkrais M. *Awareness Through Movement: Health Exercises for Personal Growth.* New York, NY: Harper & Row; 1972.
11. Hanna T. *Somatics: Reawakening the Mind's Control of Movement, Flexibility, and Health.* Cambridge, MA: DeCapo Press; 1988.
12. Hanna T. Clinical somatic education: a new discipline in the field of health care. *Somatics.* Autumn/Winter 1990–1991; VIII(1):4–10.
13. Rolf I. *Rolfing: The Integration of Human Structures.* Santa Monica, CA: Dennis-Landman; 1977.
14. Brooks C. *Sensory Awareness: Rediscovering of Experiencing Through the Workshops of Charlotte Selver.* Great Neck, NY: Felix Morrow; 1986.
15. Knaster M. *Discovering the Body's Wisdom.* New York, NY: Bantam Books; 1996.
16. Kepner JI. *Body Process: Working with the Body in Psychotherapy.* San Francisco, CA: Jossey-Bass; 1987.
17. Criswell-Hanna E. Interrelationships between somatic perception and somatic disclosure. In: Richards AC, Schumrum T, eds. *Invitations to Dialogue: The Legacy of Sidney M. Jourard.* Dubuque, IA: Kendall/Hunt; 1999: 39–50.
18. Jourard SM. Some ways of unembodiment and re-embodiment. *Somatics.* 1976;1(1):3–7.
19. Frazier AF. The phenomenon of pandiculation in the kinetic behavior of the sheep fetus. *Applied Animal Behav Sci.* 1989;24:169–182.

CHAPTER QUESTIONS

1. Somatics is:
   a. the integrated mind–body disciplines
   b. a term coined by Thomas Hanna
   c. concerned with the body only
   d. both a and b

2. Somatics research:
   a. is extensive
   b. needs further development
   c. could benefit from SEMG monitoring
   d. would be very difficult to do

3. The psychophysiology of somatics:
   a. varies depending on how the integrated mind–body is approached
   b. includes only the body
   c. includes only psychological states
   d. is not a necessary concern for somatics practitioners

4. Indications for somatics include:
   a. any condition in which sensory-motor amnesia is a factor
   b. accident recovery during the acute stage
   c. anxiety disorders
   d. chronic muscle contractions

5. Hanna Somatic Education:
   a. is the same as Functional Integration
   b. is an approach developed by Thomas Hanna
   c. uses electronic devices
   d. uptrains the muscles

6. The relationship between SEMG and somatics:
   a. is nonexistent; they are incompatible
   b. includes SEMG as a somatics discipline
   c. can demonstrate the efficacy of somatics
   d. can enhance the training of somatics practitioners

7. Somatics disciplines include:
   a. Hanna Somatic Education
   b. Functional Integration
   c. Structural Integration
   d. all of the above

8. A typical somatics and SEMG session includes:
   a. keeping the two disciplines separate
   b. assessment before and after the somatics work only
   c. somatics and SEMG assessments
   d. no talking

9. Blending somatics and SEMG includes:
   a. SEMG in the assessment phase
   b. SEMG used during the somatics session
   c. Use of SEMG to determine differential use of muscles only
   d. both a and b

10. To practice SEMG and somatics, it is necessary to:
    a. have a knowledgeable SEMG practitioner
    b. have a trained somatics practitioner
    c. have an informed and receptive client
    d. all of the above

Electromyographic Assessment of Female Pelvic Floor Disorders

Marek Jantos

INTRODUCTION

Pelvic floor disorders are a cluster of pain, incontinence, and sexual disorders that arise mainly out of dysfunctional muscle states and structural changes, rather than as a malfunction of specific pelvic organs.[1-4] The pelvic floor muscles (PFM), which make up the bulk of the pelvic soft tissue, are structurally and functionally one of the most complex muscle units in the human body.[5] Functionally, these muscles provide support to the abdominal and pelvic organs, maintain urinary and fecal continence, enable sexual intercourse, facilitate parturition, provide postural support, and assist with locomotion.[4] When pelvic floor structure and function is compromised, a range of debilitating disorders arises that have significant impact on quality of life,[6-8] lead to psychological morbidity,[9,10] and prove costly to manage.[11]

Although pelvic floor disorders affect both sexes, there is a high female-to-male ratio. One in two women, versus one in ten men, will experience some type of pelvic floor disorder during her lifetime, but the true magnitude of the problem may be unknown.[12] Although female pelvic disorders involve one of the most understudied regions of the body and are one of the most neglected areas of women's health, due to their increasing prevalence and impact on quality of life they are generating greater clinical and research interest.[4]

This is a welcome development: "It is gratifying to realize, finally, that insight into the cause and necessary treatment of disorders of the pelvis in women appears to be in a modern-day renaissance."[13]

Surface electromyography (SEMG), as the primary modality for assessment of muscle function, assists in the diagnosis and neuromuscular rehabilitation of pelvic disorders arising from dysfunctional pelvic muscle states.[14-16] The advantages of SEMG are widely acknowledged throughout this textbook, but in relation to pelvic disorders its primary benefits arise from the fact that it is a noninvasive, objective, and cost-effective assessment modality suitable for use in conservative therapy.[17] This chapter focuses on relevant SEMG research and therapeutic interventions in relation to lower tract urogenital pain, urinary incontinence (UI), and sexual dysfunction, highlighting the role of PFM and the significant cross-over of symptoms between the various disorders. To appreciate the role of SEMG in diagnostic decisions and therapeutic interventions, it is essential for clinicians to have a good knowledge of pelvic muscle anatomy and physiology.

PELVIC FLOOR ANATOMY AND PHYSIOLOGY

The pelvic floor consists of several layers of muscle tissue and supporting fasciae that span the pelvic cavity and form a strong horizontally oriented platform,[1] as shown in **Figure 13–1**. These layers of soft tissue are penetrated anteriorly by the urethra, centrally by the vagina, and posteriorly by the anorectum, in an area known as the urogenital hiatus or pelvic outlet,[1,4,18] as shown in **Figure 13–2**.

The pelvic muscles are separated into three distinct layers consisting of the superficial muscles, the urogenital diaphragm, and the pelvic diaphragm.[1,4]

1. *Superficial muscles.* This small layer of muscles assists with sexual function, but has no role in pelvic organ support. The superficial layer comprises the ischiocavernosus muscle, which assists in the erection of the penis and in the female erection of the clitoris; the bulbospongiosus muscle, which compresses the male urethra and the female vaginal orifice; and the superficial transverse perineus muscle, which helps support the perineum.
2. *Urogenital diaphragm and perineal body.* The muscles of the urogenital diaphragm and perineal body form a coordinated unit. The pelvic organ support system consists of an anterior compartment containing the urethra and bladder and a posterior compartment containing the anus and rectum. The perineal body represents the central connection between the two halves of the urogenital diaphragm.
3. *The pelvic diaphragm.* This structure comprises the levator ani muscles and their overlaying fascia, both of which are crucial to pelvic organ support in the female. The levator ani muscle has three parts:

- The pubococcygeus muscles (more correctly termed the pubovisceral for reasons discussed later) consist of paired muscles that form a "U-shaped" sling to support the anal canal and narrow the urogenital hiatus.
- The puborectalis muscles form a second pair of strap-like muscles that run from the pubic bone to the ano-rectal angle. The puborectalis is important in anal continence.
- The iliococcygeus muscle is a thin, sheet-like muscle that runs from the tendinous arch of the levator ani on each pelvic sidewall to insert into the coccyx and ano-coccygeal raphe. In contradistinction to the pubococcygeus muscle and the puborectalis, the iliococcygeus forms a "levator plate" that functions as an immovable muscular shelf (rather than as a sling mechanism). Historically, the coccygeus muscle was also considered part of the pelvic diaphragm. However, modern anatomy considers the coccygeus and piriformis to be the muscles closing the posterior pelvic walls.

The pelvic diaphragm supports the internal organs, resists surges in abdominal pressure, creates the orgasmic platform, and elevates the pelvic floor.

When viewed in cross section, the upper pelvis forms a cavity that can be visualized as consisting of an inter-

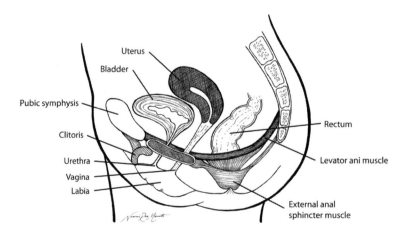

Figure 13–1 Pelvic diaphragm: medial view.
Source: Courtesy of Naomi Merritt.

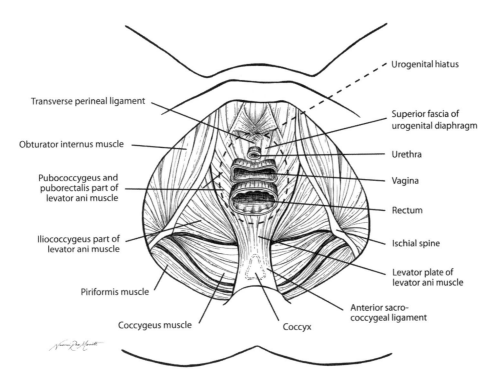

Figure 13–2 Pelvic diaphragm: superior view.

Source: Courtesy of Naomi Merritt.

nal compartment consisting of two side walls, front and back wall, and the pelvic floor,[19] as seen in Figure 13–2. The short front wall is formed by the pubic bones. The posterior walls are closed by the piriformis and coccyggeus. The two lateral walls are formed by the obturator internus, which is crossed by the muscular arch of the levator ani (from which the pelvic diaphragm arises). The floor is made up of the horizontal component of the levator ani muscles that make up the platform upon which the internal viscera rest.

The endopelvic fascia, when intact, plays an important role in pelvic organ support, by holding the viscera well back in the pelvic cavity, where the levator platform functions most efficiently.[1,20] The connective tissue of the endopelvic fascia consists of elastin (distensible tissue), collagen (noncompliant, less distensible soft tissue), and smooth muscle. Organs such as the bladder, upper vagina, cervix, and uterus are held in their positions by fascial attachments to muscles and the bony pelvis. Condensations of the endopelvic fascia form the cardinal and uterosacral ligaments, both of which serve as important landmarks in corrective pelvic surgery.

Because the fascia does not easily stretch but can readily tear, the gravitational force and intra-abdominal pressures are passed onto the pelvic musculature, sparing the endopelvic fascia from chronic overload.[21] The combined effect of the muscles and fascia spanning the pelvic outlet is to support organs and prevent them from prolapsing into the urogenital opening. The urogenital hiatus creates a central point of weakness in the pelvic floor.[18] If, as a result of trauma or injury, the integrity of the levator muscle is compromised, its function in supporting the internal organs will be weakened.[18] The muscles and fascia provide dynamic support during filling, storage, and elimination of waste, and during sexual activity.[1,21]

As shown in **Figure 13–3**, the pubococcygeus muscle originates from the pubic bone and forms the inner medial sling around the rectum and vagina, returning on the contralateral side to the pubic bone without significant anchoring to the sacrum or coccyx. The term "pubococcygeus muscle" incorrectly implies that the muscle connects between the pubis and coccyx; in fact, most of the muscle's medial fibers are inserted into the walls of the vagina, and the posterior fibers into the walls of the

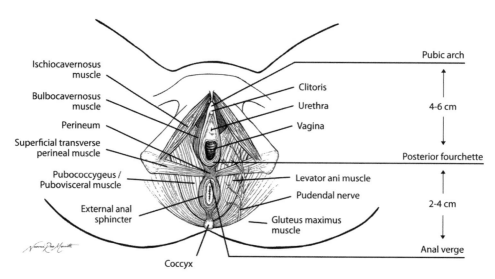

Figure 13–3 Pelvic diaphragm: superficial view.
Source: Courtesy of Naomi Merritt.

anorectum, to elevate these structures and close the genital hiatus.[4] The anterior fibers of the pubococcygeus muscle attach to the anterior walls of the vagina, forming the pubovaginal muscle. Some attach to the perineal body, and the more posterior fibers of the pubococcygeus muscle attach to the lateral walls of the rectum, forming the puborectalis muscle.[1,20]

When the pubococcygeus muscle contracts, it acts as a sling compressing the rectum, vagina, and urethra against the pubic bone, ensuring the closure of the urogenital openings.[4] An estimated 70% of the urethral closure pressure in the external sphincter muscle originates from the contraction of the levator ani muscle and the rhabdosphincter of the urethra, while the remaining 30% originates from the transverse perineal muscles.[22] The posterior portion of the levator ani, which is commonly known as the iliococcygeus, originates from the side walls of the pelvis and inserts into the outlet of the bony pelvis behind the rectum. The iliococcygeus also provides support to the internal organs and during contraction moves the viscera toward the pubic bone. These two components of the levator ani muscle comprise a single functional unit. A voluntary mass contraction of the pelvic floor muscles produces an upward lift and squeeze around the urethra, vagina, and rectum.[23]

Due to the horizontal position of the levator ani muscle, it is subject to increased gravitational forces during walking, running, and high-impact activities, and to intra-abdominal pressure associated with sneezing, coughing, or lifting.[1]

High intra-abdominal pressure is also correlated with high body mass index.[24,25] Increases in pressure stemming from coughing, Valsalva maneuvers, and straining stool have been found to be four to five times higher than increases in pressure incurred during lifting a 5-kg weight.[26] During fluctuations in gravitational force and abdominal pressure, the levator ani constantly adjusts its resting tone either by contracting and elevating the muscle or by relaxing it. During these dynamic adjustments, the levator plate will ascend or descend by 2 to 3 cm.[1] The PFMs are more suited to providing such resilient and flexible support than is the endopelvic fascia, which is susceptible to elongation and damage.[21]

Neuromuscular reflexes play an important role in regulating the resting tone of pelvic muscles. In healthy individuals, pelvic muscle SEMG activity increases before lifting, coughing, or rapid postural change.[27,28] SEMG studies of coughing show that the intra-urethral pressure and activation of the external anal sphincter muscle precedes contraction of the external intercostal and abdominal muscles by 100 to 240 milliseconds.[29] Such increases in PFM activity appear to be preprogrammed and are scaled to the intensity of the activity. Weakening or loss of such reflexes leads to delays in the preactivation of sphincteric activity and is associated with stress urinary incontinence.[28–30] Reflex-mediated adjustments are essential to preserving the integrity of pelvic function; due to trauma and overstretching of pelvic muscles, denervation may account for as many as 75% of incontinence cases in women.[22,31]

PELVIC FLOOR MICROSCOPIC ANATOMY

The microscopic anatomy of the pelvic floor also reflects its complex function. The basic functional unit of the levator ani muscle is the motor unit. A motor unit consists of an alpha neuron that descends from the anterior horn of the spine and, through its axon, connects to bundles of muscle fiber at the neuromuscular junction known as the motor end plate. Motor units in the levator ani muscle are primarily innervated by branches of the pudendal nerve.[22,32] This nerve originates from the ventral divisions of the second, third, and fourth sacral rami (S-2, S-3, and S-4), and passes between the piriformis and coccygeus muscle, exiting the pelvis through the greater sciatic foramen; it then enters the pudendal canal, where it divides into the perineal nerve and in the female to the dorsal nerve of the clitoris.[32]

The levator ani, like other skeletal muscles, is made up of a mixture of slow-twitch and fast-twitch muscle fibers.[27] Slow-twitch muscle fibers are generally small in diameter and red in color (owing to an abundance of cytochrome and myoglobin, an oxygen-storing molecule). They rely on aerobic metabolism to maintain constant muscular activity in response to the effects of gravity. The fast-twitch muscle fibers are generally larger in diameter and white in color (rich in glycogen and glycolytic enzymes), and rely on anaerobic metabolism. The larger the diameter of the fast-twitch fibers, the higher the urethral closing pressure. Proportionally, the levator muscle consists of approximately 70% slow-twitch and 30% fast-twitch muscle fibers.[27] The proportion of the two fiber types differs throughout the muscle, with a slightly higher percentage of the slow-twitch muscle fiber type being found in the perianal sections of the levator ani. In women who have pelvic floor weakness, however, the proportion of fast-twitch muscle fibers is significantly reduced, and in some cases none has been identified.[33] The slow-twitch muscle fibers are physiologically designed to maintain tone and provide ongoing resistance to gravity, opposing the tendency of the pelvic viscera to exteriorize by elevating the levator plate. Slow-twitch muscle tone in the pubococcygeus sling narrows the urogenital hiatus and maintains the urethra-vesical and ano-rectal angle.[34] The fast-twitch muscle fibers provide rapid reflex contractions to counterbalance the increased intra-abdominal pressures associated with coughing, sneezing, and lifting.

At rest, the closure pressure in the urethra must exceed bladder pressure to keep urine in the bladder. Hypothetically, if closure pressure within the mid- and proximal urethra is 60–80 cm H_2O, while bladder pressure is 10 cm H_2O, a closure pressure of 50 cm H_2O prevents urine from moving from the bladder through the urethra. However, a vigorous sneeze will generate Valsalva pressure waves greater than 200 cm H_2O. Were it not for the reflex activation of the pubococcygeus just prior to abdominal wall contraction, there would inevitably be leakage from the bladder.[4]

UROGENITAL PAIN

Chronic urogenital pain conditions are common among both women[35–38] and men.[39] Chronic pain has a significant impact on well-being and detrimentally affects quality of life.[40] The most common forms of chronic urogenital pain in women include vulvodynia, painful bladder syndrome (commonly referred to as interstitial cystitis [IC]), and vaginismus.[36–38]

Pain is a complex phenomenon in which sensory and emotional factors interact in an intricate way. The International Society for the Study of Pain defines pain as an "unpleasant sensory and emotional experience."[41] The interaction between emotions and physiology can occur at different levels of complexity. At the higher cortical level, pain activates the anterior cingulate cortex and thalamus—structures also known to be involved in the experience of conscious negative emotions.[42,43] At the peripheral sensory level, a significant interaction has been demonstrated between anxiety and pain sensitivity, with some patients who have chronic pain showing lower pain thresholds that seem to be mediated by anxiety.[44] One of the physiological correlates of anxiety is elevated muscle tension, a form of inefficient peripheral response to the hyperalertness commonly seen in chronic pain patients.[45] Muscles are the body's primary responders to pain, trauma, injury, and negative emotional states.[46–48] Sensory and emotional stimuli contribute to muscle over-activation, stiffness, spasm, and pain,[49] especially in symptomatic muscle groups.[46] The symptom-specific involvement of muscles has been extensively documented in vulvodynia,[14,15] IC,[50] and sexual dysfunction.[51]

Vulvodynia

Vulvodynia is the most common form of chronic female urogenital pain.[36] As a chronic pain syndrome, it interferes with daily activities, including sexual intercourse. Compared with other chronic vulvovaginal disorders, vulvodynia causes greater loss of quality of life and results in a higher degree of psychosocial impairment and disability.[52,53]

Vulvodynia is defined as unexplained vulvar discomfort for which there is no known physical or neurological explanation.[55] The pain is localized to the vulvar area and is most often provoked by any pressure application to the urogenital area, including tight clothing, tampon use, or attempted sexual intercourse. Once provoked, pain can be so intense as to disrupt sexual activity, arouse fear, and lead to loss of sexual desire, avoidance, or total abstinence from sexual activity. More than 80% of patients report a loss of sexual desire and a reduction in the frequency of sexual intercourse.[56]

Prevalence and Impact

Data collected from general prevalence studies on vulvodynia have varied significantly. A lack of awareness about the disorder and women's reluctance to speak about urogenital pain has resulted in the condition being frequently misdiagnosed and underdiagnosed.[36] Nevertheless, the prevalence is generally estimated to be on the order of 4% to 19%,[36,57,58] with some specialized women's clinics in Africa and Europe reporting prevalence figures as high as 22% to 34%.[59,60] Although the condition affects women of all ages, it is most prevalent among younger women.[56]

In an Australian study of 744 patients with vulvodynia, the mean age of women was 30.7 years, and 75% were younger than age 34 years.[56] The prevalence peaked at 24 years of age. The average age at onset of symptoms was 22.8 years, but ranged from 5.5 to 45.2 years. Based on these data, it is evident that chronic vulvar pain is not related to parity, nor to the commencement of sexual activity. More than 30% of patients in this study reported the onset of symptoms prior to commencement of sexual activity. The condition is known to cause notable psychological distress and affects personal relationships, sexual function, and general well-being.[53,61,62]

SEMG Studies

Several SEMG studies have confirmed an association between pelvic muscle dysfunction and symptoms of vulvar pain. The studies assessed pelvic muscle function using intravaginal probes, as shown in **Figure 13–4**.

For SEMG assessments, patients commonly rest in a semi-supine position. The tracings used as illustrations in this chapter were taken using a single-user vaginal

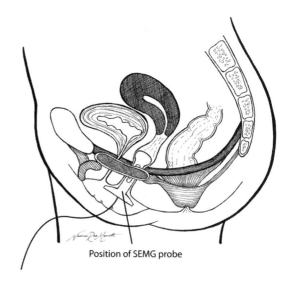

Position of SEMG probe

Figure 13–4 Pelvic diaphragm with SEMG probe.
Source: Courtesy of Naomi Merritt.

probe connected to a MyoTrac 3 encoder and analyzed by computerized software (Vaginal sensor T6065, MyoTrac 3 T9900, hardware and software manufactured by Thought Technology, Montreal, Canada). Channel bandwidth was 20–450 Hz, ± 5 Hz/± 50 Hz and the sampling rate per channel was 2000 Hz.

The earliest study highlighted pelvic floor hypertonicity and muscle instability in vulvodynia.[15] A subsequent study identified electromyographic characteristics that enabled an 88% accurate differential diagnosis of vulvodynia.[14] As compared with controls, 76% of the women demonstrated elevated resting baselines greater than 2.0 microvolts (hypertonicity); 65% showed poor contractile amplitude, defined as less than 17 microvolts (weakness); 93% showed higher resting standard deviation readings, defined as greater than 0.20 (instability); 87% demonstrated poor recruitment recovery after contraction, 0.2 second or less (irritability); and in 69%, the muscle recruitment was characterized by low-frequency muscle fiber activity, defined as less than 115 Hz (fatigue). In the same study, 88% of patients met at least three of the previously-mentioned criteria. The diagnosis could be confirmed by (1) instability of muscle; (2) irritability, as seen in poor muscle recovery after contraction; (3) hypertonicity as reflected in elevated resting baseline; plus one other optional criterion, either (4) fatigue noticeable in reduced fiber frequency or (5) weakness, as seen in low contraction amplitude. **Figure 13–5** and

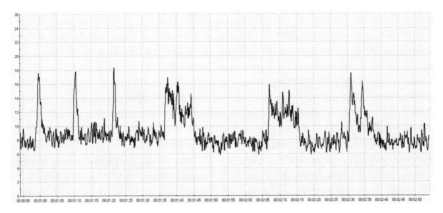

Figure 13–5 Female, nulliparous, age 29, with 12-month history of symptoms. The pre-treatment SEMG assessment shows three phasic and three tonic contractions, illustrating a very elevated resting baseline (approximately 50% of maximum voluntary contraction), instability, irritability, and fatigue. Scale range 0–26 μV.

Source: Copyright © Marek Jantos, PhD.

Figure 13–6 show average pre-treatment and post-treatment SEMG tracings, respectively.

Other SEMG studies of women with vulvodynia have confirmed similar dysfunctional patterns of muscle activation. In a comparison of women with vulvodynia with a control group, the symptomatic women were younger and of lower parity than the control group, yet showed SEMG readings inferior to those of the asymptomatic controls—the reverse pattern of what would be expected.[63]

The findings arising from SEMG assessment of patients with vulvodynia were further validated by manual assessments conducted by specially trained physical therapists.[64] This study sought to establish the differential contributions of increased tonicity, lack of pelvic muscle strength, lack of voluntary control, and the role of protective guarding contractions in response to chronic vulvar pain. Findings based on manual assessments confirmed that women with vulvar vestibulitis (currently classified as vestibulodynia) presented with superficial and deeper pelvic floor muscle hypertonicity, reduced muscle strength, and inability to relax, and demonstrated restrictions in the degree of vaginal stretch.

The same study found that 90% of the women reporting pain with intercourse demonstrated pelvic floor pathology. Other comorbidities found to be common in patients with vulvodynia, and potentially

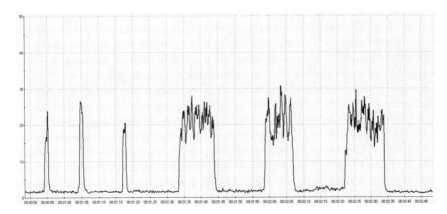

Figure 13–6 SEMG post-treatment assessment. Changes in SEMG readings reflect the normalization of muscle function associated with asymptomatic state. Scale range 0–50 μV.

Source: Copyright © Marek Jantos, PhD.

related to pelvic hypertonicity, included evacuation difficulties and anal fissures. The study suggested that addressing pelvic floor pathology needs to be the primary focus of therapy. The role of pelvic muscles was seen as central to the maintenance and exacerbation of pain, especially through reactive muscle guarding, tissue restriction, and lack of vaginal muscle control. The authors recommend that therapy should consist of conservative patient-centered protocols including pelvic exercises (also known as Kegel exercises), vaginal self-massage, stretching exercises with progressive desensitization using dilators, pain management, sex therapy, and cognitive-behavioral therapy.[64]

A more recent study, assessing the psychophysiological profile of 529 patients with vulvodynia using SEMG data, further examined the potential relationship between muscle over-activation and vulvodynia symptoms.[65] The SEMG assessments of pre-treatment, symptomatic patients were matched and compared with their post-treatment, asymptomatic assessments. The functional status of the pelvic muscle was assessed by comparing pelvic muscle resting tone, muscle stability as measured by standard deviation readings at rest, and phasic and tonic contraction amplitude pre- and post-treatment. Following SEMG-assisted retraining of

pelvic muscle function, the significant differences between pre- and post-treatment readings included (1) a decrease in muscle resting baseline, (2) a decrease in muscle instability, (3) an increase in phasic contraction amplitude, and (4) an increase in tonic contraction amplitude. These changes confirmed normalization of pelvic muscle function associated with reduction in vulvodynia symptoms, a finding consistent with earlier studies.[14,15]

The SEMG profile of patients with vulvodynia produced two other important findings.[65] First, SEMG readings did not correlate with the severity of pain symptoms. The lack of correlation between symptom severity and SEMG readings indicated that no direct inference could be made in relation to severity of pain on the basis of SEMG readings. It is important to remember that the SEMG signal is a correlate of muscle activation, but should never be seen as a measure of pain.

Second, a negative correlation was observed between resting amplitude and standard deviation readings and duration of pain, as shown in **Figure 13–7**. The finding has special significance in relation to muscle-mediated chronic pain conditions. It provides evidence that chronicity of muscle tension may be associated with a progressive reduction in muscle electrical activity as

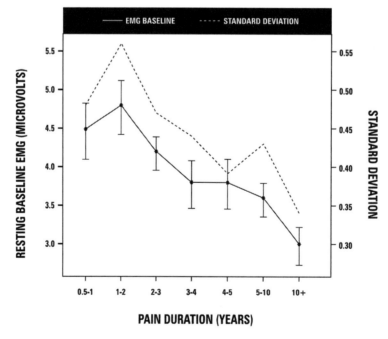

Figure 13–7 Resting amplitude and standard deviation readings in relation to duration of pain.
Source: Copyright © Marek Jantos, PhD.

measured by SEMG. In terms of muscle function, it points to a physiological quieting, or "shut-down," of chronically over-activated muscles. It is not uncommon to see patients with vulvodynia who complain of debilitating pain and severe introital muscle constriction, and who show SEMG muscle readings characterized by an exceptionally low but stable muscle tone, as illustrated in **Figure 13–8**. This anomaly may be associated with a progressive shortening of chronically over-active muscle tissue and the development of a painful muscle contracture.

Muscle contracture has been described as consisting of an electrically silent, involuntary state of maintained muscle shortness and decreased extensibility (i.e., loss of elasticity and increased rigidity) of the passive elastic properties of the connective tissue.[66] In the case of vulvodynia, pelvic muscle contracture, with its decreased extensibility, leads to a narrowing of the vaginal introitus and increased hypersensitivity to pressure.[65] Such physiological changes potentially highlight an important mechanism associated with vulvodynia.

Anatomically, when the pubococcygeus muscle contracts, the puborectalis portion of the pubococcygeal sling compresses the urethra, vagina, and rectum against the pubic bone.[4,20] Functionally, the chronic restriction of the vaginal opening and the narrowing of the urogenital hiatus mediated by hypertonic muscle not only result in narrowing of the vaginal introitus, but may also lead to ischemia and peripheral sensitization. Should the chronically over-activated muscles lose their elasticity and extensibility, this change would lead to a de-creased ability to relax sphincteric mechanisms, resulting in increased straining during bowel voiding and an increased risk of hemorrhoids and anal fissures, as previously reported.[64] Over-activation of pelvic muscles also results in inhibition of peristaltic motility in the large intestine, further complicating voiding.

Further evidence of loss of muscle extensibility, and pelvic contracture, comes from muscle assessments using graded vaginal dilators.[65] At the commencement of therapy, 75.6% of patients were able to accommodate only small-size dilators. This was true not only in the case of nulliparous patients but also in multiparous patients, and provides further evidence of shortening of muscle tissue. Following normalization of muscle function, 96.7% of asymptomatic patients were able to accommodate the larger dilator sizes. Vaginal dilation is widely used in the treatment of dyspareunia; however, the term "vaginal dilatation" is actually a misnomer, as the vagina is not physically stretched, but rather the pelvic muscles are relaxed and extended.

Muscle over-activation has been identified as a factor in a range of chronic pain syndromes. The mechanisms by which muscle over-activation gives rise to hypersensitivity have been discussed extensively in the literature.[66] Irrespective of whether muscle tension is attributable to emotional or physical triggers, ischemia, hypoxia, buildup of neurogenic metabolites (lactic acid, potassium, arachidonic acid), alterations in intramuscular blood flow, release of sensitizing agents (e.g., bradykinin, serotonin), inflammation, erythema, edema formation, or muscular rigidity, all constitute mechanisms that lead to pain.[66,67]

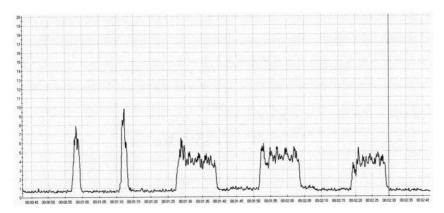

Figure 13–8 Female, nulliparous, age 33, a case of primary vulvodynia. The SEMG pre-treatment assessment shows two phasic and three tonic contractions. There is a low resting baseline, no significant instability or irritability, muscle weakness, and severe disabling pain. Scale range 0–20 μV.

Source: Copyright © Marek Jantos, PhD.

Physiological changes of this nature are associated with progressive sensitization of the peripheral and central nervous systems. Sensitization is an important property of nociceptors that manifests itself as decreased thresholds to nociceptor stimulation, increased field of nociceptor reception (from localized to generalized), nociceptor responsiveness to normally non-noxious stimuli (allodynia), increased intensity of response (hyperalgesia), prolonged post-stimulus sensations (hyperpathia), and occurrence of spontaneous pain.[45] Such sensory changes differentiate between acute and chronic pain conditions and are defining characteristics of vulvodynia.[68]

Treatment

In the context of this chapter's discussion, therapy needs to focus on SEMG-assisted normalization of pelvic muscle function. As a general rule, the normalizing of pelvic muscle function in chronic pain conditions requires downtraining and stabilizing of hypertonic muscles.[14] The specific goals of SEMG assisted therapy will be to reduce resting baselines to less than 2.0 microvolts, reduce variability in SEMG activity to less than 0.20 microvolts SD, and increase muscle responsiveness, coordination, and strength relative to the patient's assessed potential. SEMG-assisted retraining should also enable the patient to discriminate between tension holding and relaxation.

Several studies have shown SEMG-assisted rehabilitation of pelvic muscle to be effective in the treatment of vulvodynia. An early study based on the treatment of 33 patients with vulvodynia showed an average of 83% reduction in pain after 16 weeks of SEMG-assisted therapy.[15] A study of 29 patients with moderate to severe vulvodynia symptoms showed that 88.9% of patients undergoing SEMG-assisted rehabilitation of PFM reported negligible or mild pain upon completion of therapy, with 69% becoming sexually active.[69] A more recent study of 529 patients with vulvodynia focusing on SEMG-assisted normalization of PFM in conjunction with dilator-assisted therapy reported that symptoms of vulvodynia were alleviated or totally relieved, with 80% to 90% of patients resuming regular sexual activity upon conclusion of therapy.[65]

With SEMG-assisted retraining of PFM, patients follow a regular home-based protocol of twice-daily exercises, using home training SEMG units. As readings improve, muscles become more responsive to voluntary control. To restore muscle resilience and elasticity, therapy needs to incorporate elements of muscle lengthening and myofascial release.[64,70] In addition to the physiological bene-

fits derived from dilator-assisted lengthening of muscles, dilators have a desensitizing effect and can be used by the patient alone or with the help of her sexual partner.

The clinician needs to review the patient's progress every 2 to 4 weeks. Significant improvements in SEMG readings are often noted within 3 to 6 weeks of commencement of therapy. If therapy sessions are scheduled every 3 to 4 weeks, treatment requires an average of five to six consults. A follow-up appointment should be scheduled 3 to 6 months after conclusion of therapy to confirm maintenance of therapeutic gains.[65] Long-term follow-up studies have shown that SEMG-assisted PFM rehabilitation can lead to long-term resolution of vulvodynia symptoms.[71]

Vaginismus

Vaginismus is one of two sexual pain disorders included in the *Diagnostic and Statistical Manual of Mental Disorders (DSM)* published by the American Psychiatric Association.[129] This condition is defined as an involuntary spasm of the muscles surrounding the outer third of the vagina when penetration is attempted. The other sexual pain disorder in the *DSM* classification is dyspareunia, a condition also marked by painful intercourse, for which no cause is given. Several studies utilizing SEMG sought to test the validity of the muscle spasm-based diagnostic criteria for vaginismus. The SEMG findings of these studies provide clinically relevant information on the diagnosis and management of vaginismus.

Prevalence and Impact

The prevalence of dyspareunia has been estimated at 3% to 43%, and the prevalence of vaginismus at 1% to 6% of women.[72] With both conditions, sexual traumatization has been excluded as a contributing factor. As in the case of vulvodynia, the pairing of pain with sexual intercourse progressively leads to loss of desire, avoidance, and psychological distress.[56]

SEMG Studies

One of the first studies investigating the reliability of the spasm-based criterion for the diagnosis of vaginismus examined the level of voluntary control over PFM.[72] This study utilized intravaginal SEMG probes to assess pelvic muscle function and surface EMG electrodes to monitor activity in surrounding muscle groups (gluteal, adductor, and abdominal muscles). A group of 67 patients with vaginismus was compared with 43 control subjects to establish how much voluntary control each group displayed during simple flick contractions, 10-second holds, and gradual contractions. Voluntary control was defined as the ability to contract and relax the muscles when asked to do so.

The results of this study showed no differences between patients with vaginismus and control groups during resting baselines (the mean resting baseline for both groups was 1.36 microvolts); no significant difference in amplitude of flick contractions (the mean amplitude for the control group was 4.48 microvolts, SD 2.4 microvolts, and for the patient group was 3.7 microvolts, SD 2.6 microvolts); no difference in the amplitude for 10-second contractions; significant fatiguing of muscle over time in both groups; and increases in amplitude of pelvic contractions in both groups with addition of ancillary muscles. The researchers noted that in both the patient group and the control group, some women were not able to relax their pelvic floor muscles, showing a degree of muscle hyperactivity. In the vaginismus group, the muscle hyperactivity was related not only to symptoms of painful intercourse, but also to other urogenital and bowel problems, with 55% of the women also reporting hesitant micturition, bladder outlet obstruction, urinary retention, constipation, irritable bowel syndrome, and obstructed defecation. When the patient group was split into those with only vaginistic complaints and those with vaginistic symptoms and other pelvic floor complaints, and the two groups were then compared with the control group, the group with vaginistic and pelvic floor complaints and hyperactive muscles had more disturbed micturition and defecation patterns than the other two groups.

This study provided several important findings. First, there were no differences between vaginismus patients and controls in terms of resting baseline, contraction amplitude, or voluntary control of the PFM. The evidence did not provide any support for the use of muscle spasm as a defining criterion of vaginismus. The study also showed that all participants had difficulty in discerning tension in their pelvic muscles, as reflected in a notable discrepancy between subjective and physiological reports of muscle activity. It is possible that such a discrepancy may reflect either a limited level of muscle awareness or changes in muscle activity that fall below the detectable threshold of individuals. SEMG provided objective measures upon which the spasm-based criteria could be questioned, as muscle spasm did not differentiate between vaginismus cases and controls.

In a later study, the same researchers investigated the mechanisms underlying vaginismus to see if a general defense mechanism mediated muscle reflexes.[73] Patients with vaginismus and control groups were exposed to four different film excerpts that were classified as threatening, erotic, neutral, or sexually threatening. During these 5-minute video segments, pelvic floor muscle activity was measured using vaginal EMG sensors. All participants were asked to report their levels of sexual arousal and of threat during each of the excerpts. Participants felt sexually aroused during the erotic excerpt and, to a lesser degree, during the sexually threatening excerpt. The highest level of threat was reported during the threatening excerpt and the sexually threatening excerpt. The SEMG readings showed no difference in response between groups; the same changes in muscle activity were noted in women with vaginismus as in the control group. The study highlighted that it was not the sexual content that evoked the response, but rather the threatening aspect of it. It was further noted that the involuntary activation of muscles was not restricted to pelvic muscles only, but occurred in the shoulder trapezius muscle as well.

A further study examined the same parameters but also focused on a subgroup of patients with vaginismus who had reported past negative sexual experiences.[74] Women with negative experiences showed more pelvic floor muscle activity during both the sexually threatening film excerpt and the erotic excerpt. When women were specifically asked about nonsexual circumstances in which they were aware of similar reactions in their pelvic floor, they identified all stressful situations, such as getting into a traffic jam or being in a hurry. The results of this study suggest that in women who have a history of a negative sexual experience, the vaginistic reactions may be part of a general conditioned defense reaction, especially in situations where conditioning of an emotion–symptom relationship has been established. Perhaps patients associating discomfort or pain with sexual intercourse develop fear and defensive reflexes that can be activated when anticipating such an event.[74]

Further studies testing the validity of muscle spasm as a diagnostic criterion have compared patients with vaginismus and patients with vulvar vestibulitis (currently classified as vestibulodynia).[37] One study used professionals from three different specialties—gynecologists, physical therapists, and psychologists—to differentiate between the two conditions, as well as vaginal SEMG assessment and patient self-reports. The working definition of "spasm" for the gynecological examination was "an involuntary contraction of some or all of the pelvic floor muscles which prevents examination"; for the physical therapists, the definition was "a prolonged muscle contraction not relieved by reassurance"; for the psychologists, it was the *DSM-IV* criteria; and for SEMG studies, it was defined as a "sustained contraction lasting at least one minute which could not be relieved voluntarily and was accompanied by at least a 15 microvolt increase above the participant's baseline SEMG reading."

Diagnostic agreement between the two gynecologists, two psychologists, and two physical therapists was moderate (kappa values of .60, .58, and .64, respectively). Evaluating resting tone, the gynecologists and physical therapists reported that women in the vaginismus group showed higher levels of muscle tension than the vulvodynia group, with no elevated tension being observed in the no-pain group. In terms of muscle strength, the vaginismus group demonstrated less vaginal muscle strength than the vulvodynia group, and the vulvodynia group demonstrated less muscle strength than the no-pain group. In the diagnosis of vaginal spasm, SEMG testing revealed no vaginal spasms during sensor insertion by gynecologists or during testing of any of the participants. During gynecology examination, the vaginismus group demonstrated a greater frequency of vaginal spasm, but none of the women who experienced spasm during one gynecological examination experienced a spasm during the other gynecology examination. During physical therapy examinations, the therapists reported muscle spasm in 86% of women in the vaginismus group, in 93% of women in the vulvodynia group, and in 54% of the women in the no-pain group. Women in the vulvodynia group rated their pain higher than women in the vaginismus group, with more pain being experienced during physical exams than during gynecology exams. The vaginismus group was more fearful of exams; 46% of the patients with vaginismus refused to undergo an EMG assessment and 27% refused to have more than one test performed, whereas none of the patients with vulvodynia and no members of the no-pain group refused to undergo the SEMG evaluations. Women with vaginismus displayed significantly more avoidance and defensive reactions than women in the vulvodynia and the no-pain groups. From the sexual history, the study also noted that more than 70% of women in the vaginismus group reported never experiencing intercourse, had lower frequency of tampon use, and were less likely to have experienced gynecological exams.[37]

In considering the results of these studies, it is evident that vaginal spasm does not appear to be necessary or sufficient for the diagnosis of vaginismus. One of the studies concluded that muscle resting tone and muscle strength may be a more reliable diagnostic measure than spasm.[37] The most significant difference between the vaginismus, vulvodynia, and no-pain groups occurred in their level of fear and catastrophizing, suggesting that vaginismus may be a type of specific phobia characterized by significant anxiety, and in some cases panic, provoked by exposure to vaginal penetration. If vaginismus is a form of "vaginal penetration phobia," conditioned to the anticipated or real pain, therapy should address such fear and anxiety.[37]

A medical study sought to investigate the extent to which SEMG of the PFM could distinguish between women with partial vaginismus, women with vulvar vestibulitis (vestibulodynia), and asymptomatic women.[75] The study reported that SEMG was of no value in distinguishing between the three groups of women. It is noteworthy that the criticism of SEMG actually confirms the earlier reported findings, where no differences in PFM characteristic were noted between the patients with vaginismus and controls. Other recent findings have also reported that approximately 50% of patients with vaginismus met the diagnostic criteria for vulvodynia.[76] This highlights the need for more reliable and validated diagnostic criteria.

Treatment

Two important aspects of treatment potentially need to be addressed in relation to vaginismus. First, treatment needs to focus on general pain management, as many of the women experience pain that is not accounted for by spasm.[37] Because patients with vaginismus, in general, show good pelvic muscle control but demonstrate increased muscle resting tone and often coexisting weakness, treatment should focus on SEMG-assisted muscle retraining aimed at normalizing muscle tone, as in the case of vulvodynia.[37,72] In case of vaginismus where there is evidence of hypertonicity and other pelvic-related dysfunction (disturbed micturition and defecation patterns), normalizing muscle function will reduce the level of muscle-related discomfort and will enable improved voluntary muscle control. To achieve this objective, the therapist needs to customize protocols for each patient. Considering that patients with vaginismus show a lack of muscle tension awareness and tend to respond to all stressful situations with generalized pelvic bracing, biofeedback-assisted protocols may assist in improving their ability to discriminate between muscle tension levels.[72,74]

The second key aspect of vaginismus management is the need to focus on elevated anxiety levels, as reflected in increased fear and phobia in relation to penetration. Addressing anxiety-related issues in the management of vaginismus may require psychotherapeutic modalities with possible pharmacological assistance.[37]

Interstitial Cystitis, Urgency and Frequency

Interstitial cystitis (IC) is a chronic and debilitating bladder syndrome of unknown etiology, characterized by urinary frequency, urgency, nocturia, suprapubic pressure, and pain.[77] This chronic inflammatory disorder affects the lining and wall of the bladder, resulting in the constant desire to void. The lining of the bladder is known as the interstitium; hence inflammation of the lining is referred to as interstitial cystitis. Various terms are currently used for IC. The International Continence Society (ICS) refers to this condition as "painful bladder syndrome,"[78] but a more recent consensus meeting has renamed the condition to "bladder pain syndrome."[79]

IC symptoms are directly related to bladder filling and to discomfort associated with urinary urgency and frequency.[80] The condition is often misdiagnosed and generally under-diagnosed. More than 60% of patients with IC report having pain for more than 5 years and describe it as a burning, pressure pain.[80] The severity of urogenital pain associated with IC causes significant emotional distress, diminishes quality of life, and affects sexual behavior.[81–83]

Although IC was first identified by Skene in 1888,[84] its etiology is still not understood and its pathogenesis is generally considered to be multifactorial. Hypotheses to explain IC symptoms have focused on neurogenic, inflammatory, autoimmune, and psychosomatic causes.[85] No definitive evidence to support any of these hypotheses has been published, however. Some studies have shown psychological stress, bowel disorders, diabetes mellitus, and hypertension as also being correlated with the probability of IC.[82] Other reports have implicated the involvement of dysfunctional PFM.[2,50,86–93]

Prevalence and Impact

On account of the overlap between IC and various other bladder and urethral syndromes, it has been difficult to correctly estimate the true prevalence of IC.[83] The general prevalence rates cited have varied between studies.[94–96] Recent estimates based on validated questionnaires have placed the prevalence estimates for urban female populations in the range of 306 to 464 cases per 100,000 population.[82,96] The proportion of women to men with a diagnosis of IC is exceptionally high, with estimates indicating that almost 90% of IC cases occur among women, 30% of which affect women younger than the age of 30 years.[82,85] A recent analysis of the negative impact of IC on quality of life showed that 90% of affected women have impairment in daily activities, 88% report sleep disturbances, 79% have work impairment, and 70% admit problems in partnership and sexuality.[81,97] Patients with IC have also been found to experience significantly more sexual dysfunction than control groups. Sexual functioning was found to be the primary predictor of mental quality of life in women with longstanding IC.[98]

SEMG Studies

Very few studies have specifically focused on SEMG assessment and treatment of IC. Clinical evidence and assessments reveal significant similarities between IC and vulvodynia. Early studies utilizing SEMG assessments found muscle over-activation, inadequate voluntary control, muscle shortening, and trigger point referred pain to be not only associated with IC but also possibly causing its symptoms.[2,50] The individual differences in SEMG assessments of IC patients are significant. **Figure 13–9** depicts the SEMG assessment of a patient with a history of IC symptoms.

Medical examinations of the urogenital area in patients with IC show that, in addition to bladder-related symptoms, 50% of cases report vulvar pain upon cotton swab testing in the 5 and 7 o'clock positions, confirming the presence of vestibulodynia symptoms.[80] During vaginal examination of the PFM, 94.2% of patients experienced levator pain, 77% of patients reported deep pain with sexual intercourse, 69% described burning pain with or after sexual activity, and 71% indicated that the pain could last for hours or days. A recent study examining the urogynecologic features of women with IC

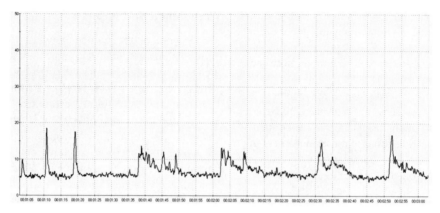

Figure 13–9 Female, nulliparous, 31 years of age with adolescent onset of IC symptoms. The pre-treatment SEMG assessment shows three phasic contractions and four tonic contractions. Scale range 0–50 µV.

Source: Copyright © Marek Jantos, PhD.

found an even higher prevalence of sexual pain.[83] This study determined that 85.1% of the patients with IC met the diagnostic criteria for localized provoked and generalized vulvodynia, whereas only 23.4% reported bladder pain and 51.1% reported urgency and frequency. The onset of vulvodynia symptoms in the IC cohort was not related to the initiation of bladder symptoms and pain.

Based on these findings, it is evident that the more prevalent symptom in IC patients is chronic vulvar pain in the form of vulvodynia. One study compared patients who have only IC symptoms with those who have both IC and vulvodynia symptoms; the latter subgroup reported significantly higher levels of levator pain.[80] This calls for a closer examination of the association between IC and vulvodynia symptoms, as the two may be one and the same condition, but varying in symptom presentation. As in the case of vulvodynia, a large percentage of patients with IC reported childhood histories of difficulties with voiding, suggestive of an early onset of pelvic floor dysfunction.[92,99]

Physical therapy of patients with IC found the levator ani muscles to be tender to palpation, producing referred pain to the suprapubic and perineal regions, rectum, glans penis in men, and labia in women.[50,92] Although the therapies focused primarily on myofascial trigger point release and pelvic muscle stretching, patients who underwent SEMG assessment showed significant changes in SEMG activity, with the average pre-treatment resting tone reduced from 9.73 microvolts to 3.61 microvolts post-treatment.[50] A 65% reduc-

tion in SEMG readings was associated with a marked improvement of IC urgency and frequency symptoms in 70% and 83% of the cases, respectively.

The link between bladder symptoms and PFM is not well understood. Neurogenic models have been proposed, on the basis of the close proximity within the spinal cord of afferent nerve endings from the pudendal nerve and parasympathetic nerves of the bladder, suggesting that painful input into spinal dorsal neurons may trigger antidromic stimulation of adjacent bladder nerves.[92] Anatomically and histologically, there are close connections among the vagina, urethra, and levator ani muscle.[1] Smooth muscle, collagen and elastin fibers of the vaginal wall, and paraurethral tissues have been shown to interdigitate with the muscle fibers of the medial portion of the levator muscle in the region of the proximal urethra. Because these structures are inseparable structurally and functionally, chronically hypertonic muscles may trigger neurogenic inflammation of the bladder wall.[91] From a myofascial perspective, overuse due to hyperactive pelvic muscles may give rise to trigger points and myofascial pain, resulting in compromised function of the pelvic floor, muscle shortening, and limited inhibition of detrusor during filling of bladder, resulting in urgency and frequency.[50,92]

Treatment

There is a lack of consensus on the best treatments for IC. Pelvic floor normalization through myofascial therapy and SEMG-assisted retraining has produced the best outcomes, with long-term benefits evident if patients maintained a home program of stress reduction and pelvic floor exercises.[50,92] Studies reporting successful treatment recommend that "as an integral part of the treatment regimen in these patients, normalization of these muscles is included by eradicating the trigger points and reeducating the pelvic floor with stretching and strengthening exercises. . . . In addition to office treatment, the patient is instructed in a home program consisting of biofeedback and Kegel instruction, external muscle stretches and strengthening, and stress reduction techniques."[50]

PFM are highly vulnerable to tension and myofascial trigger points because of their central location and involvement in transmitting forces between the upper body and the legs, and their constant supportive involvement in urinary and sexual function and high responsiveness to external stressors. Hence, "PFD [pelvic floor dysfunction] and neural upregulation may relate more appropriately to the etiology of the symptoms than an altered glycosaminoglycan layer."[80] Decreasing pelvic floor tension and eliminating trigger point activity appears to effectively ameliorate the symptoms of IC and urgency and frequency.[80,50,92] Based on these recommendations and the available evidence, SEMG management should focus on pelvic floor normalization, predominantly using downtraining protocols as described in the treatment of vulvodynia.

There is no consensus on the value of other therapies for IC but the mainstay therapy has been hydrodistention, tibial nerve stimulation, bladder training, medications, and surgery.[80] Hydrodistension has been shown to significantly reduce symptoms of pain but the benefits appear to be short lived.[99–101] Medication helps only half of the patients, and heat application and relaxation strategies provide only temporary relief in 34.6% and 25.6% of cases, respectively. Surgery is used as an absolutely last measure.[80]

URINARY INCONTINENCE

Urinary incontinence (UI) is defined by the International Continence Society as "any involuntary leakage of urine."[102] For clinical purposes, it is further described by type, frequency, severity, precipitating factors, social impact, effect on hygiene and quality of life, measures that contain the leakage, and the desire (or not) of the individual to receive help. Some patients adapt to the disorder and resign to living with the problem because they consider UI to be a part of being a woman and a conse-

quence of childbirth, while others think that it is part of growing old.[103] In reality, UI can affect women of all ages—nulliparous young women as well as parous and older women. Patients should be encouraged to be proactive and not accept UI as an inevitable fact of life. Evidence indicates that in 90% of cases it can be improved or cured with appropriate management.[103] This discussion focuses on three forms of UI: stress urinary incontinence (SUI), urge urinary incontinence (UUI), and mixed urinary incontinence (MUI).

Prevalence and Impact

A review of literature on the worldwide prevalence of urinary incontinence found the median prevalence of female UI to be 27.6% (range of 4.8% to 58.4%), with prevalence significantly increasing with age.[104] The most common cause of UI was SUI (50%), followed by MUI (32%) and UUI (14%).[104] It is generally acknowledged that the problem is far more common among women than it is among men. It is estimated that 30% to 40% of women are affected by some degree of incontinence in their lifetimes, accounting for approximately 70% of all incontinence sufferers.[105,106] A meta-analysis of 48 studies estimated the age-related prevalence of urinary incontinence to be 16% among women younger than 30 years, and 29% among women aged 30–60 years.[107] The cause of incontinence varied between age groups, with younger women being more likely to experience SUI and older women being more likely to experience UUI.[107,108]

The problem of incontinence is often not reported and is under-diagnosed. The majority of women (40% to 80%) suffering incontinence delay seeking help for more than a year after symptoms become troublesome.[109] The most common reasons given for not seeking treatment include embarrassment, fear of surgery, hope of improvement without investigation, and a belief that UI is a normal occurrence in life.

One of the exceptional trends in the prevalence of involuntary urine loss involves elite athletes. Their prevalence rates range from 0 to 67%, depending on the nature of the physical activity.[110,111] The prevalence appears to increase in proportion to the intensity of activity and the potential gravitational forces acting on the pelvic floor. When rating the risk of incontinence by particular sport, gymnastics, ballet, and aerobics are associated with the highest risk, while walking and swimming are associated with the lowest risk.

UI significantly affects sexual function in many persons, with the odds of sexual complaints being two times higher among women with incontinence problems.[112] An estimated 86% of patients with UI report some form of sexual dysfunction.[114] The most common problem reported is the loss of urine during intercourse. UI was noted by 80% of female patients during penetration and by 93% with orgasm; 92% experienced leakage with both, and 60% reported lack of orgasm.[114,115] This type of incontinence can be a source of embarrassment, and the fear of leakage may cause women to avoid sexual intercourse.[116]

The physical and emotional repercussions associated with incontinence are significant and well documented. Embarrassment, shame, depression, anger, frustration, secretiveness, loss of self-esteem, fear, guilt, and denial are some of the common responses.[117] Progressively, the problem leads to decreased social interaction and eventual withdrawal and isolation.[9]

SEMG Findings

SEMG has been frequently utilized in relation to UI for diagnosis and treatment. It is considered to be a safe, noninvasive, and cost-effective modality.[17] SEMG has been shown to differentiate between different types of incontinence, menstrual status, and parity.[4] Assessment of a group of 37 women with UI showed significant reduction in contraction strength for individuals with urinary stress and urge incontinence, as compared with continent women. Parous women showed greater weakness than nulliparous women. Perimenopausal and postmenopausal women who were not on hormone replacement therapy showed weaker PFM tone than their menopausal counterparts and postmenopausal individuals taking hormone replacement therapy. SEMG assessment of PFM demonstrated good reliability and greater predictive value than digital and manometric measures. When SEMG assessments of PFM were tested 4 weeks apart, the assessments showed a significant reliability correlation between the first and second assessments of $r = .86$ ($P < .001$).

In a study of 173 healthy and 144 women with UI, vaginal SEMG was utilized to determine changes in PFM function, in relation to age and parity.[16] The study found that women who maintained continence through the years had normal PFM function whereas women with USI, UUI, and MUI showed a successive decrease in SEMG activity with increasing age. In this study, no sig-

nificant differences could be identified between the different groups of incontinent women, leading the study authors to suggest that a common pathophysiological mechanism might exist. SEMG findings point to a progressive deterioration of the pelvic–vaginal neuromuscular function in women who develop UI.

In a well-controlled study comparing 57 women with SUI and 57 controls of the same age, body mass index, number of deliveries, and birth weight of offspring, SEMG showed significant differences in peak values for rapid contractions (14.56 microvolts in the patients with SUI versus 21.67 microvolts in the control group), work, and rest levels.[118] The authors concluded that SEMG assessment of PFM function is helpful in predicting and diagnosing SUI and, therefore, has value in clinical application.

Another study comparing 31 women with genuine stress incontinence with 35 controls likewise found significant differences in the SEMG readings during rapid contractions in both the supine and standing positions.[119] SEMG values were 17.0 microvolts among incontinent patients in the supine position and 19.5 microvolts among controls; in the standing position, they were 12.9 microvolts and 18.2 microvolts, respectively. The SEMG assessment showed lower activity in incontinent patients, especially in the standing position. On regression analysis, SEMG values were found in both groups to be dependent on age but not on parity, body mass index, or episiotomies. Other studies have shown SEMG to be sensitive to parity.[4] Differences in findings may stem from variations in study design relating to type of PFM activities measured (e.g., tonic as opposed to phasic contractions) and to the sensitivity of the equipment used.

Treatment

The goals of UI treatment should be to reduce symptoms and reestablish quality of life. In pursuing this goal, it is generally agreed that first line of treatment should be the least invasive option, with the lowest risk of complications and adverse effects. To this end, the U.S. government's *Clinical Practice Guidelines*[17] recommend that "behavioral techniques such as bladder retraining and pelvic muscle exercises are effective, low risk interventions that can reduce incontinence significantly in varied populations." In reviewing the relevant research literature, the developers of these practice guidelines found that these techniques were associated with a 54% to 95% improvement in incontinence, with a significant reduction in symptoms—if not cure—of UI. Importantly, the guidelines state, "These treatment results are obtained with no reported adverse effects or complications."

Arnold Kegel, a gynecologist and pioneer in conservative treatment of pelvic floor dysfunction, claimed that "stress incontinence of urine, uncomplicated by severe trauma or systemic disease, was cured in 86% of cases by physiologic, non-operative therapy."[120] Kegel further stated that "the common type of simple stress incontinence is a reversible neuromuscular disturbance. It can be prevented by therapeutic measures instituted at the first sign of weakness of the pubococcygeus muscle." Kegel favored conservative therapy and advocated the use of biofeedback, but did not have access to the sophisticated SEMG equipment currently available. Consequently, he used a simple manometry biofeedback device to train women to improve the tone of their pelvic floor muscles. From Kegel's protocol, the term "Kegel exercises" was derived.

A 2001 Cochrane review found that women undergoing PFM training were 7 times more likely to be cured and 23 times more likely to show improvement in symptoms as a result of PFM strengthening.[121] Studies consistently show a positive correlation between pelvic muscle strength and improvement of UI. A key to the successful retraining of PFM in relation to UI is the correct identification and activation of PFM. When comparing symptomatic incontinent women with asymptomatic continent controls, SEMG monitoring of PFM and ancillary muscles has identified distinct differences in muscle activation patterns.[122] Symptomatic women are unable to voluntarily contract PFM, but instead activate all the muscles of the chest and abdominopelvic cavity, consistently depressing the bladder base during attempted PFM contraction. Symptomatic women show a tendency to engage in muscle substitution strategies, engaging in generalized muscle activation. Inappropriate activation of muscles may exacerbate the symptoms of incontinence.

PFM retraining must focus on "specificity" of muscle activation.[123] Various studies have shown that 30% to 59% of women who receive thorough training in PFM anatomy and function are still unable to perform a correct contraction. In most cases, women attempting pelvic contractions will cocontract other skeletal muscles (especially abdominal, hip adductor, and gluteal muscles) or stretch the pelvic muscles by means of a Valsalva maneuver,

rather than contract them.[123] To this end, SEMG-assisted identification of PFM enables selective recruitment and correct sequence of muscle recruitment.

SEMG is most effective in the treatment of uncomplicated UI at time of first manifested weakness. It provides an objective assessment of pelvic muscle function, evaluating its responsiveness, contractile potential, endurance, and coordination in muscle recruitment and pelvic muscle support. Pelvic muscle retraining is recommended as first line of treatment.

In a study of 26 premenopausal women (mean age 42.5 years) with mild to moderate symptoms of SUI, patients were enrolled in a protocol of PFM exercises assisted with SEMG biofeedback.[124] All participants received individualized training and practice sessions for 40 minutes twice each week, for a total of 12 sessions. All participants performed maximum-strength phasic contractions of 3 seconds duration followed by 6 seconds of relaxation, and tonic contractions sustained for 10–20 seconds followed by 20–40 seconds of relaxation. Subjects initially performed 20 phasic and 20 tonic contractions in a supine position and then 10 phasic and 10 tonic contractions, each in a sitting and standing position, for a total of 80 contractions. From session 2 to session 7, there was a progressive increase in the number of contractions until the women were able to complete a total of 200 contractions. No additional home exercises were prescribed. Based on objective and subjective measures, significant improvements were noted. Objective cure was achieved in 61.5% of the cases, with the remainder achieving a 75% improvement. Among the group of participants, 92.3% showed a significant strengthening of muscles. SEMG amplitudes for all types of contractions improved significantly throughout the intervention.

The largest follow-up study of SEMG-assisted treatment of SUI and MUI highlighted the short- and long-term effectiveness of treatment.[125] In the sample of 390 women, 80% presented with SUI and 20% with MUI. The mean age of participants was 52 years, and 50% of them were classified high-grade SUI (stage III on stress provocation test). Vaginal surface EMG electrodes were used to obtain an objective measurement of pelvic floor contraction strength. Patients were trained to perform one to two 10-minute training sessions per day at home for 3 to 6 months and were seen in the clinic every 4 to 12 weeks. SEMG assessments showed a doubling of PFM strength as measured by SEMG (from 11.2 microvolts to 21.5 microvolts), and a 94%

rate of improvement was self-reported by participants. This gave rise to a high level of patient satisfaction with the therapeutic result. At the 3-year follow-up, 71% of all women reported maintaining improvement in their UI symptoms.[125]

PFM retraining has been shown to be effective in treatment of female SUI. It increases muscle volume and structural support, and it improves muscle recruitment coordination.[23] Meta-analyses of research on adding biofeedback to PFM retraining have shown this combination to be superior to muscle training alone.[121] Utilizing SEMG-assisted protocols of PFM retraining produces better outcomes in treatment of UI and leads to high satisfaction rates among patients.[126] Treatment of UI, however, needs to be implemented at three different levels: SEMG-assisted pelvic muscle training, lifestyle change, and behavioral bladder retraining.

SEXUAL DYSFUNCTION

Human beings inherently seek self-fulfilment through intimate pleasurable activities. Yet, in some instances, pleasurable sensations may be diminished, if not altogether absent, during sexual activity. Sexual function is an important dimension of adult life and a significant aspect of women's health.[112] Considering how prevalent sexual dysfunction is in women, it is surprising that so little research effort has been devoted to the relationship between sexual dysfunction and pelvic floor disorders.[112,127] Estimates of sexual difficulties among women range from 19% to 50% in "normal" patient populations, and increase to 68% to 75% when sexual dissatisfaction problems are included.[128]

The most common forms of female sexual dysfunction include low desire (hypoactive sexual desire disorder—77%), low sexual arousal (sexual arousal disorder—62%), and inability to achieve or difficulty in achieving orgasm (orgasmic disorder—56%).[129] These disorders have a detrimental effect on women's quality of life and lead to significant psychological distress.[130] Clinicians involved in the management of pelvic floor disorders should be aware of the association with sexual disorders, and are in a position to address these issues through therapy and counseling.

Several studies have confirmed that sexual dysfunction increases in conjunction with the presence of other pelvic floor disorders.[112,115,131] For example, women with a higher scores on the Pelvic Floor Disorders Inventory are significantly more likely to report decreased arousal, infrequent orgasm, and increased dys-

pareunia.[112] Although prevalence of pelvic floor disorders in women increases with age, many of the changes in sexual function cannot be accounted for by age-related variables alone.[112]

In one study, of patients presenting with urinary, gastric, or sexual complaints, 77.2% had measurable SEMG pelvic floor dysfunction, with 70% presenting with over-active muscle resting tone and 8% with under-active resting tone.[3] Although a causal relationship is difficult to establish, there may be direct links between anatomical and physiological aspects of PFM and sexual function.[51,131] Psychological variables such as body image, self-esteem, and general well-being are also important, however, and must not be overlooked.[131]

The sexual pain disorders have been addressed earlier in this chapter. This section focuses specifically on female orgasmic disorder, a condition mediated by a hypotonic PFM.[131-133] The essential feature of this disorder is a recurrent delay or absence of orgasm.[71] While recognizing the complexity of human sexual response and the role of psychological and social factors in sexual arousal and orgasm, the role of PFM has direct bearing on the individual's potential to experience the rhythmic contractions associated with orgasm.[131]

In 1952, Arnold Kegel identified a link between pelvic muscle weakness and orgasmic dysfunction. Kegel wrote, "I find a deficiency in the pubococcygeal muscle in 40% of anorgasmic women."[134] Where anorgasmia is primarily due to pelvic muscle deficiency, SEMG assessments can assist with identifying and correcting muscle weakness, as illustrated in **Figure 13–10**.

Prevalence and Impact

Female orgasmic disorder is the second most frequently reported sexual problem, with approximately 24% of randomly sampled women in the United States reporting orgasmic dysfunction.[135] However, data from a web-based survey of 3807 women found a much higher prevalence, with 62% of respondents reporting an inability to achieve or difficulty in achieving orgasm.[129] Although web-based surveys may reflect a certain degree of self-selection, this statistic nevertheless shows a high prevalence of the problem. The same survey found that 40% of the women did not seek help for the problem, although 54% reported that they would like to do so. In general, women internalized their lack of sexual fulfilment as negative emotions of shame, devaluation, or disgust. Orgasmic dysfunction was never considered

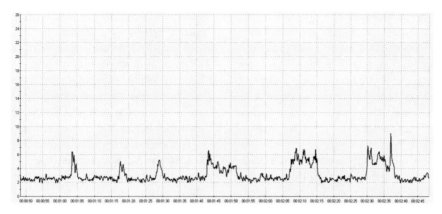

Figure 13–10 Female, nulliparous, 28 years of age with a history of primary orgasmic dysfunction. The pre-treatment SEMG assessment shows three phasic and three tonic contractions. Scale range 0–26 µV.

Source: Copyright © Marek Jantos, PhD.

emotionally positive, and high levels of frustration and anxiety were reported in relation to treatment options for the disorder.

The prevalence of orgasmic disorder increases significantly in certain subgroups of women. Women with stress urinary incontinence are particularly susceptible, with 86% reporting sexual dysfunction and 60% specifically reporting anorgasmia.[113] Obese women are also at a greater risk of sexual dysfunction, which is strongly correlated with body mass index (BMI). On a multivariate analysis, age and BMI explained 68% of variance in female sexual function index scores.[136] The possible common mechanism by which high BMI, stress urinary incontinence, and anorgasmia are linked may be PFM weakness.

A number of studies have highlighted a link between parity, gynecological surgery, and sexual dysfunction. Short-term sexual difficulties are experienced by 22% to 86% of women, most of whom report short-term changes in sexual function postpartum.[137] Studies have found a close relationship between the method of delivery and sexual dysfunction, with assisted vaginal delivery resulting in greater mechanical trauma than spontaneous vaginal delivery, and an increased incidence of sexual dysfunction. No significant differences have been noted between spontaneous vaginal delivery and cesarean delivery, but assisted delivery is known to increase the risk of injury to the pudendal nerve, perineum, and anal sphincter muscle. Pelvic floor injury commonly arises from excessive pelvic muscle fiber stretch during the second stage of labor.[12] Women with third- and fourth-degree anal sphincter tears during de-

livery are five times less likely to be sexually active one year after childbirth as compared with women with an intact perineum.[138] Some studies examining specific postpartum defects report a high prevalence of denervation in relation to incontinence and anorgasmia.[139]

Uncomplicated pregnancy itself does not appear to cause changes in sexual function, with some findings showing multiparous women having fewer orgasm-related problems than nulliparous women.[140] Nulliparous women have more pain-related problems and report being sexually less satisfied as compared to women with children.

Likewise, sexual function in women after general gynecological surgeries, such as hysterectomy, has been found either not to change or to improve on measures of frequency of orgasm and degree of orgasm.[141] From these findings, it is evident that PFM weakness arising from involuntary relaxation of the muscle and from muscle injury, more so than parity or general surgery, is a significant factor in relation to sexual dysfunction.

SEMG Studies

As yet, no structured studies have established the validity of SEMG assessments in relation to sexual arousal and orgasm. However, orgasm has always been defined as a pleasurable sensation directly associated with the rhythmic contractions of pelvic muscles.[71,135] A strong pelvic muscle was traditionally seen as necessary for attainment of orgasm, whereas a deconditioned muscle was considered to inhibit orgasmic potential.[133,134]

Masters and Johnson identified two principal physiological changes during sexual arousal: vasoconstriction and myotonia.[142] Their early findings have since been supported by more recent studies utilizing SEMG and photoplethysmography.[143] Vasoconstriction refers to the congestion of blood vessels in the genital area as it becomes engorged with venous blood, and myotonia refers to increased muscle tension in response to sexual stimulation.

Masters and Johnson identified four phases in the sexual response cycle: excitement, plateau, orgasm, and resolution.[142] During the excitement phase, the clitoral glans in the female becomes tumescent and the clitoral shaft increases in diameter and elongates. The vaginal barrel expands and lengthens. Maintaining tumescence in the clitoral tissue requires a degree of muscle tension to compress and prevent the return of venous blood; this pressure is provided by tension in the ischiocavernous muscle, which attaches to the clitoral hood. During the plateau phase, the clitoris retracts underneath the clitoral hood, while vasocongestion of the outer third of the vagina and the labia majora continues and tension in the pubococcygeus muscle is increased by means of voluntary and involuntary mechanisms. During the orgasmic phase, the PFM that surround the lower third of the vagina and form the orgasmic platform contract against the engorged tissue at 0.8-second intervals for 5 to 12 contractions, producing a sense of heightened pleasure. The muscle contractions are felt strongly around the vaginal introitus and the anal sphincter. During the resolution phase, the vasoconstriction and tumescence of the clitoris dissipate slowly and the vagina and labia majora return to their pre-excitement state, although the myotonia persists for a few minutes.

A study of 100 female health professionals found that 80% reported experiencing accompanying PFM contractions with orgasm, while others reported only occasional contractions.[144] In a study utilizing SEMG vaginal and anal probes to monitor pelvic contractions associated with self-stimulated orgasm in nulliparous women, synchronized vaginal and anal contractions were noted, with progressively increasing amplitude during the first half of orgasmic contractions, followed by a gradual decrease during the second half.[132] Women in the study group showed marked differences in orgasm duration and the number of contractions. Two out of 11 women did not show any contractions during reported orgasms.

There is considerable evidence highlighting individual differences in the experience of orgasm. Women differ widely in terms of preferred types of stimulation and mental activities to facilitate orgasm, but also experience orgasm in more than one anatomical site.[145] For many individuals, the orgasmic experience is more related to cognitive-affective aspects and relationship satisfaction rather than anatomical site.[146] These findings are an important reminder of the importance of psychosocial factors in the experience of orgasm.

Further research is needed to more clearly explore the relationship between pelvic muscle tone and different aspects of orgasm. What is evident is that throughout the individual phases of sexual arousal, good muscle tone enhances the level of sexual pleasure,[131] whereas vaginal hypotonia accentuates hyposensitivity.[147] It logically follows that strengthening of pelvic floor muscles has the potential to improve sexual function, whereas weakness has been shown to be associated with an increased incidence of anorgasmia.[3,112]

Treatment

Biofeedback-assisted strengthening of pelvic muscles has been shown to improve sexual function.[148] In contrast, involuntary relaxation of muscles, or trauma arising from assisted deliveries, impairs sexual functioning.[137–139] To the extent that multiple pregnancies may increase the risk of PFM weakness, parity has been negatively related to pubococcygeal strength.[149] Using perineometry, one study found no direct relationship between muscle strength and frequency or intensity of orgasm, although muscle strength was found to be related to the pleasurability of orgasm through clitoral stimulation. The weight of the evidence, though, points to muscle weakness being associated with anorgasmia, and good muscle tone with enhanced capacity for arousal and orgasmic potential. One of the evident mechanisms by which pleasure can be enhanced is well outlined in a treatment proposal:

> The vagina has mechanoreceptors which, when stimulated by the penis during intercourse, cause reflex contraction of the musculature, thus improving vaginal sensory perception. In patients with hypotonia, these receptors can never be activated and this accentuates the hyposensitivity.[147]

To this end, biofeedback can be used not only to improve pelvic muscle tone, but also to assist the patient in gaining awareness, improve the quality of the pelvic–perineal contraction, and enhance the quality of the orgasmic experience.[147]

SEMG-assisted muscle retraining needs to be incorporated as part of the overall therapy, but its efficacy will be enhanced when it is provided in conjunction with counseling that aims to restore a healthy mind–body link and a positive subjective appraisal of self-image and self-esteem. Psychological therapy needs to focus on promoting positive attitude and sexually relevant thought changes, reduction of anxiety, sex education, and improved communication.

RESPONSIBILITY AND COMPETENCE IN TREATING PELVIC DISORDERS

Contributions to the research and clinical work reviewed in this chapter have been sourced from a network of professionals representing the fields of behavioral science, medicine, and allied health. Specialist associations continue to focus on the treatment of pelvic disorders and seek to bridge some of the traditional professional boundaries that have hindered progress in this area in the past. A multidisciplinary interest in pelvic disorders will ensure that knowledge and management are no longer limited to any one specialty.[13]

The need for multidisciplinary input also reflects the complex nature of pelvic disorders, which are characterized not only by anatomical and physiological changes but also by psychological distress, behavioral changes, and loss of quality of life. In addressing the multifaceted aspects of pelvic disorders, the questions of professional boundaries, qualifications, ethics, and scope of practice are pertinent.

SEMG as a modality is used by professionals of various disciplines. In the context of this chapter's discussion, the question of qualifications arises. What qualifies a clinician to use SEMG in the treatment of pelvic disorders and which ethical issues do clinicians need to be aware of? There is no simple answer to these questions. In relation to training, it is essential that the clinician, if not a medical practitioner, have advanced training in health-related disciplines such as psychology, behavioral medicine, physical therapy, sex therapy, nursing, or other allied health streams. In addition, a good knowledge of pelvic anatomy and physiology is essential. In the clinical application of SEMG, the clinician must have a high level of proficiency in its use and advanced applications.

Clinical work with pelvic floor disorders can pose a certain challenge for therapists coming from a background in traditional talk-oriented therapies such as psychology. In the clinical and academic spheres, where applied psychophysiology has not been widely recognized, traditional disciplines and statutory licensing bodies may not be open and accepting of therapies addressing disorders linked to pelvic dysfunction and human sexuality. It is not uncommon for conservative statutory bodies to perceive pelvic disorders as "closet" diseases not falling within the scope of practice of a given profession. By anticipating such barriers and participating in specialist professional associations, clinicians can gain support and enjoy the range of benefits that such membership bestows. Examples of these associations include the Association for Applied Psychophysiology and Biofeedback, pain societies, continence nurses' associations, pelvic floor special-interest groups, sexual medicine organizations, and the International Society for the Study of Vulvovaginal Diseases.

Another important area of professional development is participation in professional meetings that focus on pelvic dysfunction. Sharing of ideas and seeking feedback and input from those who share a common interest is invaluable. Engaging in research, publishing papers in peer-reviewed journals, and subscribing to relevant journals all create opportunities to remain abreast of developments and to constantly reevaluate current practice and progress of clinical work. Arranging joint consultations and seeking supervision from peers are other important activities in developing professional competence.

In the management of pelvic floor disorders, it is important to always ensure that all patients first undergo proper medical screening and diagnosis. The medical practitioner should always be the primary case manager, not only referring patients but also overseeing treatment and advising on all medical matters. Ultimately, it is the patient, as the consumer, who has the right to choose the best treatment available and who should give informed consent to any proposed therapy. To this end, the patient needs to be briefed on the nature of the treatment, the goals of therapy, the expected outcomes, the duration of time required to achieve the stated goals, and the alternative treatments available.

As with any clinical work, adherence to professional and ethical codes of conduct is essential. In proceeding with treatment, the patient's privacy rights need to be respected, the rationale for each aspect of treatment explained, and the assessments and results of therapy always made available and explained. The patient should be provided with an opportunity to have a support person available throughout therapy, and to have the option to review the course of therapy or to terminate therapy at any point. The clinician should always remember that an empowered and motivated patient, when cooperatively engaged in therapy, can enhance the clinical outcomes and contribute to the clinician's professional satisfaction.

Several articles have been published focusing on practice guidelines in the assessment and treatment of pelvic floor disorders. The most recent was published in the *Journal of Applied Psychophysiology and Biofeedback* and addresses a number of pertinent issues.[150] As there are no simple answers to many questions being asked, the clinician must always remain abreast of current issues and developments.

REFERENCES

1. DeLancey J. Functional anatomy of the pelvic floor and urinary continence mechanisms. In: Schussler B, Laycock J, Norton P, Stanton S, eds. *Pelvic Floor Re-education: Principles and Practice.* London: Springer-Verlag; 1994:9–27.

2. Bernstein AM, Philips HC, Linden W, et al. A psychophysiological evaluation of female urethral syndrome: evidence for a muscular abnormality. *J Behav Med.* 1992;15:299–312.

3. Voorham-van der Zalm PJ, Lycklama A Nijeholt GA, Elzevier HW, et al. Diagnostic investigation of the pelvic floor: a helpful tool in the approach in patients with complaints of micturition, defecation, and/or sexual dysfunction. *J Sex Med.* 2008;5:864–871.

4. Ashton-Miller JA, DeLancey JOL. Functional anatomy of the female pelvic floor. *Ann NY Acad Sci.* 2007;1101: 266–296.

5. Dickinson RL. Studies of the levator ani muscle. *Am J Dis Wom.* 1889;22:897–917.

6. Jelovsek JE, Walters MD, Barber MD. Psychosocial impact of chronic vulvovaginal conditions. *J Reprod Med.* 2008;53:75–82.

7. Valezquez-Magana M, Rodriguez-Purata JM, Oviedo-Ortega G, et al. Prevalence and quality of life in women with urinary incontinence (abstract). 32nd Annual Meeting of the International Urogynecological Association. *Int Urogynecol J.* 2007;18 suppl 1:S201–S202.

8. Haessler AL, Hguyen JN, Bhatia NN. Urinary incontinence diagnosis and their impact on quality of life symptom scores in women (abstract). 32nd Annual Meeting of the International Urogynecological Association. *Int Urogynecol J.* 2007;18 suppl 1:S99–S100.

9. Jamison MG, Weidner AC, Romero AA, Amundsen CL. Lack of psychological resilience: an important correlate for urinary incontinence. *Int Urogynecol J.* 2007;18: 1127–1132.

10. Aston R, Barnick C, Porrett T, Roberts C. Levels of anxiety and depression in women attending a designated pelvic floor dysfunction clinic (abstract). 32nd Annual Meeting of the International Urogynecological Association. *Int Urogynecol J.* 2007;18 suppl 1:S98–S99.

11. Subak L, Van Den Eeden S, Thom D, et al. Urinary incontinence in women: direct costs of routine care. *Am J Obstet Gynecol.* 2007;197:596.e1–596.e9.

12. Parente MPL, Natal Jorge RM, Mascarenhas AA, et al. Deformation of the pelvic floor muscles during a vaginal delivery. *Int Urogynecol J.* 2008;19:65–71.

13. Economou SG. Forward. In: Brubaker LT, Saclarides TJ, eds. *The Female Pelvic Floor: Disorders of Function and Support.* Philadelphia, PA: F.A. Davies; 1996:vii.

14. White G, Jantos M, Glazer HI. Establishing the diagnosis of vulvar vestibulitis. *J Reprod Med.* 1997;45:157–160.

15. Glazer HI, Rodke G, Swencionis C, et al. Treatment of vulvar vestibulitis syndrome with electromyographic biofeedback of pelvic floor musculature. *J Reprod Med.* 1995;40:283–290.

16. Gunnarsson M, Mattiasson A. Female stress, urge, and mixed urinary incontinence are associated with a chronic and progressive pelvic floor/vaginal neuromuscular disorder: an investigation of 317 healthy and incontinent women using vaginal surface electromyography. *Neurourol Urodynam.* 1999;18:613–621.

17. Agency for Health Care Policy and Research, Urinary Incontinence Guideline Panel. *Urinary Incontinence in Adults: Clinical Practice Guidelines* (AHCPR Publication No. 96-0682). Rockville, MD: U.S. Department of Health and Human Services; March 1996.

18. Dietz HP. Levator trauma in labour: how common is it, do we need to know and does it matter? *ANZ Cont J.* 2005;11:105–107.

19. Rogers RM. Basic pelvic neuroanatomy. In: Steege JF, Metzger DA, Levy BS, eds. *Chronic Pelvic Pain: An Integrated Approach.* Philadelpia, PA: W.B. Saunders; 1998.

20. DeLancey JO. Structural anatomy of the posterior pelvic compartment as it relates to rectocele. *Am J Obstet Gynecol.* 1999;180:815–823.

21. Schussler B, Anthuber C, Warrell D. The pelvic floor before and after delivery. In: Schussler B, Laycock J, Norton P, Stanton S, eds. *Pelvic Floor Re-education: Principles and Practice.* London: Springer-Verlag; 1994: 105–110.

22. Junemann K, Thuroff J. Innervation. In: Schussler B, Laycock J, Norton P, Stanton S, eds. *Pelvic Floor Re-education: Principles and Practice.* London: Springer-Verlag; 1994:22–27.

23. Bo K. Pelvic floor muscle training is effective in treatment of female stress urinary incontinence, but how does it work? *Int Urogynecol J.* 2004;15:76–84.

24. Noblett KL, Jensen JK, Ostergard R. The relationship of body mass index to intraabdominal pressure measured by multichannel cystometry. *Int Urogynecol J Pelvic Floor Dysfunct.* 1997;8:323–326.

25. Mommsen S, Foldspang A. Body mass index and adult female urinary incontinence. *World J Urol.* 1994;12: 319–322.

26. Mouristan L, Hulbaek M, Brostrom S, et al. Vaginal pressure during daily activities before and after vaginal repair. *Int Uregynecol J.* 2007;18:943–948.

27. Dixon J, Gosling J. Histomorphology of pelvic floor muscle. In: Schussler B, Laycock J, Norton P, Stanton S, eds. *Pelvic Floor Re-education: Principles and Practice.* London: Springer-Verlag; 1994:28–33.

28. Smith MD, Coppieters MW, Hodges PW. Postural activity of the pelvic floor muscles is delayed during rapid arm movements in women with stress urinary incontinence. *Int Urogynecol J.* 2007;18:901–911.

29. Deffieux X, Hubeaux K, Porcher R, et al. External muscle and external anal sphincter electromyographic recordings during cough in healthy volunteers and in women presenting with stress and urinary incontinence. *Int Urogynecol J.* 2007;18 suppl 1:S9–S10.

30. Amarenco G, Ismael SS, Lagauche D, et al. Cough anal reflex: strict relationship between intravesical pressure and pelvic floor muscle electromyographic activity during cough: urodynamic and electrophysiological study. *J Urol.* 2005;173:149–152.

31. van der Kooi JB, van Wanroy PJ, De Jonge MC, Kornelis JA. Time separation between cough pulse in bladder, rectum and urethra in women. *J Urol.* 1984;132: 1275–1278.

32. Grigorescu BA, Lazarou G, Olsen TR. Innervation of the levator ani muscles: description of the nerve branches to the pubococcygeus, iliococcygeus, and puborectalis muscles. *Int Urogynecol J.* 2008;19:107–116.

33. Sayer T, Smith T. Pelvic floor biopsy. In: Schussler B, Laycock J, Norton P, Stanton S, eds. *Pelvic Floor Re-education: Principles and Practice.* London: Springer-Verlag 1994:98–101.

34. Dietz HP, Clark B, Herbison P. Bladder neck mobility and urethral closure pressure as predictors of genuine stress incontinence. *Int Urogynecol J.* 2002;13:289–293.

35. Laumann EO, Paik A, Rose RC. Sexual dysfunction in the United States: prevalence, predictors and outcomes. *JAMA.* 1999;281:537–545.

36. Harlow BL, Stewart EG. A population-based assessment off chronic unexplained vulvar pain: have we underestimated the prevalence of vulvodynia? *J Am Med Women Assoc.* 2003;58:82–88.

37. Reissing ED, Binik YM, Khalife S, et al. Vaginal spasm, pain and behaviour: an empirical investigation of the diagnosis of vaginismus. *Arch Sex Behav.* 2004;33:3–17.

38. Gardella B, Porru D, Ferdeghini F, et al. Insight into urogynecologic features of women with interstitial cystitis/painful bladder syndrome. *Euro Urol.* 2008;54: 1145–1153.

39. Egan KJ, Krieger JL. Chronic abacterial prostatitis: a urological chronic pain syndrome? *Pain.* 1997;69:213–218.

40. Hay-Smith EJ, Boberghmans LC, Hendriks HJ, et al. Pelvic floor muscle strengthening for urinary incontinence in women. *Cochrane Database Syst Rev.* 2001;1:CD001407.

41. Merskey H, Bogduck N, eds. *Classification of Chronic Pain.* 2nd ed. Washington, DC: IASP Press; 1994.

42. Coghill RC, Sang CN, Maisog JM, et al. Pain intensity processing within the human brain: a bilateral, distributed mechanism. *J Neurophysiol.* 1999;82:1934–1943.

43. Hofbauer RK, Olausson HW, Bushnell MC. Thermal and tactile sensory deficits and allodynia in a nerve-injured patient: a multimodal psychophysical and functional magnetic resonance imaging study. *Clin J Pain.* 2006;22: 104–108.

44. Granot M, Friedman M, Yarnitsky D, et al. Enhancement of the perception of systemic pain in women with vulvar vestibulitis. *BJO.* 2002;109:863–866.

45. Hawthorn J, Redmond K. The physiology of pain. In: Hawthorn J, Redmond K, eds. *Pain: Causes and Management.* Oxford, UK: Blackwell Science; 1998:7–28.

46. Flor H, Miltner W, Birbaumer N. Psychophysiological recording methods. In: Turk DC, Melzack R, eds. *Handbook of Pain Assessment.* New York, NY: Guilford; 1992:169–190l or 1992a.

47. McNulty WH, Gevirtz RN, Hubbard DR, et al. Needle electromyographic evaluation of trigger point response to a psychological stressor. *Psychophysiology.* 1994;31:313–316.

48. Gevirtz RN, Hubbard DR, Harpin RE. Psychological treatment of chronic lower back pain. *Prof Psychol Res Prac.* 1996;27:561–566.

49. Miller TM, Layzer RB. Muscle cramps. *Muscle Nerve.* 2005; 32:431–442.

50. Weiss JM. Pelvic floor myofascial trigger points: manual therapy for interstitial cystitis and the urgency–frequency syndrome. *J Urol.* 2001;166:2226–2231.

51. Rosenbaum TY, Owens A. The role of pelvic floor physical therapy in the treatment of pelvic and genital pain-related sexual dysfunction. *J Sex Med.* 2008;5:513–523.

52. Arnold LD, Backmann GA, Rosen R, et al. Vulvodynia: characteristics and associations with comorbidities and quality of life. *Obstet Gynecol.* 2006;107:617–624.

53. Ponte M, Klemperer E, Sahay A, et al. Effects of vulvodynia on quality of life. *J Amer Acad Dermatol.* 2009;60: 70–76.

54. Cantin-Drouin M, Damat D, Turcotte D. Une recension des écrits concernant la réalité psychoaffective des femmes ayant une vulvodynia: difficultes rencontrées et strategies développées (abstract). *Pain Res Manage.* 2008;13:255–263.

55. Moyal-Barracco M, Lynch PJ. 2003 ISSVD terminology and classification of vulvodynia: a historical perspective. *J Reprod Med.* 2004;49:772–777.

56. Jantos M, Burns NR. Vulvodynia: development of a psychosexual profile. *J Reprod Med.* 2007;52:63–71.

57. Bachmann GA, Rosen R, Arnold LD, et al. Chronic vulvar and other gynecologic pain: prevalence and characteristics in a self-reported survey. *J Reprod Med.* 2006;51:3–9.

58. Goetsch MF. Vulvar vestibulitis: prevalence and historic features in a general gynecologic practice population. *Am J Obstet Gynecol.* 1991;164:1609–1616.

59. Berglund AL, Nigaard L, Rylander E. Vulvar pain, sexual behavior and genital infections in a young population: a pilot study. *Acta Obstet Gynecol Scand.* 2002;81:738–742.

60. Adanu RM, Haefner HK, Reed BD. Vulvar pain in women attending a general medical clinic in Accra, Ghana. *J Reprod Med.* 2005;50:130–134.

61. Jantos M, White G. The vestibulitis syndrome: medical and psychosexual assessment of a cohort of patients. *J Reprod Med.* 1997;42;145–151.

62. Masheb RM, Wang E, Lozano C, et al. Prevalence and correlates of depression in treatment-seeking women with vulvodynia. *J Obstet Gynaecol.* 2005;25:786–791.

63. Glazer HI, Jantos M, Hartman EH, et al. Electro-myographic comparisons of the pelvic floor in women with dysesthetic vulvodynia and asymptomatic women. *J Reprod Med.* 1998;43:959–962.

64. Reissing ED, Brown C, Lord MJ, Binik YM, Khalife S. Pelvic floor muscle functioning in women with vulvar vestibulitis syndrome. *J Psychosom Obstet Gynecol.* 2005; 26:107–113.

65. Jantos M. Vulvodynia: A psychophysiological profile based on electromyographic assessment. *Appl Psychophysiol Biofeedback.* 2008;33:29–38.

66. Cailliet R. *Soft Tissue Pain and Disability.* 3rd ed. Philadelphia, PA: F.A. Davis; 1996.

67. Cram JR, Kasman GS, Holtz J. *Introduction to Surface Electromyography.* Gaithersburg, MD: Aspen; 1998.

68. McKay E, Kaufman RH, Doctor U, et al. Treating vulvar vestibulitis with electromyographic biofeedback of pelvic floor musculature. *J Reprod Med.* 2001;46: 337–342.

69. Murina F, Bernorio R, Palmiotto R. The use of amielle vaginal trainers as adjuvant in the treatment of vestibu-lodynia: an observational multicentric study. *Medscape J Med.* 2008;10:23.

70. Glazer HI. Dysesthetic vulvodynia: long term follow-up after treatment with surface electromyography-assisted pelvic floor muscle rehabilitation. *J Reprod Med.* 2000;45: 798–802.

71. American Psychiatric Association. *Diagnostic and Statistical Manual of Mental Disorders.* 4th ed., text rev. Washington, DC: Author; 2000.

72. Van der Velde J, Everaerd W. Voluntary control over pelvic floor muscles in women with and without vaginistic reactions. *Int Urogynecol J.* 1999;10:230–236.

73. Van der Velde J, Laan E, Everaerd W. Vaginismus, a component of a general defensive reaction: an investi-gation of pelvic floor muscle activity during exposure to emotion-inducing film excerpts in women with and without vaginismus. *Int Urogynecol J.* 2001;12:328–331.

74. Van der Velde J, Everaerd W. The relationship between involuntary pelvic floor muscle activity, muscle awareness and experienced threat in women with and without vaginismus. *Behav Res Ther.* 2001;39:395–408.

75. Engmann M, Lindehammar H, Wijma B. Surface electro-myography diagnosis in women with partial vaginismus with or without vulvar vestibulitis and in asymptomatic women. *J Psychosom Obstet Gynecol.* 2004;25: 281–294.

76. Ter Kuile MM, van Lankveld JJ, Vlieland C V, et al. Vulvar vestibulitis syndrome: an important factor in the evalua-tion of lifelong vaginismus? *J Psychosom Obstet Gynecol.* 2005;26:245–249.

77. Gillenwater JY, Wein AJ. Summary of the National Institute of Arthritis, Diabetes, Digestive and Kidney Diseases workshop on interstitial cystitis, National Institute of Health, Bethesda, Maryland, August 28–29, 1987. *J Urol.* 1988;140:203–206.

78. Abrams P, Cardozo L, Fall M, et al. The standardization of terminology in lower urinary tract function: report from the standardization sub-committee of the International Continence Society. *Urology.* 2003;61:37–49.

79. Joop P, van de Merwe, Jorgen Nordling, et al. Diagnostic criteria, classification, and nomenclature for painful bladder syndrome/interstitial cystitis: an ESSIG proposal. *Eur Urol.* 2008;53:60–67.

80. Peters KM, Carrico DJ, Ibrahim IA, et al. Characterization of a clinical cohort of 87 women with interstitial cystitis/painful bladder syndrome. *Urology.* 2008;71: 634–640.

81. Koziol JA. Epidemiology of interstitial cystitis. *Urol Clin North Am.* 1994;21:7–20.

82. Temml C, Wehrberger C, Reidl C, et al. Prevalence and correlates for interstitial cystitis symptoms in women participating in a health screening project. *Eur Urol.* 2007; 51:803–809.

83. Gardella B, Porru D, Ferdeghini F, et al. Insight into uro-gynecologic features of women with interstitial cystitis/painful bladder syndrome. *Eur Urol.* 2008 Nov; 54(5): 1152–1153.

84. Skene AJC. *Treatise on the Diseases of Women, for the Use of Students and Practitioners.* New York, NY: Appleton; 1888.

85. Peters-Gee JM. Bladder and urethral syndrome. In: Steege JF, Metzger DA, Levy B, eds. *Chronic Pelvic Pain: An Integrated Approach.* Philadelphia, PA: W.B. Saunders; 1998:197–204.

86. Schmidt RA, Vapnek JM. Pelvic floor behaviour and interstitial cystitis. *Sem Urol.* 1991;9:154–159.

87. Schmidt RA, Tanagho EA. Urethral syndrome or urinary tract infection? *Urology.* 1981;18:424–427.

88. Chaiken DC, Blaivis JG, Blaivis ST. Behavioral therapy for the treatment of refractory interstitial cystitis. *J Urol.* 1993;149:1445–1448.

89. Whitmore KE. Self care regimens for patients with interstitial cystitis. *Urol Clin North Am.* 1994;21:121–130.

90. Costello K. Myofascial syndrome. In: Steege JF, Metzger DA, Levy B, eds. *Chronic Pelvic Pain: An Integrated Approach.* Philadelphia, PA: W.B. Saunders; 1998: 251–266.

91. Webster DC. Sex and interstitial cystitis: explaining the pain and self care. *Urol Nurs.* 1993;13:4–11.

92. Fitzgerald MP, Kotarinos R. Rehabilitation of the short pelvic floor. I: Background and patient evaluation. *Int Urogynecol J Pelvic Floor Dysfunct.* 2003;14:261–268.

93. Peters KM, Carrico DJ, Kalinowski SE, et al. Prevalence of pelvic floor dysfunction in patients with interstitial cystitis. *Urology.* 2007;70:16–18.

94. Oravisto KJ. Epidemiology of interstitial cystitis. *Ann Chir Gynaecol Fenn.* 1975;64:75–77.

95. Curhan GC, Speizer FE, Hunter DJ, et al. Epidemiology of interstitial cystitis: a population based study. *J Urol.* 1999;161:549–552.

96. Leppilahti M, Tammela TL, Huhtalia H, et al. Prevalence of symptoms related to interstitial cystitis in women: a population based study in Finland. *J Urol.* 2002;168:139–143.

97. Michael YL, Kawachi I, Stampfer MJ, et al. Quality of life among women with interstitial cystitis. *J Urol.* 2000;164:423–427.

98. Held PJ, Hanno, PM, Wein AS, et al. Epidemiology of interstitial cystitis. In: Hanno PM, Staskin DR, Krane RJ, et al. *Interstitial Cystitis.* New York, NY: Springer-Verlag; 1990:24–48.

99. Hsieh CH, Chang CH, Chang ST, et al. Treatment of interstitial cystitis with hydrodistension and bladder training. *Int Urogynecol J.*, 2008;19(10):1379–1384.

100. Yamada T, Murayama T, Andoh M. Adjuvent hydrodistension under epidural anaesthesia for interstitial cystitis. *Int J Urol.* 2003;10:463–468.

101. Parsons M, Toozs-Hobson P. The investigation and management of interstitial cystitis. *J Br Menopause Soc.* 2005;11:132–139.

102. Abrams P, Cardozo L, Fall M, et al. The standardisation of terminology of lower urinary tract function. *Neurol Urodyn.*, 2002;21:167–178.

103. Retzy SS, Rogers RM. Urinary incontinence in women. *Ciba Clin Sympos.* 1995;47:2–32.

104. Minassian V. Urinary incontinence as a worldwide problem. *Int J Gynecol Obstet.* 2003;82:327–338.

105. Olsen AL, Smith VJ, Bergstrom JO, et al. Epidemiology of surgically managed pelvic organ prolapsed and urinary incontinence. *Obstet Gynecol.* 1997;89:501–506.

106. Thom D. Variations in estimates of urinary incontinence prevalence in the community: effects of difference in definition, population characteristics, and study type. *J Am Geriatr Soc.* 1998;4:473–480.

107. Hampel C, Weinhold N, Eggersmann C, Thuroff JW. Definition of overactive bladder and epidemiology of urinary incontinence. *Urology.* 1997;50(suppl 6A):4–14.

108. Luber KM. The definition, prevalence, and risk factors for stress urinary incontinence. *Rev Urol.* 2004;6:S3–S9.

109. Norton PA, MacDonald LD, Sedgwick PM, et al. Distress and delay associated with urinary incontinence, frequency and urgency in women. *Br Med J.* 1988;297:1187–1189.

110. Nygaard IE, Thompson FL, Suengalis SH, et al. Urinary incontinence in elite nulliparous athletes. *Obst Gynecol.* 1994;84:183–187.

111. Thyssen HH, Clevin L, Olesen S, et al. Urinary incontinence in elite female athletes and dancers. *Int Urogynecol J.* 2002;13:15–17.

112. Handa VL, Cundiff G, Chang HH, et al. Female sexual function and pelvic floor disorders. *Obstet Gynecol.* 2008;111:1045–1052.

113. Amareco G, Le Cocquen A, Bosc S. Stress urinary incontinence and genito-sexual conditions: study of 35 cases. *Prog Urol.*, 1996;6:913–919.

114. Moran PA, Dwyer PL, Ziccone SP. Urinary leakage during coitus in women. *J Obstet Gynaecol.* 1999;19:286–288.

115. Achtari C, Dwyer PL. Sexual function and pelvic floor disorders. *Best Pract Res Clin Obstet Gynaecol.* 2005;19:993–1008.

116. Wymen JE. The psychiatric and emotional impact of female pelvic floor dysfunction. *Curr Opini Obstet Gynecol.* 1994;6:336–339.

117. Weidner AC, Myers ER, Visco AG, et al. Which women with stress incontinence require evaluation? *Am J Obstet Gynecol.* 2001;184:20–27.

118. Zhang Q, Wang L, Zheng W. Surface electromyography of pelvic floor muscles in stress urinary incontinence. *Int J Gynecol Obstet.* 2006;95:177–178.

119. Aukee P, Penttinen J, Airaksinen O. The effect of aging on the electromyographic activity of pelvic floor muscles: a comparative study among stress incontinent patients and asymptomatic women. *Maturita.* 2003;44:253–257.

120. Kegel AH. Stress incontinence of urine in women: physiologic treatment. *J Int Coll Surg.* 1956;25:487–499.

121. Hay-Smith EJ, Berghamans LC, Hendriks HJ, et al. Pelvic floor muscle training for urinary incontinence in women. *Cochrane Database Syst Rev.* 2001;1:CD001407.

122. Thompson JA, O'Sullivan PB, Briffa NK, et al. Altered muscle activation patterns in symptomatic women during pelvic floor muscle contraction and Valsalva manoeuvre. *Neurol Urodyn.* 2006;25:268–276.

123. Bo K. Isolated muscle exercises: technique. In: Schuessler B, Laycock J, Norton P, eds. *Pelvic Floor Re-education: Principles and Practice.* London: Springer; 1994:134–139.

124. Rett MT, Simoes JA, Herrmann V, et al. Management of stress urinary incontinence with surface electromyography-assisted biofeedback in women of reproductive age. *Phys Ther.* 2007;87:136–142.

125. Dannecker C, Wolf V, Raab R, et al. EMG-biofeedback assisted pelvic floor muscle training is an effective therapy of stress urinary or mixed oncontinence: a 7-year experience with 390 patients. *Arch Gynecol Obstet.* 2005;273:93–97.

126. Vico CMT, Segal HS, Sanchez TM, et al. Level of satisfaction and of subjective clinical improvement after pelvic floor muscle training and treatment of urinary incontinence. *Int Urogynecol J.* 2007;18(suppl 1):S187.

127. Verit FF, Verit A, Yeni E. The prevalence of sexual dysfunction and associated risk factors in women with chronic pelvic pain: a cross-sectional study. *Arch Gynecol Obstetarit.* 2006;274:297–302.

128. Phillips NA. Female sexual dysfunction: evaluation and treatment. *Am Family Phys.* 2000;62:127–136, 141–142.

129. Berman L, Berman J, Felder S, et al. Seeking help for sexual function complaints: what gynecologists need to know about the female patient's experience. *Fertil Steril.* 2003;79:572–576.

130. Aslan E, Fynes M. Female sexual dysfunction. *Int Urogynecol J Pelvic Floor Dysfunct.* 2008;19:293–305.

131. Rosenbaum TY. Pelvic floor involvement in male and female sexual dysfunction and the role of pelvic floor rehabilitation in treatment: a literature review. *J Sex Med.* 2007;4:4–13.

132. Bohlen JG, Held JP, Sanderson MO, et al. The female orgasm: pelvic contractions. *Arch Sex Behav.* 1982;11: 367–386.

133. Graber G, Kline-Graber G. Female orgasm: Role of the pubococcygeus muscle. *J Clin Psychiatry.* 1979;40: 348–351.

134. Kegel AH. Sexual function of puboccygeus muscle. *West J Surg Obstet Gynecol.* 1952;60:521–524.

135. Meston CM, Hull E, Levin RJ, et al. Disorders of orgasm in women. *J Sex Med.* 2004;1:66–68.

136. Esposito K, Ciotola M, Giugliano F, et al. Association of body weight with sexual function in women. *Int J Impot Res.* 2007;19:353–357.

137. Hicks TL, Forrester Goodall S, Quattrone EM, et al. Postpartum sexual functioning and method of delivery: summary of the evidence. *J Mid Women's Health.* 2004; 49:430–436.

138. Van Brummen HJ, Bruinse HW, van de Pol G, et al. Which factors determine the sexual function 1 year after childbirth. *BJOG.* 2006;113:914–918.

139. Ismael SS, Amarenco G, Bayle B, et al. Postpartum lumbosacral plexopathy limited to autonomic and perineal manifestations: clinical and electrophysiological study or 19 patients. *J Neurol Neurosurg Psychiatry.* 2000;68:771–773.

140. Whiting K, Santtila P, Alanko K, et al. Female sexual function and its association with number of children, pregnancy, and relationship satisfaction. *J Sex Marital Ther.* 2008;34:89–106.

141. Kim DH, Lee YS, Lee ES. Alterations of sexual function after classic intrafascial supracervical hysterectomy and total hysterectomy. *J Am Assoc Gynecol Laparosc.* 2003; 10:60–64.

142. Masters W, Johnson V. *Human Sexual Response.* Boston, MA: Little, Brown; 1966.

143. Both S, Laan E. Simultaneous measurement of pelvic floor muscle activity and vaginal blood flow: a pilot study. *J Sex Med.* 2007;4:690–701.

144. Kratochivil S. Vaginal contractions in female orgasm. *Cesk Psychiatr.* 1994;90:28–33.

145. Sholty MJ, Ephross PH, Plaut SM, et al. Female orgasmic experience: a subjective study. *Arch Sex Behav.* 1984;13: 155–164.

146. Mah K, Binik YM. Are orgasms in the mind or the body? Psychosocial versus physiological correlates of orgasmic pleasure and satisfaction. *J Sex Marital Ther.* 2005;31: 187–200.

147. Pigne A, Oudin G. Treatment of sexual dysfunction. In: Schussler B, Laycock J, Norton P, Stanton S, eds. *Pelvic Floor Re-education: Principles and Practice.* London: Springer-Verlag; 1994:126–129.

148. Bo K, Talseth T, Visnes A. Randomized controlled trial on the effect of pelvic floor muscle training on quality of life and sexual problems in genuine stress incontinent women. *Acta Obstet Gynecol Scand.* 200;79: 598–603.

149. Chambless DL, Stern T, Sultan FE, et al. The pubococcygeus and female orgasm: a correlational study with normal subjects. *Arch Sex Behav.* 1982;11:479–490.

150. Striefel S, Glazer HI. A proposed set of ethical guidelines in the assessment and treatment of pelvic disorders. *Appl Psychophysiol Biofeedback.* 2008;33: 181–193.

CHAPTER QUESTIONS

1. Pelvic floor disorders include:
   a. malfunction of specific pelvic organs
   b. incontinence
   c. sexual disorders
   d. pain conditions
   e. b, c, and d

2. The primary function of pelvic floor muscles is to assist with:
   a. urinary and fecal continence
   b. parturition
   c. sexual intercourse
   d. postural support
   e. all of the above

3. SEMG assessment of pelvic muscle function is:
   a. cost-effective
   b. noninvasive
   c. objective
   d. helpful in the diagnosis of neuromuscular disorders
   e. all of the above

4. Which of the following structures connects the anterior and posterior compartments of the urogenital diaphragm?
   a. anal sphincter muscle
   b. urogenital hiatus
   c. perineal body
   d. coccyx
   e. none of the above

5. The pubococcygeus (more correctly termed the pubovisceral) muscle attaches to which of the following structures?
   a. coccyx
   b. pubis
   c. ischial spine
   d. both a and b
   e. none of the above

6. Which of the following statements is true about the nature and function of slow-twitch muscle fibers?
   a. They make up 30% of the levator ani muscle.
   b. They provide ongoing resistance to gravity.
   c. They are red in color and rely on aerobic metabolism.
   d. They are rich in glycogen and glycolytic enzymes.
   e. They are large in diameter as compared to fast-twitch muscle fibers.

7. Based on SEMG studies, vulvodynia is best classified as:
   a. a sexual dysfunction
   b. a somatoform disorder
   c. an anxiety disorder
   d. a chronic pain syndrome
   e. none of the above

8. SEMG muscle assessment of conditions like vulvodynia reveal:
   a. hypertonicity
   b. irritability
   c. instability
   d. fatigue
   e. weakness
   f. all of the above

9. Which of the following risk factors contributes to onset of urinary incontinence?
   a. lifting of heavy objects
   b. straining while voiding
   c. obesity
   d. age
   e. all of the above

10. Studies of vaginismus have revealed:
    a. involuntary spasm of pelvic floor muscles
    b. disturbed micturition and increased prevalence of irritable bowel syndrome symptoms
    c. generalized muscle bracing under stress
    d. increased levels of catastrophizing and fear
    e. half of the patients meet the diagnostic criteria for vulvodynia
    f. answers b through e

11. Interstitial cystitis (IC) or "bladder pain syndrome" is characterized by:
    a. inflammation of the lining of the bladder (known as the interstitium)
    b. urgency and frequency
    c. painful sexual intercourse as in the case of vulvodynia
    d. hypertonicity and levator pain
    e. myofascial trigger points
    f. all of the above

Surface Electromyography Past, Present, and Future

Eleanor Criswell

Since the first edition of the *Introduction to Surface Electromyography*, there have been numerous developments in research and instrumentation. The Association for Applied Psychophysiology and Biofeedback and the Biofeedback Foundation of Europe have continued to evolve, and an increasing number of international research articles are being published. Surface electromyography (SEMG) research during the past 10 years can be grouped under following topics: SEMG physiological mechanisms, SEMG monitoring, and SEMG feedback (rehabilitation and special applications). This chapter looks at the development of surface electromyography past, present, and future.

SEMG PAST

In evaluating SEMG studies, it is important to consider the research design; random selection and assignment of research participants; participant selection criteria, sample size, use of control groups, and control group conditions; SEMG experimenter qualifications (How trained and experienced was the person conducting the measurements or training?); length, number, and spacing of training sessions (Did the participant train to criterion?); the research environment; instrumentation specifications and electrode placement sites; adequacy of performance evaluations (not just subjective reports of performance); whether SEMG was combined with other experimental treatments; data analysis approach or technique; and whether the data warrant the conclusions and discussion. Learning how to read and evaluate SEMG research articles enhances the ability to use the information wisely. There is a trend toward evidence-based practice in many fields, including SEMG feedback. Research is a key source of evidence. Therefore, the practitioner needs to be a good research consumer. SEMG research can make key contributions to that trend. A great deal of SEMG research remains to be done. That is part of the excitement of this growing field.

Locations and affiliations of the principal authors of the research articles discussed in this chapter as well as the years of publication are included to illustrate the global nature of SEMG research and to give a sense of its current evolution.

Physiological Mechanisms

The comparison between functional magnetic resonance imaging (fMRI) of the brain and muscle activity (EMG and force) is a very promising area of SEMG research. Dai et al.[1] (2001, Cleveland Clinic Foundation, Cleveland, Ohio) explored the relationship between muscle activity and fMRI-measured brain activation.

Specifically, this study looked at the relationship "between fMRI-measured brain activity and handgrip force and between fMRI-measured brain signal and SEMG of extrinsic finger muscles."[1 (p. 290)] Dai et al. designed a system that records joint force and surface EMG online along with fMRI data. The authors state, "The degree of muscle activation, which includes force and EMG, is directly proportional to the amplitude of the brain signal recorded by a fMRI of the entire brain. . . ."[1 (p. 299)] A number of motor "function-related" cortical fields (including the primary motor area, sensory regions, supplementary motor area, premotor, prefrontal, parietal, and cingulate cortices, and cerebellum) showed activation. These areas are all involved with motor function. All of the examined brain areas demonstrated a similar relationship between the fMRI signal and force.

The authors speculated that "a stronger fMRI signal during higher force indicates that more cortical output neurons and/or interneurons may participate in generating descending commands and/or processing additional sensory information."[1 (p. 290)] This furthers the understanding of "the control mechanisms of voluntary motor actions."[1(p. 290)] The authors discovered that "from 65% to 80% force level, the number of activated fMRI pixels did not increase."[1 (p. 297)] It seems that the brain does not recruit additional neurons in the primary motor and sensory cortices at a force higher than 65% maximum voluntary contraction (MVC) level. The firing rate of the neurons continues to increase, however.

The discovery that after 65% of the MVC had been reached no further cortical activation and no increase in force occurred is very useful information. It opens a very promising avenue for understanding motor function, determining which kinds of activities will be useful in therapy, and refining the motor tasks assigned. This understanding may lead to more specific and intelligent training and treatment protocols because it refines the sense of how much muscle force is needed to work functionally.

MRI/SEMG

Price et al.[2] (2003, Department of Diagnostic Radiology, Yale University School of Medicine) compared MRI and SEMG. The muscles of choice in their study were the plantar flexors of the ankle. These authors studied the muscle activity during dynamic plantar flexion. In this study, magnetic resonance imaging (MRI) and SEMG were compared to evaluate the effect of knee angle on plantar flexion activity in the triceps surae muscles (medial and lateral gastrocnemius [MG, LG] and the soleus [SOL]). It was determined that the MRI and SEMG "produce similar results from different physiological sources, and are therefore complementary tools for evaluating muscle activity."[2 (p. 853)] This finding underlines the "efficacy of MRI for simultaneously detecting activity of groups of muscles."[2 (p. 854)] Price et al. concluded that MRI and SEMG measures are complementary: They give a three-dimensional sense of what is going on in a muscle or muscle group.

The authors further concluded that "plantar flexion is a shared phenomenon, with the degree of contribution of the plantar-flexor muscles influenced by the degree of flexion of the knee joint."[2 (p. 860)] The MRI shows the configuration of muscle groups, but does not show how the somatic nervous system and muscle contractions contributed to that configuration. The MRI of an area provides an invaluable (although expensive relative to SEMG) look at muscle activity.

Acoustic Startle

The acoustic startle was used in an innovative way to look at reticulospinal activity and its effects on movement and particular diseases in a study by Grosse and Brown[3] (2003, Sobell Department of Motor Neuroscience and Movement Disorders, Institute of Neurology, London). They demonstrated that the human reticulospinal tract activity caused by the acoustic startle response was correlated with a characteristic synchronization pattern of bilateral motor unit firing. There was coherence (i.e., a continuous-phase relationship of the waves) in the 10- to 20-Hz EMG frequency band between comparable muscles. The researchers speculated that this measure could be used to determine the contribution of the reticulospinal system to movement. They found that the proximal muscles of the upper limbs showed the strongest synchronizing influence of the startle response.

In conclusion, due to the evidence, the authors ascribed the common oscillatory drive of both sides of the body to the reticulospinal system. Historically, access to reticulospinal function has been limited. The authors concluded that they had demonstrated a pattern of EMG–EMG coherence; they associated the coherence with human nonrespiratory reticulospinal activity.

Gaze Direction

SEMG research can clarify the understanding of which muscles are involved in which movements. Bexander, Mellor, and Hodges[4] (2005, Division of Physiotherapy,

University of Queensland, Brisbane, Australia) looked at gaze direction and neck muscle EMG activity during cervical rotation. They found that rotation of the head to the right increased EMG activity for the right splenius capitus (SC) and left sternocleidomastoid (SCM) muscles, the obliquus capitis inferior (OI) muscle EMG increased in both directions, and the multifides (MF) EMG did not change from the recording at rest.

EMG levels were higher when the eyes moved with the direction of the head movement. The authors suggested that the relationship between eye position and neck muscle EMG activity may contribute to neck posture and movement. Their hypothesis that the position of the eyes contributed to the SCM EMG activity caused by cervical rotation was confirmed. These findings can be used to increase the effectiveness of therapeutic interventions and treatment outcomes.

Motor Unit Activation

Suzuki et al.[5] (2002, Department of Rehabilitation Medicine, Dokkyo University School of Medicine, Tochigi, Japan) conducted a study of surface-detected EMG signals and motor unit activation, using an indwelling concentric needle electrode. They discovered that S-MUAP (motor unit action potential) size of the vastus medialis (VM) increased with increasing force. This finding suggests that there was a recruitment of larger motor units during the mean firing rate increase up to at least 50% MVC. As a consequence, Suzuki et al. suggested that motor unit recruitment may be the primary way that the VM increases muscle force.

In sum, these authors found that with increasing force generation and sustained submaximal contractions, the mean absolute SEMG amplitude increased. In addition, they indicated that the number, size, and firing rates of activated motor units determine the mean absolute SEMG amplitude during different levels of force. The motor units also contribute to the mean absolute SEMG amplitude of sustained contraction.

Another study utilized a combination of wire electrodes and surface electrodes. Hansen et al.[6] (2001, Division of Neurophysiology, Department of Medical Physiology, Panum Institute, Copenhagen University, Copenhagen, Denmark) looked at lower-limb motor unit activity during human walking. In this study, wire electrodes were placed in and surface electrodes place over the tibialis anterior; surface electrodes were placed over the "soleus, gastrocnemius lateralis, gastrocnemius medialis, biceps femoris, vastus lateralis, and vastus

medialis"[6 (p. 1266)] muscles. An important finding of this study is that "motor units within a muscle as well as synergistic muscles acting on the same joint receive a common synaptic drive during human gait."[6 (p. 1266)]

This study primarily investigated neuromuscular activity during tonic muscle contractions. The authors observed that "central peaks are likely to reflect some central process that synchronizes the discharges of motor units during gait."[6 (p. 1274)]

Cortical Potential

The following example describes combined SEMG and electroencephalograph (EEG) research. It demonstrates the potential of EEG/SEMG research. It is also an example of how researchers find out more definitively what is going on during typical human movement function.

Fang et al.[7] (2001, Department of Biomedical Engineering, Lerner Research Institute, Cleveland Clinic, Cleveland, Ohio) looked at the difference between human eccentric and concentric muscle contractions as measured by the EEG-derived movement-related cortical potential (MRCP). Concentric (toward the center) muscle contractions result in the shortening of the muscle fibers; eccentric (away from the center) muscle contractions result in the lengthening of contractions. During eccentric contractions, the muscle maintains the contraction while allowing its muscle fibers to lengthen. Although different nervous system control strategies have been suggested for human concentric and eccentric muscle contractions, Fang et al. state that there are no data indicating that brain signals for eccentric versus concentric muscle actions differ. The purpose of their study was to look at the electroencephalography (EEG)-derived movement-related cortical potential level during two types of muscle activities.

The study revealed that during eccentric contraction, the elbow flexor muscle activity (EMG) was lower than during concentric contraction. Conversely, the amplitude of the major MRCP components (during movement planning and execution) and the feedback from the peripheral systems were significantly greater for eccentric versus concentric contractions. Further, the authors observed that the onset time for the eccentric task MRCP occurred before the concentric contraction. It has been observed that the motor cortex inhibits the antagonist muscle before the agonist muscle contracts. This outcome might be expected because eccentric, lengthening contractions are created by a decrease in motor unit recruitment and firing as the contraction/force is maintained. The decrease in antagonist contraction allows for agonist muscle contraction. The authors concluded that the programming is different for eccentric versus concentric muscle tasks, with the eccentric contraction requiring a greater cortical signal. They speculated that a larger amount of sensory information is being processed in the brain during eccentric contractions, in addition to the reflex-induced feedback from stretched muscles.

Another eccentric versus concentric contraction study was conducted by McHugh et al.[8] (2002, Nicholas Institute of Sports Medicine and Athletic Trauma, Lenox Hill Hospital, New York, New York). They looked at the activation patterns of eccentric and concentric quadriceps contractions. Their main finding was that the eccentric contractions of the quadriceps femoris had a higher mean SEMG frequency than the concentric contractions. The authors used a range of submaximal contractions, suggesting that this research design represented the greater proportion of fast-twitch motor units activated during submaximal eccentric contractions and might yield higher mean SEMG frequencies. They concluded that this approach has implications for sports training, especially for sports that use fast-twitch muscle fibers, and for rehabilitation of injuries that affected fast-twitch fibers.

Stretching

The stretch reflex is a monosynaptic reflex that occurs when a muscle is stretched. The neuromuscular spindles within the muscle are sensitive to stretch. When the muscle is stretched, a signal is sent to the spinal cord along the dorsal root ganglion to synapse on the alpha motor neuron, causing the muscle fibers to contract. Myriknas, Beith, and Harrison[9] (2000, Department of Physiology, University College London, London) conducted a study of the stretch reflexes of the human rectus abdominus (RA) muscle. They used a mechanical tap to the muscle to induce the stretch. Tapping the RA muscle revealed local stretch reflexes in both the ipsilateral and contralateral muscles. Both sides showed early and late responses. A 2–millisecond delay in response for both muscles was reported. Both early and late reflexes had a reduced amplitude during vibration. The Jendrassik maneuver (a technique of increasing muscle tonicity to enhance a reflex response) increased their amplitudes. The researchers concluded that a crossed monosynaptic (a single neuron synapse) pathway might be present. The late response seen in both muscles and the increase in amplitude during vibration suggest the involvement of a polysynaptic pathway.

A study by Cramer et al.[10] (2005, Department of Kinesiology, Exercise Science Research Laboratories, University of Texas at Arlington, Texas) looked at static stretching (peak torque, mean power output, electromyography, and mechanomyography). Mechanomyography uses a piezoelectric accelerometer to measure muscle activity. The researchers found that static stretching decreases the force-producing capabilities of a muscle. The primary findings were that stretching decreased peak torque (PT) and EMG amplitude for the vastus lateralis and rectus femoris muscles of the stretched limb. This was also true of the unstretched limbs.

Stress

Stress has become an increasingly significant aspect of contemporary life. In a study by Krantz, Forsman, and Lundberg[11] (2004, Centre for Health Equity Studies, Stockholm, Sweden), male and female participants were exposed to stress. Their physiological stress responses and electromyographic activity were then compared. The physiological responses during mental and physical stressors that were measured included systolic and diastolic blood pressure, heart rate, urinary levels of epinephrine and norepinephrine, salivary levels of cortisol, and trapezius muscle SEMG activity. The results showed significant increases in the activity of all measures except cortisol level. Statistically significant correlations were noted between sympathetic nervous system arousal and SEMG activity.

This study is important because of the correlation between sympathetic nervous system arousal and muscle activity, which has been found to contribute to musculoskeletal complaints in physically undemanding but mentally stressful jobs. The differences between men and women included a higher blood pressure level and increased epinephrine (adrenalin) output for men; women had a higher heart rate. Another important finding was that the sympathetic nervous system seemed to be more sensitive to moderate stress exposure than the pituitary (e.g., salivary cortisol did not increase). The hypothalamic–pituitary–adrenal (HPA) axis, as measured by salivary levels of cortisol, was not activated. Men produced more epinephrine than women during performance stress. This finding has wide implications for stress-related conditions affecting men and women. Both men and women responded to stress exposure with sympathetic arousal and trapezius muscle activity.

Isometric Muscle Contractions

Steingrímsdóttir, Knardahl, and Vollestad[12] (2004, Department of Physiology, National Institute of Occupational Health, Oslo, Norway) looked at the effect of postal workers' muscloskeletal and psychological complaints on electromyographic activity during isometric muscular contractions. They measured the SEMG activity of the trapezius, deltoid, and forearm extensor muscles because of the high prevalence of muscle complaints regarding these areas of the body. Inability to relax after muscle contractions has long been considered a contribution to musculoskeletal disorders. The data analysis showed that postal workers with a history of musculoskeletal complaints or shoulder pain had lower trapezius EMG activity during submaximal contraction. This study is an example of EMG data yielding findings that are the opposite of the initial expectations (counter-intuitive). The authors found "no relation between a history of psychological complaints and the investigated muscle responses."[12 (p. 418)] Perhaps the lower trapezius EMG activity represents protective holding that avoids the activation of key muscles.

Pain

Pain is a very important facet of rehabilitation and of life. Pain is particularly bothersome for persons with fibromyalgia, for whom the cause is elusive. The question is: Is fibromyalgia a special condition or is it comparable to other pain syndromes?

In their study, Nilsen et al.[13] (2006, Norwegian University of Science and Technology, Department of Neurosciences, Trondheim, Norway) looked at patients with fibromyalgia (FMA) and patients with chronic shoulder/neck pain (SNP) during low-grade stress-induced pain using surface electromyography. The authors observed that the patients with FMA and SNP recovered from the stress-induced pain more slowly than the healthy participants in the control group. The subjective variables of pain, tension, and fatigue did not correlate with SEMG activity (temporalis muscle EMG was the exception). Generalized pain responses were more characteristic of the FMS patients than of the SNP patients. The authors concluded that there was no significant difference between the muscular or subjective responses to the low-grade, 60-minute mental stress condition. For both groups, SEMG data during the stressful task did not correlate with the induced pain, tension, and fatigue. The authors speculated that the disease-related sensitization of pain pathways may have contributed to the longer pain responses of patients with FMS and SNP compared to healthy control group members.

In a pilot study, Donaldson et al.[14] (2002, Myosymmetries, Calgary, Canada) looked at the diffuse muscular coactivation (DMC) in persons with fibromyalgia. They examined the electrical characteristics (root mean square [RMS] and median frequency) of diffuse muscular coactivation (DMC) associated with the tender points of FMA. Donaldson et al. define DMC as "an increase from resting levels (tonus) in the electrical activity of any muscle during a movement which does not involve that muscle and is not part of the agonist–antagonist unit."[14 (p. 41)] This is a very useful distinction, especially in looking at the experience of the patient with FMA. The researchers found an increase in RMS responses for patients with FMA as compared to the control group. Coactivation of muscles was stronger closer to the neck, but decreased in intensity as more distant areas were recorded. The authors noted that there was unusual muscle activity occurring in all patients with FMA: Movement of the head correlated with increased muscle electrical activity throughout the body.

Acute whiplash injury that results in chronic neck pain disability was studied by Nederhand et al.[15] (2003, Roessingh, Research and Development, Netherlands). Contrary to expectations, their results showed no elevated SEMG activity in the acute stage of this condition or during the follow-up. Their important observation was that in the case of future disability, the acute stage includes a reorganization of neck and shoulder muscle use. They speculated that this is probably an attempt to avoid muscle pain.

Tai Chi

Chan, Luk, and Hong[16] (2003, Department of Sports Science and Physical Education, Chinese University of Hong Kong, Hong Kong) conducted a study of the push movement in tai chi using kinematic and electromyographic measures. Their work is an example of phenomenological study of the muscle contraction patterns of an accomplished participant. Many studies use naive subjects or participants. In sports and other physical disciplines, different muscular organization patterns are typically observed at different stages of development within the discipline. This is a valuable contribution to the understanding of SEMG activity during complex movement patterns.

Golf

Watkins et al.[17] (1996, Kerlan Jobe Orthopaedic Clinic, Los Angeles, California) looked at trunk musculature of professional golfers using a dynamic electromyographic analysis. Their work demonstrates the usefulness of dynamic SEMG data. In this study, the right abdominal oblique, left abdominal oblique, right gluteus maximus, left gluteus maximus, right erector spinae, left erector spinae, upper rectus abdominis, and lower rectus abdominis muscles were measured by SEMG electrodes during the golfer's swing.

Five phases of golf swing were monitored with SEMG: "take away," "forward swing," "acceleration," "early follow-through," and "late follow-through."[17(p. 535)] The authors stated that although there were unique golfers' swings, reproducible patterns of trunk muscle SEMG activity occurred through all stages of the golf swing. They concluded that the trunk muscles are important for stabilizing and controlling the load response for maximal power and accuracy during the golf swing. These findings can be used to enhance rehabilitation programs for golfers. An emphasis on strength of trunk muscles and coordination exercises is recommended.

The following statements reflect the authors' more detailed observations of the data: Potential energy to kinetic energy occurs most in the acceleration phase of the golf swing; all trunk muscles are active during this phase. The left gluteus maximus muscle is more activated than the corresponding right muscle during the "pushing-off" effect during the acceleration. The developed athlete has refined cooperation of all muscle groups.

Musicians

A great deal of research needs to be conducted concerning use of SEMG with musicians. This need reflects the large number of neuromuscular complaints musicians often develop over time. Chan et al.[18] (2000, Department of Rehabilitation Sciences, Hong Kong Polytechnic University, Hung Hom, Hong Kong) measured the self-perceived exertion level and objective evaluation of neuromuscular fatigue (upper trapezius muscle) of orchestral violin players following a training session. The fatigue rate of the upper trapezius was measured by median frequency of the EMG signals. The use of median frequency for muscle fatigue assessment is common in SEMG research. Because the violinists did not show elevated median frequencies in this study, the authors concluded that multiple factors contribute to the violinist's self-perceived exertion. Because playing-related musculoskeletal complaints (PRMCs) are highly prevalent among musicians, further ergonomic investigations of the work-related risk factors for musicians are warranted. The training of musicians and the field of arts medicine could benefit greatly from this information.

Work

In a prospective study of postal workers, Steingrímsdóttir, Vollstad, and Knardahl[19] (2005, Department of Physiology, National Institute of Occupational Health, Oslo, Norway) looked at performance of standardized cognitive and motor tasks in relationship to musculoskeletal and psychological complaints and muscular responses. Higher SEMG levels and a steeper increase in the activity of muscles not engaged in the task seemed to relate to psychological complaints from the previous four months. During complex choice/reaction time tasks, the psychological complaints of the previous four months predicted lower SEMG levels. These complaints predicted an EMG temporal increase for longer-duration tasks. Further, the authors observed that the strongest individual predictor of increased SEMG responses was sleep disturbance. They found that the muscle-activity responses to the standardized tasks did not predict changes in severity of musculoskeletal or psychological complaints during the following one-year period.

The main findings were that postal workers responded to cognitive and motor tasks, similar to their everyday work tasks, with elevated SEMG activity both during the tasks and during the rest periods. Due to the orienting reflex (the physiological responses of the organism to new stimuli), there is the possibility that the responses were greater than they would have been to habitual tasks.

SEMG Feedback Studies

The studies described in this section feature SEMG feedback as the independent variable—that is, the use of SEMG feedback to modify muscle usage.

Computer

An important consideration at this time in history is the neuromuscular response to computer work. A number of SEMG studies have looked at this issue. For example, Madeleine et al.[20] (2006, Center for Sensory–Motor

Interaction, Department of Health Science and Technology, Aalborg University, Aalborg, Denmark) looked at electromyographic and mechanomyographic biofeedback of the upper trapezius muscle activity. Standardized computer work was the task selected for scrutiny. The authors discovered that audio or visual biofeedback using the surface EMG or MMG signal helped lower the contraction level of the upper trapezius. Surface EMG and MMG were confirmed as valuable methods to lower the upper trapezius muscle static load during computer work. The authors suggested that this approach may also change the muscle synergies involved and help prevent work-related musculoskeletal disorders.

Sports Performance

The use of SEMG feedback to enhance sports performance has been explored in numerous studies, frequently by using a single measure or modality of biofeedback. In one study, Kavussanu, Crews, and Gill[21] (1998, Loughborough University, Department of Physical Education, Sport Science and Recreation Management, Loughborough, Great Britain) explored basketball free-throw shooting performance using single versus multiple measures of biofeedback. The researchers used EMG, EEG, and HR (heart rate) bidirectional biofeedback training with one group; the second group received bidirectional EMG only. The secondary purpose of the study was to look at perceived control and self-efficacy as they might contribute to the biofeedback/performance outcomes. In the statistical analysis, self-efficacy was the only predictor of performance according to a stepwise multiple regression of the data. It accounted for "approximately 60% and 46% of the variance in pre- and post-test performance scores respectively."[21 (p132)] The authors quote Bandura[22] as suggesting "that biofeedback can be used as a method to help people control emotional arousal and subsequently enhance self-efficacy."[21 (p. 141)]

Reinforcement Schedules

To date, many elements of SEMG biofeedback have not been researched to determine the best approach. For example, analog or digital feedback has historically been the norm. If you consider biofeedback from the operant conditioning paradigm, as many do, what is the ideal reinforcement schedule?

Cohen et al.[23] (2001, Bloomsburg University of Pennsylvania, Bloomsburg, Pennsylvania) looked at potential EMG biofeedback reinforcement schedules. Reinforcement is said to occur when behavior happens again or increases. In the SEMG feedback process, the feedback signal is considered a reinforcer. This study examined continuous reinforcement (CRF) as well as fixed ratio (FR), variable ratio (VR), fixed interval (FI), and variable interval (VI) reinforcement schedules during the acquisition and extinction of forearm muscle tension increases. The FR schedule generated the highest response rate; the VR schedule was next. A higher sustained muscle contraction level was engendered by the CRF schedule. A contraction–relaxation action was more likely to be encouraged by the FR and VR schedules. A high sustained EMG level was created by the CRF schedule; this level also proved least resistant to extinction. If a response is not reinforced, after a period of time it is extinguished or is less likely to occur. Most resistant to extinction in this study were the VI and VR schedules. These results represent highly useful information both for understanding the effect of SEMG feedback and for planning home practice and self-reinforcing schedules for compliance.

SEMG and Physical Therapy

Can SEMG feedback supplement physiotherapy programs, particularly in the case of patellofemoral pain syndrome? In patellofemoral pain syndrome, the patella is not tracking properly and pain ensues. Weakness of the vastus medialis obliquus muscle is implicated in the patellofemoral syndrome.

To explore this issue, Yip and Ng[24] (2006, Department of Rehabilitation Sciences, Hong Kong Polytechnic University, Hong Kong) looked at a rehabilitation program for patellofemoral pain syndrome with SEMG feedback as a supplement to a physiotherapy exercise program. This is an example of the use of SEMG feedback in refining exercises—that is, increasing the specificity of function so that learning is speeded up. The authors' objectives were to investigate the "effect" on perceived pain, patellar tracking, and isokinetic knee extension strength of the addition of SEMG to the rehabilitation program. Data revealed that the SEMG feedback group changed patellar rotation faster than the exercise-only group. The authors suggested that the correct muscle recruitment pattern allowed the SEMG feedback group of subjects to achieve an earlier patellar alignment than the exercise-only group. This study used a standard rehabilitation exercise program for patients with patellofemoral pain syndrome; clinical pain measurements showed no additional effect from the combination of SEMG and exercises.

In another study, researchers explored chronic whiplash symptoms. Voerman, Vollenbroek-Hutton, and Hermens[25] (2006, Roessingh Research and Development, Netherlands) looked at ambulant myofeedback training as an intervention for pain, disability, and muscle activation patterns in patients with chronic whiplash. This was an exploratory study—an example of instrument and protocol innovation. The study featured ambulatory myofeedback training. The authors recorded the upper trapezius muscle continuously for four weeks and the data were processed. There was no control group. The authors considered their approach to be Cinderella-based myofeedback training. "Cinderella-based" refers to biofeedback addressing low threshold motor units that are recruited first, but are often neglected in SEMG, and whose activity levels do not decrease until the muscle fully relaxes. The authors found a "clinically relevant decrease in pain in a substantial number of patients."[25 (p. 661)]

Dystonia

Hand dystonia is an important repetitive-use symptom for musicians, computer technicians, and many other people whose hands are an important part of their professional and other endeavors. Dystonia is a movement disorder characterized by chronically contracted muscles and difficulty in using muscles.

Deepak and Behari[26] (1999, Department of Physiology, All India Institute of Medical Sciences, New Delhi, India) looked at hand dystonia (writer's cramp) and the use of EMG biofeedback for rehabilitation. They observed that a number of muscles not ordinarily involved in writing received an "uncontrolled outflow of abnormal involuntary efferent output."[26 (p. 268)] These were nontargeted muscle groups. Following SEMG feedback, nine patients ($N = 13$) showed a 37% to 93% improvement in their handwriting and a decrease in discomfort and pain. Pain level was assessed using a visual analogue scale.

The authors speculated that this abnormal efferent outflow might cause the key symptoms of dystonia, which are "dystonic posture, discomfort, fatigue and pain, labored writing, and finally, hypertrophy of the proximal muscles."[26 (p. 268)] They concluded that SEMG biofeedback decreases the excessive outflow to the hand muscle groups responsible for the posture of dys-

tonia, which reduces dystonic symptoms. According to Deepak and Behari, SEMG feedback helps the subject become more aware of the "abnormal contractions" and the decreasing "cocontractions of the involved muscle groups."[26 (p. 279)]

Another study focused on cervical dystonia. Smania et al.[27] (2003, Center of Functional Reeducation, G. B. Rossi Hospital, Verona, Italy) looked at two different rehabilitation treatments for idiopathic cervical dystonia (ICD) or spasmodic torticollis, a condition characterized by abnormal turning of the head and other postural distortions. The research design was a behavioral analysis of single cases. Four patients participated in the study.

The authors stated that dystonia can be central or peripheral nervous system mediated, as well as mediated by bone, joint, or muscle disease or imbalances. Physical activity, fatigue, and emotional distress can exacerbate the condition. The researchers quote Berardelli et al.[28] as suggesting that "dystonia may result from functional disturbance of the basal ganglia, possibly involving striatal control of the globus pallidus and, consequently, thalamic control of cortical motor planning and execution."[28 (p. 219)]

The sternocleidomastoid, scalenes, levator scapulae, and upper trapezius muscles were targeted in this study. Given that ICD cannot be controlled easily with medication, SEMG is a frequently used intervention. SEMG biofeedback and a novel physiotherapy program consisting of "postural reeducation exercises and passive elongation of myofascial cervical structures"[28 (p. 219)] were compared in this study. The authors did not specify the novel physiotherapy program. In future SEMG research, greater specificity in the description of all interventions would be helpful.

Headache (Chronic Tension)

Years ago, research showed that raising hand skin temperature contributed to decreasing migraine headache symptoms. Subsequent research showed the opposite: Decreasing hand skin temperature through biofeedback training helped decrease the incidence of migraine headaches. It was speculated that the change in awareness was the factor that contributed to the outcomes.

In a study by Rokicki et al.[29] (1997, Department of Psychology and Institute of Health and Behavioral Sciences, Ohio University, Athens, Ohio), a significant relationship was found between self-efficacy and decreasing headache activity at the end of treatment and at post-treatment for follow-up participants who received the experimental treatment. The experimental treatment was relaxation/SEMG feedback. The authors suggested that the cognitive changes that accompanied the EMG feedback training, rather than the EMG training itself, made the difference. Although this finding has huge implications for future SEMG applications, changes were based on the perceived ability to self-regulate physiological function. Looking at this research, it appears that the self-regulation of neurological and physiological changes made the difference, not the sense of self-efficacy per se. A complex set of factors is clearly involved.

Essential Tremor

In developing a new application area, investigators with small participant samples are a first step, letting researchers and clinicians know what may be possible. Many older adults experience essential tremor, a shaking of the arms and sometimes the legs that subsides at rest. Medication is frequently prescribed to deal with this condition. A study by Lundervold and Poppen[30] (2004, Central Missouri State University, Warrensburg, Missouri) used relaxation and dynamic EMG biofeedback training with three participants having essential tremor. The authors concluded that this combination—relaxation and dynamic SEMG training—holds promise for the older population who must cope with tremor and compromised functional movements.

Gait

A preliminary study by Bolek[31] (2003, Cleveland Clinic Children's Hospital for Rehabilitation, Cleveland, Ohio) used real-time SEMG to modify gait. Two children with cerebral palsy were the participants. The goal was to recruit the tibialis anterior using SEMG-assisted learning. Knowledge of performance was the focus, rather than knowledge of the results. Removing the goal-directed nature of movements enhances progress, demonstrating what is possible with dynamic SEMG feedback during movement. Following the SEMG-assisted learning intervention, the authors observed a decrease in "toe-dragging and hip-hiking during gait."[31 (p. 133)] Endurance was remarkably improved. This "real-time"[31 (p. 136)] rehabilitation experience is an example of the many rehabilitation and enhanced-performance possibilities using SEMG.

Another SEMG biofeedback study featuring gait and children with cerebral palsy was conducted by Dursun, Durson, and Alican[32] (2004, Kocaeli University Faculty of Medicine, Department of Physical Medicine and Rehabilitaton, Kocaeli, Turkey). A total of 36 children with spastic cerebral palsy and dynamic equinus deformity (a condition in which the foot is plantar flexed) participated in the study. The study featured SEMG feedback versus a conventional exercise program. The authors found that the co-activation of the agonist and antagonist muscle groups contributed to the spasticity.

In the study, subjects were asked to contract the tibialis anterior muscle and relax the chronically contracted triceps surae muscles (gastrocnemius and soleus muscles). SEMG feedback from those muscles was simultaneously displayed. A notable conclusion was that SEMG feedback was probably enhanced by the exercise program. The applications of this finding to many rehabilitation settings would be very productive.

The authors further concluded that this important finding causes a reversal of the conventional approach—that is, to relax the triceps surae and "strengthen" the tibialis anterior. "Deficient motor control may be secondary to inadequate inhibition of muscular contraction of antagonists and weakness of agonists."[32 (p. 120)] It is the overall organization of the movement that is important. Using systems theory, repetitive practice of "functional and goal-directed activities"[32 (p. 120)] leads to integrated, organized, and normal movement. This follows the concept developed by Hans Weber—namely, that differentiation leads to integration and a higher level of organization. The repetitive and concentrated practice of SEMG feedback may also contribute to brain plasticity. Gait function improved statistically significantly for both groups in the Durson et al. study, but the SEMG feedback group made more progress.

SEMG PRESENT

Currently, therapeutic modalities are moving toward evidence-based therapy and treatment for assessment, evaluation, and therapeutic interventions. SEMG is valuable in assessment, training, reporting, and determining outcomes. This technology is poised to play a large role in evidence-based treatment. As always, more research is needed. Clinicians, educators, and researchers need to partner to increase the research into the various applications of SEMG.

In *EEG/EMG/Brain Function Monitoring*, a market research report, Global Industry Analysts (2007) reported that more than 66 EEG/EMG/brain functioning instrument manufacturers exist, many offering SEMG as part of their systems, in approximately 20 countries. The

United States is the largest market; outside the United States, Europe is the fastest-growing market. With this large number of manufacturers, there must be a correspondingly large number of practitioners worldwide.

Currently, SEMG instrument manufacturers are expanding their systems' data acquisition and analysis capabilities. They are also expanding SEMG feedback capabilities to include a vast array of images, sounds, and other software interfaces (see **Table 14–1**).

SEMG FUTURE

The Future of SEMG Research

The future of SEMG research might include the following developments:

- An increase in fMRI and SEMG research
- An increase in MRI and SEMG research
- Greater awareness of neural plasticity and the value of SEMG-enhanced performance in neural activity and development
- More SEMG research emphasizing frequency characteristics of the EMG signal
- fMRI and SEMG research on the role of imagery and guided imagery in muscle function
- Increased statistical analysis of the amplitude and frequency of SEMG waveforms and the timing of muscle use
- More research combining SEMG with other data-gathering systems

Future Applications of SEMG Feedback and Monitoring

Future applications of SEMG might include the following:

- Use of SEMG in educational settings so that children can gain a greater understanding of their bodies and learn how to self-regulate them to achieve goals such as stress management and preparation for events
- Preincident training so that accidents have less impact and recovery can be faster
- Use of SEMG in arts medicine and arts education
- Greater use of SEMG training in sports conditioning and performance
- Greater use of SEMG in rehabilitation to speed up the patient's connection to the appropriate muscles for a function
- Increased use of SEMG by the educated layperson using personal computers and portable systems

Table 14–1 A Sampling of Surface Electromyography Instrument Manufacturers

The Biocomp Research Institute
    Biocomp 2010
    www.biocompresearch.org
BioResearch Institute
    Bio Integrator Version 7.0
        Bio Integrator
        Bio Integrator Phoenix
    www.7hz.com
Delsys, Inc.
    Myomonitor® Wireless EMG System
    Myomonitor® IV Wireless Transmission and Data Logging System
    Bagnoli™ Desktop EMG Systems
    Bagnoli™ Handheld EMG Systems
    Trigno™ Wireless
    www.delsys.com
J&J Engineering
    J&J 1-220-C2 + 12 channel
    J&J 1-330-C2 + 6 channel
    www.jjengineering.com
Mind Media, Inc. (Netherlands)
    NeXus-32A
    NeXus-16 A & B
    Wireless NeXus-10
    NeXus-4 (portable)
    RSI Protector® (home trainer)
    www.mindmedia.nl
NeuroDyne Medical Group
    Monitor Series (home care)
    Clinical Series
    System/3 Series
    System/4 Series
    www.neumed.com
Noraxon
    MyoTrace™ 400
    MlyoSystem™1200
    MyoSystem™ 1400A
    MyoSystem™1400L
    www.noraxon.com
SRS Medical
    Orion® Biofeedback
    SRS Medicine Orion® Platinum X
    Regain™ 2020
    www.srsmedical.com
Thought Technology, Ltd.
    ProComp® Infiniti System
    ProComp 2™ (home use or second system in lab)
    ProComp 5
    Myotrac Infiniti U-Control TM
    FlexComp® Infiniti
    MyoTrac 3™ Infiniti System
    U-Control™ Home Trainer
    www.thoughttechnology.com

In selecting SEMG instruments, make sure that the instrument specifications fit your needs and that technical support is available.

- Use of SEMG in psychotherapy
- Further SEMG technological innovations
- Enhanced patient feedback options, such as more elaborate visual feedback displays and more contingent auditory feedback
- Miniaturization of SEMG systems for a variety of uses
- Advances in SEMG telemetry systems
- Increased use of online Internet SEMG training
- A merger of neurofeedback and SEMG assessment and feedback

Future Benefits of SEMG Feedback and Monitoring

The following are some of the benefits of SEMG that might be enjoyed in the future:

- The awareness of precise SEMG work for managing and reversing some of the negative effects of aging
- Fewer sports injuries due to misuse of the body and greater actualization of the athlete's potential
- Fewer workplace accidents and injuries due to greater body awareness and enhanced coordination
- The realization that greater self-awareness accompanies the self-regulation of muscles
- The integration of SEMG with other disciplines
- More frequent blend of SEMG and somatics

- The continued development of mind–body potential through SEMG training

CONCLUSION

Kasman and Wolf[33] state that "emergent themes today involve use of SEMG with functional movement tasks, sophisticated exercise prescription, and a muscle imbalance perspective."[33 (p. 45)] Ideally, future themes will include these aspects, but move beyond them into prevention, education, and general actualization of full movement potential. SEMG can increase precision in the use of muscles and enhance cooperation among muscle groups in the context of many other treatment/training protocols and activities. Humans have tremendous somatic potential, and SEMG can help them achieve that potential.

Surface EMG is an exciting and evolving field. Although research has continued to develop globally and to expand the application areas, much research remains to be done. The field will reap the benefits of worldwide research and the new innovations and application areas in the coming years. Future applications of SEMG will likely be far reaching. Realization of these applications rests heavily on the awareness of the decision makers in the relevant settings and the economic support provided for the endeavors. SEMG has huge potential for human development and welfare, but training of SEMG professionals and wider public education about the benefits of SEMG are important parts of actualizing its potential.

REFERENCES

1. Dai TH, Liu JZ, Sahgal, V, Brown RW, Yue GH. Relationship between muscle output and functional MRI-measured brain activation. *Experi Brain Res.* 2001; 140(3):290–300.
2. Price TB, Kamen G, Damon BM, Knight CA, Applegate B, Gore JC, Eward K, Signorile JF. Comparison of MRI with EMG to study muscle activity associated with dynamic plantar flexion. *Magnetic Resonance Imaging.* 2003;21: 853–861.
3. Grosse P, Brown P. Acoustic startle evokes bilaterally synchronous oscillatory EMG activity in the healthy human. *J Neurophysiol.* 2003;90(3):1654–1661.
4. Bexander CSM, Mellor R, Hodges PW. Effect of gaze direction on neck muscle activity during cervical rotation. *Experi Brain Res.* 2005;167(3):422–432.
5. Suzuki H, Conwit RA, Stashuk D, Santarsiero L, Metter EJ. Relationships between surface-detected EMG signals and motor unit activity. *Med Sci Sports Exercise.* 2002;34(9): 1509–1517.

6. Hansen NL, Hansen S, Christensen LOD, Petersen NT, Nielsen JB. Synchronization of lower limb motor unit activity during walking in human subjects. *J Neurophysiol.* 2001;86(3):1266–1276.
7. Fang Y, Siemionow V, Sahgal V, Xiong F, Yue GH. (2001). Greater movement-related cortical potential during human eccentric versus concentric muscle contractions. *J Neurophysiol.* 2001;86(4):1764–1772.
8. McHugh MP, Tyler TF, Greenberg SC, Gleim, GW. Differences in activation patterns between eccentric and concentric quadriceps contractions. *J Sports Sci.* 2002; 20(2):83–91.
9. Myriknas SE, Beith ID, Harrison PJ. Stretch reflexes in the rectus abdominis muscle in man. *Experi Physiol.* 2000; 85(4):445–450.
10. Cramer JT, Housh TJ, Weir JP, Johnson GO, Coburn, JW, Beck TW. The acute effects of static stretching on peak torque, mean power output, electromyography, and mechanomyography. *Eur J Applied Physiol.* 2005;93(5–6):530–539.

11. Krantz G, Forsman M, Lundberg U. Consistency in physiological stress responses and electromyographic activity during induced stress exposure in women and men. *Integrative Physiol Behav Sci.* 2004;39(2): 105–118.

12. Steingrímsdóttir OA, Knardahl S, Vollestad NK. Prospective study of the relationship between musculoskeletal and psychological complaints and electromyographic activity during isometric muscular contractions in a working population. *Scand J Work Environ Health.* 2004;30(5);410–420.

13. Nilsen KB, Westgaard R H, Stovner LJ, Helde G, Ro M, Sand TH. Pain induced by low-grade stress in patients with fibromyalgia and chronic shoulder/neck pain, related to surface electromyography. *Eur J Pain.* 2006;10(7): 615–627.

14. Donaldson CCS, MacInnes AL, Snelling LS, Sella GE, Mueller HH. Characteristics of diffuse muscular coactivation (DMC) in persons with fibromyalgia: part 2. *NeuroRehabilitation.* 2002;17(1):41–48.

15. Nederhand MJ, Hermens HJ, Ijzerman MJ, Turk DC, Zilvold G. Chronic neck pain disability due to an acute whiplash injury. *Pain.* 2003;102(1–2):63–71.

16. Chan SP, Luk TC, Hong Y. Kinematic and electromyographic analysis of the push movement in tai chi. *Brit J Sports Med.* 2003;37(4):339–344.

17. Watkins RG, Uppal GS, Perry J, Pink M, Dinsay, JM. Dynamic electromyographic analysis of trunk musculature in professional golfers. *Am J Sports Med.* 1996;24(4):535–538.

18. Chan RFM, Chow C, Lee GPS, To L, Tsang XYS, Yeung SS, Yeung EW. Self-perceived exertion level and objective evaluation of neuromuscular fatigue in a training session of orchestral violin players. *Applied Ergonomics.* 2000; 31(4):335–341.

19. Steingrímsdóttir OA, Vollestad NK, Knardahl S. A prospective study of the relationship between musculoskeletal or psychological complaints and muscular responses to standardized cognitive and motor tasks in a working population. *Eur J Pain.* 2005;9(3): 311–324.

20. Madeleine P, Vedsted P, Blangsted AK, Sjogaard G, Sjogaard K. Effects of electromyographic and mechanomyographic biofeedback on upper trapezius muscle activity during standardized computer work. *Ergonomics.* 2006;49(10):921–933.

21. Kavussanu M, Crews DJ, Gill DL. The effects of single versus multiple measures of biofeedback on basketball free throw shooting performance. *Int J Sport Psychol.* 1998;29(2):132–144.

22. Bandura A. Self-efficacy: Toward a unifying theory of behavioral change. *Psychol Rev.* 1977;84:191–215.

23. Cohen SL, Richardson J, Klebez J, Febbo S, Tucker, D. EMG biofeedback: the effects of CRF, FR, FI, VI schedules of reinforcement on the acquisition and extinction of increases in forearm muscle tension. *Applied Psychophysiol Biofeedback.* 2001;26(3):179–194.

24. Yip SLM, Ng GYF. Biofeedback supplementation to physiotherapy exercise programme for rehabilitation of patellofemoral pain syndrome: a randomized controlled pilot study. *Clin Rehab.* 2006;20(12):1050–1057.

25. Voerman GE, Vollenbroek-Hutten MMR, Hermens HJ. Changes in pain, disability, and muscle activation patterns in chronic whiplash patients after ambulant myofeedback training. *Clin J Pain.* 2006;22(7):656–663.

26. Deepak KK, Behari M. Specific muscle EMG biofeedback for hand dystonia. *Applied Psychophysiol Biofeedback.* 1999;24(4):267–280.

27. Smania N, Corato E, Tinazzi M, Montagnana B, Fiaschi A, Aglioti SM. The effect of two different rehabilitation treatments in cervical dystonia: preliminary results in four patients. *Functional Neurol.* 2003;18(4):219–226.

28. Berardelli A, Rothwell JC, Hallett M, Thompson PD, Manfredi M, Marsden CD. The pathophysiology of primary dystonia. *Brain.* 1998;121:1195–1212.

29. Rokicki LA, Holroyd KA, France CR, Lipchik GL, France JL, Kvaal SA. Change mechanisms associated with combined relaxation/EMG biofeedback training for chronic tension headache. *Applied Psychophysiol Biofeedback.* 1997;22(1): 21–41.

30. Lundervold DA, Poppen R. Biobehavioral intervention for older adults coping with essential tremor. *Applied Psychophysiol Biofeedback.* 2004;29(1):63–73.

31. Bolek JE. A preliminary study of modification of gait in real-time using surface electromyography. *Applied Psychophysiol Biofeedback.* 2003;28(2):129–138.

32. Dursun E, Dursun N, Alican D. Effects of biofeedback treatment on gait in children with cerebral palsy. *Disability Rehab.* 2004;26(2):116–120.

33. Kasman G, Wolf S. *Surface EMG Made Easy: A Beginner's Guide for Rehabilitation Clinicians.* Scottsdale, AZ: Noraxon; 2002.

Conclusion

Jeffrey R. Cram, Glenn S. Kasman, and Eleanor Criswell

Surface electromyography (SEMG) has come quite a long way. It appeals to any professional who works with muscles. This technology is attractive because it is non-invasive; it is like an electronic stethoscope for muscles. Practitioners find SEMG attractive because it examines muscle function rather than structure. Surface EMG has evolved from the days when it was conducted from within copper cages. While it began in the halls of scientific inquiry into muscle and muscle function, it has clearly found its way into clinical practice. Although this book has explored some of the scientific foundations of SEMG, its primary focus has been clinical.

This book is an introductory text, which means it only begins to scratch the surface of what we know about muscle energy and how it can be used clinically to assess and treat musculoskeletal disorders and pain. It presents an initial exploration of the anatomy and physiology of muscle. A vast amount of information is available on this topic—from introductory texts such as *Job's Body*, by Juhan,[1] to advanced texts such as *Principles of Neural Science*, edited by Kandel, Schwartz, and Jessell.[2]

Part I of this book presented a brief introduction to the electrical concepts, the instrumentation, and the technology behind SEMG. For a more in-depth look at the basics, consider reading Peek's chapter on instrumentation in *Biofeedback: A Practitioner's Guide*, edited by Schwartz.[3] For a more sophisticated presentation, con-

sider the first chapters of *Muscles Alive* (fifth edition) by Basmajian and DeLuca.[4]

Part II included "The History of Muscle Dysfunction and Surface Electromyography" by Jeffrey Cram and Maya Durie, "Somatics and Surface Electromyography" by Eleanor Criswell, "Electromyographic Assessment of Female Pelvic Floor Disorders" by Marek Jantos, and "Surface Electromyography Past, Present, and Future" by Eleanor Criswell. Cram and Durie overviewed muscle dysfunction and approaches to changing those conditions; Criswell presented the field of somatics and described how it relates to SEMG; Jantos reviewed SEMG and female pelvic floor disorders; and the final chapter explored the field's progress since publication of the first edition of Cram's *Introduction to Electromyography* and considered its future potential. Part II revealed a vast vista of opportunities for SEMG. It is up to the researchers, clinicians, and interested patients and students to actualize the potential of this field.

The electrode atlas in Part III of this book provides information concerning the placement of electrodes, along with the types of recruitment patterns one might see using such placements. In addition, it recommends clinical uses for the various placements and provides clinical information relevant to each site. Only 69 electrode placement sites for the more than 600 muscles of the human body are explored, representing only a small portion (10%) of the total muscle energy of the human body. Fortunately, many of the muscles we currently can observe using SEMG are major muscles of the human body. Unfortunately, many troublesome muscles (such as the levator scapulae) cannot be seen with today's instruments.

The assessment chapters emphasize normal resting tone and provide representative samples of the types of recruitment patterns seen on a very small subset of "normal" individuals. We encourage practitioners to think about what type of recruitment pattern they would expect to see for a given muscle and then to test out those assumptions using SEMG. Through this type of inquiry, practitioners will expand their knowledge of

how SEMG can aid in the understanding of muscle function and its applications to clinical problems.

To conclude, this book has introduced the practitioner to the foundations and clinical uses of SEMG. It is our hope that practitioners will recognize and appreciate that SEMG is a very powerful and exciting tool. Along with its uses, however, come its abuses. We hope that practitioners take a conservative stance toward the use of this technology, in particular toward the interpretations of clinical study results. Finally, the use of SEMG for treatment is very promising, but practitioners must be careful about the claims they make. Surface EMG is but a tool to enhance the already existing skills of the provider. If nothing else, it turbocharges providers' treatment efforts.

REFERENCES

1. Juhan D. *Job's Body.* 3rd ed. New York, NY: Midpoint Trade Books; 2002.
2. Kandel E, Schwartz E, Jessen T. *Principles of Neural Science.* 4th ed. New York, NY: McGraw-Hill; 2000.
3. Peek CJ. A primer of biofeedback instrumentation. In: Schwartz M, ed. *Biofeedback: A Practitioner's Guide.* New York, NY: Guilford Press; 1987.
4. Basmajian J, DeLuca CJ. *Muscles Alive.* 5th ed. Baltimore, MD: Williams & Wilkins; 1985.

ATLAS FOR ELECTRODE PLACEMENT

Jeffrey R. Cram and Glenn S. Kasman with Jonathan Holtz

Electrode Atlas Overview

INTRODUCTION

The placement of the electrodes for surface electromyography (SEMG) recordings will, in large part, determine the quality of the recordings. Because the SEMG can "listen" only so deep and the SEMG signal is frequently contaminated by cross-talk from neighboring muscles, practitioners must decide whether they are interested in a specific or general recording and place the electrodes accordingly.

For a general recording, it is recommended that practitioners place the electrodes with a wide spacing. This positioning will capture all of the muscle energy contributions between the two active electrodes, and more. For recording from a specific muscle group, the practitioner must know specifically where the muscle is located, the direction of its muscle fibers, and its depth. Palpation of the surface muscles is essential to ensure accurate placement. A general rule of thumb is that the depth and area of the SEMG recording are directly proportional to the interelectrode distance.[1] This relationship is illustrated in **Figure 16-1**, where the darker fibers contribute more heavily than the lighter ones. This concept may be seen in cross section in Figure 3-3. For both superficial and slightly deeper muscles, the practitioner must ask the patient to do the primary

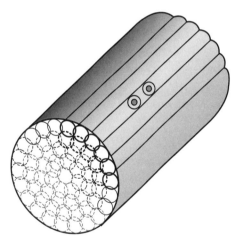

Figure 16-1 Relationship of interelectrode distance and depth of SEMG recordings.

movement of the muscle, either through its active range of motion or in a resisted isometric fashion. In this way, the practitioner can verify that placement is correct. Finally, it is often useful to monitor simultaneously the targeted muscle's synergist or antagonist so as to appreciate more fully the functional nature of the movement pattern.

INFORMATION CONTAINED IN ELECTRODE ATLAS

Type of Placement

This section describes general, specific, and quasi-specific electrode placements. Each description incorporates a variety of sources of information.

Some electrode placements monitor the muscular energy in a *general* region, while others are more *specific*. This atlas also includes a number of placements that are considered to be controversial; although SEMG recording from these controversial placements might appear to be specific, the muscles commonly lie beneath or adjacent to other muscles and, therefore, are fraught with the possibility of cross-talk. These placements are called *quasi-specific*.

General Placement

This electrode placement strategy takes advantage of volume conduction and records from a general region rather than a specific muscle. For example, the frontalis (wide) placement is specifically designed to record from muscle activity of the upper and, perhaps, lower face (rather than specifically monitoring from the frontalis muscle).

Specific Placement

This electrode placement strategy attempts to detect the activity of a specific muscle group. Usually, these muscles are close to the surface and relatively easy to isolate. The position for placement and the spacing and orientation of the electrodes can play a significant role in determining the practitioner's success in recording from a specific muscle. The type of movement associated with a muscle recording may help isolate the muscle activity or contaminate it through volume conduction. For example, smaller movements that require less recruitment tend to necessitate few synergists and, therefore, produce less volume conduction. As in muscle testing, correct positioning and instruction to the subject are necessary to ensure specificity in SEMG recordings.

Quasi-Specific Placement

This electrode placement strategy uses the strategies of the specific placement, such as closely spaced elec-

trodes oriented to record from specific muscles. However, specific recordings for certain muscles are difficult to complete because of the proximity of neighboring muscles (particularly in the extremities) or the depth of the muscle from the surface (as in the axial muscles). In both cases, it is difficult to identify clearly which muscle is contributing to the SEMG signal. Superficial muscles are typically easy to palpate and identify, but they may be difficult to isolate using SEMG techniques if they are packed closely together. Cross-talk from neighboring muscles may contaminate your confidence in a specific recording, such as a forearm recording. Recordings from deep muscles are difficult, because the source SEMG must pass through the more superficial layers of muscles to reach the recording electrodes. It is impossible to state that the recording is primarily from the deeper muscle, because the SEMG recording could easily be contaminated by the more superficial layers of muscle. The proof of specificity of recording resides in demonstrating that the SEMG signal is activated during the movements ascribed to the muscle of interest and not during contraction of neighboring muscles.

Action or Purpose

For both specific and quasi-specific sites, this section lists the primary function or action of the muscle. For general sites, it refers to the purpose of the SEMG recording.

Clinical Uses

This section highlights some of the conditions or procedures for which SEMG recordings at a particular site might be considered useful.

Muscle Insertions

This section describes the origins and insertions of the muscles of interest. This information may be important in understanding the direction of the muscle fibers, because surface electrodes are commonly oriented in the direction of these fibers.

Innervation

In cases where specific and quasi-specific muscle sites are described, this section identifies the motor nerves associated with the muscle group.

Joint Considerations

When appropriate, the joints considered pertinent to and possibly affecting the SEMG recordings are highlighted.

Location

This section describes the actual placement of the electrodes in verbal terms. This verbal description augments the graphical description provided on the same page. *Experience with muscle testing and palpation will help the practitioner to place the electrode over the correct muscle group.* Information on muscle testing and palpation is available in *Muscles: Testing and Function* by Kendall, Kendall, and McCreary.[2] It is recommended that the practitioner palpate the described area during a muscle testing procedure to locate the exact position of the muscle belly and to assist in placing the electrode. Better-quality SEMG recordings are obtained when the SEMG electrodes are placed parallel to the muscle fibers and slightly off center of the belly of the muscle.

Behavioral Test

Whenever electrodes are placed over a muscle group, the practitioner should ask the patient to engage in a specific movement to determine whether the electrodes are over the muscle of interest. This section describes at least one of the main movements associated with the muscle. The SEMG tracing shown for the site usually reflects one or more of these movements.

Tracing Comment

These tracings illustrate the SEMG recording seen during one of the movements described in the "Behavioral Test" section. Most of these tracings are presented in the raw SEMG format.* Whenever possible, this format was selected because it provides the clearest view of the SEMG activity. In addition, a pre-gelled, recessed electrode at a fixed interelectrode distance (center to center) was used for many of the recordings to help obtain

a clean signal and to provide a standard for later replication. These tracings are not intended to represent the "ideal" recruitment pattern, but rather what one would commonly see in the "normal" population. The tracings presented in this section are representative samples of SEMG tracings observed at a given site, on a given individual, using a given movement. The tracings are intended as a conceptual aid to electrode placement. They should not be taken as templates on which to base clinical decisions. No attempt has been made to evaluate systematically the variability of recruitment across a large population of normal subjects or patients. Simply put, these tracings demonstrate some of the expected recruitment patterns for the area of interest. Given the richness of human movement, it is important to note that these tracings do not represent a comprehensive study of an area. Slight variations in electrode placement and movement patterns may produce different recruitment patterns.

Clinical Considerations

This section identifies some of the potential postural or positional elements that might affect the recordings. The SEMG activity may vary dramatically with the body in a different posture owing to the effects of gravity on the more axial muscles or changes in SEMG activity levels because of small changes in the elements of the kinetic chain. In addition, a natural repositioning of the surface electrodes in relationship to the muscles beneath them may occur during movement of an extremity. For example, placement of electrodes on the triceps muscle should be done with the arm in the position or plane in which the training will be taking place, because supination and pronation of the arm can alter the position of the electrodes in relation to the muscle belly.

In addition, the SEMG recording may be affected by dysfunctions in the joints and fascia. Comments regarding the effects of these restrictions are supplied, when appropriate. Finally, this section lists some of the common clinical uses for certain placements. Such descriptions are not intended to be exhaustive, nor are they intended to limit SEMG uses for a given muscle site.

Volume Conduction

This section identifies the muscles that might commonly contaminate the specificity of the recording through volume conduction.

---

*The SEMG recordings were made using a Norodyn 8000 SEMG instrument (raw) or J&J I-330 M-501 SEMG instrument (processed). All recordings, unless otherwise specified, were conducted using the Norotrode 2.0 electrode. This electrode is a pre-gelled, recessed, or floating electrode with a 1.0-cm pellet and an interelectrode distance of 200 cm (center to center).

Other Sites of Interest

This section identifies other sites that the practitioner may want to monitor concurrently with the muscle of interest. These additional sites may be synergists, agonists, or antagonists that participate with the muscle of interest in a given movement. Although this concept of relatedness is self-evident for kinesiologically oriented practitioners, there is no common term for it. Travell and Simons[3] have referred to this concept as a *myotatic unit*. The additional sites may be part of a larger mass-action pattern, a kinetic chain, or simply some form of coordinated movement. This section helps the practitioner to see the "bigger picture" of muscle interaction patterns.

Referred Pain Considerations

Trigger points in a muscle group may affect features of the SEMG recording.[4, 5] When appropriate, the pain referral pattern for a trigger point located in the muscle group of interest is provided.[3]

Artifacts

This section identifies common artifacts associated with a given electrode placement.

Benchmark

This section provides a reference SEMG value for resting values. Such information is provided for some sites but not others. The issues pertaining to dynamic SEMG recordings preclude meaningful benchmark values at this time. For example, it is unclear whether these values should be taken as an average of the entire tracing, the peak of the movement, the recovery back to baseline, the concentric component, the eccentric component, and so on. In addition, the anthropomorphic variables may make absolute SEMG data less meaningful than normalized values. Normalized values may provide a more accurate picture of SEMG activity when one is comparing one muscle group to another. The percentage of asymmetry between the right and left homologous muscles of a particular group during a given movement may yield more meaningful information than absolute SEMG values.

The SEMG values associated with rest are considered meaningful. However, these values should be seen as guidelines rather than absolutes (see Chapter 6). Nearly all values have been converted to the J&J M-501 standard benchmark value; the benchmark values have been computed using the conversion factors listed in Table 3–1. To convert the benchmark value to a figure that is compatible with a particular instrument, simply multiply the benchmark value by the ratio associated with the particular SEMG instrument. For example, if the benchmark value is 5.0 microvolts and the practitioner is using a Davicon SEMG instrument, the practitioner would multiply 5.0 by 1.67 to obtain a Davicon equivalent value (or 8.35 microvolts). If a particular instrument is not listed in Table 3–1, record root mean square (RMS) values during rest from several muscle groups and compare the SEMG values to the benchmark value. If they consistently differ from the benchmark value by some factor (e.g., if they are twice as high), then use that factor to convert the benchmark values to ones relevant to the SEMG system.

REFERENCE PLANES AND MOVEMENT DESCRIPTIONS

Certain terms are used to describe dynamic movements. Descriptions of some of the movements are provided here to help practitioners replicate these procedures during the studies of muscle function. For a more extensive review of descriptions of movement, see Gowitzke and Milner's, *Scientific Basis of Human Movement,*[6] or Kendall, Kendall, and McCreary's *Muscles: Testing and Function.*[2]

Three cardinal reference planes of movement exist. The *frontal plane* divides movement toward the front and the back of the body. The *sagittal plane* divides the movement into right and left planes. The *horizontal* or *transverse plane* refers to the upper and lower portions of the body. These planes are shown in **Figure 16–2**.

Flexion, *extension*, *rotation*, and *side bending* are attributes used in movement of the head. These movements are clearly depicted in **Figure 16–3**. Flexion of the head brings the head forward, away from midline, chin to chest. The term *return* indicates a movement back to midline. Formal extension is movement backward, away from midline, letting the head fall back over the shoulders. Axial rotation of the head is associated with turning the head to look over the shoulder. Side bending involves bringing the ear toward the shoulder.

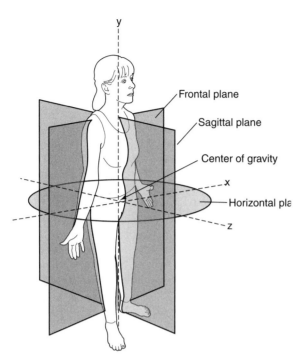

Figure 16–2 The primary cardinal reference planes.

Source: Reprinted with permission from Gowitzke B, Milner M, *Scientific Basis of Human Movement*, p. 9, © 1988, Williams & Wilkins.

Movement of the jaw may also be described. In addition to opening and closing the jaw, the jaw may be laterally deviated to the left or right and may be protruded outward from the cranium or retracted back toward the neck.

The study of shoulder functions is rather complex. Several forms and planes of movement are possible. *Shoulder abduction*, *adduction*, *flexion*, and *extension* are shown in **Figure 16–4**. Flexion and extension of the arm move in the sagittal plane out in front of the chest (as if walking in one's sleep) and backward (as if to dive). Abduction moves the arm laterally out to the side, as if to form a T with the body. Many of the shoulder and arm movements presented in the atlas limit abduction and flexion to 90 degrees, while others entail the full range of motion with the hands fully overhead. Adduction is associated with movement in toward the center of the body. *Scaption*, which is not shown in Figure 16–4, entails raising the arm out away from the body at an oblique 45-degree angle halfway between the frontal and sagittal planes—in other words, halfway between flexion and abduction. *Internal* and *external rotation* of the shoulder are presented in **Figure 16–5**. Internal rotation rounds the shoulder in, while external rotation rounds the shoulder back. *Shoulder girdle elevation*, *depression*, *retraction*, and *protraction* reflect another dynamic range of motion for the shoulder. With elevation, one raises the shoulder up around the ears; with depression, one pulls the shoulders down; with retraction, one pulls the shoulders back as if to stand in a military posture; with protraction, one moves the shoulders forward.

Movement of the upper extremities involves many aspects. *Elbow flexion* and *extension* are probably the easiest to define. The flexion component is presented in **Figure 16–6**. Here the biceps and brachialis shorten as the elbow bends. With elbow extension, the triceps shortens while the arm straightens. The forearm may also rotate. External rotation with the palm up is termed

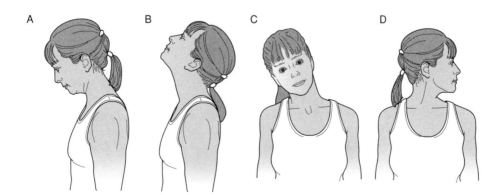

Figure 16–3 Cervical spine movements: **(A)** flexion, **(B)** extension, **(C)** lateral bending, and **(D)** rotation.

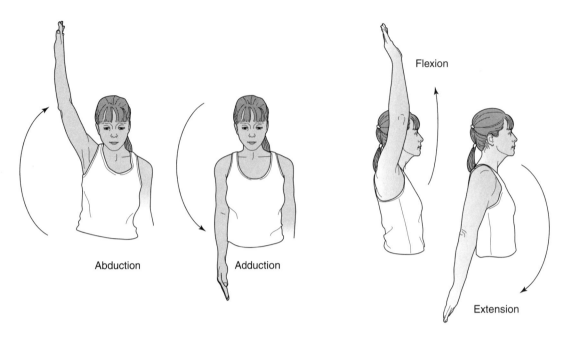

Figure 16–4 Primary movements of the shoulder.

supination, while internal rotation with the palm down is termed *pronation*. These terms are graphically depicted in **Figure 16–7**. Wrist movements also need to be defined. Wrist extension (*dorsiflexion*) cocks the wrist up, wrist flexion (*palmar flexion*) curls the wrist down, radial abduction (*deviation*) moves the wrist toward the thumb side, and ulnar adduction (*deviation*) moves the wrist toward the little finger side. These movements are depicted in **Figure 16–8**. Movement of the fingers and thumb may be isolated on SEMG recordings, as shown in **Figure 16–9** and **Figure 16–10**. Flexion and extension of the thumb allow one to hitchhike, while abduction and adduction of the thumb allow one to cut with scissors. Extending the fingers opens the hand, while flexing the fingers makes a fist.

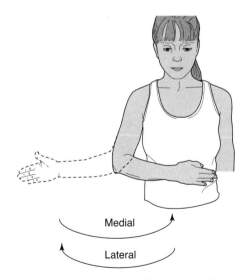

Figure 16–5 External (lateral) and internal (medial) rotation of the shoulder.

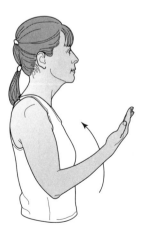

Figure 16–6 Elbow flexion.

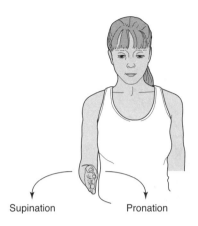

Figure 16–7 Pronation and supination at the radioulnar joint.

Supination   Pronation

Trunk movements have been studied primarily in terms of *flexion*, *extension*, *side bending*, and *rotation*. Flexion of the trunk brings one forward as if to touch the toes, while extension occurs when one leans back. The term *return of the trunk* indicates a return to midline from a flexed position. Side bending occurs when the subject bends to the side while sliding the hand down the leg. Axial rotation of the trunk entails rotation of the chest relative to the pelvis. In some cases, the hips must be stabilized to facilitate and isolate rotation of the torso. Flexion and extension of the trunk are illustrated in **Figure 16–11**.

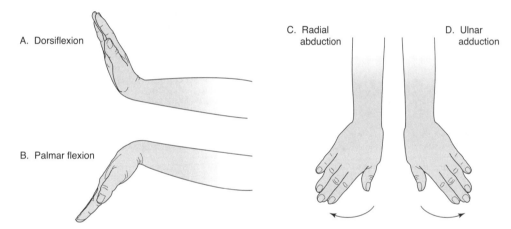

A. Dorsiflexion

B. Palmar flexion

C. Radial abduction

D. Ulnar adduction

Figure 16–8 Function of muscles acting on the wrist. **(A)** Extension, **(B)** flexion, **(C)** radial abduction, and **(D)** ulnar adduction.

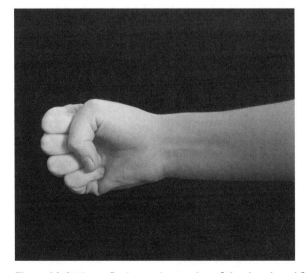 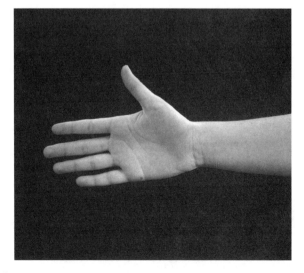

Figure 16–9 Finger flexion and extension of the thumb and fingers.

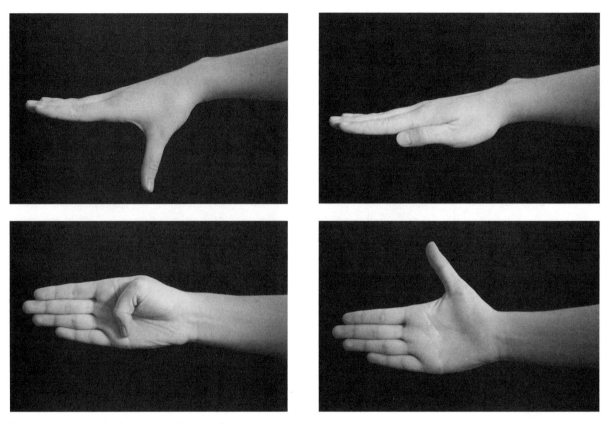

Figure 16–10 Thumb abduction, adduction, flexion, and extension.

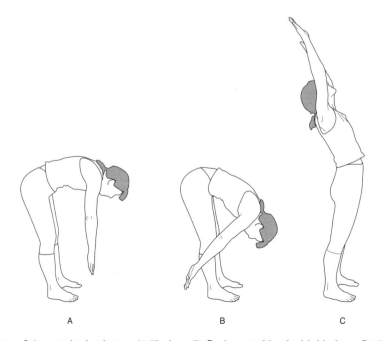

Figure 16–11 Movement of the vertebral column. (**A**) Flexion, (**B**) flexion combined with hip hyperflexion, and (**C**) extension.

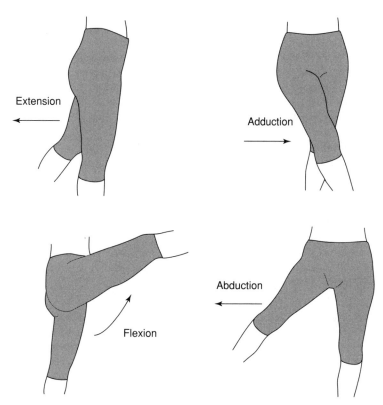

Figure 16–12 Muscle function and movement of the hip.

Hip and lower extremity movements are relatively straightforward. **Figure 16–12** shows *hip flexion*, *extension*, *abduction*, and *adduction*. Hip flexion and extension occur when the leg moves forward and backward in the sagittal plane. One flexes the leg, moving it forward to take a step, and then extends the leg backward to push off to move the leg forward. Abduction moves the leg out to the side, while adduction moves the leg in toward midline. *Internal rotation* rotates the foot/knee in toward midline, while *external rotation* rotates the foot/knee out away from midline. *Knee flexion* occurs when hamstrings shorten and the knee bends; *extension* occurs when the rectus femoris shortens and the leg straightens. *Plantar flexion* occurs when the toe is pointed. *Dorsiflexion* occurs when the toes are pointed toward the knee. *Inversion* and *eversion* of the foot are illustrated in **Figure 16–13**. The foot is rolled inward to invert and rolled outward to evert it.

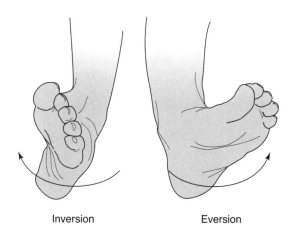

Inversion   Eversion

Figure 16–13 Inversion and eversion of the left foot.

REFERENCES

1. Lynn PA, Bettles ND, Hughes AD, Johnson SW. Influence of electrode geometry on bipolar recordings of the surface electromyogram. *Med Biol Eng Comput.* 1978;16:651–660.

2. Kendall FP, Kendall E, McCreary BA. *Muscles: Testing and Function.* 3rd ed. Baltimore, MD: Williams & Wilkins; 1983.

3. Travell J, Simons D. *Myofascial Pain and Dysfunction: A Trigger Point Manual, I and II.* Baltimore, MD: Williams & Wilkins; 1983.

4. Donaldson S, Skubick D, Donaldson M. *Electromyography, Trigger Points and Myofascial Syndromes.* Calgary, Alberta: Behavioral Health Consultants; 1991.

5. Donaldson S, Skubick D, Clasby B, Cram J. The evaluation of trigger-point activity using dynamic EMG techniques. *Am J Pain Manage.* 1994;4:118-122.

6. Gowitzke B, Milner M. *Scientific Basis of Human Movement.* 3rd ed. Baltimore, MD: Williams & Wilkins; 1988.

Electrode Placements

FRONTAL (WIDE) PLACEMENT

Type of Placement: General.

Purpose: General recording of facial muscle activity; favors upper face.

Clinical Uses: Psychophysiology, stress profiling, general relaxation.

Location: Electrodes are placed on the forehead, with the ground electrode in the center and the two active electrodes one-quarter inch above the eyebrow, directly above the iris of the eyes (**Figure 17–1A**).

Behavioral Test: Ask the patient to raise the eyebrows, frown, clench teeth, and swallow. All of these movements will be seen by this wide placement.

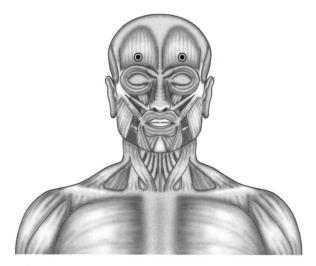

Figure 17–1A Electrode placement for the frontal site.
Source: Copyright © Clinical Resources, Inc.

Tracing Comment: In **Figure 17–1B**, the upper tracing shows surface electromyography (SEMG) from the wide frontal placement, while the lower tracing shows SEMG from the masseter muscle site. Following recording of the baseline, the patient is asked to raise the brow. Here, a clear separation between the frontal lead and the masseter may be seen. Next, the subject is asked to clench the teeth. Clenching of the jaw (masseteric activity) may be seen in frontal leads. This is an excellent example of volume conduction (processed: full-wave rectified recording).

Clinical Considerations: This site is considered a good barometer of general emotional state.[1,2] It is one of the original sites used in psychophysiological research,[3] particularly in assessing physiological responses to stress.[2] It is considered useful in the assessment of stress-related disorders such as anxiety, autonomic nervous system symptomology (e.g., asthma, irritable bowel syndrome), headache, and temporal mandibular joint dysfunction.[4,5] This site has been used extensively to study and treat headache.[6] Biofeedback from this site is commonly used as an adjunct to general relaxation training.

Volume Conduction: Primarily frontalis, temporalis, corrugator, nasalis, and masseter.

Other Sites of Interest: Temporal/mastoid, midcervical paraspinal, upper trapezius (wide), and forearm to assess and facilitate generalization.

Artifacts: Swallowing, talking.

Benchmark: Relaxed (N = 46): 2.5 µV (RMS) ($\pm$0.63). Stressful image (N = 46): 3.6 (V (RMS) ($\pm$0.78). Recorded using Autogen 1700 set at 100- to 200-Hz filter.[7]

TEMPORAL/MASTOID (WIDE) PLACEMENT

Type of Placement: General.

Purpose: General recordings from the cephalic musculature. Accesses facial, cervical, and temporal muscle sets. Four sets of recordings may be taken from these electrodes.

Clinical Uses: Headache, tinnitus, other cephalgia.

Location: Four electrodes are placed. An electrode is placed over the right and left anterior temporal muscles. Go lateral to the orbit of the eye, placing the electrodes approximately 3 cm above the zygomatic arch, just lateral to the eyebrow. The practitioner should palpate the muscle by placing the fingers in the temple area, just lateral to the eyebrow. Have the patient clench his or her teeth. The practitioner will feel the muscle bulge. Stay forward of the hairline. The other two electrodes are placed on the mastoid process, just below the hairline behind the ear (**Figures 17–2A** and **17–2B**).

As a variation to this placement, two electrodes can be placed at each of the four sites mentioned earlier. Two electrodes with a 2-cm spacing can be placed at the temporal sites so that one electrode is on the temporal location, and the second of the electrode pair is oriented obliquely toward the frontalis muscle. In addition, two electrodes with a 2-cm spacing can be placed at the

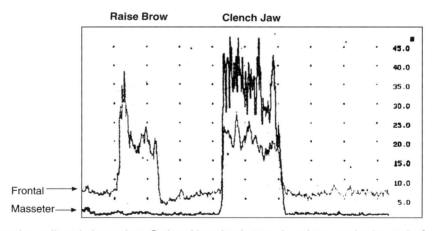

Figure 17–1B Frontal recordings during eyebrow flash and jaw clench. Note the volume conduction to the frontal leads during jaw clench.

Source: Copyright © Clinical Resources, Inc.

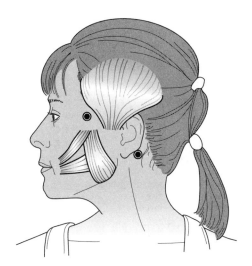

Figure 17–2A Electrode placement for the temporal/mastoid (wide) site. The temporal mastoid placements are shown from the side.

Source: Copyright © Clinical Resources, Inc.

mastoid site so that one of the electrode pairs is placed over the mastoid process, and the second pair is oriented obliquely toward the cervical paraspinals. In this way, four leads can be monitored simultaneously, as is depicted in the tracing in **Figure 17–2C**.

Behavioral Test: Raise brow, frown, clench teeth, cervical flexion, extension and rotation of the head, wiggle ears.

Tracing Comment: In Figure 17–2C, all four sets of recordings are shown simultaneously during eyebrow raise (F), head rotation (R), and ear wiggling (W). The top tracing is from the wide temporal leads, the second tracing is from the left temporal mastoid leads, the third tracing is from the right temporal mastoid leads, and the bottom tracing is from the wide mastoid leads. The mild asymmetry between the right and left temporal/mastoid recordings during ear wiggling is considered abnormal. To display all four recordings simultaneously may require a special cable or a variation of the electrode placement. These recordings were done using the variation of the electrode placement described previously. In addition, recording the frontal and cervical leads separately (i.e., at a later point in time) from right and left temporal/mastoid leads is acceptable (full-wave rectified recording).

Clinical Considerations: This placement was originally presented by Schwartz,[5] and was examined in the field by Hudzynski and Lawrence.[8] Its beauty lies in its ability to sample from the cephalic musculature, front and

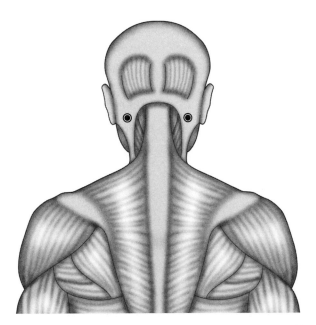

Figure 17–2B Electrode placement for the temporal/mastoid (wide) placement. The mastoid leads are shown from a posterior view.

Source: Copyright © Clinical Resources, Inc.

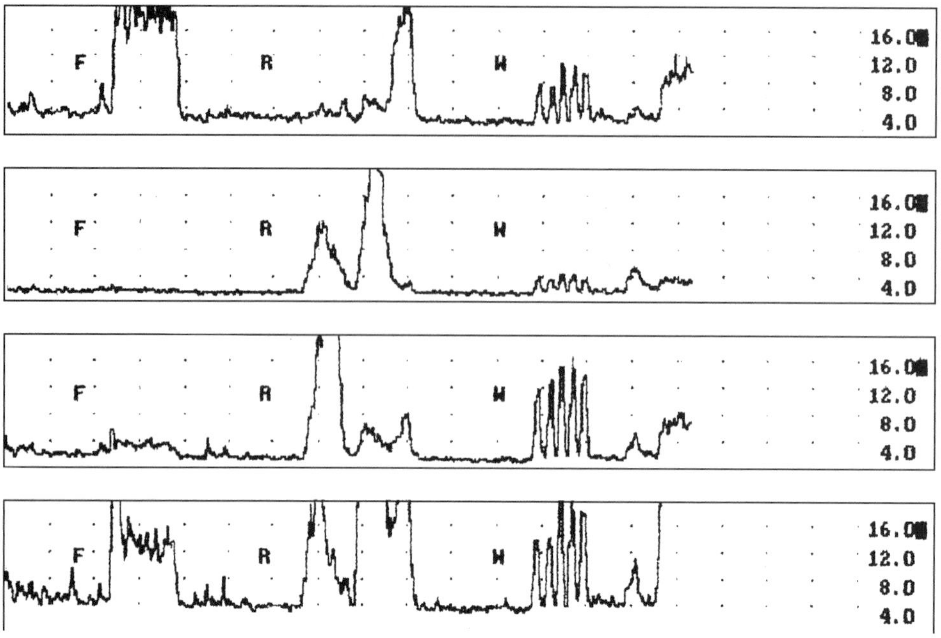

Figure 17–2C Surface EMG recordings using four leads from the temporal/mastoid electrodes. The top tracing is from the wide temporal leads, the second tracing is from the left temporalis/mastoid leads. The third tracing is from the right temporal/mastoid lead. The bottom tracing is from the wide mastoid leads. All four sets of recordings are shown simultaneously during (**F**) eyebrow raise, (**R**) head rotation, and (**W**) ear wiggling.

Source: Copyright © Clinical Resources, Inc.

back and both sides, rather than relying on a single indicator such as the wide frontal placement. A comparison of the facial versus cervical activity is accomplished by monitoring the widely spaced temporal electrodes with one set of leads, and with the widely spaced cervical electrodes using the second set of leads. As an alternative or in addition to the frontal–cervical comparisons, the right and left cephalic muscles may be monitored by simultaneously recording from the temporalis and mastoid leads on the right and left sides independently.

Volume Conduction: Frontalis-occipitalis, temporalis (anterior and posterior), corrugator, orbicularis oculi, masseter, capitis muscle groups, levator scapulae, sternocleidomastoid, and scalene.

Other Sites of Interest: Upper trapezius (wide), forearm extensor bundle (wide) to promote generalization.

Artifacts: Swallowing, breathing, talking.

Benchmark: Left frontal cervical placement (N = 25): 3:32 μV (RMS) (±1.22).

Right frontal cervical placement (N = 25): 3.09 μV (RMS) (±1.12).

Recorded during quiet sitting using J&J M-57 set at 100- to 200-Hz filter.[8]

TEMPORAL/MASSETER (WIDE) PLACEMENT

Type of Placement: General.

Purpose: General recording of mastication and facial muscles.

Clinical Uses: Temporomandibular joint (TMJ) dysfunction and other oral facial pain disorders.

Location: Right and left aspects are monitored separately. One electrode is placed on the anterior temporalis muscle, and a second electrode is placed on the masseter muscle. The anterior temporalis muscle is located in the temple region. Go lateral to the orbit of the eye, placing the electrodes approximately 3 cm above the zygomatic arch, just lateral to the eyebrow. Place fingers on the temple area and ask the patient to clench his or her teeth. Feel the muscle bulge and place electrode there. The masseter muscle group is located between the cheek bone and the corner of the jaw. Palpate the location by placing the fingers over that area; ask the patient to clench the teeth. Feel the muscle bulge. Place the electrode in the center of the muscle mass (**Figure 17–3A**).

Behavioral Test: Clench teeth, lateral excursion of the jaw, protraction and retraction of the jaw.

Tracing Comment: In **Figure 17–3B**, recordings are from the right and left aspects of the temporal/masseter site. A brief rest is followed by clenching the teeth together. Note the symmetry of recruitment. The next four movements entail left lateral excursion, right lateral excursion, retraction, and protraction of the jaw. Note the asymmetrical recruitment during the asymmetrical movements of right and left lateral excursion. Also note the symmetrical recruitment during the symmetrical movement of protraction and retraction (processed: full-wave rectified recording).

Clinical Considerations: This placement records from both the upper and lower face, providing a very global

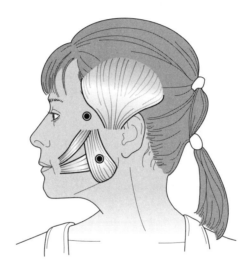

Figure 17–3A Electrode placement for the temporal/masseter (wide) site.
Source: Copyright © Clinical Resources, Inc.

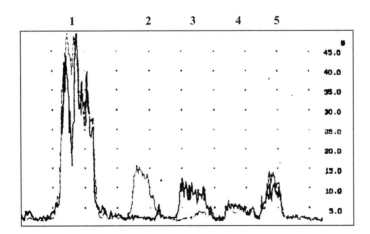

Figure 17–3B Surface EMG tracing for right and left temporal/masseter placement during (**1**) clench, lateral excursion of the jaw (**2**) to the left and then (**3**) to the right, followed by (**4**) protraction and (**5**) protrusion.
Source: Copyright © Clinical Resources, Inc.

view of functioning for the right and left aspects. Symmetry of electrode placement must be emphasized if one is concerned with asymmetrical patterns observed during movement. As a treatment site, it can provide the basis for a well-directed, general relaxation training protocol,[5] or it can be used for feedback for quiet movements of the jaw.[9]

Volume Conduction: Anterior and posterior temporalis, masseter, frontalis, corrugator, orbicularis oculi, orbicularis oris, buccinator, zygomaticus.

Other Sites of Interest: Temporal mylohyoid, midcervical paraspinal, upper trapezius (wide) to assess and promote generalization.

Artifacts: Swallowing, talking.

TEMPORAL/SUPRAHYOID (WIDE) PLACEMENT

Type of Placement: General.

Purpose: To monitor general facial and perioral muscle activity.

Clinical Uses: TMJ dysfunction, oral facial pain, and anxiety-related disorders.

Location: An active electrode is placed on the anterior temporalis. Palpate the muscle belly by placing the fingers lateral to the notch in the eye and asking the patient to clench his or her teeth. Go lateral to the orbit of the eye, placing the electrode approximately 3 cm above the zygomatic arch, just lateral to the eyebrow. To locate the area of the mylohyoid/digastric muscles, palpate the area by placing the fingers under the patient's chin and asking the patient to open the jaw wide several times. Place the electrode over the muscle mass that is felt toward the anterior lateral border of the underside of the chin (**Figure 17–4A**).

Behavioral Test: Ask the patient to move the jaw through its range of motion (open, close/clench, lateral, protrusion, retraction), frown, raise the brow, smile. Any facial movement should be seen.

Tracing Comment: **Figure 17–4B** presents SEMG recordings from the right and left temporal/suprahyoid placement during teeth clench, mouth opening, and left and right lateral deviations. Symmetry is noted during symmetrical movements and separation of function during lateral deviations (full-wave rectified recording).

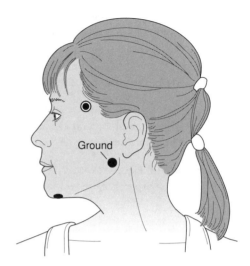

Figure 17–4A Electrode placement for the temporal suprahyoid (wide) site.

Source: Copyright © Clinical Resources, Inc.

Clinical Considerations: This placement was introduced by Schneider and Wilson,[10] and Hudzynski and Lawrence[8] elaborated on a clinical protocol for its use. It provides a very general neuromuscular assessment of the perioral muscles for stress-related and movement components. As a treatment site, it can provide the basis for a well-directed, general relaxation training protocol, or it may be used for feedback for quiet movements of the jaw.[9]

Volume Conduction: Frontalis, corrugator, anterior temporalis, orbicularis oculi, orbicularis oris, masseter, buccinator, mentalis, depressor, digastric, hyoid muscles, and tongue.

Other Sites of Interest: Midcervical paraspinals, upper trapezius (wide) to assess and promote generalization.

Artifacts: Swallowing, talking.

SUPRAHYOID PLACEMENT

Type of Placement: Quasi-specific.

Purpose: To record general muscle activity from the muscles that open the mouth, move the tongue, and elevate the larynx.

Clinical Uses: Dysphagia, TMJ dysfunction.

Muscle Insertions: The suprahyoid muscles (mylohyoids, digastrics, geniohyoids) originate on the mandible

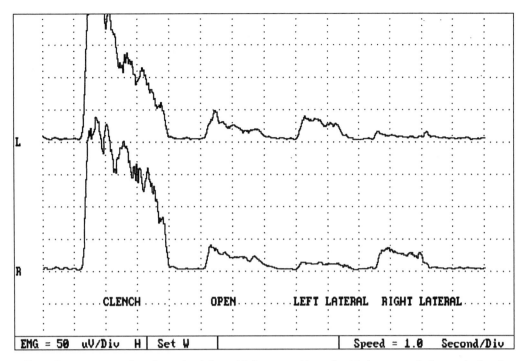

Figure 17–4B Surface EMG recordings from the right and left temporal/suprahyoid placement during teeth clench, mouth opening, and left and right lateral deviations.

Source: Copyright © Clinical Resources, Inc.

and insert on the hyoid bone. They primarily raise the hyoid bone in swallowing and/or opening the jaw.

Location: One set of electrodes is placed under the chin in the midline, running in the anterior-to-posterior di-

rection. Palpate the area by placing the fingers under the chin; ask the patient to swallow a few times. Place the electrodes in the center of that mass (**Figure 17–5A**).

Behavioral Test: Swallowing, jaw opening.

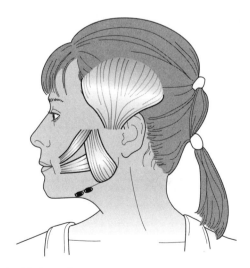

Figure 17–5A Placement of the suprahyoid electrode.

Source: Copyright © Clinical Resources, Inc.

Tracing Comment: **Figure 17–5B** presents SEMG recordings from the right and left aspects of the suprahyoid site during swallowing, protruding of the tongue, and speaking (saying the alphabet). The amplitudes and derecruitment patterns are typical for the site (processed SEMG).

Figure 17–5C presents SEMG recording from the temporalis and suprahyoid sites during teeth clench, mouth opening, and left and right lateral deviations. Symmetry is noted during the symmetrical movements (e.g., clench), and separation of function is noted during the lateral excursions. One can also see the role that the

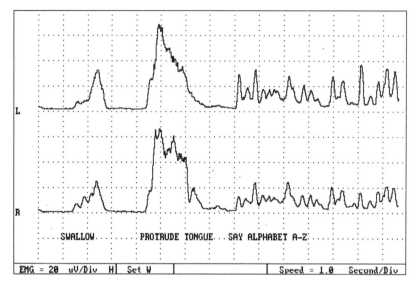

Figure 17–5B Surface EMG recordings from the right and left aspects of the suprahyoid site during swallowing, protruding of the tongue, and speaking (saying the alphabet).

Source: Copyright © Clinical Resources, Inc.

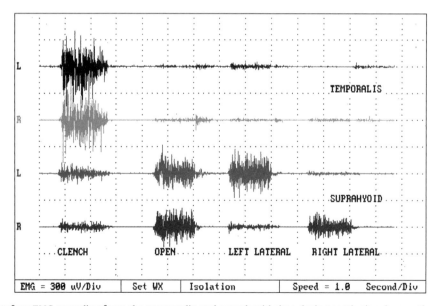

Figure 17–5C Surface EMG recording from the temporalis and suprahyoid sites during teeth clench, mouth opening, and left and right lateral deviations.

Source: Copyright © Clinical Resources, Inc.

temporalis plays in clenching and the suprahyoids play in mouth opening (raw SEMG).

Also see the tracings for the temporalis/suprahyoid site (Figure 17–4B).

Clinical Considerations: This site is useful in the treatment of dysphagia.[11,12] An emphasis is placed on shaping and training the correct muscle recruitment pattern during swallowing.

Volume Conduction: Platysma, sternocleidomastoid.

Other Sites of Interest: Masseter, buccinator, orbicularis oris during oral movements; temporal, midcervical paraspinal, upper trapezius (wide) to assess and treat generalized tension.

Artifacts: Talking.

CERVICAL TRAPEZIUS (WIDE) PLACEMENT

Type of Placement: General.

Purpose: To monitor general muscle activity from the upper back and neck, while assessing right- and left-side differences.

Clinical Uses: Headaches, shoulder pain, upper quarter pain, repetitive strain injury (RSI), tension myalgias.

Location: Two sets of electrodes are used: one for the right aspect and one for the left. For each side, one electrode is placed in the middle cervical area (approximately at C-4) and about 1 cm from midline over the muscle mass. Palpate to locate the muscle mass that parallels the spine. The second electrode is placed over the upper fibers of trapezius, along the ridge of the shoulder, approximately half the distance between the cervical vertebra at C-7 and the acromion. Palpate the muscle mass and place the electrode slightly lateral to that center point. See **Figure 17–6A**.

Behavioral Test: Shoulder elevation, retraction, protraction, cervical rotation, flexion, and lateral bending.

Tracing Comment: Figure 17–6B provides a view of SEMG recorded from the cervical trapezius sites using both a 25- to 1000-Hz band pass filter (wide), which shows the ECG artifact, and a 100- to 200-Hz filter (narrow). Notice how low and balanced the SEMG is for the 100- to 200-Hz filter setting. A noteworthy respiration artifact is present throughout. This is abnormal. When the 25- to 1000-Hz filter is used, the ECG artifact is quite striking on the left aspect for this subject. The respiration artifact continues to be clearly seen through the troughs of the recording. The amplitude attributed to the tracing would be determined by reading the value at

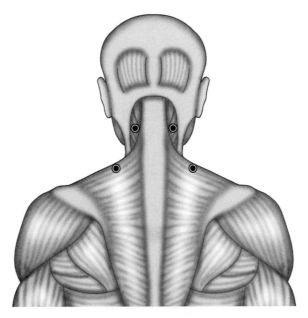

Figure 17–6A Electrode placement for the cervical trapezius (wide) site.
Source: Copyright © Clinical Resources, Inc.

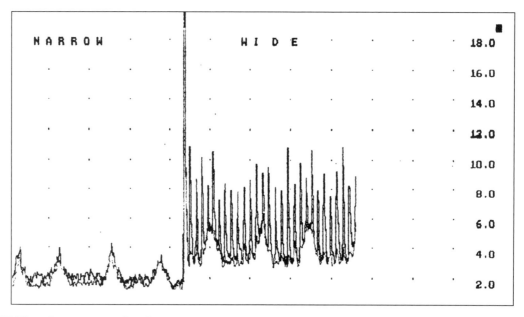

Figure 17-6B Surface EMG recordings from the cervical trapezius at rest. The right aspect of the tracing was conducted using a 25- to 1000-Hz band pass filter (wide) while the left aspect was conducted using a 100- to 200-Hz filter (narrow). Notice how the 100- to 200-Hz filter eliminates the ECG artifact, while the right aspect of the cervical trapezius leads shows a striking ECG artifact. Also note that the respiratory artifact is present in both types of filtering. This is considered abnormal.

Source: Copyright © Clinical Resources, Inc.

the trough of the tracing. Because of the marked ECG artifact, using an integrated SEMG value would provide an inaccurate estimate of the SEMG amplitude for the left aspect (full-wave rectified recording).

Figure 17–6C presents SEMG recordings from cervical trapezius placement using the 100- to 200-Hz filter during head rotation to the right and left, followed by a shoulder girdle elevation (full-wave rectified recording).

Figure 17–6D presents right and left recordings from the placement sites using the 100- to 200-Hz filter during quiet sitting, standing, walking in place, standing a second time, and returning to the sitting posture.[13] Notice how quiet the SEMG recordings are except during the movements associated with the transition from one posture to another and during walking in place (full-wave rectified recording).

Also see the tracings for cervical dorsal (Figures 17–18B and 17–18C) and dorsal lumbar (Figure 17–47B) placements for extensions of this wide placement strategy.

Clinical Considerations: Because this site monitors from the neck and upper back in general, it is particularly

useful for assessing general levels of tension (resting levels).[14] This site is useful in teaching and reinforcing general relaxation skills. In addition, it is particularly useful as an indicator of how these muscles are affected by posture. Ettare and Ettare[13] have developed extensive clinical protocols for the use of this site in training patients to return to healthy levels of rest following changes in posture or movement.

Volume Conduction: Upper, middle, and lower trapezius; capitis muscle groups; levator scapulae; rhomboid; and scalene.

Other Sites of Interest: Frontal (wide), temporalis (wide), forearm extensors (wide), wrist-to-wrist site to assess and promote generalization.

Artifacts: ECG, breathing.

Benchmark: Sitting quietly: 2.0 μV (RMS).
Standing, arms at sides: 2.0 μV (RMS).
Walking in place: 5.0 (±1.0) μV (RMS).
Values from Ettare and Ettare[13] using J&J M-501 with 100- to 200-Hz filter.

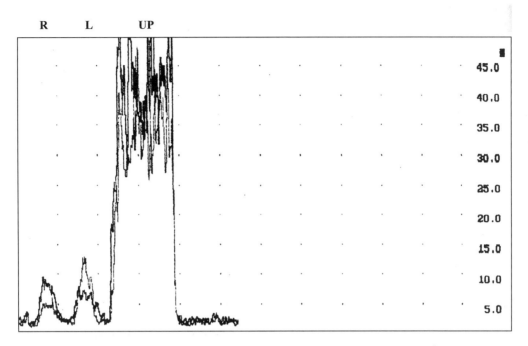

Figure 17-6C Surface EMG recordings from cervical trapezius placement using the 100- to 200-Hz filter during head rotation to the right and left, followed by a **(UP)** shoulder girdle elevation. There is separation of recruitment during rotation, and symmetry during elevation.

Source: Copyright © Clinical Resources, Inc.

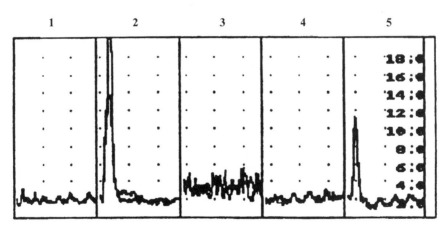

Figure 17-6D Surface EMG recording from the right and left cervical trapezius electrode placement during **(1)** sitting, **(2)** standing, **(3)** walking in place, **(4)** standing again, and **(5)** sitting.

Source: Copyright © Clinical Resources, Inc.

UPPER TRAPEZIUS (WIDE) PLACEMENT

Type of Placement: General.

Purpose: General recording of muscles of the upper back and neck.

Clinical Uses: Headache, neck, shoulder pain, upper quarter pain, tension myalgias.

Location: Electrodes are placed on the upper back, with the two active electrodes placed at the upper crest of the shoulder, halfway between the spine (C-7) and the acromion of the shoulder. Palpate the muscle at the crest and place the electrode over the area of largest mass (**Figure 17–7A**).

Behavioral Test: Ask the patient to raise the shoulders, rotate the head, and pull the shoulder blades together.

Tracing Comment: **Figure 17–7B** presents SEMG recordings from a wide upper trapezius placement during resting baseline, shoulder elevation (up), and retraction (back). The left aspect of the tracing, which was collected using a 25- to 1000-Hz band pass filter, shows the ECG artifact. The right side of the tracing used a 100- to 200-Hz band pass filter, which elimi-nated the ECG artifact. This may be seen during the rest periods between movements (full-wave rectified recording).

Clinical Considerations: This site is a good barometer of the shoulder elevation associated with an aroused emotional state.[3] It is useful in assessing and treating stress-related disorders, anxiety, asthma, hyperventilation syndromes, and headache.[5] It is also useful as part of an evaluation of neck and shoulder pain and RSI.[15]

Volume Conduction: Upper, middle, and lower trapezius; rhomboids; capitis muscle groups; levator scapulae; posterior deltoids.

Other Sites of Interest: Frontal (wide), temporal (wide), forearm extensors (wide), wrist-to-wrist site to assess and promote generalization.

Artifacts: ECG, breathing.

Benchmark: At rest (sitting quietly): 3.3 (±0.64) µV (RMS).
Stressful imagery: 3.8 (±0.37) µV (RMS).
Recorded using Autogen 1700 with 100- to 200-Hz filter.

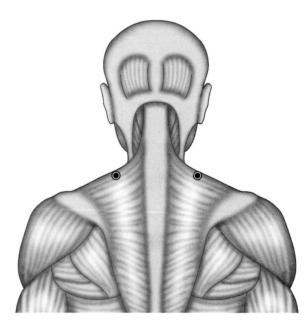

Figure 17–7A Electrode placement for the upper trapezius (wide) site.
Source: Copyright © Clinical Resources, Inc.

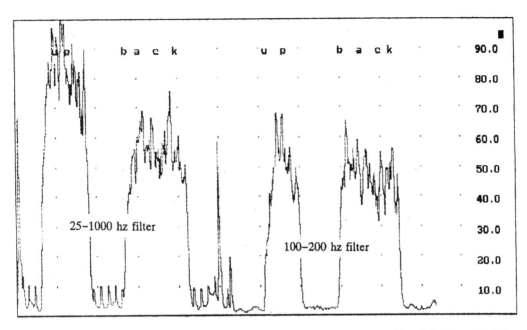

Figure 17–7B Surface recordings from upper trapezius leads using both a 25- to 1000-Hz filter (left side) and a 100- to 200-Hz filter (right side) during a shoulder elevation and retraction. Notice how the 100- to 200-Hz filter eliminates the ECG artifact during the resting baseline periods.

Source: Copyright © Clinical Resources, Inc.

ANTERIOR TEMPORALIS PLACEMENT

Type of Placement: Specific.

Action: Elevation of the mandible, retraction and lateral deviation of mandible, assistance in chewing.

Clinical Uses: TMJ dysfunction and related disorders.

Muscle Insertions: The anterior temporalis arises from the temporal fossa and inserts on the coronoid process of the mandible.

Innervation: Mandibular branch of the trigeminal nerve (fifth cranial nerve).

Location: To monitor the anterior portion of temporalis, palpate the temple region while the patient clenches his or her teeth. Two active electrodes, approximately 2 cm apart, are placed over the muscle mass so that they run parallel to the muscle fibers. The lowest electrode of the pair is placed just above the zygomatic arch or opposite the notch of the eye (**Figure 17–8A**).

Variations: The temporalis muscle also has posterior fibers, which are more consistently involved in retraction (retrusion) and lateral deviation of the mandible.[4,16] This placement is located on the lateral aspect of the head, behind the ear. Electrodes are placed on the bare skin, behind the flap of the ear.

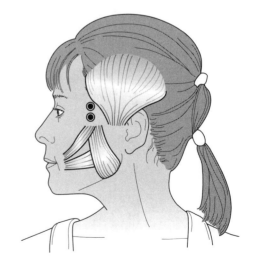

Figure 17–8A Electrode placement for the anterior temporalis site.

Source: Copyright © Clinical Resources, Inc.

Behavioral Test: Clenching of the jaw, lateral deviation of the jaw, protraction and retraction of the jaw, swallowing.

Tracing Comment: In **Figure 17–8B**, tracings of the temporalis (top two tracings) and the masseter (bottom two tracings) show synergistic functions during jaw clenching and chewing (raw SEMG).

Clinical Considerations: With normal dentition, gentle closure of the jaw is primarily associated with the anterior fibers of the temporalis.[4] The temporalis muscle is responsible for keeping the mandible in the rest position while in the upright posture.[16] The patient may need to separate the teeth and intentionally relax the jaw musculature before quiet levels of recording are seen at this site with surface electrodes. Placing the tip of the tongue on the roof of the mouth just behind the front teeth can help quiet the perioral musculature. In addition, with patients who cannot intentionally relax the muscles at this site in the upright posture, the practitioner can attempt to do the procedure with the patient supine. Any training in the supine posture would then need to be generalized to the upright posture.

Volume Conduction: Posterior temporalis, frontalis, corrugator, orbicularis oculi, masseter.

Other Sites of Interest: Masseter, posterior temporalis, suprahyoid sites to assess other potential muscles associated with movement; midcervical to assess the effects that chewing has on neck muscles.

Referred Pain Considerations: Trigger points may refer pain to the temporal region, the eyebrow, and the upper teeth.[17]

Artifacts: Swallowing, talking.

Benchmark: Sitting quietly (N = 104): 2.4 (±2.1) µV (RMS).
Standing quietly (N = 104): 2.3 (±2.1) µV (RMS).
Values taken using a J&J M-501 EMG set with a 100- to 200-Hz filter.[18]

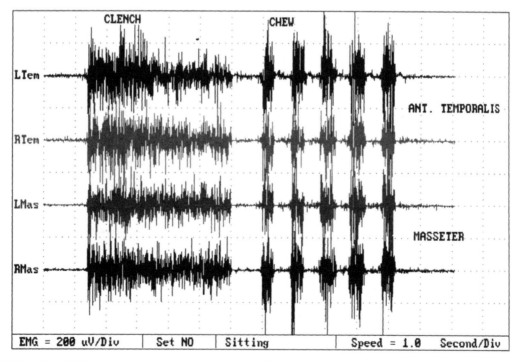

Figure 17–8B Surface EMG recordings from the anterior temporalis and the masseter during a clench and chewing.
Source: Copyright © Clinical Resources, Inc.

MASSETER PLACEMENT

Type of Placement: Specific.

Action: Elevation of the mandible; closure/grinding of jaw; mastication.

Clinical Uses: TMJ dysfunction and oral–facial disorders.

Muscle Insertions: The masseter muscle arises from the zygomatic arch (cheek bone) and inserts on the superior half of the lateral surface of the ramus of the mandible (corner of the jaw).

Innervation: The masseter is innervated by the masseteric aspect of the trigeminal nerve (fifth cranial nerve).

Location: Two active electrodes, approximately 2 cm apart, are placed along the direction of the fibers of the masseter muscle. Palpate the area while asking the patient to clench his or her teeth. Identify the muscle belly. Electrodes are placed over the belly of the muscle. If symmetry of SEMG recording is an issue, the practitioner should be aware that slight differences in electrode placement and spacing may radically alter the SEMG recordings and conclusions regarding symmetry (**Figure 17–9**). Note that a forward head position may affect the resting value of the recordings.

Behavioral Test: Clench teeth, swallow, talk.

Tracing Comment: In Figure 17–8B, the temporalis (top two tracings) and the masseter (bottom two tracings) show synergistic functions during jaw clenching and chewing (raw SEMG).

Clinical Considerations: Generally, the masseter and the temporalis are synergists and function concurrently. While the temporalis provides a basis for mandibular balance and postural control, the masseter is used during grinding and chewing.[19] During chewing, the masseter responds before the temporalis. The masseter, unlike the temporalis, is not thought to be required to maintain the resting position of the mandible,[16] and it does not change its tonic levels as a person moves from the sitting posture to the supine posture.

Volume Conduction: Lateral pterygoid, buccinator, zygomaticus.

Other Sites of Interest: Temporalis and suprahyoids to assess other potential muscles involved in movement of the mandible; midcervical paraspinals to assess for chewing in the neck.

Referred Pain Considerations: Trigger points in the superficial layer of masseter may be projected to the eyebrow, maxilla, mandible, and upper or lower molar teeth.[17]

Artifacts: Swallowing, talking.

Benchmark: Sitting quietly ($N = 104$): 1.7 (± 1.3) μV (RMS).
Standing quietly ($N = 104$): 1.6 (± 1.5) μV (RMS).
Values taken using a J&J M-501 with a 100- to 200-Hz filter.[18]

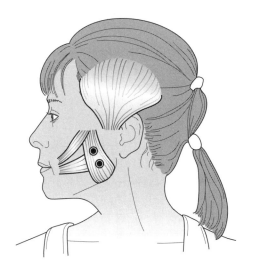

Figure 17–9 Electrode placement for the masseter site.
Source: Copyright © Clinical Resources, Inc.

CHEEK (ZYGOMATICUS) PLACEMENT

Type of Placement: Quasi-specific.

Action: Retraction and elevation of the lips, smiling.

Clinical Uses: Psychophysiological studies, rehabilitation of facial muscles.

Muscle Insertions: The zygomaticus arises from the zygomatic bone. The major aspect inserts on the corner of the mouth, while the minor aspect inserts on the upper portion of the lip.

Innervation: Facial nerve (seventh cranial nerve).

Location: Two active electrodes are placed so that they run parallel to the muscle fibers (cheek bone to corner of the mouth) and are placed at the midpoint (**Figure 17–10A**). A gross recording was obtained by using 1-cm

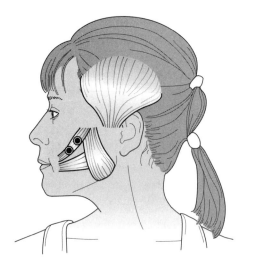

Figure 17–10A Electrode placement for the zygomaticus site.

Source: Copyright © Clinical Resources, Inc.

electrodes placed 2 cm apart (**Figure 17–10B**). Recordings using 1-cm spacings did not improve the specificity of the recording dramatically (see also Figure 17–12B).

Behavioral Test: Smile.

Tracing Comment: In Figure 17–10B, recordings with electrodes with 2-cm spacing are taken from the orbicularis oculi, zygomaticus, and buccinator during a smile. Note the continual activation of the orbicularis oculi throughout the tracing, indicating that the patient tends to squint, with an increased level during the smile itself. During the intentional smile, a very strong synergistic pattern occurs between zygomaticus and orbicularis oculi and buccinator. Note that a slightly different smiling expression could potentially bring out a different synergistic pattern. In addition, the smaller and more closely spaced electrodes seen in Figures 17–11B and 17–12B suggest that one cannot easily isolate the SEMG activity for zygomaticus, even with a more specific electrode placement (raw SEMG).

Clinical Considerations: The primary use of this site is in psychophysiological studies.[20] It has recently found its way into clinical use during anesthesia procedures.[21]

Volume Conduction: Masseter, buccinator, orbicularis oculi, and orbicularis oris.

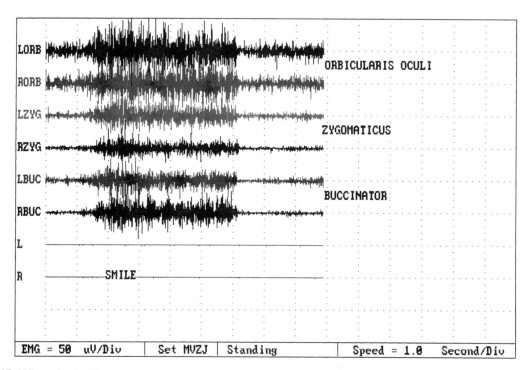

Figure 17–10B Surface EMG recordings from the orbicularis oculi, zygomaticus, and buccinator using 1-cm electrodes 2 cm apart. The action is smiling.

Source: Copyright © Clinical Resources, Inc.

Other Sites of Interest: Orbicularis oculi, corrugator, frontal, and depressor anguli oris to study facial expressions.

Referred Pain Considerations: Trigger points in the zygomaticus major refer pain in an arch close to the side of the nose and reaching the forehead.[17]

Artifacts: Swallowing, talking.

ORBICULARIS OCULI PLACEMENT

Type of Placement: Specific.

Action: Eye closure and squinting.

Clinical Uses: Psychophysiological studies of emotions.

Muscle Insertions: The orbital portion of this muscle wraps broadly around the orbit of the eye.

Innervation: Facial nerve (seventh cranial nerve).

Location: This muscle is most easily monitored by placing two closely spaced electrodes horizontally on the zygomatic bone just below the lower eyelid and toward the lateral aspect of the eye (**Figure 17–11A**). As can be seen in **Figure 17–11B**, the best recordings are obtained using miniature electrodes placed 1 cm apart. A grosser recording may be obtained by using 1-cm electrodes placed 2 cm apart (see **Figure 17–12C**). Compare the tracings seen in Figure 17–12C with those seen in Figure 17–11B.

Behavioral Test: Squint.

Tracing Comment: Figure 17–11B presents SEMG recordings from the zygomaticus and the orbicularis oculi during smiling and squinting. In this individual, both muscles are active during smiling, but only the orbicularis oculi is active during squinting. Compared to Figure 17–12C, there is a slight improvement with narrowly spaced electrodes and the specificity of the SEMG recording (raw SEMG). See also the tracings for the zygomaticus (Figure 17–10B) and the buccinator (Figure 17–12C).

Clinical Considerations: The primary use of this site is in psychophysiological studies.[20] It has recently found its way into clinical use during anesthesia procedures.[21]

Volume Conduction: Masseter, temporalis, zygomaticus, corrugator.

Other Sites of Interest: Corrugator, frontal, and zygomaticus to study emotional displays.

Artifacts: Eye blinking, swallowing, talking.

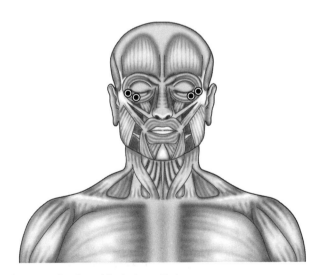

Figure 17–11A Surface EMG placement for the orbicularis oculi site.
Source: Copyright © Clinical Resources, Inc.

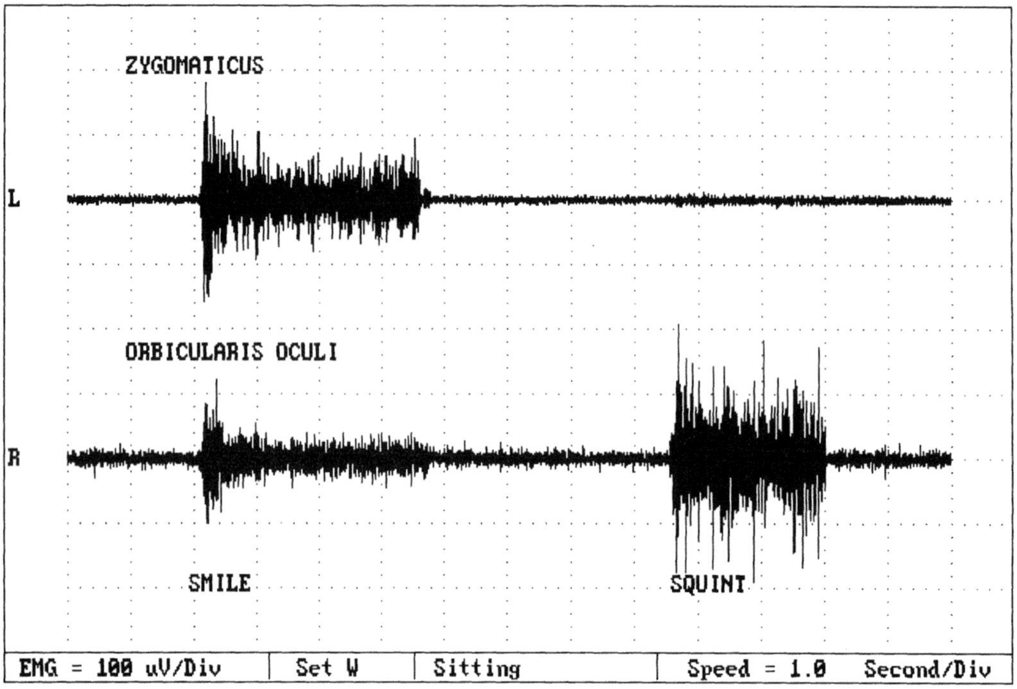

Figure 17–11B Surface EMG recordings from the zygomaticus and the orbicularis oculi during smiling and squinting using miniature electrodes and 1-cm spacing.

Source: Copyright © Clinical Resources, Inc.

BUCCINATOR PLACEMENT

Type of Placement: Specific.

Action: Retraction of cheek toward mandible; assists in chewing.

Clinical Uses: Bell's palsy, dysphagia.

Muscle Insertions: The buccinator arises from the mandible in the region of the first and second molars and extends to the corner of the mouth, blending with the orbicularis oris.

Innervation: Facial nerve (seventh cranial nerve).

Location: Two active electrodes are placed parallel to the muscle fibers. One electrode is placed just lateral to the corner of the mouth, with the second one just lateral to it (**Figure 17–12A**). As can be seen in a comparison of **Figure 17–12B** with **Figure 17–12C**, the best recordings are obtained using miniature electrodes placed 1 cm apart. A grosser recording may be obtained by using 1-cm electrodes placed 2 cm apart.

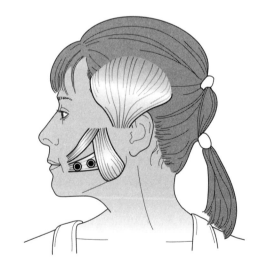

Figure 17–12A Electrode placement for the buccinator site.

Source: Copyright © Clinical Resources, Inc.

Behavioral Test: Press the cheeks against the sides of the teeth and pull the corners of the lips back as if to play a trumpet (buccinating).

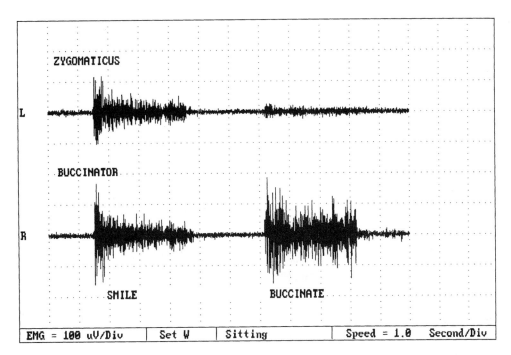

Figure 17–12B Surface EMG recordings from the zygomaticus and the buccinator using miniature electrodes and 1-cm spacing. The actions are smiling and buccinating.

Source: Copyright © Clinical Resources, Inc.

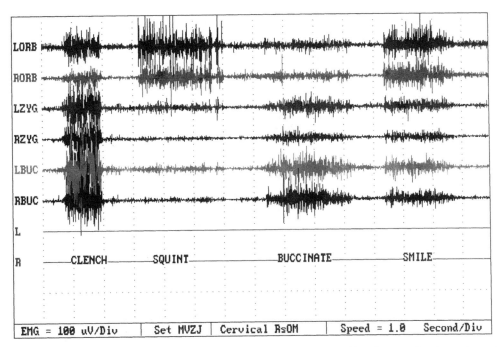

Figure 17–12C Surface EMG recordings from the orbicularis oculi, zygomaticus, and buccinator using 1-cm electrodes at 2-cm spacings. The actions are clenching, squinting, buccinating, and smiling.

Source: Copyright © Clinical Resources, Inc.

Tracing Comment: Two tracings are shown with different levels of specificity. Figure 17–12B shows the zygomaticus and buccinator using miniature electrodes set 1 cm apart, while Figure 17–12C shows the zygomaticus, orbicularis oculi, and buccinator using larger and more widely spaced electrodes.

In Figure 17–12B, the buccinator recordings are clearly differentiated from the zygomaticus recordings during buccinating but not during smiling (raw SEMG).

Figure 17–12C shows recordings from the orbicularis oculi, zygomaticus, and buccinator during clenching, squinting, retracting the lips as if to play the trumpet (buccinating), and smiling. Note the volume conduction that appears on all channels during a jaw clench. The closer to the SEMG source, the larger the volume conduction.

During the retraction of the lips, a strong burst of SEMG may be seen at the buccinator site. Collateral activity is also noted in the zygomaticus (raw SEMG).

Clinical Considerations: This site may be useful in retraining the lips and cheek in patients with dysphagia and Bell's palsy.

Volume Conduction: Masseter, orbicularis oris, risorius, zygomaticus, depressor.

Other Sites of Interest: Zygomaticus, depressor, orbicularis oris, and mentalis to study other muscles associated with lip and cheek movement.

Artifacts: Swallowing, talking.

FRONTALIS (NARROW) PLACEMENT

Type of Placement: Specific.

Action: Elevates the brow.

Clinical Uses: Psychophysiological recordings of emotions (surprise, anger, sadness, fear).

Muscle Insertions: This muscle arises from the skin and subcutaneous tissue at the eyebrow and extends up over the crown of the head, joining the fibers of the occipitalis muscle.

Innervation: Facial nerve (seventh cranial nerve).

Location: Two active electrodes (2 cm apart) are placed vertically, half the distance between the eyebrow and the hairline, just lateral of midline and parallel to the muscle fibers of interest (**Figure 17–13A**). As can be seen in Figure 17–14B, the best recordings are obtained using miniature electrodes placed 1 cm apart. A grosser recording (see **Figure 17–13B**) may be obtained by using 1-cm electrodes placed 2 cm apart.

> *Variations:* Due to the high innervation ratio of this muscle, the degree of lateral placement from midline may allow the practitioner to record different aspects of emotional displays.[22]

Behavioral Test: Raise the brow as if in surprise.

Tracing Comment: Figure 17–13B shows recordings from two sets of electrodes, 2 cm apart, which have

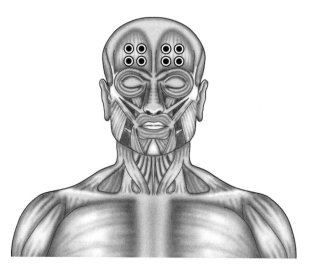

Figure 17–13A Electrode placement for the frontalis (narrow) site. These electrodes are placed vertically so as to follow the direction of the muscle fibers.

Source: Copyright © Clinical Resources, Inc.

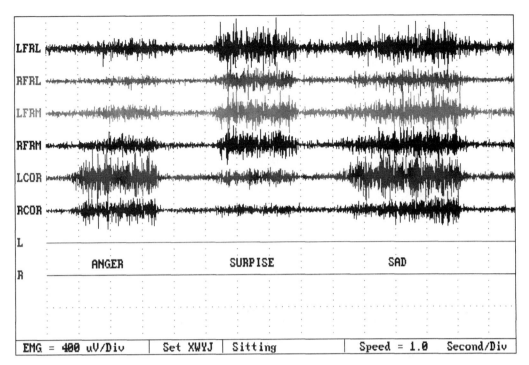

Figure 17–13B Surface EMG recordings using electrodes 2 cm apart placed on the (FRL) lateral and (FRM) medial frontalis, along with the (COR) corrugator. The subject is asked to display anger, surprise, and sadness.

Source: Copyright © Clinical Resources, Inc.

been placed over the frontalis. The most lateral electrodes were placed above the iris of the eye, and the medial electrodes were placed just lateral of midline. In addition, the corrugator is monitored. Three emotional displays are studied: anger, surprise, and sadness. Note that the frontalis muscle is active during surprise and sadness, but only minimally active during anger. During sadness, there is a strong synergy pattern noted with the corrugator. The practitioner should note that slight variations in the emotional expression could result in slightly different synergistic patterns. The specificity of the recordings is improved slightly with more narrowly spaced electrodes (see Figure 17–14B).

Clinical Considerations: Systematic study of the right and left aspects of the frontalis muscle may yield information concerning the emotionality of an individual. Sackeim and his colleagues[23] found that the left aspect of the frontalis is more active during emotional events. In addition, this site has recently been used by Bennett and Kornhauser[21] as part of an algorithm for assessing nociception and consciousness during anesthesia.

Volume Conduction: Corrugator, temporalis, and masseter.

Other Sites of Interest: Corrugator, orbicularis oculi, zygomaticus, depressor to study emotional displays; midcervical, upper trapezius, forearm extensor bundle (wide) to assess for general tension levels.

Referred Pain Considerations: Trigger points in the belly of the frontalis muscle project pain diffusely over the local muscle belly.[17]

Artifacts: Swallowing, nonverbal communication.

CORRUGATOR PLACEMENT

Type of Placement: Specific.

Action: Frowning at the brow.

Clinical Uses: Psychophysiological studies of emotional displays.

Muscle Insertions: This small muscle arises from the superciliary arch of the frontal bone (just above the nose) and inserts on the skin of the middle third of the supraorbital margin, at the eyebrow.

Innervation: Facial nerve (seventh cranial nerve).

Location: Two active electrodes are placed over the eyebrow, just lateral of midline and at a slightly oblique angle (**Figure 17–14A**). As can be seen in **Figure 17–14B**, the best recordings are obtained using miniature electrodes placed 1 cm apart. Compare this to Figure 17–13B, in which a grosser recording is obtained by using 1-cm electrodes placed 2 cm apart.

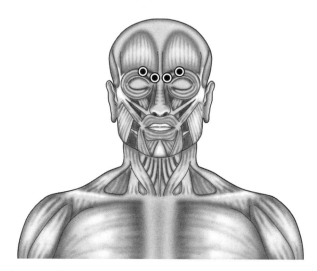

Figure 17–14A Surface EMG placement for the corrugator site.

Source: Copyright © Clinical Resources, Inc.

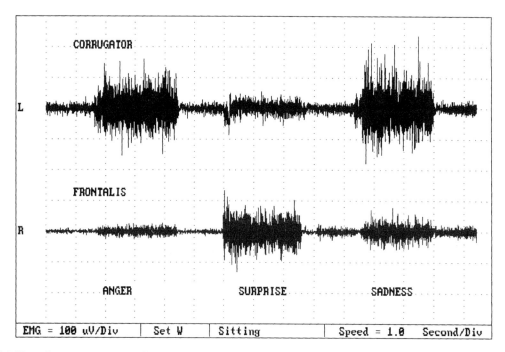

Figure 17–14B Surface EMG recordings from miniature electrodes, 1 cm apart, placed on the (medial) frontalis and corrugator muscles. The actions are anger, surprise, and sadness.

Source: Copyright © Clinical Resources, Inc.

Behavioral Test: Furrow the brow, frown.

Tracing Comment: Figure 17–14B presents SEMG recordings using 1-cm spacings from the corrugator and (medial) frontalis during the three facial expressions of anger, surprise, and sadness. The corrugator is more active during anger and sadness than surprise, while the frontalis is most active during surprise and modestly active during sadness. Both corrugator and frontalis are active during expressions of sadness. By comparing Figure 17–13B with Figure 17–14B, one can note that the more narrowly spaced electrodes (Figure 17–14B) provide a cleaner recording and separation of muscle function. Slight changes in any of the emotional expressions can result in changes in the synergistic patterns (raw SEMG).

Clinical Considerations: The corrugator is responsible for the furrowing of the brow, as in the display of anger. In addition, this site has recently been used by Bennett and Kornhauser[21] as part of an algorithm for assessing nocioception and consciousness during anesthesia.

Volume Conduction: Procerus, frontalis, orbicularis oculi.

Other Sites of Interest: Frontalis, orbicularis oculi, zygomaticus, depressor to study emotional displays; masseter, temporalis, midcervical, and upper trapezius to assess generalized tension.

Artifacts: Eye blink, nonverbal communication.

STERNOCLEIDOMASTOID (SCM) PLACEMENT

(Also known as sternomastoid.)

Type of Placement: Specific.

Action: Rotation of the head to the contralateral side, ipsilateral side bending, and forward flexion.

Clinical Uses: Neck and shoulder pain and headache.

Muscle Insertions: This two-bellied muscle arises by one head from the sternum and the other head from the clavicle. It inserts on the mastoid process.

Innervation: The accessory nerve; via the cervical plexus, the ventral rami of the C-2 and C-3 spinal nerves.

Joint Considerations: The SCM is attached to the anterior and superior surfaces of the sternum, and the superior border of the proximal third of the clavicle. The upper attachments include the mastoid process of the temporal bone and the lateral portion of the superior nuchal line of the occipital bone. Thus, the joints directly related to the muscle length include the S-C joint, the cervical joints as a group, and the O/A joint in particular.

Location: Palpate the large muscle belly on the anterior lateral aspect of the neck. Two active electrodes (2 cm apart) are placed half the distance between the mastoid process and the sternal notch, slightly posterior to the center of the muscle belly so that they run parallel to the muscle fibers. If the practitioner asks the patient to rotate the head to identify the muscle belly, electrodes should be placed once the patient has returned to the midline position (**Figure 17–15A**).

Behavioral Test: Rotate, side bend, or flex the head.

Tracing Comment: In **Figures 17–15B** and **17–15D**, the SCM, scalene, and C-4 paraspinals are monitored; in **Figure 17–15C**, the upper trapezius (narrow) placement has been added.

In Figure 17–15B, a comfortable, self-limited axial rotational pattern is studied. Note the cooperative functions between SCM and C-4 paraspinal during rotation. The left SCM is activated first to provide movement during right rotation; the right C-4 paraspinal is activated a little later. The opposite is true for left rotation. Also note how quiet the scalene muscles are during this

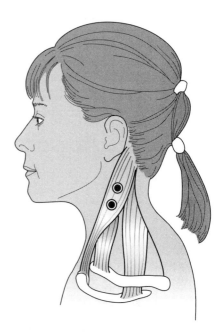

Figure 17–15A Electrode placement for the SCM site.

Source: Copyright © Clinical Resources, Inc.

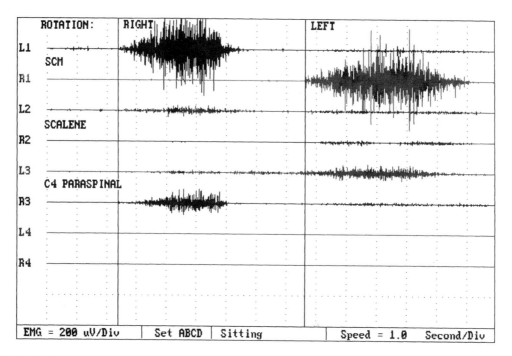

Figure 17–15B Surface EMG tracings during head rotation for the SCM, midcervical (C-4) paraspinals, and scalene muscles.

Source: Copyright © Clinical Resources, Inc.

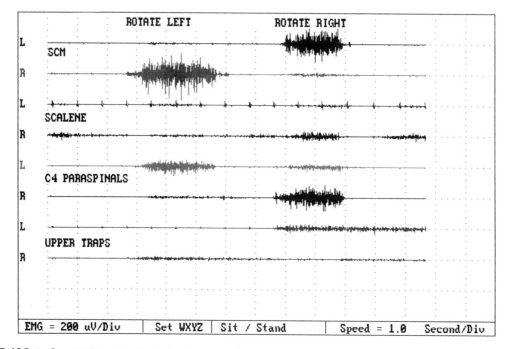

Figure 17–15C Surface EMG tracings during head rotation for the SCM, scalene, midcervical (C-4) paraspinals, and upper trapezius.

Source: Copyright © Clinical Resources, Inc.

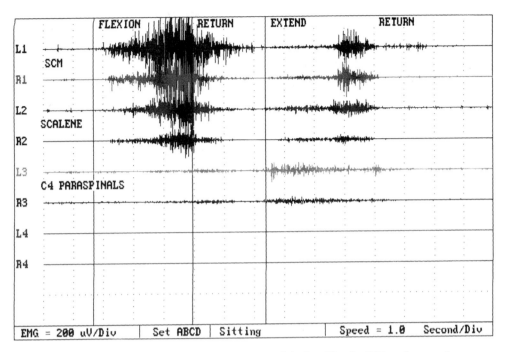

Figure 17–15D Surface EMG tracings during flexion and extension of the head for the SCM, scalene, and midcervical paraspinals.

Source: Copyright © Clinical Resources, Inc.

movement, showing good isolation of the SEMG recordings for these sites in this individual (raw SEMG).

In Figure 17–15C, rotational patterns are studied again, but this time with the inclusion of the upper trapezius muscle. This tracing is similar to Figure 17–15B, in that the scalene remains relatively quiet (as does the upper trapezius). If the end range of motion is pushed a little bit, there will be an increase in the activity of trapezius. This may be seen in Figure 17–17B (raw SEMG).

In Figure 17–15D, flexion of the head at the uppermost cervical segment is followed by a return to midline. This is then followed by extension and return back to midline. Note how the SCM and the scalene work synergistically during flexion. The recruitment of the left SCM during the return to midline is mildly abnormal. The C-4 paraspinal site shows minimal recruitment during the return to midline compared to extension of the head back over the shoulders. Here, a mild symmetry is also noted. Note how the scalene site shows activity during this movement, while it did not during rotation (see Figure 17–15B). Examination of these two movement patterns allows for an assessment for synergistic movement patterns versus cross-talk. In this case, it ap-

pears that the scalene muscle participates in flexion but not rotation. The practitioner should note that the pattern of recruitment is radically altered when the flexion is conducted at the lowest possible cervical segment. The SCM muscle group would be less active, while the C-4 paraspinal site would be more active (raw SEMG).

Also note the tracings for the scalene (Figure 17–16B) and midcervical paraspinals (Figure 17–17B).

Clinical Considerations: Bilateral contraction of the SCM results in flexion of the lower cervical spine and extension of the upper cervical spine.[24] Limitations in the ability of the upper cervical spine to flex will affect the ability of the lower cervical spine to extend. The converse is true for the impact of restricted extension in the lower cervical spine on the ability of the upper cervical spine to flex. Passive insufficiency (restricted excursion due to contracture or contraction) of the SCM can account for limited upper cervical spine flexion.[23]

The SCM muscles are phasic muscles that should show distinct patterns of activity associated with discrete motion. Their total amplitude is affected by the range of motion and the degree of excursion the muscle experiences in its motion. Postural forward head position is endemic to our sedentary society. Concomitant with this posture is the tendency for the SCM to shorten, thereby altering the normal amount of excursion the muscle experiences in rotation and flexion/extension. Any additional increase in the gamma gain of a given SCM could have a significant effect on the physiologically paired muscles, including the sternalis, scalene, cervical paraspinal, upper trapezius, deep cervical flexors, clavicular portion of pectoralis, and platysma. Forward head posture with dysfunctional overlay in the SCM can be responsible for inhibited lower trapezius, cervical paraspinals, and other postural/functional problems.

The upper cervical spine has a unique morphology that allows for postural adaptations that return the eyes to the horizontal, regardless of the position of the neck and torso, via the righting reflex. Joint/muscle dysfunctions that limit the ability of the upper cervical spine to perform this function (e.g., an O/A joint stuck in relative extension, causing side flexion left and rotation right) should be compensated at C-1 or C-2, preferably, or in the upper thoracic spine and/or lower cervical spine. This will tend to shorten the ipsilateral SCM and lengthen the contralateral SCM. Because the SCM is an accessory respiratory muscle, visceral and mechanical restrictions to respiration may cause increased SCM activity with inspiration. In craniomandibular dysfunctions, increased SCM activity can be related to a dysfunctional resting posture of the tongue[25] or cranial faults.[26]

Volume Conduction: Upper fibers of the trapezius, scalene, cervicis, and capitis groups.

Other Sites of Interest: Ipsilateral cervical paraspinals and upper trapezius during lateral bending and rotation, as well as scalene during deep inspiration.

Referred Pain Considerations: Trigger points in the sternal division of the SCM refer pain to the vertex, to the occiput, across the cheek, and over the eye. Trigger points in the clavicular division commonly refer pain to the frontal region (frontal headaches) or the ear (earaches).[17]

Artifacts: ECG (this is augmented if electrodes are placed too far to the front).

Benchmark: Sitting quietly at midline ($N = 104$): 1.3 (± 1.5) μV (RMS).
Values taken using a J&J M-501 with a 100- to 200-Hz filter.[18]

SCALENE (ANTERIOR) PLACEMENT

Type of Placement: Specific.

Action: Lateral cervical flexor and stabilizer; assists in forward flexion; may play a role as an accessory muscle of respiration.

Clinical Uses: Headache, repetitive strain injury.

Muscle Insertions: The anterior scalene arises from the anterior tubercle of the C-3, C-4, and C-5 vertebrae and inserts on the scalene tubercle of the first rib.

Innervation: The motor branch of the spinal nerves C-2 to C-7, depending on the location of attachment.

Location: Palpate the SCM just lateral and above its attachment to the clavicle. Move posteriorly toward the outer superior edge of upper trapezius. Find the hollow triangle that lies just posterior to the SCM, just above the clavicle and anterior to the upper trapezius. Isolation of the scalene is better when the electrodes are placed in the hollow by the clavicle than when they are placed higher up on the neck. Two active electrodes (2 cm apart) are placed on a slightly oblique angle just above the clavicle in the hollow triangle, so that they run parallel to the muscle fibers (**Figure 17–16A**).

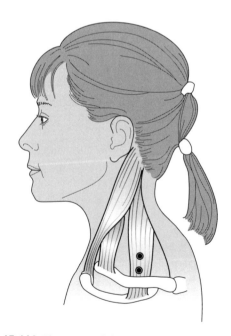

Figure 17–16A Placement of electrodes for the scalene site.
Source: Copyright © Clinical Resources, Inc.

Behavioral Test: Side bending of the neck, deep inspiration.

Tracing Comment: In **Figure 17–16B**, the SCM, midcervical paraspinals at C-4, scalene, and upper trapezius are monitored during a deep inspiration. Three of the four muscle groups participate in this movement. Note the ECG artifact on the LSCA and LUTR sites (raw SEMG).

In **Figure 17–16C**, the SCM, scalene, C-4, paraspinals, and upper trapezius are monitored during lateral bending. The sternocleidomastoid and scalene are active, while the C-4 paraspinals and upper trapezius (narrow) are relatively quiet.

Figure 17–16D illustrates a synergy pattern between the scalene and the serratus anterior. During the first movement for flexion of the arms, the serratus anterior is activated while scalene remains relatively quiet. During the second movement of a sitting push-up, a clear synergy pattern between the serratus anterior and the scalene is noted because the scalene group is being placed on stretch due to torsion on the rib cage by the serratus anterior (raw SEMG).

Also note the tracings for the SCM (Figure 17–15D) and the midcervical paraspinals (Figure 17–17B).

Clinical Considerations: The scalene muscles should be studied during deep inspiration as well as during movement. The scalene is seen as an ancillary muscle of respiration by some,[27] and a primary muscle of respiration by others.[28] A nice, symmetrical recruitment pattern should be observed or cultivated during treatment.

Volume Conduction: SCM, upper fibers of trapezius, and omohyoid.

Other Sites of Interest: SCM during elevation of the chest and flexion of the head; upper trapezius during elevation of the shoulder; serratus anterior in resisted flexion of the arm.

Referred Pain Considerations: Trigger points in all three aspects of the scalene muscles can radiate pain into the pectoral region, laterally down to the front and back of the arm or into the thumb and index finger, and posteriorly to the upper vertebral border of the scapula.[17]

Artifacts: ECG, breathing.

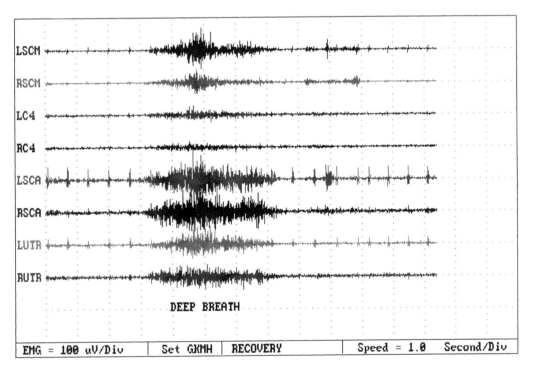

Figure 17–16B Surface EMG readings from the sternocleidomastoid, midcervical paraspinals at C-4, scalene, and upper trapezius are presented during a deep inspiration.

Source: Copyright © Clinical Resources, Inc.

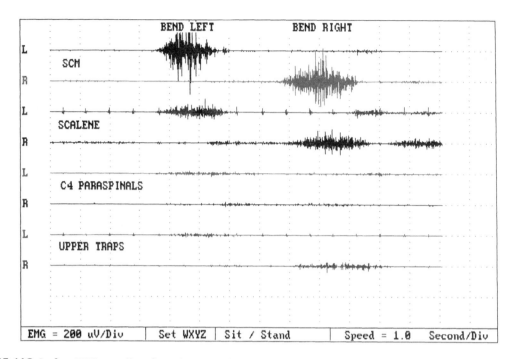

Figure 17–16C Surface EMG recordings from the sternocleidomastoid, scalene, C-4 paraspinals, and upper trapezius are presented during lateral bending.

Source: Copyright © Clinical Resources, Inc.

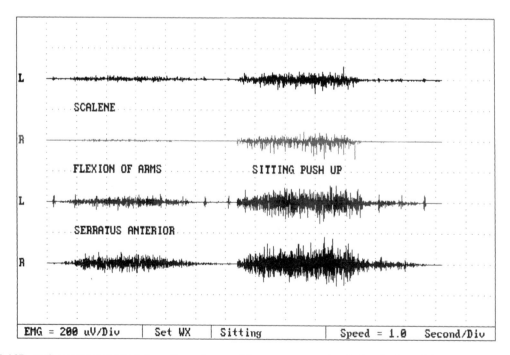

Figure 17–16D Surface EMG recordings from the scalene and the serratus anterior during flexion of the arms and push-up from a chair (sitting).

Source: Copyright © Clinical Resources, Inc.

MIDCERVICAL (C-4) PARASPINAL PLACEMENT

Type of Placement: Quasi-specific.

Action: Stabilizes and extends the neck.

Clinical Uses: Headache, neck pain, flexion/extension injuries, and TMJ dysfunction.

Muscle Insertions: This placement will record from the fibers of upper trapezius, along with the capitis and cervicis groups.

Innervation: Dorsal rami of the spinal nerves of the middle and lower cervical segments (C-3 to C-8). The dorsal ramus wraps around the articular pillar of the joint that makes up the posterior wall of the foramen. Arising off the dorsal ramus is the recurrent meningeal nerve; it retraces its path back into the spinal foramen and innervates the sensitive structures of the spinal segment as well as portions of the segments above and below, creating redundant innervation.[29]

Joint Considerations: When cervical segments are restricted due to postural habit, they are generally more symmetrical than those that are restricted due to trauma. In the middle and lower cervical spine, the motions of rotation and side flexion are conjoined. The resulting side flexion/rotation must be compensated for in the vertebral column, especially at the upper cervical spine.

Location: Palpate for the spinous processes of the cervical spine and the two muscle bellies that lie just lateral to it. Two active electrodes (approximately 2 cm apart) are placed so that they run parallel to the spine, approximately 2 cm from the midline, over the muscle belly at approximately C-4. Avoid the hairline (**Figure 17–17A**).

Behavioral Test: Cervical flexion and extension, lateral bending, and cervical rotation.

Tracing Comment: In **Figure 17–17B**, the SCM, scalene, and C-4 paraspinals are monitored. In this tracing, rotational patterns are studied during rotation to the physiologic end of the range of motion. Note the cooperative functions between SCM and C-4 paraspinals during rotation. The left SCM activates to provide movement during right rotation, with the right C-4 paraspinals stabilizing. The opposite is true for left rotation. The scalene muscles are quiet during this movement, showing little cross-talk for the SEMG recordings for these three sites (raw SEMG).

Figure 17–17C monitors the same muscle sites during resisted rotation. The recruitment pattern for resisted

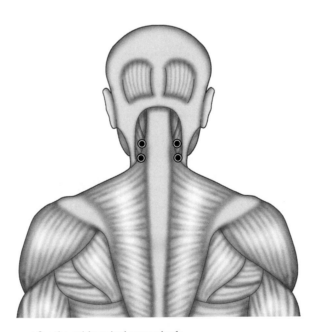

Figure 17–17A Electrode placement for the midcervical paraspinals.
Source: Copyright © Clinical Resources, Inc.

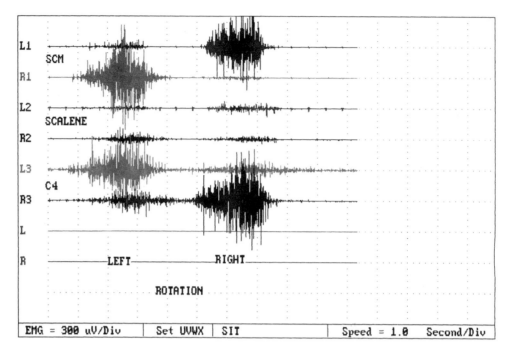

Figure 17–17B Surface EMG recordings from the SCM, scalene, and cervical paraspinals during head rotation to full range of motion.

Source: Copyright © Clinical Resources, Inc.

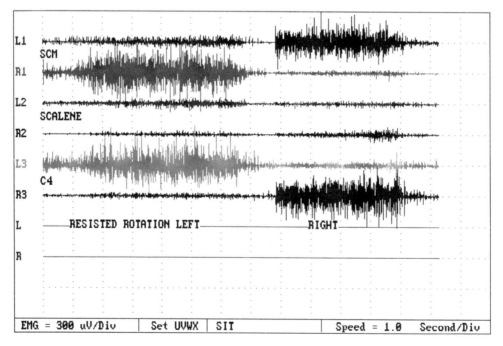

Figure 17–17C Surface EMG recordings from the SCM, scalene, and cervical paraspinals during resisted head rotation.

Source: Copyright © Clinical Resources, Inc.

rotation is very similar to the one collected during full range of motion (Figure 17–17B).

Also note the tracings for the SCM site (Figures 17–15B and 17–15C).

Clinical Considerations: The cervical paraspinals are made of groups of muscle; the most superficial is the splenius capitis, but these muscles include many others. These muscles have differing responsibilities regarding the motion of the head, neck, ribs, and thoracic spine. They can act in concert as cervical extensors. The practitioner should distinguish which layer of muscle and which direction of motion are most affected. As a whole, these muscles span many levels of the neck into the thoracic spine. They create functional links between distant regions of seemingly unrelated problems. A common example is the pulling and pain that many patients feel in the thoracic or lumbar region upon cervical flexion following a motor vehicle accident. This effect may be structural, as in restrictions in the free glide of the aponeurosis and fascia, or neurologically mediated, as in reflexive muscle contraction somewhere along the line of myofascium. Neurologically mediated restriction in multiple areas can also occur due to the redundant innervation within the spinal column. Palpation may reveal a motion segment responsible for the patient's symptoms, because unilateral pressure over one of the posterior vertebral joints of that segment reproduces the patient's symptoms, and perhaps some guarding muscle spasm is noted during palpation. However, passive motion testing may reveal restricted motion in the segment above or below.[24] The segment with restricted motion may actually be located several segments away from the irritable segment.

Volume Conduction: Upper fibers of trapezius, deep cervical muscles, and levator scapulae.

Other Sites of Interest: Upper trapezius and SCM during extension and rotation of the neck.

Referred Pain Considerations: Trigger points in the splenius capitis muscle refer pain to the vertex of the head, while trigger points in the splenius cervicis refer pain intensely to the back of the orbit or downward toward the shoulder girdle and the angle of the neck.[17]

Artifacts: Respiration, electrode slippage during movement.

Benchmark: Sitting quietly at midline (*N* = 104): 1.9 (±2.2) μV (RMS).
Values taken using a J&J M-501 with a 100- to 200-Hz filter.[18]

CERVICAL DORSAL (WIDE) PLACEMENT

Type of Placement: General.

Purpose: Monitor all cervical, shoulder, and thoracic movements.

Clinical Uses: Headache; neck, shoulder, and arm pain.

Location: The active electrodes are placed at the C-4 and T-10 levels, approximately 2 cm out from the spine over the muscle mass of the paraspinals (**Figure 17–18A**).

Behavioral Test: Flex, extend, and rotate the head; elevate, retract, and protract the shoulders; abduct and flex the arms.

Tracing Comment: **Figure 17–18B** shows SEMG tracings from the cervical dorsal site during transitions between sitting and standing and forward flexion of the head. Note the general symmetry of the tracing, along with the activation that occurs during flexion of the head (processed SEMG).

Figure 17–18C shows SEMG activity from cervical dorsal leads during repeated sitting, walking, and sitting activities. The tracings are from a patient who has been trained to use minimal muscular effort in this region[13] (processed SEMG).

Also note the tracings for the cervical trapezius placements (Figures 17–6B, 17–6C, and 17–6D).

Clinical Considerations: This site is particularly influenced by posture, with higher SEMG values commonly seen as patients go from sitting to standing. Patients may be taught, however, to rapidly quiet this region following movement.[13] This task involves intentionality (i.e., becoming aware that the muscles remain active following a postural change) and postural adjustments of the rib cage (sternal lift) and head position (better alignment of the head over the shoulders).

Volume Conduction: Cervical and thoracic paraspinals; upper, middle, and lower trapezius; levator scapulae; rhomboids; and scalene.

Other Sites of Interest: SCM and scalene to assess other muscles that contribute to cervical motion; dorsal lumbar (wide) to consider movement of the spine as a whole. More specific monitoring sites should be considered if these more generalized treatments are ineffective.

Artifacts: ECG, breathing.

Benchmark: Sitting: 2.0 μV (RMS).
Standing: 2.0 μV (RMS).
Values based on the observation of Ettare and Ettare.[13]

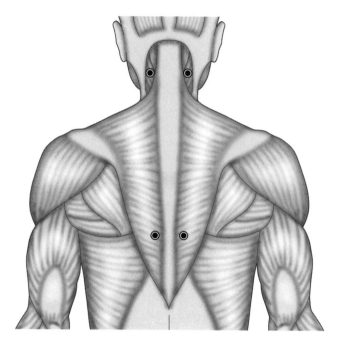

Figure 17–18A Electrode placement for the cervical dorsal (wide) site.

Source: Copyright © Clinical Resources, Inc.

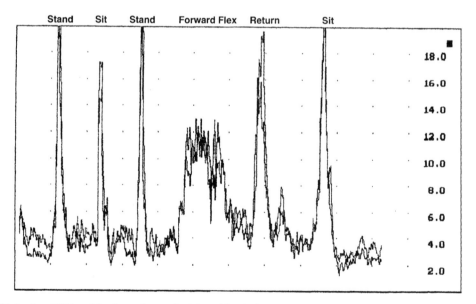

Figure 17–18B Surface EMG activity from the cervical dorsal leads during sitting–standing transitions and forward flexion of the head.

Source: Copyright © Clinical Resources, Inc.

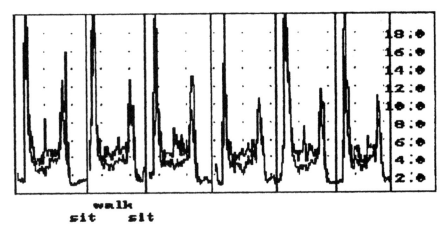

Figure 17–18C Surface EMG activity from the cervical dorsal leads during repeated sitting, walking, and sitting activities.
Source: Copyright © Clinical Resources, Inc.

UPPER TRAPEZIUS (NARROW) PLACEMENT

Type of Placement: Specific.

Action: Adduction, upward rotation, and elevation of the scapula; side bending of head.

Clinical Uses: Headaches, shoulder pain, upper quarter pain, repetitive strain injury, tension myalgia.

Muscle Insertions: The upper fibers of the trapezius arise from the superior nuchal line, the external occipital protuberance, and the ligamentum nuchae. They insert on the lateral third of the clavicle and the spine of the scapula.

Innervation: C-3, C-4 myotome via sensory nerves of the ventral rami of the C-3 and C-4 spinal nerves.

Joint Considerations: O/A; C-6 through T-3 spinous process; acromioclavicular and sternoclavicular joints.

Location: Place two active electrodes (2 cm apart) so that they run parallel to the muscle fibers (origins and insertions) of the upper trapezius, along the ridge of the shoulder, slightly lateral to and one-half the distance between the cervical spine at C-7 and the acromion. Palpate the muscle mass and place the electrodes over the muscle belly (**Figure 17–19A**).

Variations: Due to the broad nature of the trapezius muscle, the farther the electrode placement is moved down from the crest of the shoulder, the more the SEMG recording will register the actions associated with scapular adduction.

Behavioral Test: Shoulder elevation/shrug, lateral bending of the head.

Tracing Comment: **Figure 17–19B** shows upper and lower trapezius recruitment during shoulder girdle elevation (shrug). The upper trapezius shows a large recruitment pattern as the shoulder girdle is raised (raw SEMG).

Figure 17–19C shows the upper trapezius, supraspinatus, infraspinatus, posterior deltoids, and latissimus dorsi during the movements of shoulder girdle elevation, external rotation, and extension of the arm. Shoulder girdle elevation brought about the largest recruitment pattern for the upper trapezius tracing. The infraspinatus was most active during external rotation. The posterior deltoid and latissimus dorsi were more active during extension of the arm. The electrodes placed above the supraspinatus fossa (upper trapezius and supraspinatus) did not differentiate during any of the movements (raw SEMG).

See also the tracings for the lower trapezius (Figures 17–21B, 17–21C, 17–21D, and 17–21E) and suprascapular/supraspinatus site (Figures 17–23C and 17–23D).

Clinical Considerations: Sitting unsupported may yield higher values than when the back is supported.

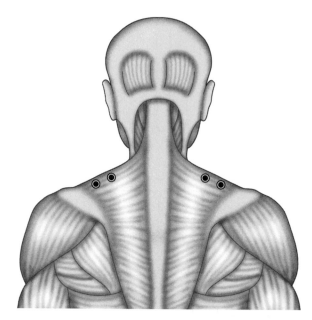

Figure 17–19A Electrode placement for the upper trapezius site.

Source: Copyright © Clinical Resources, Inc.

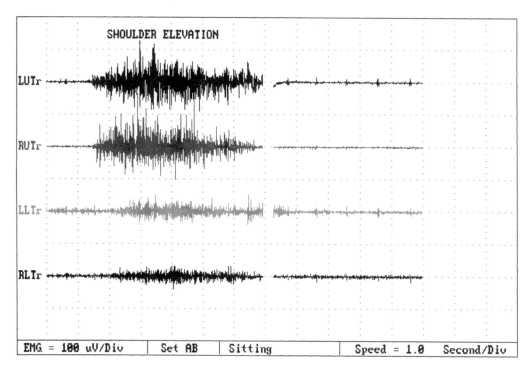

Figure 17–19B Surface EMG activity from the upper and lower trapezius during shoulder girdle elevation.

Source: Copyright © Clinical Resources, Inc.

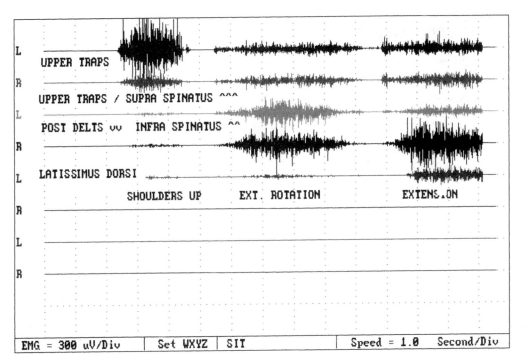

Figure 17-19C Surface EMG activity from the upper trapezius, supraspinatus, infraspinatus, posterior deltoids, and latissimus dorsi during shoulder girdle elevation, external rotation, and extension of the arm.

Source: Copyright © Clinical Resources, Inc.

Arms in the lap may yield lower values than when arms are at the sides. Standing values are commonly higher than sitting values.[18] Acting unilaterally, the upper trapezius bends the neck and head toward the same side.[16] Working synergistically with other muscles, it assists in the abduction and flexion of the arm. Bilateral activation may be seen during resisted extension of the head.

The upper trapezius could be affected by dysfunction in segments C-3 through T-2 because of its insertions on the ligamentum nuchae. Forward head posture and associated changes in the positions of the scapula, ribs, O/A joints, and other cervical structures may also cause upper trapezius dysfunction. An irritable contralateral scalene, possibly due to underlying cervical joint structures, may create hypertonicity in the upper trapezius. Myofascial restrictions in the latissimus dorsi, deltoids, and biceps may affect upper trapezius recordings. Finally, elevations in the upper trapezius have been noted in multidirectional instabilities of the shoulder.

Cook, Gray, Savinar-Nogue, and Madeiros monitored the SEMG activity of shoulder muscle during the throwing of a ball in pitchers and non-pitchers.[30]

Volume Conduction: Middle fibers of trapezius, levator scapulae, supraspinatus.

Other Sites of Interest: Lower trapezius, middle trapezius, serratus anterior, supraspinatus, biceps, deltoid, infraspinatus, teres major, and pectoralis major during movements of the upper extremities.

Referred Pain Considerations: Trigger points in the upper trapezius characteristically refer pain along the posterolateral aspect of the neck behind the ear and up into the temple.[17]

Artifacts: ECG, breathing.

Benchmark: Sitting quietly at midline (*N* = 104): 2.2 (±2.6) μV (RMS).

Standing quietly at midline (*N* = 104): 3.1 (±3.1) μV (RMS).

Values taken using a J&J M-501 with a 100- to 200-Hz filter.[18]

INTERSCAPULAR (MIDDLE TRAPEZIUS) PLACEMENT

Type of Placement: Quasi-specific.

Action: Scapular stabilization; adduction, retraction, and upward rotation of the scapula during flexion and abduction of the arms, especially near its full range of motion.

Clinical Uses: Shoulder rehabilitation.

Muscle Insertions: These fibers arise from the spinal processes of C-6 to T-3 and insert on the acromion and superior lip of the spine of the scapula.

Innervation: Spinal portion of the accessory nerve (eleventh cranial nerve), and the ventral ramus C-2, C-3, and C-4.

Location: To place the electrodes, locate the medial border of the spine of the scapula (root). The electrodes are placed horizontally, 2 cm apart, next to the root (**Figure 17–20A**).

Behavioral Test: Retract the scapula and abduct the arms through the full range of motion.

Tracing Comment: **Figure 17–20B** shows recordings from the interscapular site during shoulder retraction.

While middle trapezius fibers are thought to contribute to this recording, it is difficult to separate out this muscle's SEMG contribution from the SEMG contributions of rhomboid (raw SEMG). Also see the tracings for the lower trapezius (Figure 17–21B).

Clinical Considerations: The middle fibers of the trapezius are known to adduct and retract the scapula.[31] They are thought to play a larger role in abduction of the arm near its full range.[32]

Volume Conduction: Upper trapezius, levator scapulae, rhomboids, erector spinae.

Other Sites of Interest: Upper trapezius, lower trapezius, serratus anterior, supraspinatus, biceps, deltoid, infraspinatus, teres major, and pectoralis major during movements of the upper extremities and shoulder girdle.

Referred Pain Considerations: Trigger points in this region tend to refer pain toward the vertebrae and the interscapular region in general.[17]

Artifacts: ECG, breathing.

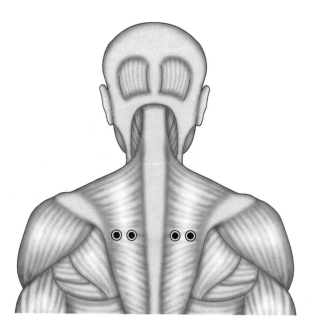

Figure 17–20A Electrode placement for the interscapular (middle trapezius) site.
Source: Copyright © Clinical Resources, Inc.

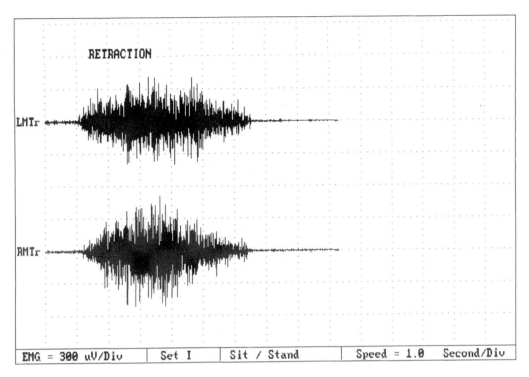

Figure 17–20B Surface EMG recordings from the middle trapezius site during scapular retraction.

Source: Copyright © Clinical Resources, Inc.

LOWER INTERSCAPULAR (LOWER TRAPEZIUS) PLACEMENT

Type of Placement: Quasi-specific.

Action: Scapular stabilization; upward rotation, retraction, and depression of the scapula during abduction, flexion, and scaption of the arms.

Clinical Uses: Shoulder, neck, and upper quarter pain; repetitive strain injury.

Muscle Insertions: The fibers arise from the third to the twelfth thoracic vertebrae (T-3 through T-12) and insert on the scapular spine.

Innervation: Spinal portion of the accessory nerve (eleventh cranial nerve), and the ventral ramus C-2, C-3, and C-4.

Location: Palpate the interscapular region. Have the patient retract and depress the scapula and then flex the arm to at least 90 degrees. Palpate the inferior medial border of the scapula for the muscle mass that emerges. Place the electrodes on an oblique angle, approximately 5 cm down from the scapular spine. The two active elec-trodes (2 cm apart) are placed next to the medial edge of the scapula at a 55–degree oblique angle (**Figure 17–21A**).

Behavioral Test: Abduction of arms; retraction of the shoulder back and down at a 45–degree angle.

Tracing Comment: Four tracings are shown for a variety of muscle groups and movements to provide the practitioner with an appreciation of the complexity of recruitment patterns and synergy at this site.

Figure 17–21B shows a normal tracing of abduction through 90 degrees, followed by an isolated movement of retraction and depression of the scapula. Both upper and lower trapezius muscles are roughly equally active during the abduction. In this example, during the return phase, the lower trapezius continues in its recruitment pattern slightly longer than the upper trapezius. The key attribute of a normal synergy pattern during this movement is symmetry between the right and left trapezius and the upper and lower trapezius. Isolation of the lower trapezius is also presented and is characterized by active retraction and depression of the scapula.

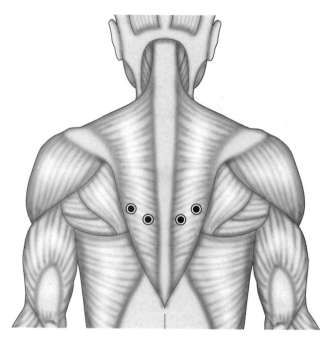

Figure 17–21A Electrode placement for the lower interscapular (lower trapezius) site.

Source: Copyright © Clinical Resources, Inc.

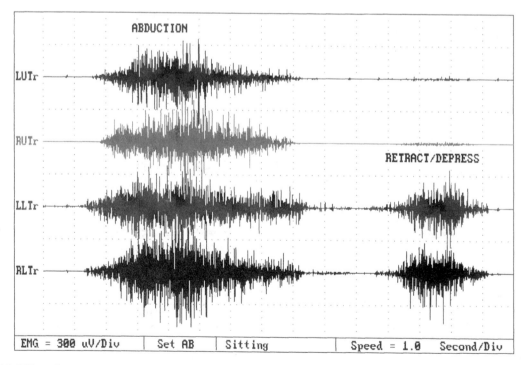

Figure 17–21B Surface EMG recordings from the upper and lower trapezius sites during abduction and retraction. Note the balance of recruitment between upper and lower trapezius during abduction, while only the lower trapezius muscles are active during retraction.

Source: Copyright © Clinical Resources, Inc.

Figure 17–21C represents an abnormal recruitment pattern during abduction to 90 degrees. The lower trapezius is dominant, which suggests excessive scapular depression. Normally, during the last third of the active recruitment, the lower trapezius has a slightly greater activation associated with the return phase of the movement. As a rough rule of thumb, when abduction is done to 90 degrees, the upper trapezius to lower trapezius ratio should be less than 1.0. An abnormal synergy is noted when activation of upper fibers of trapezius exceeds activation of lower fibers at 90 degrees.[33]

Figure 17–21D shows SEMG recordings from the upper trapezius, middle trapezius, lower trapezius, and serratus anterior. The first half of the tracing represents abduction to 180 degrees for the right arm. A separate, isolated flexion of the right arm to 180 degrees follows. The lower trapezius is activated more briskly during abduction, while the upper trapezius and serratus anterior are activated more briskly during flexion of the arm.

Figure 17–21E shows the upper trapezius, middle trapezius, lower trapezius, and serratus anterior during three isolated movements of abduction, scaption, and flexion for the right upper extremity only. The recruit-

ment pattern in this example is slightly different from that in Figure 17–21D. All three of the trapezius recording sites play a role in controlling the scapula. The role of the upper trapezius gradually diminishes as one moves from abduction through scaption to flexion of the arm, as does the role of the middle trapezius. The lower trapezius appears to be constant across all three movements, while the recordings at the serratus anterior site increase across the three movements (raw SEMG).

Also see the tracings for the suprascapular/supraspinatus site (Figures 17–23C and 17–23D).

Clinical Considerations: The lower trapezius interacts with the upper trapezius through the process of reciprocal inhibition.[33] Whenever the upper trapezius is found to be hyperactive, it is worthwhile to monitor the lower trapezius simultaneously; it is commonly found to be inhibited. When uptraining the lower trapezius, it is useful to explore how the position of the sternum affects the muscle recruitment patterns. Allowing the person to engage in a sternal lift prior to attempted isolation of the lower trapezius may enhance the probability of successful isolation of recruitment.

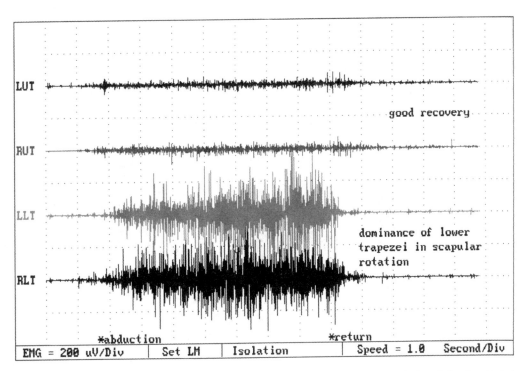

Figure 17–21C Abnormal surface EMG recordings from the upper and lower trapezius sites during abduction. Note how the lower trapezius appears to be dominant.

Source: Copyright © Clinical Resources, Inc.

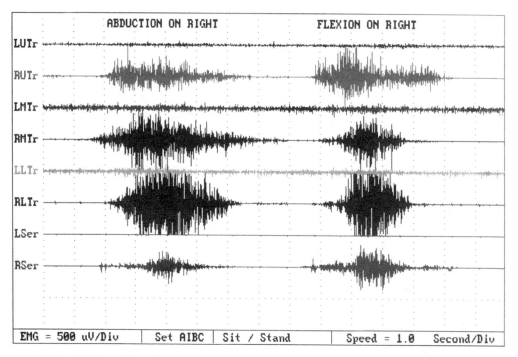

Figure 17–21D Surface EMG recordings from the upper (UTr), middle (MTr), and lower (LTr) trapezius sites, along with the serratus anterior (Ser) during abduction and flexion for the right side only.

Source: Copyright © Clinical Resources, Inc.

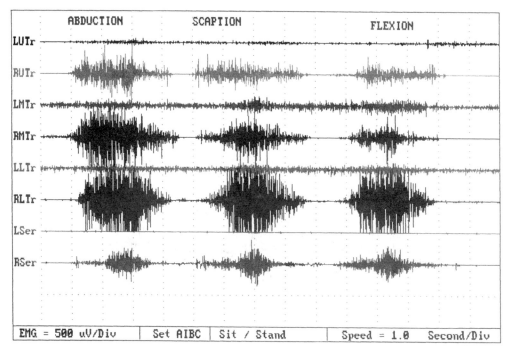

Figure 17–21E Surface EMG recordings from the upper (UTr), middle (MTr), and lower (LTr) trapezius sites, along with the serratus anterior (Ser) during abduction, scaption, and flexion.

Source: Copyright © Clinical Resources, Inc.

Volume Conduction: Middle trapezius, rhomboids, and erector spinae.

Other Sites of Interest: Upper trapezius, middle trapezius, serratus anterior, supraspinatus, biceps, deltoid, infraspinatus, teres major, and pectoralis major during movements of the upper extremities and shoulder girdle.

Referred Pain Considerations: Trigger points in this muscle group refer pain sharply to the upper cervical region of the paraspinal muscles.[17]

Artifacts: ECG, breathing.

Benchmark: Sitting quietly at midline ($N = 104$): 2.3 (±2.3) μV (RMS).
Standing quietly at midline: 2.5 (±2.5) μV (RMS).
Values taken using a J&J M-501 with a 100- to 200-Hz filter.[18]

SERRATUS ANTERIOR (LOWER FIBERS) PLACEMENT

Type of Placement: Specific.

Action: Upward rotation, depression, and abduction of the scapula during abduction and flexion of the arm; protraction of scapula during pushing activities.

Clinical Uses: Upper quarter, neck, and headache pain (i.e., with upper trapezius placements in overuse syndromes).

Muscle Insertions: The fibers of this multibellied muscle usually arise by nine slips from the first to ninth ribs. The lowest portion of this muscle inserts on the costal surface of the inferior angle of the scapula.

Innervation: The anterior rami of the C-5 through C-8 spinal nerves.

Location: Have the patient flex the arm against resistance. Palpate this contraction in an area just anterior to the border of the latissimus dorsi muscle at the level of the inferior tip of the scapula. Place two active electrodes horizontally (2 cm apart) just below the axillary area, at the level of the inferior tip of the scapula, and just medial of the latissimus dorsi. It is important that the electrodes are anterior to the latissimus dorsi muscle (**Figure 17–22A**).

Behavioral Test: Forward flexion of the arms, protraction of the shoulders, push-ups.

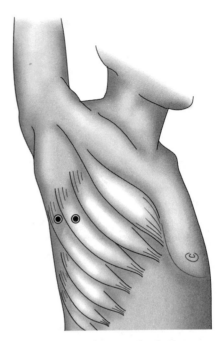

Figure 17–22A Electrode placement for the serratus anterior site.
Source: Copyright © Clinical Resources, Inc.

Tracing Comment: **Figure 17–22B** shows recordings from the serratus anterior during a series of push-up maneuvers: wall push-up, knee push-up, and floor push-up. Note the increasing level of recruitment associated with the increasing efforts. Also note a mildly abnormal asymmetry between the right and left aspects (raw SEMG).

Figure 17–22C shows SEMG recordings from the upper trapezius, lower trapezius, pectoralis (clavicular head), and serratus anterior during flexion of the arms. The pectoralis group shows the greatest activation pattern. The serratus anterior also recruits during this movement for this subject, while the upper and lower trapezius do not (raw SEMG).

Also see the tracings for scalene placement (Figure 17–16D).

Clinical Considerations: The EMG activity of this muscle during a neutral rest position should be quiet.[16] Protraction of the scapula has been noted along with SEMG activity during forward pushing movements.[32,34] The portion of the serratus anterior monitored using the site described in this section is most active during flexion of the arm, and slightly less active during abduction.[16]

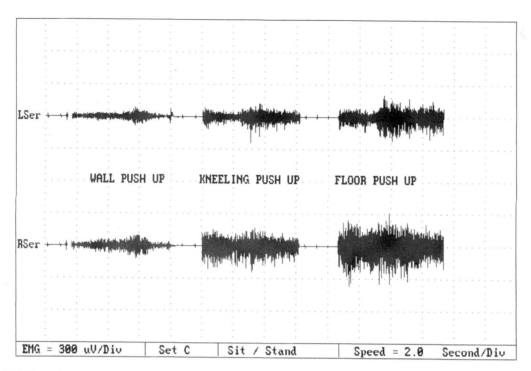

Figure 17–22B Surface EMG recordings from the serratus anterior during wall push-up, kneeling push-up, and floor push-up.
Source: Copyright © Clinical Resources, Inc.

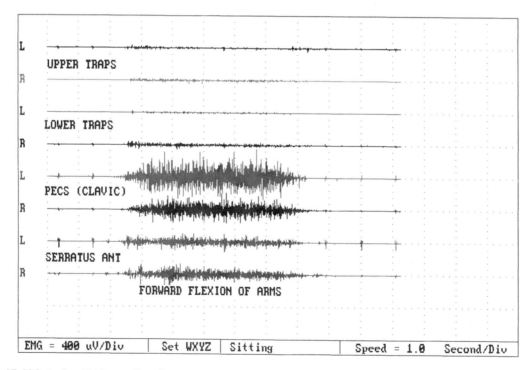

Figure 17–22C Surface EMG recordings from the upper trapezius, lower trapezius, pectoralis (clavicular head), and serratus anterior during flexion of the arms.
Source: Copyright © Clinical Resources, Inc.

Volume Conduction: Latissimus dorsi, intercostal muscles, costal portion of pectoralis.

Other Sites of Interest: Upper trapezius, middle trapezius, lower trapezius, supraspinatus, biceps, deltoid, infraspinatus, teres major, latissimus dorsi, and pectoralis major during movements of the upper extremities and shoulder girdle.

Referred Pain Considerations: Trigger points refer pain to the side and back of the chest.[17]

Artifacts: ECG, respiration.

SUPRASCAPULAR FOSSA (UPPER TRAPEZIUS/SUPRASPINATUS) PLACEMENT

Type of Placement: Quasi-specific.

Action: Abduction of the arm; controls the head of the humerus in the glenoid fossa.

Clinical Uses: Shoulder rehabilitation.

Muscle Insertions: The fibers of supraspinatus lie beneath middle and upper fibers of the trapezius. They arise from the supraspinatus fossa and insert on the greater tubercle of the humerus.

Location: Palpate the spine of the scapula, locating its lateral distal aspect. The electrodes are placed there 2 cm apart, directly above the spine of the scapula, over the suprascapular fossa (**Figure 17–23A**).

Behavioral Test: Abduction of the arm.

Tracing Comment: **Figure 17–23B** shows recordings taken from the right side only of the upper trapezius, supraspinatus, infraspinatus, and middle deltoid during shoulder elevation (shrug) and abduction with the thumb in the down and then up positions. Shoulder elevation is associated with contractions at the upper trapezius and supraspinatus site but does not involve the middle deltoid. The recruitment pattern noted during abduction indicates that the deltoid fires first during the initiation of the movement. The contraction of the upper trapezius is thought to facilitate a stable length–tension relationship for the deltoid. Note that the thumb-up and thumb-down portions of the tracing are very similar for all sites for this subject (raw SEMG).

In **Figures 17–23C and 17–23D**, two studies were conducted on the right side of another subject during abduction with the thumb up, palm down, and thumb down. The upper trapezius (narrow), suprascapular/ supraspinatus, middle deltoid, infraspinatus, lower interscapular (lower trapezius), and latissimus dorsi

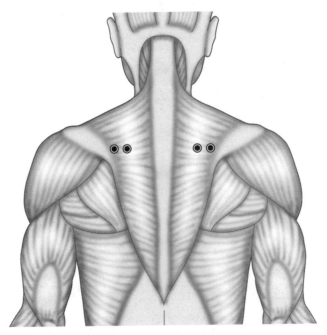

Figure 17–23A Electrode placement for the upper suprascapular fossa (trapezius/supraspinatus) site.
Source: Copyright © Clinical Resources, Inc.

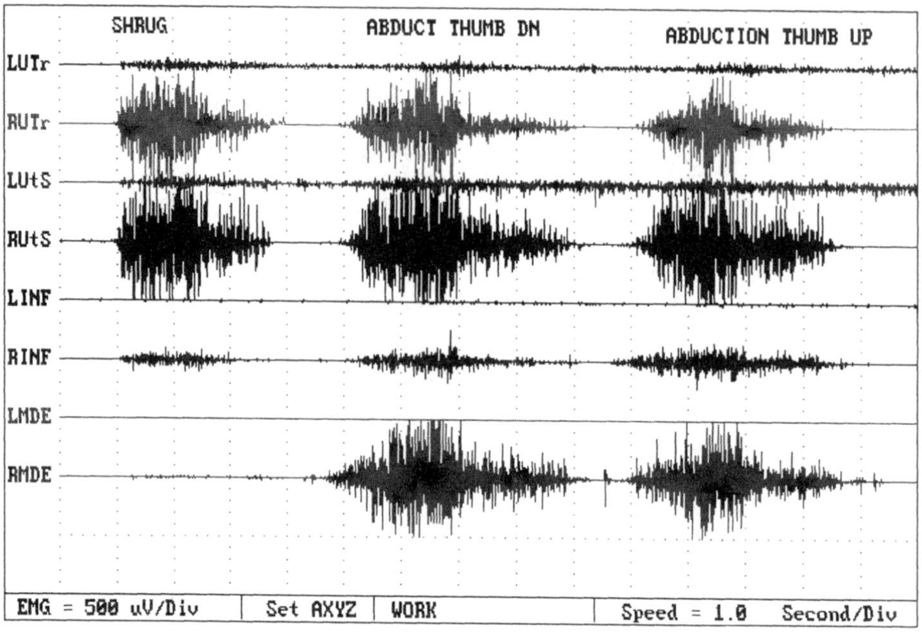

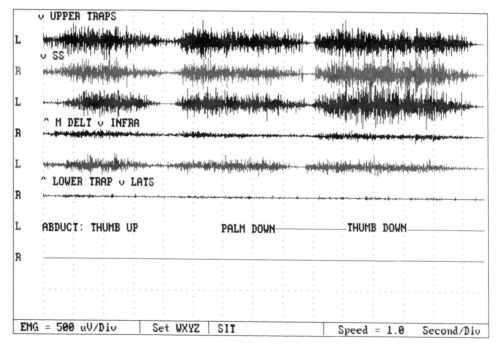

Figure 17–23B Surface EMG recordings from the upper trapezius, suprascapular (upper trapezius/supraspinatus), infraspinatus, and middle deltoid sites during a shoulder shrug, abduction of the arm with the thumb down, and abduction with the thumb up.

Source: Copyright © Clinical Resources, Inc.

Figure 17–23C Surface EMG recordings from the upper trapezius (narrow), suprascapular/supraspinatus, middle deltoid, infraspinatus, lower interscapular (lower trapezius), and latissimus dorsi placement sites during abduction with thumb up, palm down, and thumb down, and with a slightly flexed upper back.

Source: Copyright © Clinical Resources, Inc.

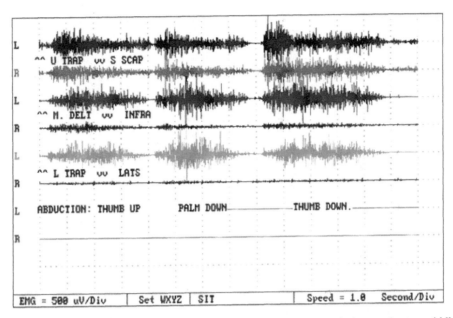

Figure 17–23D Surface EMG recordings from the upper trapezius (narrow), suprascapular/supraspinatus, middle deltoid, infraspinatus, lower interscapular (lower trapezius), and latissimus dorsi placement sites during abduction with thumb up, palm down, and thumb down following a sternal lift.

Source: Copyright © Clinical Resources, Inc.

placement sites were monitored. In Figure 17–23C, the subject was standing with a slight flexion to the upper back during the movement patterns of abduction. In Figure 17–23D, these movements were conducted during a sternal lift, raising the rib cage and upper torso into a more upright posture. By comparing the recruitment patterns for a given muscle under the two different postural loads, one can see that during the sternal lift (Figure 17–23D), the suprascapular/supraspinatus site shows a stronger distinction between the thumb-up and thumb-down movements, with a more robust recruitment pattern during the thumb-down abduction. The thumb-down movement is predicted to augment recruitment of the supraspinatus. Such augmentation, however, may not be seen unless the rib cage is in the proper position. In addition, the sternal lift brings about a stronger recruitment pattern for the lower trapezius during all three abduction movements. Using the rules regarding relationships for upper and lower trapezius presented in Chapter 7, the level of recruitment during abduction should be approximately the same for both the upper and lower trapezius sites. In Figure 17–23C, when abduction is conducted with a slightly flexed upper back, the lower trapezius recruitment pattern appears slightly abnormal because it is so much smaller

than the upper trapezius pattern. In Figure 17–23D, however, the sternal lift augments the recruitment of the lower trapezius, making the abduction movement look more normalized (raw SEMG).

Clinical Considerations: The supraspinatus muscle is extremely difficult to monitor electromyographically using surface electrodes because the middle and upper trapezius muscles overlie it. To record from the supraspinatus, indwelling electrodes are needed. For the most part, recordings from this site correlate remarkably well with those of middle and upper trapezius. However, under isolated circumstances, using particular movements and with the correct posture (such as the ones seen in Figures 17–23C and 17–23D), recruitment from the supraspinatus can be inferred.

Volume Conduction: Major problems of cross-talk arise from the middle and upper fibers of the trapezius. It is impossible to isolate EMG activity from the supraspinatus (relative to the upper trapezius) with surface electrodes. These muscles are layered next to each other and function synergistically. Movements that attempt to separate out differential muscle function fail to show differential recruitment patterns from the upper trapezius at this site.

Other Sites of Interest: Upper trapezius, middle trapezius, lower trapezius, serratus anterior, biceps, deltoid, infraspinatus, teres major, and pectoralis major during movements of the upper extremities and shoulder girdle.

Referred Pain Considerations: Trigger points at this site refer pain to the middle deltoid region and may include the lateral epicondyle region.[17]

Artifacts: ECG.

INFRASPINATUS PLACEMENT

Type of Placement: Specific.

Action: Lateral rotation of the shoulder joint, along with stabilization of the head of the humerus in the glenoid cavity.

Clinical Uses: Treatment of stroke patients to facilitate use of the upper extremities; treatment of shoulder instability and orthopedic impingement syndromes.

Muscle Insertions: The fibers arise from the infraspinatus fossa, below the spine of the scapula, and insert on the greater tubercle of the humerus.

Innervation: The superior cord of the brachial plexus, from the spinal nerves of segments C-4, C-5, and C-6.

Joint Considerations: The joints of the cervical spine related to the muscle (C-4, C-5, and C-6) may affect the SEMG resting or recruitment patterns, along with the glenohumeral joint (particularly the anterior glide stability and the inferior glide capacity) and the acromioclavicular (AC) joint.

Location: Palpate the spine of the scapula. Two closely spaced electrodes (2 cm apart) are placed parallel to and approximately 4 cm below the spine of the scapula, on the lateral aspect, over the infrascapular fossa of the scapula. Avoid placement over the posterior deltoid (**Figure 17–24A**).

Behavioral Test: Elbow bent to 90 degrees with lateral (external) rotation of the bent arm out to the side; abduction of the arm.

Tracing Comment: **Figure 17–24B** shows SEMG tracings from infraspinatus and posterior deltoid during lateral rotation with the right arm flexed at the elbow, and external rotation and extension of the right arm with the elbow extended. During lateral rotation, the activity at the infraspinatus site is greater. During lateral rotation

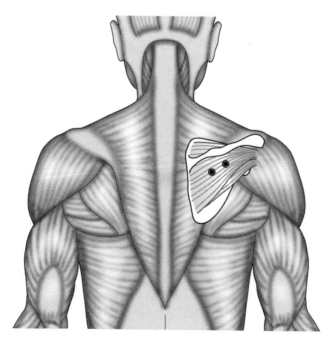

Figure 17–24A Electrode placement for the infraspinatus site.
Source: Copyright © Clinical Resources, Inc.

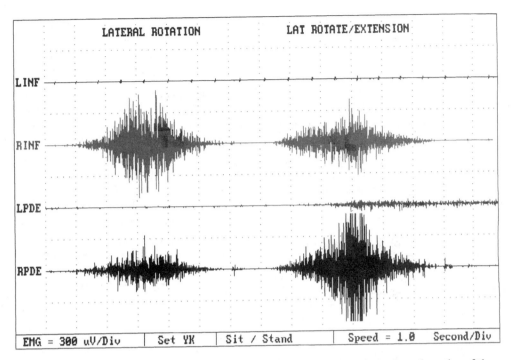

Figure 17–24B Surface EMG recordings from the infraspinatus and posterior deltoid during lateral rotation of the arm and lateral rotation and extension of the shoulder.

Source: Copyright © Clinical Resources, Inc.

with extension of the shoulder, the SEMG activity of the posterior deltoid site is greater (raw SEMG).

Also see the tracings from the upper trapezius (Figure 17–19C) and the triceps (Figure 17–34B).

Clinical Considerations: Forward head posture and thoracic kyphosis, with the downward pull of the rib cage, may allow the internal rotators of the shoulder (both scapular and glenohumeral) to shorten, altering the normal length–tension relationship for the infraspinatus.

During abduction, the supraspinatus requires external rotation of the humeral head to clear the greater tubercle from impinging against the coracoacromial ligament. With slight dysfunction (e.g., tightness of the supraspinatus muscle, slight anterior capsule laxity, excessive tightness of the internal rotators, spurring of the AC joint), the infraspinatus overworks and develops triggers.

In full overhead elevation, as in throwing, the lower trapezius is in a functional line with the infraspinatus and posterior deltoids. Inhibition of the lower trapezius alters the ability of the scapula stabilizers to protect the length–tension advantage of the deltoids. With the deltoids working at a disadvantage and the lower trapezius dysfunctional, the infraspinatus is asked to overwork.

Volume Conduction: Posterior deltoid, teres major, and teres minor.

Other Sites of Interest: Upper trapezius, middle trapezius, lower trapezius, serratus anterior, supraspinatus, biceps, deltoid, teres major, and pectoralis major during movements of the upper extremities and shoulder girdle.

Referred Pain Considerations: Trigger points at this site refer pain to the anterior deltoid region and the shoulder joint.[17]

Artifacts: ECG.

ANTERIOR DELTOID PLACEMENT

Type of Placement: Specific.

Action: Forward flexion, medial rotation, and abduction of the arm.

Clinical Uses: Shoulder rehabilitation.

Muscle Insertions: This muscle arises from the lateral third of the clavicle and inserts on the deltoid tuberosity of the humerus.

Innervation: Via the axillary nerve from the posterior cord of the brachial plexus (these carry fibers from the spinal nerves of segments C-5 and C-6).

Joint Considerations: Deltoid muscle dysfunctions can arise from neurogenic causes from the cervical spine (C-5 primarily, but also C-6, C-7, C-8, and T-1). Joint motion dysfunctions that would affect the tension of the posterior cord of the plexus (namely, the costovertebral articulations of the first rib, the sternocostal junctions, and the scapulothoracic positioning as seen via the acromioclavicular joints, the sternoclavicular joints, and the posture of the scapula) could also affect SEMG recordings.

Location: Palpate the clavicle. Two active electrodes, 2 cm apart, are placed on the anterior aspect of the arm, approximately 4 cm below the clavicle, so that they run parallel to the muscle fibers (**Figure 17-25A**).

Behavioral Test: Forward flexion, abduction, and horizontal adduction of the arm.

Tracing Comment: **Figure 17-25B** shows SEMG recordings from the anterior, middle, and posterior deltoids monitored during flexion, abduction, and extension of the right side only. The largest recruitment of the anterior

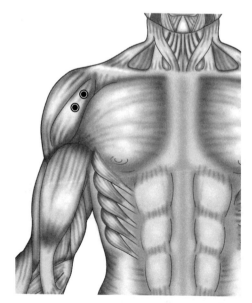

Figure 17–25A Electrode placement for the anterior deltoid site.

Source: Copyright © Clinical Resources, Inc.

deltoid is seen during flexion of the arm. It also contributes during abduction (raw SEMG).

Also see the tracings from the triceps (Figure 17–34B) and the pectoralis major (Figure 17–28B).

Clinical Considerations: Simultaneous activation of the anterior, middle, and posterior deltoids abducts the arm.[16] The anterior portion flexes the arm,[16] and also plays a role in the horizontal flexion of the arm across the chest.[32] Movement of the hand to the face requires adequate function of anterior deltoids and serratus anterior muscles.[31]

The position of the humeral head in the glenohumeral joint, and that of the scapula on the chest wall, are important to the function of the deltoids. Behavioral nuances of movement strategy in the initiation of elevation of the upper extremity are also important. It is necessary to attempt to control and standardize these factors to ensure successful testing at this site.

Myofascial factors that would tend to activate the neural pathway of the deltoids and dysfunction include the scalene, latissimus dorsi, teres minor, and the muscles of the arm and forearm supplied by the radial nerve. Factors from the contralateral side that activate the neural tree also must be considered. Inhibition of the lower trapezius with hyperactivity of the upper trapezius could affect the functions of elevation, reaching, and weight bearing through the upper extremity. Elevation of the arm into abduction is normally a result of the force couple of the scapular rotators (upper trapezius, lower trapezius, serratus anterior) and the force couple of the supraspinatus and deltoids. Imbalance in the shoulder elevator group could be related to imbalance between elements of the elevators and the supraspinatus/deltoid force couple.

Volume Conduction: Medial deltoid, biceps, and pectoralis major.

Other Sites of Interest: Clavicular aspect of pectoralis, long head of biceps, serratus anterior, upper and lower trapezius, suprascapular fossa site, and middle and posterior deltoid during movements of the upper extremities.

Referred Pain Considerations: Trigger points at this site refer pain locally.[17]

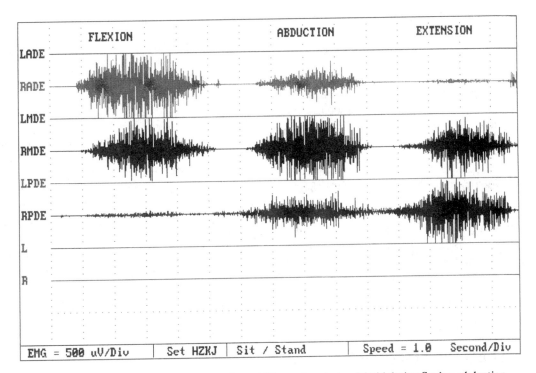

Figure 17–25B Surface EMG recordings from the anterior, middle, and posterior deltoid during flexion, abduction, and extension.

Source: Copyright © Clinical Resources, Inc.

MIDDLE DELTOID PLACEMENT

Type of Placement: Specific.

Action: Abduction of the arm.

Clinical Uses: Shoulder rehabilitation.

Muscle Insertions: This muscle arises from the acromion and inserts on the deltoid tuberosity of the humerus.

Innervation: The axillary nerve, spinal segments C-5 and C-6.

Location: The active electrodes are placed on the lateral aspect of the upper arm, 2 cm apart, and approximately 3 cm below the acromion, over the muscle mass so that the electrodes run parallel to the muscle fibers (**Figure 17–26**).

Behavioral Test: Abduction of the arm.

Tracing Comment: Figure 17–25B for the anterior deltoid shows how the middle deltoid is active during all

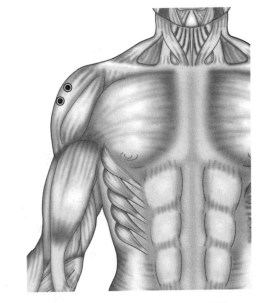

Figure 17–26 Electrode placement for the middle deltoid site.

Source: Copyright © Clinical Resources, Inc.

three phases of movement: flexion, abduction, and extension. Also see Figure 17–23B (suprascapular fossa), where timing issues relative to other synergists are highlighted.

Clinical Considerations: Simultaneous activation of the anterior, middle, and posterior deltoids abducts the arm.[16] Abduction is the primary function of the middle deltoid, and this muscle is also active during flexion and extension of the arm.

Volume Conduction: Anterior and posterior deltoids, biceps, and triceps.

Other Sites of Interest: Suprascapular fossa site; anterior and posterior deltoids; upper, lower, and middle trapezius; pectoralis; teres major; and latissimus dorsi during movements of the upper extremities.

Referred Pain Considerations: Trigger points at this site refer pain locally.[17]

POSTERIOR DELTOID PLACEMENT

Type of Placement: Specific.

Action: Extension, lateral (external) rotation, and abduction of the arm.

Clinical Uses: Shoulder rehabilitation.

Muscle Insertions: This muscle arises from the lower border of the spine of the scapula and inserts on the deltoid tuberosity of the humerus.

Innervation: The axillary nerve, spinal segments C-5 and C-6.

Joint Considerations: Deltoid muscle dysfunctions can arise from neurogenic causes from the cervical spine (C-5 primarily, but also C-6, C-7, C-8, and T-1). Joint motion dysfunctions that affect the tension of the posterior cord of the plexus (namely, the costovertebral articulations of the first rib, the sternocostal junctions, and the scapulothoracic positioning as seen via the acromioclavicular joints, the sternoclavicular joints, and the posture of the scapula) could also affect SEMG recordings.

Location: Palpate the spine of the scapula. Two active electrodes are placed 2 cm apart and approximately 2 cm below the lateral border of the spine of the scapula and angled on an oblique angle toward the arm so that they run parallel to the muscle fibers (**Figure 17–27**).

Behavioral Test: Extension, abduction, and lateral rotation of the arm.

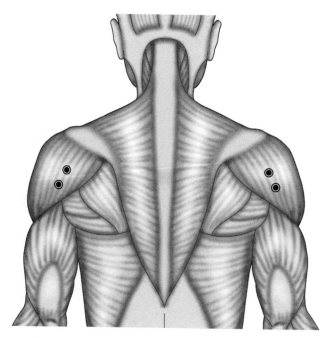

Figure 17–27 Electrode placement for the posterior deltoid site.
Source: Copyright © Clinical Resources, Inc.

Tracing Comment: Figure 17–25B (anterior deltoid) shows that for the posterior deltoid the largest recruitment occurs during extension, but that the posterior deltoid also contributes to abduction. Figures 17–19C (upper trapezius) and 17–24B (infraspinatus) indicate that the posterior deltoid is active during lateral rotation of the arm and extension of the shoulder.

Clinical Considerations: Simultaneous activation of the anterior, middle, and posterior deltoids abducts the arm.[16] The posterior deltoid, however, is primarily active in extension of the arm.

The posterior deltoid seems to be hypoactive more often than the anterior deltoid, possibly because it gets fatigued and stretched; there is currently no scientific evidence to support this theory. Documentation indicates that the internal rotators are naturally stronger than the external rotators.[35]

Compared to the anterior and middle compartments, there is almost always more atrophy and less SEMG of the posterior deltoid. Clinically, this outcome might be due to the increased length of the posterior deltoid with anterior translated head of the humerus associated with forward shoulders. In patients with multidirectional shoulder instability, the posterior deltoid is the most important muscle to train. In these patients, the deltoid should be trained isometrically to restore its ability to approximate the glenoid into the fossa to prevent excessive caudal glide.[36]

Volume Conduction: Middle deltoid, infraspinatus, teres major, and triceps.

Other Sites of Interest: Long head of triceps, latissimus dorsi, teres major, middle and anterior deltoid, and upper and lower trapezius during movements of the upper extremities.

Referred Pain Considerations: Trigger points at this site refer pain locally.[17]

PECTORALIS MAJOR (CLAVICULAR AND STERNAL) PLACEMENT

Type of Placement: Specific.

Action: Medial (internal) rotation and flexion of the shoulder; horizontal adduction of the arm; depression of the shoulder (sternal aspect).

Clinical Uses: Shoulder and arm rehabilitation.

Muscle Insertions: The clavicular aspect arises from the medial third of the clavicle. The sternal aspect arises from the sternal membrane and the cartilage of the second to sixth ribs. Both insert on the greater tubercle of the humerus.

Innervation: This area is innervated by the medial and lateral pectoralis nerves. The clavicular aspect is innervated mainly via the C-5 and C-6 spinal nerves; the sternal aspect is innervated mainly via the C-6 and C-7 spinal nerves.

Joint Considerations: In addition to the spinal joints that might affect the nerve roots (C-5 through T-1), other joints that should be cleared of problems include the sternoclavicular joint (and thus the AC joint), the sternomanubrial joint, the costocartilaginous and costosternal junctions, and the second through sixth ribs.

Location: For clavicular placement, palpate the clavicle. Two active electrodes (2 cm apart) are placed on the chest wall at an oblique angle toward the clavicle, approximately 2 cm below the clavicle, just medial to the axillary fold (**Figure 17–28A**).

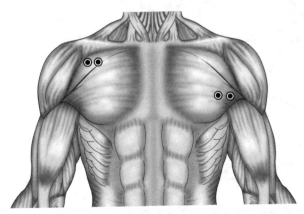

Figure 17–28A Electrode placement for the pectoralis major clavicular (right side) and sternal (left side) sites.
Source: Copyright © Clinical Resources, Inc.

For sternal placement, locate the anterior axillary fold (armpit). Palpate just medial to the fold while the patient medially rotates the arm against resistance. Place two active electrodes (2 cm apart) horizontally on the chest wall over the muscle mass that arises (approximately 2 cm out from the axillary fold) (Figure 17–28A).

Behavioral Test: Flexion of the arm, abduction of the arm above 90 degrees, medial rotation, and horizontal adduction of arm.

Tracing Comment: **Figure 17–28B** shows SEMG recordings from the clavicular and sternal pectoralis sites, along with anterior deltoids and posterior deltoids. The motions of right arm flexion, chair push-up, and right palm to left ear (medial rotation and adduction) are represented. Note the primary role of anterior deltoid and the clavicular aspect of pectoralis during forward flexion. During a chair push-up, all muscle groups are used for movement and stabilization. When the right palm is moved toward the left ear, both clavicular and sternal aspects are active, with the sternal aspect coming into play toward the end of the movement pattern.

The anterior deltoid also contributes to this movement (raw SEMG).

Also see the tracings for the serratus anterior (Figure 17–22C).

Clinical Considerations: Chronically protruded shoulders can lead to shortening of the internal rotators of the shoulder, which include the pectoralis major. Thoracic kyphosis leads to shortening of the pectoralis.

The brachial plexus, with its diverse connections, is complex. The suprascapular nerve leaves the anterior division of the superior trunk and goes cranially and posteriorly; a short distance more distally, the lateral pectoral nerve goes in the opposite direction. The pectoralis major has many fascial connections to the neck, abdomen, lateral trunk, and upper extremity. The clavicular portion can be seen as an extension of the clavicular portion of the sternocleidomastoid, particularly if the upper extremity is in slight depression/extension and the face is rotated away.

The distal insertion of the clavicular portion is immediately adjacent to the fibers of the anterior deltoid muscle. These muscles are strong synergists and are often

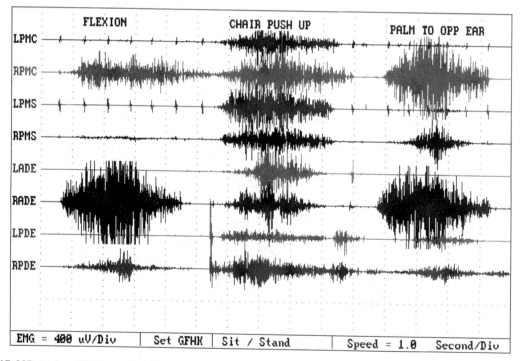

Figure 17–28B Surface EMG recordings from the clavicular (PMC) and sternal (PMS) aspects of pectoralis major, along with anterior (ADE) and posterior (PDE) deltoid during flexion of the arm, chair push-up, and movement of the right palm to left ear during horizontal adduction.

Source: Copyright © Clinical Resources, Inc.

dysfunctional in shoulder conditions. The sternal portion's tendinous insertion can blend into the shoulder capsule. The lower portion of the pectoralis major arises off the aponeurosis of the external obliques. This may be a connection in addition to the latissimus dorsi for the many myofascial patients who complain of shoulder and pelvic pain.

The pectoralis is an accessory respirator, particularly if the upper extremities are weight bearing. Care should be taken to assess breathing habits and correct dysfunctional patterns.

Volume Conduction: Anterior deltoid, sternal or clavicular aspect of pectoralis major, pectoralis minor.

Other Sites of Interest: Deltoids, upper trapezius, lower trapezius, serratus anterior, teres major, the long head of the triceps during movements of the upper extremities; SCM, scalene with extreme respiration.

Artifacts: ECG.

WRIST-TO-WRIST (WIDE) PLACEMENT

Type of Placement: General.

Purpose: General index of tension in the upper extremity, shoulders, neck, and torso.

Clinical Uses: Commonly used in relaxation-based treatments for headache and upper extremity, neck, and chest wall pain.

Location: The active electrodes are placed on a more distal part of the arm. The wrists or backs of the hands are convenient locations. The ground electrode is placed next to one of the active electrodes (**Figure 17–29A**).

Behavioral Test: Systematically ask the patient to tense and relax the muscles of the arm, shoulder, and torso (forearm flexors, extensors, biceps, shoulder elevation, shoulder retraction). The farther away the contracting muscles are from the active electrodes, the lower the recorded SEMG level should be.

Tracing Comment: In **Figure 17–29B** (top to bottom), the wrist-to-wrist placement, upper trapezius (wide) placement, and upper trapezius (narrow) placement on the right side were monitored simultaneously. The left half of the tracing was recorded using a narrow 100- to 200-Hz band pass filter, while the right half was conducted using a wide 25- to 1000-Hz band pass filter. ECG artifact is present during the second half of the

tracing for the two upper panels, but not for the lower panel (narrow upper trapezius placement). ECG artifact is more problematic when the two recording electrodes cross the midline and are placed farther apart. Surface EMG recordings from the left side of the upper back, even when using narrow placements, are typically more contaminated with ECG artifact compared to right-sided placements. In addition, the wider 25- to 1000-Hz filter passes more of the SEMG spectrum along for amplification and, therefore, shows a higher level of RMS microvolts. This is most clearly seen in the lower panel. Although the tracing does not show the heart rate artifact once the filters are changed to 25- to 1000-Hz range, it does show an increase in the SEMG levels (processed SEMG).

Figure 17–29C presents recordings from (top to bottom) the wrist-to-wrist placement, the cervical trapezius (wide) placement for the right side only, and the upper trapezius (narrow) placement for the left side only. The 100- to 200-Hz band pass filter is used, which is usually recommended for the wrist-to-wrist placement. Three sets of activation patterns are seen in the tracing. The

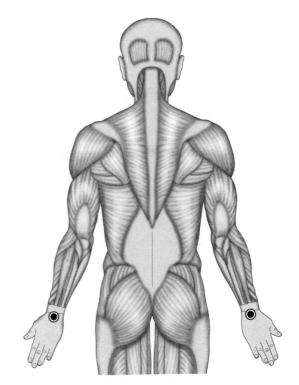

Figure 17–29A Electrode placement for the wrist-to-wrist site.

Source: Copyright © Clinical Resources, Inc.

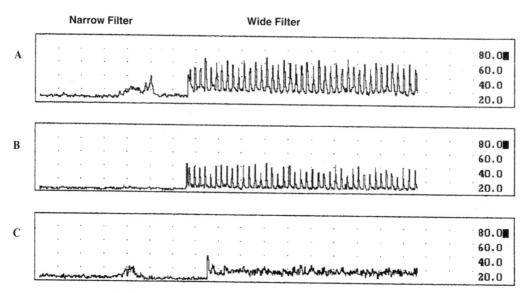

Figure 17–29B Surface EMG recordings from (**A**) wrist-to-wrist placement, (**B**) upper trapezius (wide) placement, and (**C**) upper trapezius (narrow) placement on the right side were monitored simultaneously. The first half of the tracing was recorded using 100- to 200-Hz band pass filter; the second half was conducted using a 25- to 1000-Hz band pass filter.

Source: Copyright © Clinical Resources, Inc.

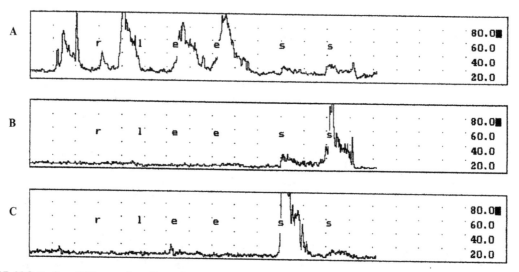

Figure 17–29C Surface EMG recordings from (**A**) wrist-to-wrist placement, (**B**) cervical trapezius (wide) placement for the right side only, and (**C**) upper trapezius (narrow) placement for the left side only are shown using the 100- to 200-Hz band pass filter. Three sets of activation patterns are seen in the tracing. The first set (**r** and **l**) represents right and then left wrist extension. The second (**e** and **e**) represents right and then left elbow flexion. The third (**s** and **s**) represents right and then left shoulder girdle elevation.

Source: Copyright © Clinical Resources, Inc.

first set represents right and then left wrist extension. The second represents right and then left elbow flexion. The third represents right and then left shoulder girdle elevation. Note how the wrist-to-wrist leads pick up volume-conducted SEMG activity from the forearm extensors during wrist extension, from the biceps during elbow flexion, and to a lesser extent from the upper trapezius during shoulder girdle elevation (processed SEMG).

Clinical Considerations: Head, shoulder, arm, hand, and finger position can alter the resting levels. One can readily demonstrate how this placement records from all of the muscles in both upper extremities and upper torso by asking the patient to systematically tense and release each major muscle group in the left upper extremity, left shoulder, right shoulder, and right lower extremity. If the SEMG system allows a choice of filters, the narrow 100- to 200-Hz band pass filter will eliminate the ECG artifact.

Volume Conduction: This placement detects SEMG activity from all of the muscles of the arm, shoulder, and upper back.

Other Sites of Interest: Frontalis (wide) and ankle-to-ankle (wide) to assess and promote generalization. ,

Artifacts: ECG, breathing.

FOREARM FLEXOR/EXTENSOR (WIDE) PLACEMENT

Type of Placement: General.

Purpose: To monitor the general level of muscle tension in the forearm bundles.

Clinical Uses: To study general tension of the body, and the forearm in particular; to assess and treat arm-related pains such as repetitive strain injury; for use in industrial medicine and ergonomics.

Location: One active electrode is placed over the wrist extensor bundle (top of the arm) and the other is placed over the flexor bundle (bottom of the arm). The extensor site is found on the dorsal aspect of the arm, approximately 5 cm distal from the elbow. The practitioner should place the fingers on that surface and ask the patient to extend his or her wrist. Place the electrode in the center of the muscle mass that emerges. The flexor site is located on the ventral aspect of the arm, approximately 5 cm distal from the elbow. Ask the patient to flex his or her wrist. Place the electrode in the center of the muscle mass that emerges (**Figure 17–30A**).

Behavioral Test: Flexion, extension, pronation, and supination of the wrist and hand.

Tracing Comment: In **Figure 17–30B**, SEMG recordings from the wide flexor extensor site are presented along with recordings from wide placements for the flexor and the extensor. Activation patterns during wrist extension, flexion, and cocontraction (making a fist) are

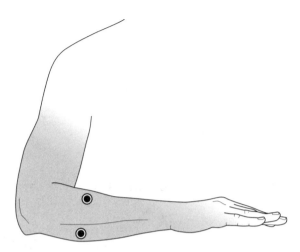

Figure 17–30A Electrode placement for the forearm flexor/extensor (wide) site.

Source: Copyright © Clinical Resources, Inc

presented. This wide placement shows recruitment for all movements, while the wide extensor and wide flexor sites show specificity of function and recruitment only during their movement (processed SEMG).

Clinical Considerations: The SEMG values may change radically as a function of the arm/wrist being supported. Sitting with arms in the lap provides different values than standing with arms at the sides. Degree of pronation/supination or ulnar deviation can also alter resting levels.

This site is commonly used to monitor the upper extremity in cases involving repetitive strain injury or carpal tunnel syndrome. Lundervold[37] studied a large number of normal subjects and patients with occupational myalgias using needle EMG recordings and noted that patients showed increased and prolonged recruitment patterns during typing compared to normal subjects. He observed that activity in the asymptomatic arm could cause recruitment in the symptomatic arm while at rest and that forearm muscle activity could be readily induced by physical or emotional stress. Skubick, Clasby, Donaldson, and Marshall[38] noted that in patients with carpal tunnel syndrome, the forearm flexors and extensors tend to become active during cervical rotation. They attributed this outcome to a return of the tonic neck reflex in these symptomatic individuals. In addition, the SEMG levels of distal segments increase when scapular instability is present. Singh and Karpovich[39] also provide information concerning isotonic and isometric contractions in the flexors and extensors.

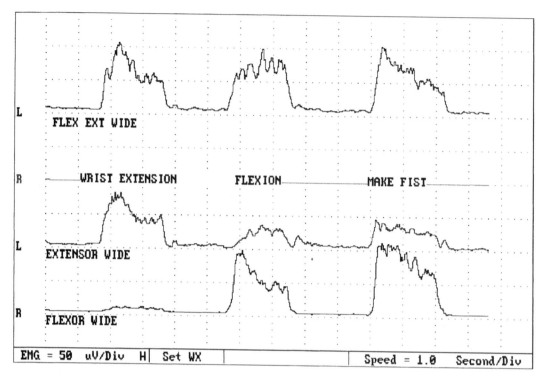

Figure 17–30B Surface EMG recordings from the forearm flexor/extensor site, along with recordings from wide placements of the flexor and extensor sites during the movements of wrist extension, flexion, and cocontraction (making a fist).

Source: Copyright © Clinical Resources, Inc.

Volume Conduction: All of the muscles of the forearm; to a lesser extent, muscles of the upper arm.

Other Sites of Interest: Biceps, triceps, deltoids, upper trapezius, midcervical paraspinals, SCM.

FOREARM EXTENSOR BUNDLE (WIDE) PLACEMENT

Type of Placement: Quasi-specific.

Purpose: To measure the muscle bundle associated with wrist extension (primarily extensor digitorum).

Clinical Uses: Rehabilitation of the wrist and hand, assessment and treatment of repetitive strain injury, industrial medicine, ergonomics.

Location: The extensor site is found on the dorsal aspect of the arm, approximately 5 cm distal from the elbow. The practitioner should place the fingers on that surface and ask the patient to extend his or her wrist. Place the electrodes 3 to 4 cm apart in the center of the muscle mass that emerges, with the electrodes oriented in the direction of the muscle fibers. The wide place-

ment will ensure volume-conducted pickup from the extensor carpi radialis and extensor carpi ulnaris, as well as the extensor digitorum (**Figure 17–31A**).

Behavioral Test: Extension of the wrist.

Tracing Comment: In **Figure 17–31B**, SEMG recordings for both the wide forearm extensor site (upper) and the wide forearm flexor site are presented during left and right wrist flexion. The extensor groups recruit vigorously during wrist extension (raw SEMG).

In **Figure 17–31C**, the flexor and extensor sites for the left arm are monitored. The subject first makes a fist, coactivating both the extensor and flexor groups. This action is followed by wrist extension, and then wrist flexion in the neutral position.

Also see the tracings from the wrist flexors (Figure 17–32B).

Clinical Considerations: Resting values may be affected by arm, wrist, and finger positions, along with the degree of pronation and supination.

This site is commonly used to monitor the upper extremity in cases involving repetitive strain injury or carpal

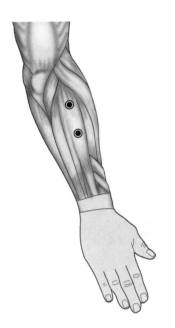

Figure 17–31A Electrode placement for the forearm extensor (wide) site.

Source: Copyright © Clinical Resources, Inc.

tunnel syndrome. Lundervold[37] studied a large number of normal subjects and patients with occupational myalgias, using needle EMG recordings, and he noted that patients showed increased and prolonged recruitment patterns in the extensor carpi radialis during typing compared to normal subjects. He observed that activity in the asymptomatic arm could cause recruitment in the symptomatic arm while at rest and that forearm muscle activity could be readily induced by physical or emotional stress. Skubick et al.[38] noted that in patients with carpal tunnel syndrome, the forearm flexors and extensors tend to become active during cervical rotation. They attributed this effect to a return of the tonic neck reflex in these symptomatic individuals. In addition, the SEMG levels of distal segments increase when scapular instability is present. Singh and Karpovich[39] also provide information concerning isotonic and isometric contractions in the flexors and extensors.

Volume Conduction: Extensor digitorum, brachioradialis, extensor carpi radialis (longus and brevis), and pronator teres.

Other Sites of Interest: Forearm flexor (wide) placement, biceps, triceps, deltoids, upper trapezius, midcervical paraspinals, SCM.

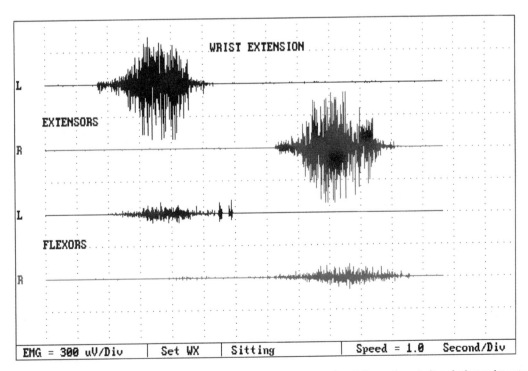

Figure 17–31B Surface EMG recording from the wide forearm extensor (upper) and flexor (lower) sites during wrist extension.

Source: Copyright © Clinical Resources, Inc.

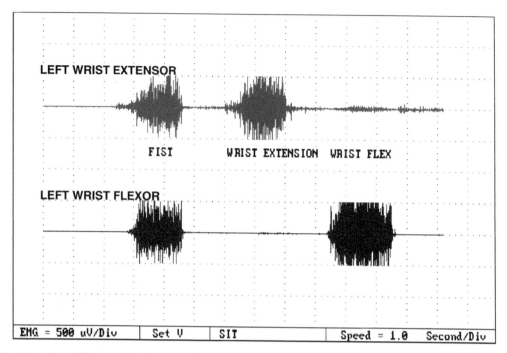

Figure 17–31C Surface EMG recordings from the forearm extensor and flexor (wide) sites during making a fist, wrist extension, and wrist flexion.

Source: Copyright © Clinical Resources, Inc.

FOREARM FLEXOR BUNDLE (WIDE) PLACEMENT

Type of Placement: Quasi-specific.

Purpose: To monitor the muscles associated with wrist flexion.

Clinical Uses: To assess and treat arm pain and repetitive strain injury; used in industrial medicine and ergonomics.

Location: The flexor site is located on the ventral aspect of the arm, approximately 5 cm distal from the elbow. Hold the patient's dorsal side of the arm. Ask the patient to flex his or her wrist, and palpate the muscle mass that emerges. Place two active electrodes 3 to 4 cm apart over the belly of the muscle in the direction of the muscle fibers (**Figure 17–32A**).

Behavioral Test: Flexion of the wrist.

Tracing Comment: In **Figure 17–32B**, both the flexor and extensor bundles are monitored simultaneously during flexion of the left and right wrists (raw SEMG).

Also see the tracings from the wrist extensors (Figure 17–31B).

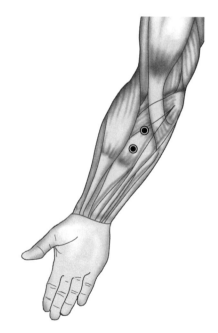

Figure 17–32A Electrode placement for the forearm flexor bundle (wide) site.

Source: Copyright © Clinical Resources, Inc.

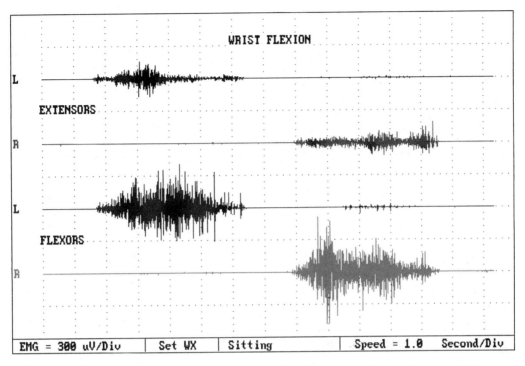

Figure 17–32B Surface EMG recordings from forearm extensor (wide) placement and forearm flexor (wide) placement during left and right wrist flexion.

Source: Copyright © Clinical Resources, Inc.

Clinical Considerations: Position and support of the hand, fingers, and arm may affect SEMG values. The resting tone is greatly affected by arm, finger, and wrist position. Degree of supination or pronation during flexion may affect the readings, depending on electrode placement.

This site is commonly used to monitor the upper extremity in cases involving repetitive strain injury or carpal tunnel syndrome. Lundervold[37] studied a large number of normal subjects and patients with occupational myalgias, using needle EMG recordings, and he noted that patients showed increased and prolonged recruitment patterns during typing compared to normal subjects. He observed that activity in the asymptomatic arm could cause recruitment in the symptomatic arm while at rest and that forearm muscle activity could be readily induced by physical or emotional stress. Skubick et al.[38] noted that in patients with carpal tunnel syndrome, the forearm flexors and extensors tend to become active during cervical rotation. They attributed this effect to a return of the tonic neck reflex in these symptomatic individuals. Singh and Karpovich[39] also provide information concerning isotonic and isometric contractions in the flexors and extensors.

Volume Conduction: Flexor digitorum (superficialis and profundus), flexor carpi (ulnaris and radialis), and flexor pollicis longus.

Other Sites of Interest: Forearm extensor (wide) placement, biceps, triceps, deltoids, upper trapezius, midcervical paraspinals, SCM.

BICEPS–BRACHIUM PLACEMENT

Type of Placement: Specific.

Action: Forearm flexion, supination, and shoulder flexion.

Clinical Uses: Rehabilitation.

Muscle Insertions: The biceps is a two-bellied muscle. The long head arises from the superior margin of the supraglenoid tubercle of the scapula and passes over the head of the humerus. The short head arises from the coracoid process of the scapula. Both insert into the tuberosity of the radius.

Innervation: The musculocutaneous nerve via the lateral cord and spinal nerves C-5 and C-6.

Location: Ask the patient to flex his or her forearm in the supinated position. Palpate the muscle mass in the dorsal aspect of the upper arm that emerges. Place two active electrodes (2 cm apart) parallel to the muscle fibers and in the center of the mass (**Figure 17–33A**, left arm).

> *Variations:* Due to the compartmentalization of this muscle, placing the active electrodes more laterally will emphasize detection of shoulder flexion (in addition to forearm flexion), and placing the electrodes more medially will emphasize detection of adduction and internal rotation. If electrodes are placed too distally with the lateral placement, there will be volume conduction from the brachialis (Figure 17–33A, right arm).

Behavioral Test: Flex the forearm. Resisted flexion augments the signal.

Tracing Comment: The tracings for the biceps also include recordings from other related muscles, such as the triceps, deltoids, brachioradialis, and pronator teres. Refer to the tracings for these sites as well.

For biceps/triceps isolation, see **Figure 17–33B**, in which three sites for placement of electrodes on the biceps and triceps are used. The top three tracings show the lateral, intermediate, and medial aspects of the biceps. The lower three tracings show the lateral, intermediate, and medial aspects of the triceps. Two movements are depicted: resisted elbow flexion in the supinated position and resisted elbow extension. Here, there is clear isolation of the biceps during flexion and fairly clear isolation of the triceps during extension.

There is minor cross-talk to the lateral and medial biceps (raw SEMG).

For the biceps during supination, see **Figure 17–33C**, in which the intermediate biceps and pronator teres are studied during supination and pronation. During supination, the biceps is active while the pronator is quiet. However, during pronation, the pronator teres is active while the biceps is quiet (raw SEMG).

For the biceps during elbow flexion, see **Figure 17–33D**, in which the brachioradialis (top) and the biceps (bottom) are studied during elbow flexion in three positions. During elbow flexion with supination (palm up), both muscles recruit briskly. In the neutral position (thumb up), the muscles display the same pattern, only more reduced. During flexion with pronation (palm down), the biceps is no longer involved and the brachioradialis does all of the work of flexion (raw SEMG).

In **Figure 17–33E**, elbow and shoulder flexion are shown while monitoring the biceps (intermediate), anterior deltoids, long head of triceps, lateral triceps, posterior deltoids, and latissimus dorsi. During elbow flexion, the biceps show a very strong recruitment pattern. During shoulder flexion, the anterior deltoid recruits robustly, with some recruitment seen in the biceps.

Clinical Considerations: Positioning of the arm can dramatically alter the resting tone and recruitment patterns. Consider how the arm is supported while in the seated position. As seen in Figure 17–33D, the degree of supination/pronation is important. Length–tension relationships that are altered by the amount of flexion at the elbow can dramatically alter biceps recruitment patterns.

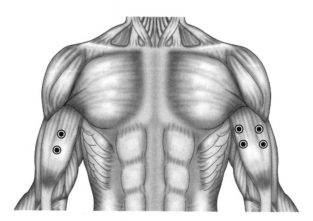

Figure 17–33A Electrode placement for the biceps-brachium site.
Source: Copyright © Clinical Resources, Inc.

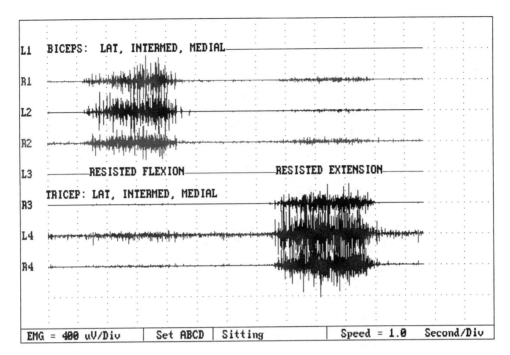

Figure 17–33B Surface EMG recordings from the biceps and triceps are presented. The top three tracings show the (**R1**) lateral, (**L2**) intermediate, and (**R2**) medial aspects of the biceps. The lower three tracings show the (**R3**) lateral, (**L4**) intermediate, and (**R4**) medial aspects of the triceps. Resisted elbow flexion and extension are presented.

Source: Copyright © Clinical Resources, Inc.

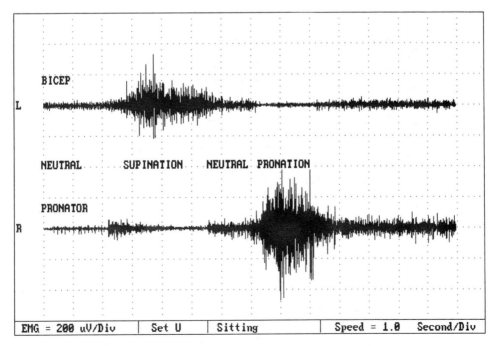

Figure 17–33C Surface EMG recordings from the biceps and the pronator teres are presented during supination and pronation.

Source: Copyright © Clinical Resources, Inc.

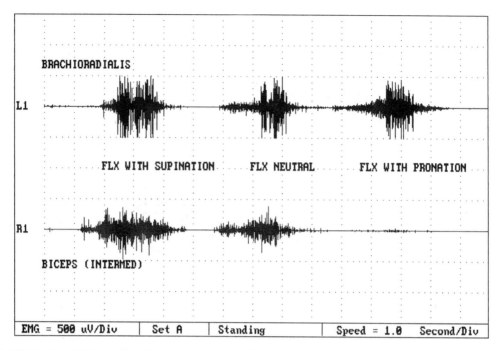

Figure 17–33D Surface EMG recordings from the brachioradialis and the biceps are shown during elbow flexion in the supinated and pronated positions. Note the absence of biceps recruitment during pronated elbow flexion.

Source: Copyright © Clinical Resources, Inc.

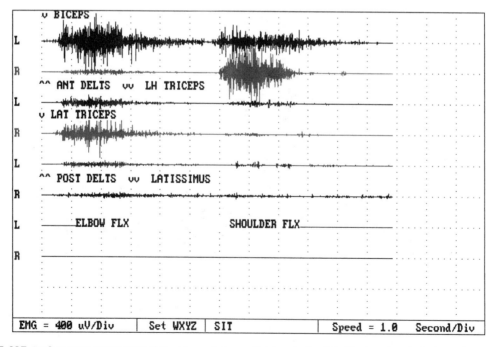

Figure 17–33E Surface EMG monitoring of the biceps (intermediate), anterior deltoids, long head of triceps, lateral triceps, posterior deltoids, and latissimus dorsi during elbow and shoulder flexion.

Source: Copyright © Clinical Resources, Inc.

Recruitment of the biceps during elbow flexion is enhanced during supination and diminished during pronation.[16,40]

Volume Conduction: Brachialis, deltoids, triceps, forearm, extensors.

Other Sites of Interest: Brachioradialis during flexion of the forearm; brachioradialis, anterior deltoid, suprascapular fossa site (supraspinatus) during abduction of the arm; triceps.

Referred Pain Considerations: Trigger points in this muscle refer pain mainly upward, to the anterior deltoid region.[17]

TRICEPS PLACEMENT

Type of Placement: Specific.

Action: Extension of the elbow and adduction and extension of the shoulder.

Clinical Uses: Rehabilitation.

Muscle Insertions: The long head of this three-bellied muscle arises from infraglenoid lip of the scapula; the medial and lateral heads arise from the medial and lateral aspects of the radial groove of the humerus, respec-

tively. All three fuse together and insert on the olecranon process of the ulna via a common tendon.

Innervation: Branches of the radial nerve via the posterior cord and the spinal nerves C-7 and C-8.

Location: To monitor from the long head of the triceps, two active electrodes (2 cm apart) are placed parallel to the muscle fibers, 2 cm medial from midline of the arm, approximately 50% of the distance between the acromion and the olecranon or elbow. Caution should be exercised not to place the electrodes too distally. Because electrode position on the skin relative to the muscles below may change as a function of arm/palm position, palpate and place the electrodes in the arm position to be studied. To place the electrode on the lateral aspect of the triceps muscle, palpate the lateral aspect of the triceps region during an isometric contraction. As with the long head placement, two active electrodes (2 cm apart) are placed parallel to the muscle fibers, approximately 2 cm lateral from the midline of the arm, approximately 50% of the distance between the acromion and the olecranon or elbow (**Figure 17–34A**).

Behavioral Test: Extension of the forearm (resistance of this movement augments the SEMG signal).

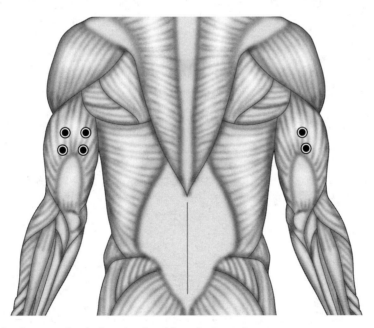

Figure 17–34A Electrode placement for the long head and lateral triceps sites.
Source: Copyright © Clinical Resources, Inc.

Tracing Comment: In **Figure 17–34B**, SEMG recordings from the right posterior deltoid, medial triceps, lateral triceps, and infraspinatus are shown during isometric extension with the elbow at 90 degrees with three angles of shoulder flexion, and again with the elbow at 0 degrees and resisted extension of the shoulder and arm. The posterior deltoid appears to be deactivated when the shoulder is at 160 degrees of flexion; it becomes more active as the shoulder reaches 90 degrees of flexion. Both aspects of triceps are active during all four movements. The level of recruitment is stronger when the arm is straight than when it is bent, and particularly when the shoulder and elbow are extended. The infraspinatus is active primarily during the shoulder and arm extension (raw SEMG).

Figure 17–34C presents SEMG recordings from the right posterior deltoid, general triceps, and infraspinatus during resisted elbow flexion at 90 degrees, with the shoulder flexed to 90 degrees. This level of shoulder flexion allows recruitment of the triceps to be seen (raw SEMG).

See the biceps tracings for additional tracings of the triceps (Figure 17–33B).

Clinical Considerations: Surface EMG values may differ when the patient is sitting with the arm supported versus when the patient is standing. Arm position may affect the recordings and should be noted.

Although the medial head of triceps is the main "workhorse" for elbow extension,[16,41] the long head of the triceps is strongly involved in adduction.[31]

Volume Conduction: Biceps, posterior and medial deltoids.

Other Sites of Interest: Forearm extensors; latissimus dorsi and teres major during adduction and extension of the shoulder.

Referred Pain Considerations: Trigger points in this muscle project primarily up and down the posterior aspect of the arm and to the lateral epicondyle, with potential spillover into the fourth and fifth digits.[17]

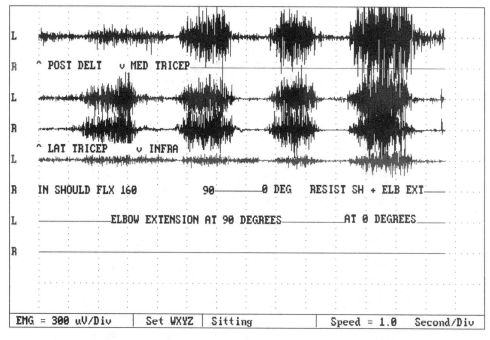

Figure 17–34B Surface EMG recordings from the right posterior deltoid, medial triceps, lateral triceps, and infraspinatus are shown during isometric extension with the elbow at 90 degrees with three angles of shoulder flexion and again with the elbow at 0 degrees and resisted extension of the shoulder and arm.

Source: Copyright © Clinical Resources, Inc.

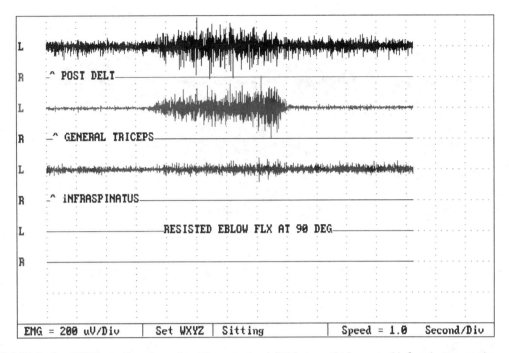

L

R _^ POST DELT

L

R _^ GENERAL TRICEPS

L

R _^ INFRASPINATUS

L _____RESISTED EBLOW FLX AT 90 DEG_____

R

| EMG = 200 uV/Div | Set WXYZ | Sitting | Speed = 1.0   Second/Div |

Figure 17–34C Surface EMG recordings from the right posterior deltoid, general triceps, and infraspinatus are shown during resisted elbow flexion at 90 degrees, with the shoulder flexed to 90 degrees.

Source: Copyright © Clinical Resources, Inc.

BRACHIORADIALIS PLACEMENT

Type of Placement: Quasi-specific.

Action: Elbow flexion.

Clinical Uses: Rehabilitation.

Muscle Insertions: This muscle arises from the lateral supracondylar ridge of the humerus and the related intermuscular septum and inserts on the tendinous attachments of the styloid process of the wrist.

Innervation: The radial nerve from the posterior cord and spinal nerves C-5 and C-6.

Location: Palpate the muscle mass just distal to the elbow while resisting elbow flexion with the wrist in the neutral position (thumb up). Two active electrodes, 2 cm apart, are placed approximately 4 cm distally from the lateral epicondyle of the elbow on the medial fleshy mass that covers that area, so that they run parallel to the muscle fibers (**Figure 17–35A**).

Behavioral Test: Flex the forearm.

Tracing Comment: In **Figure 17–35B**, three muscle sites are monitored: extensor carpi ulnaris, extensor

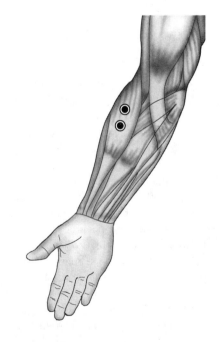

Figure 17–35A Electrode placement for the brachioradialis site.

Source: Copyright © Clinical Resources, Inc.

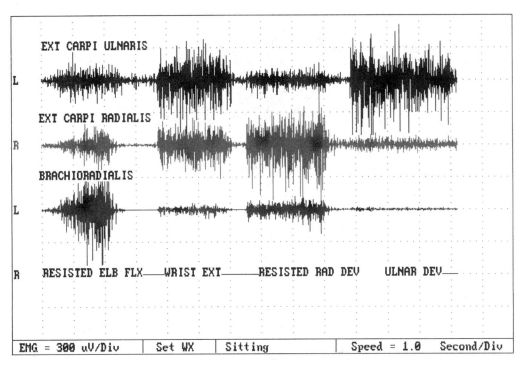

Figure 17–35B Surface EMG recordings from the extensor carpi ulnaris, extensor carpi radialis, and brachioradialis during resisted elbow flexion, wrist extension, resisted radial deviation, and ulnar deviation.

Source: Copyright © Clinical Resources, Inc.

carpi radialis, and brachioradialis. Four isolated movements are shown with the elbow at 90 degrees, thumb up. During resisted elbow flexion with the wrist relaxed, brachioradialis shows the strongest activation pattern with suspected cross-talk at the extensor carpi ulnaris and extensor carpi radialis sites. During wrist extension with the rest of the arm well supported and relaxed, the extensor carpi ulnaris and extensor carpi radialis sites show strong burst patterns. Activation in the brachioradialis site during this movement probably reflects minor cross-talk. During resisted radial deviation, the extensor carpi radialis shows its strong recruitment pattern, with minor cross-talk or compensatory stabilization activity noted at the extensor carpi ulnaris and brachioradialis sites. During ulnar deviation, the extensor carpi ulnaris shows its strongest recruitment pattern, with minor cross-talk or stabilization activity noted at the extensor carpi radialis site. There is little or no cross-talk or activation noted at the brachioradialis site during this movement (raw SEMG).

Also see the tracings for the biceps (Figure 17–33D), the flexor carpi radialis (Figure 17–40B), and the flexor carpi ulnaris (Figure 17–41B).

Clinical Considerations: The position of the wrist can affect the level of recruitment, as is seen in Figure 17–33D. The degree of elbow flexion can affect the amplitude and time of recruitment due to length–tension relationships. The activity of this muscle is augmented during quick elbow flexion movements, when a weight is to be lifted, and when the arm is in the neutral position.[16]

Volume Conduction: Volume conduction is a major problem. Signals from extensor carpi radialis (longus and brevis) and brachioradialis are common.

Other Sites of Interest: Biceps brachium during forearm flexion, and extensor carpi radialis (longus and brevis) during wrist extension and grasping.

Referred Pain Considerations: Trigger points in this muscle refer pain primarily to the lateral epicondyle, as well as down the length of the muscle to the web of the hand.[17]

VENTRAL FOREARM (PRONATOR TERES) PLACEMENT

Type of Placement: Quasi-specific.

Action: Pronation of the arm.

Clinical Uses: Rehabilitation.

Muscle Insertions: The pronator teres arises from the humeral head of the epicondyle and the ulnar head of the coronoid process, and inserts on the middle of the lateral surface of the radius.

Innervation: The median nerve through spinal nerves C-6 and C-7.

Location: Support the arm in the palm-up (supinated) position. Palpate in the soft valley in the middle of the ventral aspect of the forearm just below the elbow. Ask the patient to pronate (palm up to palm down) the arm and feel for the muscle mass. Place two active electrodes (2 cm apart) on an oblique angle so that they run parallel to the muscle fibers (**Figure 17–36A**).

Behavioral Test: Pronate the arm.

Tracing Comment: In **Figure 17–36B**, recordings are made from the flexor carpi radialis and pronator teres

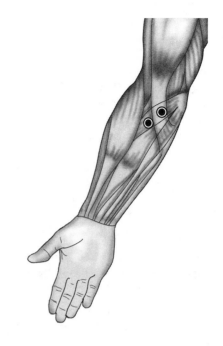

Figure 17–36A Electrode placement for the pronator teres site.

Source: Copyright © Clinical Resources, Inc.

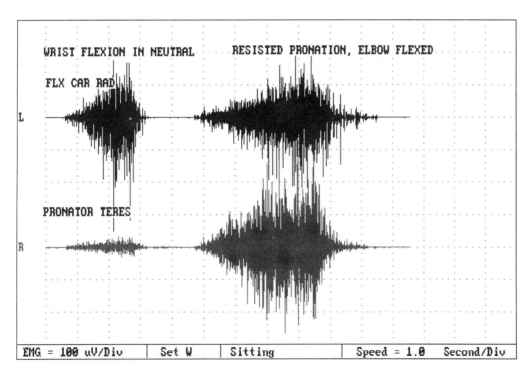

Figure 17–36B Surface EMG recordings from the flexor carpi radialis and the pronator teres during neutral wrist flexion and resisted pronation.

Source: Copyright © Clinical Resources, Inc.

placement. The elbow is bent at 90 degrees with the wrist in a neutral position (thumb up). Two isolated movements are shown. During wrist flexion in the neutral position, the flexor carpi radialis shows a clear burst pattern. Minor cross-talk is suspected at the pronator site. Resisted pronation was accomplished by securing the patient's wrist, then asking the patient to rotate the arm toward the palm-down position while keeping the fingers relaxed. Note the poor separation of these two recording sites, suggesting cross-talk between recording sites (raw SEMG).

Also see the tracings for the biceps (Figure 17–33B).

Clinical Considerations: Support of the arm may affect the initial resting tone of the muscle. The beginning wrist position would, of course, affect the observed recruitment pattern. The degree of elbow flexion does not appear to affect the activity in this muscle.[16]

Volume Conduction: Expect considerable cross-talk from the flexor carpi radialis, palmaris longus, and brachioradialis.

Other Sites of Interest: Brachioradialis.

Referred Pain Considerations: Trigger points in this muscle commonly refer pain to the base of the thumb.[17]

EXTENSOR CARPI ULNARIS PLACEMENT

Type of Placement: Quasi-specific.

Action: Wrist extension, ulnar deviation.

Clinical Uses: Hand rehabilitation, industrial ergonomics.

Muscle Insertions: This muscle arises from the common extensor tendon from the lateral epicondyle of the humerus and the aponeurosis from the border of the ulna, and inserts on the pisiform bone in the hand and the fifth metacarpal.

Innervation: The radial nerve from spinal nerves C-6, C-7, and C-8.

Location: Support the patient's arm in the palm-down position. Palpate the ulnar (little finger) side of the arm a few centimeters below the elbow. Have the patient do an ulnar deviation of the wrist, and palpate for the active muscle mass. Place two active electrodes 2 cm apart in the direction of the muscle fibers (**Figure 17–37A**).

Behavioral Test: Ulnar deviation of the wrist.

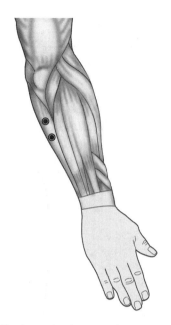

Figure 17–37A Electrode placement for the extensor carpi ulnaris.

Source: Copyright © Clinical Resources, Inc.

Tracing Comment: In **Figure 17–37B**, extensor carpi radialis and extensor carpi ulnaris sites are monitored while the wrist is supported in the neutral position (thumb up), and the hand is out over the edge of the table. Radial deviation is resisted to augment and isolate the recruitment pattern. Note the burst of activity at the extensor carpi radialis site. Next, an unresisted ulnar deviation is conducted. Clear isolation of the extensor carpi ulnaris is present. Finally, an unresisted wrist extension is examined, with both sites showing a synergy pattern (raw SEMG).

Also see the brachioradialis tracings (Figure 17–35B).

Clinical Considerations: The degree of support of the arm affects the resting tone. Wrist position alters initial resting amplitudes and recruitment patterns.

Volume Conductor: Extensor carpi radialis, brachioradialis, and extensor digitorum.

Other Sites of Interest: Extensor carpi radialis, brachioradialis, flexor carpi ulnaris.

Referred Pain Considerations: Trigger points in this muscle refer pain to the dorsal side of the wrist.[17]

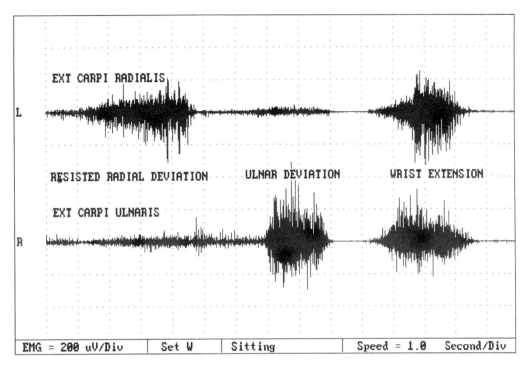

Figure 17–37B Surface EMG recordings from the extensor carpi radialis and extensor carpi ulnaris sites during resisted radial deviation, unresisted ulnar deviation, and wrist extension.

Source: Copyright © Clinical Resources, Inc.

EXTENSOR CARPI RADIALIS (LONGUS AND BREVIS) PLACEMENT

Type of Placement: Quasi-specific.

Action: Wrist extension, abduction, radial deviation.

Clinical Uses: Hand rehabilitation, industrial ergonomics.

Muscle Insertions: The brevis component arises from the common head of the lateral epicondyle of the humerus and related ligaments and inserts on the base of the third metacarpal. The longus component arises from the margin of the humerus and related septum and inserts on the base of the second metacarpal.

Innervation: The radial nerve via the spinal nerves at C-6 and C-7.

Location: Ask the patient to flex the wrist and palpate the muscle mass approximately 5 cm distal from the lateral epicondyle of the elbow, on the dorsal side of the arm just lateral to the brachioradialis. Place two active electrodes 2 cm apart over the muscle mass that emerges, with the electrodes running in the direction of the muscle fibers (**Figure 17–38A**).

Behavioral Test: Wrist extension and radial deviation.

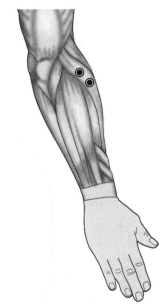

Figure 17–38A Electrode placement for the extensor carpi radialis (longus and brevis) site.

Source: Copyright © Clinical Resources, Inc.

Tracing Comment: In **Figure 17–38B**, SEMG recordings from the extensor carpi radialis, extensor indicis proprius, and abductor pollicis sites while the wrist was supported in the neutral position (thumb up) are presented. Three movements were studied in isolation:

1. During wrist extension with the fingers remaining relaxed, the extensor carpi radialis shows clear isolation.
2. During extension of the first finger with the wrist in the neutral position, a clear burst pattern is seen at the extensor indicis proprius site not involving abductor pollicis. Some activity is also noted in the extensor carpi radialis. It is uncertain as to whether this is a synergy pattern or cross-talk.
3. During thumb and finger extension (spreading the palm), a clear burst pattern is seen from the abductor pollicis site, along with strong activity from extensor indicis proprius. Extensor carpi radialis shows some minor activity (raw SEMG).

Also see the tracings for the brachioradialis (Figure 17–35B), the extensor carpi ulnaris (Figure 17–37B), and the extensor digitorum (Figure 17–39B).

Clinical Considerations: The way in which the wrist is supported may affect SEMG values associated with resting tone. Because finger extension activity is noted at this site (Figure 17–38B), finger position may also affect recording levels. This site is known to play a role in the power grip.[42]

Volume Conduction: Brachioradialis and extensor digitorum.

Other Sites of Interest: Extensor carpi ulnaris and finger extensors during extension; flexor carpi radialis during ulnar deviation; flexor carpi ulnaris during flexion.

Referred Pain Considerations: Trigger points in these muscles refer pain primarily to the lateral epicondyle, lightly over the dorsum of the arm, and the dorsal aspect of the web of the thumb.[17]

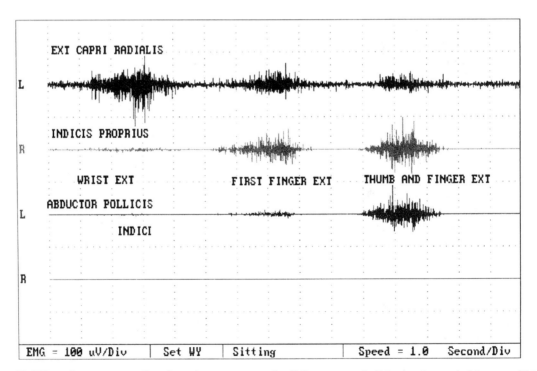

Figure 17–38B Surface EMG recordings from the extensor carpi radialis, extensor indicis proprius, and abductor pollicis during wrist extension, first-finger extension, and thumb and finger extension.

Source: Copyright © Clinical Resources, Inc.

EXTENSOR DIGITORUM PLACEMENT

Type of Placement: Quasi-specific.

Action: Finger extension.

Clinical Uses: Hand rehabilitation.

Muscle Insertions: This muscle arises from the lateral epicondyle of the humerus, the lateral collateral ligament, and the annular radial ligament and related fascia, and joins the common extensor tendon of the second to fifth fingers.

Innervation: The radial nerve via the posterior cord and the spinal nerves C-6, C-7, and C-8.

Location: Palpate the middle of the forearm approximately three quarters of the distance between the elbow and the wrist while the patient extends his or her fingers. Place two active electrodes, 2 cm apart, over the palpable muscle mass, placing them in the direction of the muscle fibers (**Figure 17–39A**).

Behavioral Test: Finger extension.

Tracing Comment: **Figure 17–39B** shows recordings from the extensor digitorum and extensor carpi radialis

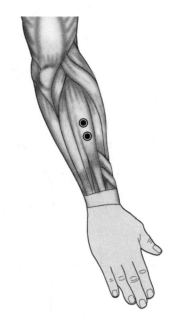

Figure 17–39A Electrode placement for the extensor digitorum site.

Source: Copyright © Clinical Resources, Inc.

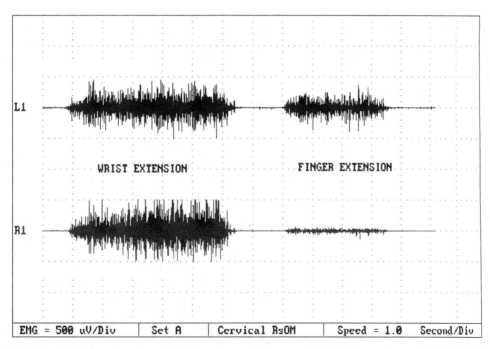

Figure 17–39B Surface EMG recordings from (**L1**) the extensor digitorum and (**R1**) the extensor carpi radialis during wrist extension and finger extension.

Source: Copyright © Clinical Resources, Inc.

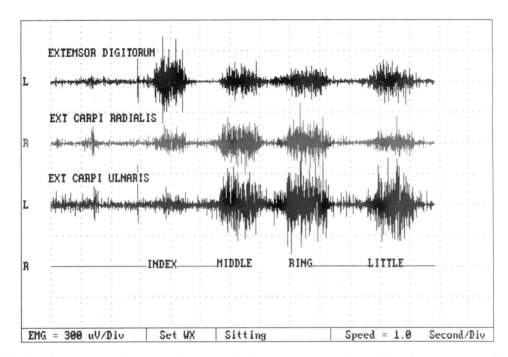

Figure 17–39C Surface EMG recordings from the extensor digitorum, extensor carpi radialis, and extensor carpi ulnaris with the wrist in neutral, with resisted solitary extension of the index, middle, ring, and little fingers.

Source: Copyright © Clinical Resources, Inc.

sites during two movements while the arm and hand are fully supported.

1. During wrist extension, recruitment from both sites is noted.
2. During finger extension, isolation at the extensor digitorum site is noted (raw SEMG).

In **Figure 17–39C**, three muscle sites are monitored (top down): extensor digitorum, extensor carpi radialis, and extensor carpi ulnaris. In this tracing, each finger is extended individually against resistance while the hand is supported in the neutral position in the lap. Under these conditions, the extensor digitorum placement now shows recruitment during extension of each of the four fingers. The extensor radialis and extensor carpi radialis are also active during each movement. Note that unresisted extension of the fingers yields a different pattern of recruitment (raw SEMG).

Also see the tracings for the extensor carpi radialis (Figure 17–38B).

Clinical Considerations: The level of support for the arm, wrist, and fingers can affect the resting tone. Wrist position (deviation) can affect the magnitude of recruitment during finger movement.

Volume Conduction: By placing the electrodes distally, one can better isolate the finger extensors from the wrist flexors. However, volume conduction from extensor digiti minimi and extensor carpi ulnaris may be a problem.

Other Sites of Interest: The finger flexors during a strong palmar grasp.

Referred Pain Considerations: Trigger points in this muscle project pain down the forearm to the back of the hand and sometimes to the ring or middle finger. Projections to the lateral epicondyle are known to occur from trigger points in the ring and little finger extensors.[17]

FLEXOR CARPI RADIALIS AND PALMARIS LONGUS PLACEMENT

Type of Placement: Quasi-specific.

Action: Wrist flexion and radial deviation.

Clinical Uses: Hand rehabilitation.

Muscle Insertions: The flexor carpi radialis muscle arises from the medial epicondyle of the humerus and related superficial fascia, and inserts on the palmar surface of the base of the second metacarpal. The palmaris longus muscle arises from the medial epicondyle of the humerus and radiates into the palmar aponeurosis.

Innervation: The median nerve via the spinal nerves C-6 and C-7.

Location: Support the arm with the fingers while palpating the ventral aspect of the forearm near the elbow on the medial (little finger) side of the arm. Ask the patient to flex the wrist. Place two active electrodes, 2 cm apart, over that muscle mass so that they run in the direction of the muscle fibers (**Figure 17–40A**).

Behavioral Test: Wrist flexion.

Tracing Comment: In **Figure 17–40B**, the flexor carpi radialis and brachioradialis sites are examined while the elbow is flexed to 90 degrees and the thumb is up. First, the wrist is in radial deviation with slight flexion. A very clear separation of recordings is noted between the two sites, with the flexor carpi radialis showing a strong burst of activity. Next, the elbow flexion is resisted at

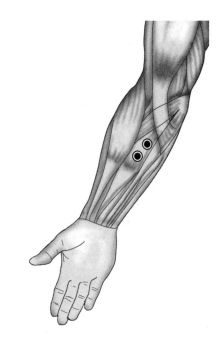

Figure 17–40A Electrode placement for the flexor carpi radialis and palmaris longus site.

Source: Copyright © Clinical Resources, Inc.

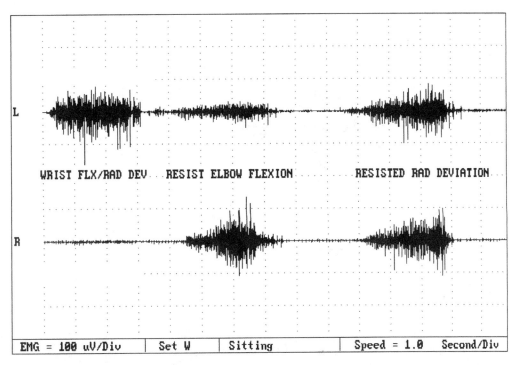

Figure 17–40B Surface EMG recordings from (**L**) the flexor carpi radialis and (**R**) the brachioradialis during wrist flexion and radial deviation, resisted elbow flexion, and resisted radial deviation.

Source: Copyright © Clinical Resources, Inc.

the forearm. Here the brachioradialis shows a strong burst of activity, with minor activity at the flexor carpi radialis site. Finally, an isolated radial deviation is studied with resistance applied to the top of the thumb. Note the coactivation (raw SEMG).

In **Figure 17–40C**, both the flexor carpi radialis and flexor digitorum superficialis sites are studied. Simple wrist flexion with fingers relaxed is conducted from the neutral position. Clear separation between the wrist flexors and finger flexors is noted (raw SEMG).

In **Figure 17–40D**, the flexor carpi radialis and flexor carpi ulnaris sites are studied with the wrist supported in the neutral position. Flexion in midline, with ulnar deviation, and with radial deviation are studied. In the midline movement, both muscle sites are activated. During the flexion with ulnar deviation, only the flexor carpi ulnaris is activated. During the flexion with radial deviation, only the flexor carpi radialis is activated (raw SEMG).

Also see the tracings for the flexor digitorum superficialis (Figure 17–42B).

Clinical Considerations: Support of the arm and the hand may affect resting baseline levels. Deviation of the wrist can alter recruitment patterns. Interesting information regarding the compartmentalization of this muscle is available in the chapter by McMahon et al. in Anderson, Hobart, and Danoff's book.[43]

Volume Conduction: Even with closely spaced miniature electrodes, it is impossible to separate the SEMG activity of the flexor carpi radialis from that of the palmaris longus. This placement may also record from the pronator teres.

Other Sites of Interest: Flexor digitorum superficialis and flexor carpi ulnaris during wrist flexion; extensor carpi radialis (longus and brevis) during abduction of the wrist; wrist extensor muscle groups during extension.

Referred Pain Considerations: Trigger points in this muscle project pain to the center of the volar wrist crease.[17]

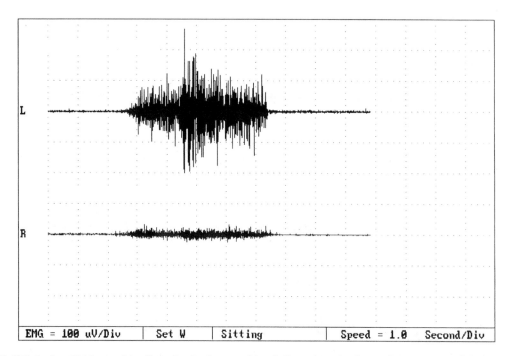

| EMG = 100 uV/Div | Set W | Sitting | Speed = 1.0 Second/Div |

Figure 17–40C Surface EMG recordings from (**L**) the flexor carpi radialis and (**R**) the flexor digitorum superficialis during wrist flexion with fingers very relaxed.

Source: Copyright © Clinical Resources, Inc.

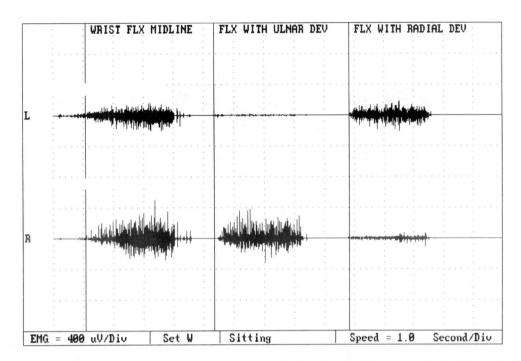

Figure 17–40D Surface EMG recordings from (**L**) the flexor carpi radialis and (**R**) the flexor carpi ulnaris during wrist flexion at midline, wrist flexion with ulnar deviation, and wrist flexion with radial deviation.

Source: Copyright © Clinical Resources, Inc.

FLEXOR CARPI ULNARIS PLACEMENT

Type of Placement: Quasi-specific.

Action: Flexion and adduction of the wrist.

Clinical Uses: Hand rehabilitation.

Muscle Insertions: This muscle arises from the medial epicondyle of the humerus and the olecranon and upper two thirds of the ulna, and inserts on the pisiform bone of the wrist and extends down to the fifth metacarpal.

Innervation: The ulnar nerve via the spinal nerves at C-8 and T-1.

Location: Support the arm while palpating the medial (little finger) aspect of the forearm, approximately 2% of the distance from the elbow to the wrist. Ask the patient to deviate the hand toward the little finger side. Place two active electrodes, 2 cm apart, over the palpable muscle mass in the direction of the muscle fibers (**Figure 17–41A**).

Behavioral Test: Adduction and flexion of the wrist.

Tracing Comment: **Figure 17–41B** is recorded from the flexor carpi ulnaris, flexor carpi radialis, and brachiora-

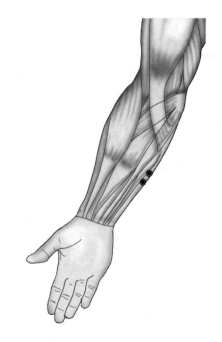

Figure 17–41A Electrode placement for the flexor carpi ulnaris site.

Source: Copyright © Clinical Resources, Inc.

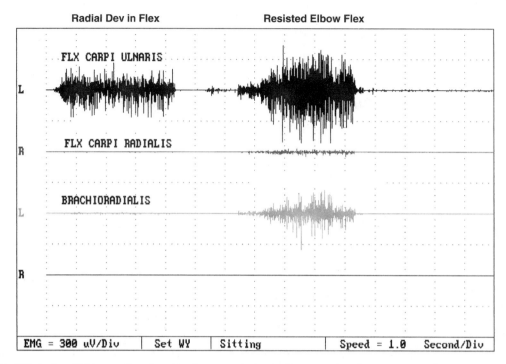

Figure 17–41B Surface EMG recordings from the flexor carpi ulnaris, flexor carpi radialis, and brachioradialis during radial deviation in flexion and resisted elbow flexion.

Source: Copyright © Clinical Resources, Inc.

dialis sites. Two movements are studied with the arm supported and the elbow flexed at 90 degrees with the thumb up. Radial deviation of the wrist during flexion is contrasted to resisted elbow flexion. The flexor carpi ulnaris shows a strong burst of activity during the first movement. During resisted elbow flexion, the ulnaris site shows a very strong burst pattern, along with the brachioradialis (raw SEMG).

Also see the tracing for the flexor carpi radialis (Figure 17–40D).

Clinical Considerations: Adequate support of the arm may play a role in resting SEMG levels. Wrist position affects recruitment patterns.

Volume Conduction: Flexor digitorum superficialis.

Other Sites of Interest: Extensor carpi ulnaris, flexor carpi radialis, and brachioradialis sites.

Referred Pain Considerations: Trigger points in this muscle project pain to the ulnar side of the volar aspect of the wrist.[17]

FLEXOR DIGITORUM SUPERFICIALIS PLACEMENT

Type of Placement: Quasi-specific.

Action: Flexor of the wrist and the second through fifth fingers.

Clinical Uses: Hand rehabilitation.

Muscle Insertions: This muscle arises from the medial epicondyle of the humerus, the coronoid process of the ulna, and the radius. The muscle ends in four tendons, which insert on the lateral bony crests in the center of the middle phalanges of the second to fifth digits.

Innervation: The median nerve via the spinal nerves C-7, C-8, and T-1.

Location: With the wrist supported, palpate in the middle of the forearm on the ventral side, approximately three quarters of the distance from the elbow to the wrist. Ask the patient to flex only the fingers and not the wrist. Place two active electrodes, 2 cm apart, over the area where the greatest movement is felt, in the direction of the muscle fibers (**Figure 17–42A**).

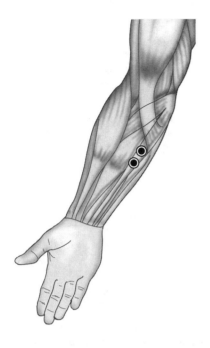

Behavioral Test: Finger flexion, while avoiding wrist flexion.

Tracing Comment: In **Figure 17–42B**, recordings are taken from the flexor carpi radialis and the flexor digitorum superficialis. The arm is supported up to the wrist, and wrist flexion is studied in the neutral position with the fingers relaxed. The fingers are then flexed without moving the wrist (raw SEMG).

Also see the tracing from the flexor carpi radialis (Figure 17–40C).

Clinical Considerations: Adequate support of the arm and wrist may affect resting levels.

Volume Conduction: If placed too close to flexor carpi radialis, cross-talk will occur.

Other Sites of Interest: Wrist flexors during grasping; finger extensors.

Referred Pain Considerations: Trigger points in the radial head of the flexor digitorum superficialis project pain down to the middle finger, while a trigger point in the humeral head projects pain into the ring and little fingers.[17]

Figure 17–42A Electrode placement for the flexor digitorum superficialis site.

Source: Copyright © Clinical Resources, Inc.

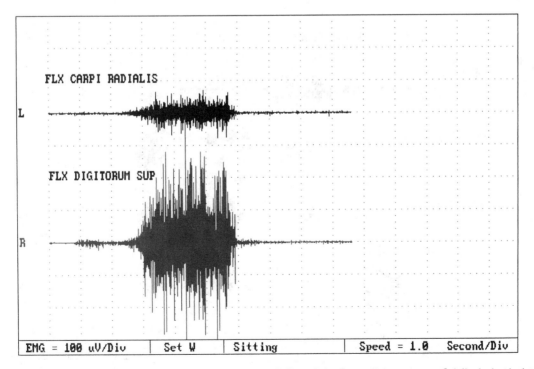

Figure 17–42B Surface EMG recordings from the flexor carpi radialis and the flexor digitorum superficialis during isolated flexion of the fingers.

Source: Copyright © Clinical Resources, Inc.

ABDUCTOR POLLICIS LONGUS AND EXTENSOR POLLICIS BREVIS PLACEMENT

Type of Placement: Quasi-specific.

Action: Abduct and extend the thumb.

Clinical Uses: Hand rehabilitation.

Muscle Insertions: The abductor pollicis longus arises from the dorsal surface of the ulna and radius, along with the interosseous membrane, and inserts on the base of the first metacarpal. The extensor pollicis brevis arises more distally from the ulna and radius, along with the associated interosseous membrane, and inserts on the base of the proximal phalanx of the thumb.

Innervation: The radial nerve from the spinal nerves C-6, C-7, and C-8.

Location: Palpate the dorsal aspect of the forearm just above the wrist on the thumb side while the patient abducts the thumb. Two active electrodes, 2 cm apart, are placed on an oblique angle approximately 4 cm above the wrist on that palpable muscle mass (**Figure 17–43A**).

Behavioral Test: Abduction of the thumb (thumb up).

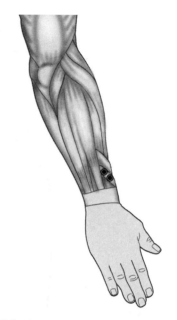

Figure 17–43A Electrode placement for the abductor pollicis longus and extensor pollicis brevis site.
Source: Copyright © Clinical Resources, Inc.

Tracing Comment: In **Figure 17–43B**, four muscle sites were monitored (top to bottom): abductor pollicis

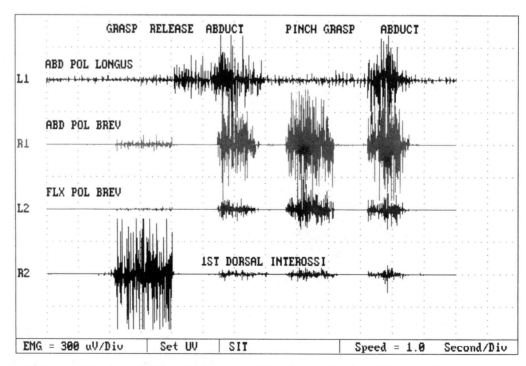

Figure 17–43B Surface EMG recordings from the abductor pollicis longus, abductor pollicis brevis, flexor pollicis brevis, and first dorsal interosseus are presented during a grasp, release, abduction, pincher grasp, and second abduction.
Source: Copyright © Clinical Resources, Inc.

longus, abductor pollicis brevis, flexor pollicis brevis, and first dorsal interosseus. The hand and wrist are supported in the neutral position (thumb up). Five movements were studied.

1. With grasping a cup, the first dorsal interosseus shows a strong burst of activity with minor activity in the abductor pollicis longus and brevis.
2. With releasing the cup, a small burst of activity from abductor pollicis longus is seen.
3. When the thumb is abducted, the abductor pollicis brevis and longus show a strong burst of activity, with minor recruitment noted at the flexor pollicis brevis.
4. With a pincher grasp, the abductor pollicis brevis shows a strong burst of activity, along with a moderate burst from the flexor pollicis brevis.
5. With the final abduction of the thumb, the same pattern of recruitment is seen as during the earlier abduction (raw SEMG).

Clinical Considerations: Adequate support of the arm and the wrist may affect resting levels. Without needle EMG recordings, it would be difficult to isolate specific movements of the different elements of the thumb and its joints. This SEMG recording reflects general movements of extension of the thumb.

Volume Conduction: If the electrodes are placed too close to the extensor digitorum and extensor digiti minimi, cross-talk will occur.

Other Sites of Interest: Adductor pollicis brevis and flexor pollicis brevis.

FIRST DORSAL INTEROSSEUS PLACEMENT

Type of Placement: Specific.

Action: Index finger abductor.

Clinical Uses: Hand rehabilitation.

Muscle Insertions: This muscle arises from the first phalanx of the thumb and index finger and inserts on the second phalanx of the index finger.

Innervation: The ulnar nerve via spinal nerves C-8 and T-1.

Location: Two active electrodes are placed on the dorsal surface of the hand in the web space between the index finger and the thumb, parallel to the direction of the finger. This muscle can easily be palpated during the pincher grasp (thumb opposes index finger) (**Figure 17–44**).

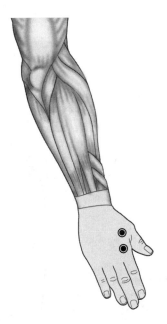

Figure 17–44 Electrode placement for the first dorsal interosseus site.

Source: Copyright © Clinical Resources, Inc.

Behavioral Test: Pincher grasp of the index finger opposing the thumb.

Tracing Comment: See the abductor pollicis longus tracing (Figure 17–43B).

Clinical Considerations: The degree of support of the arm and the hand may alter the resting tone. Surface recordings from this site primarily look at gross movement of the index finger, such as opposition of the thumb.

Volume Conduction: Flexor and abductor pollicis brevis.

Other Sites of Interest: Thumb adductor during grasping.

Referred Pain Considerations: Trigger points in the first interosseus project pain down into the index finger.[17]

FLEXOR POLLICIS BREVIS PLACEMENT

Type of Placement: Quasi-specific.

Action: Thumb flexion and opposition.

Clinical Uses: Hand rehabilitation, pincher grasp.

Muscle Insertions: The superficial aspect of this muscle arises from the flexor retinaculum. The muscle inserts on the radial sesamoid bone.

Innervation: The superficial head is innervated via the median nerve via spinal nerves C-6, C-7, C-8, and T-1. The deep head of this muscle is innervated by the ulnar nerve via spinal nerves C-8 and T-1.

Location: Palpate the medial aspect of the thenar eminence while the patient abducts the thumb. Two active electrodes, 2 cm apart, are placed on the medial aspect of the thenar eminence, parallel to the direction of the thumb (**Figure 17–45**). Smaller, more closely spaced electrodes will provide for greater specificity of recordings.

Behavioral Test: Pincher grasp, thumb opposed to index finger.

Tracing Comment: See the abductor pollicis longus tracing (Figure 17–43B).

Clinical Considerations: The degree of support of the wrist and the arm may alter resting levels. Surface recordings from this site primarily look at gross movement of the thumb (such as during opposition).

Volume Conduction: Abductor pollicis brevis, adductor pollicis.

Other Sites of Interest: Adductor pollicis brevis; abductors of the thumb.

ABDUCTOR POLLICIS BREVIS PLACEMENT

Type of Placement: Quasi-specific.

Action: Abduction of the thumb.

Clinical Uses: Hand rehabilitation.

Muscle Insertions: This muscle arises from the scaphoid tubercle and the flexor retinaculum and inserts on the radial sesamoid bone and the proximal phalanx of the thumb.

Innervation: The median nerve via spinal nerves C-6, C-7, C-8, and T-1.

Location: Two active electrodes, 2 cm apart, are placed in the center of the largest mound of the thenar eminence, running in the same direction as the thumb (**Figure 17–46**). Smaller, more closely spaced electrodes may provide for greater specificity of recordings.

Behavioral Test: Abduct the thumb. Lay the hand palm up. Move the thumb from the side of the index finger, out away from the fingers.

Tracing Comment: See the abductor pollicis longus tracing (Figure 17–43B).

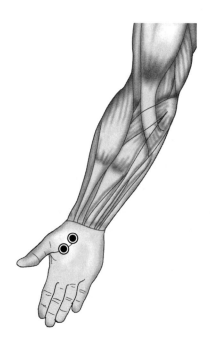

Figure 17–45 Electrode placement for the flexor pollicis brevis.

Source: Copyright © Clinical Resources, Inc.

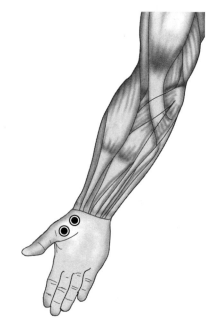

Figure 17–46 Electrode placement for the abductor pollicis brevis.

Source: Copyright © Clinical Resources, Inc.

Clinical Considerations: Adequate support of the wrist and the arm may alter the resting levels. The initial thumb position may affect the recruitment pattern.

Volume Conduction: Flexor pollicis brevis, opponens pollicis.

Other Sites of Interest: Flexor pollicis brevis during abduction of the thumb; adductor muscles of the thumb.

DORSAL LUMBAR (WIDE) PLACEMENT

Type of Placement: General.

Purpose: To monitor from the general region of the low back, the erector spinae.

Clinical Uses: Assessing and treating back pain; teaching the patient to deactivate muscle activation patterns.[13]

Location: The right and left aspects of the paraspinals are monitored separately. Two active electrodes are placed, one at the T-10 level and one at the L-3 level of the spine, approximately 2 cm lateral from the spine over the muscle belly (**Figure 17–47A**).

Behavioral Test: Walking, forward flexion, and extension.

Tracing Comment: **Figure 17–47B** shows SEMG recordings from the right and left aspects of the dorsal lumbar

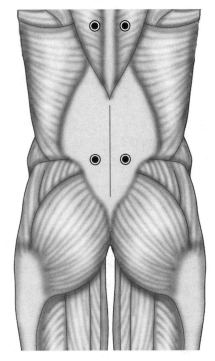

Figure 17–47A Electrode placement for the dorsal lumbar site.

Source: Copyright © Clinical Resources, Inc

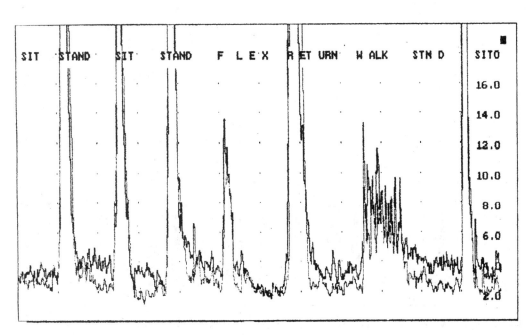

Figure 17–47B Surface EMG recordings from the right and left aspects of the dorsal lumbar site during sit-stand transitions, forward flexion, and walking.

Source: Copyright © Clinical Resources, Inc.

site during sit–stand transitions, forward flexion and return, and walking. Note the symmetry of recruitment during the various activities. Following the transitions, the recruitment patterns quiet down quickly. There is a flexion–relaxation response during forward flexion (processed SEMG).

Figure 17–47C shows an assessment and treatment technique developed by Ettare and Ettare.[13] Here, the ideal pattern is displayed during walking and quiet standing with 14 replications (processed SEMG).

Also note the tracings from the cervical trapezius (Figures 17–6B, 17–6C, and 17–6D) and cervical dorsal (Figures 17–18B and 17–18C) sites.

Clinical Considerations: Resting levels may be affected by the posture of sitting versus standing. Pelvic tilt may lower values. Scoliosis may be associated with asymmetry of resting values. Leg-length discrepancy may play a role as well.

Volume Conduction: Erector spinae, latissimus dorsi, quadratus lumborum.

Other Sites of Interest: Cervical dorsal recordings to obtain a larger view of spinal support; gluteus maximus during walking.

Artifacts: ECG, electrode slippage during forward flexion.

Benchmark: Sitting: 2 µV (RMS).
Standing: 2 µV (RMS).
Walking: 4–6 µV (RMS).
These values are based on a J&J M-501 EMG.[13]

T-12 PARASPINAL PLACEMENT

Type of Placement: Quasi-specific.

Action: To monitor the thoracic paraspinal stabilizers. These muscles are thought to be important due to the transition of the mechanical stability of the spine at the T-12 level.

Clinical Uses: Assessment and treatment of back pain.

Muscle Insertions: This placement is thought to monitor from the iliocostalis thoracis, longissimus thoracis, and spinalis thoracis. In general terms, it monitors from the erector spinae group.

These muscles can be anatomically separated into intersegmental muscles, acting on single and two-level joint movements (those that anchor the spine to the pelvis, the multifidus and lumbar fibers of the longissimus and the iliocostalis, and those that span the vertebral column, the thoracic fibers of the longissimus and the iliocostalis).[17] Most medial to the spinous process are the thoracic fibers of the iliocostalis, the thoracic fibers of the longissimus, and the multifidus. More lateral are the lumbar fibers of the longissimus and the lumbar fibers of the iliocostalis.

Innervation: The ventral and lateral intertransversarii receive their nerve supply from the lumbar ventral rami, while the more dorsal fibers receive their supply from the dorsal ramus.

The multifidi are innervated by the medial branch of the dorsal ramus of the spinal nerve that issues from below the particular vertebrae. The dorsal ramus separates into medial and lateral branches, with the lateral

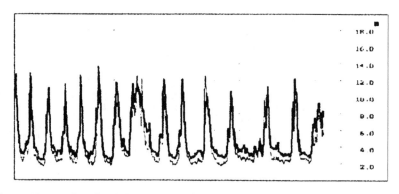

Figure 17–47C Surface EMG recordings from the right and left aspects of the dorsal lumbar site with 14 replications of standing and walking in place. The normal recordings indicate that the right and left aspects are symmetrical, and the activation pattern associated with walking quiets down quickly when the person stands.

Source: Copyright © Clinical Resources, Inc.

branch innervating the more lateral and superficial muscles. It runs obliquely downward and laterally, crossing one or two segments before terminating in muscle fibers.[17]

Joint Considerations: The complex nature of the functional anatomy of the paraspinal muscle group defies easy association of muscle dysfunction to underlying articular disturbances. Certainly, the spinal joints associated with the related spinal nerve should be assessed (T-10 through L-1), as should the joints and structures related to the insertions of the longer longissimus and spinalis fibers. However, this assessment should be made in the context of the posture and motion of the entire vertebral column and lower kinetic chain.

Location: To find T-12, have the patient forward flex, and palpate where the lowest rib joins the spine. Going laterally from the spine approximately 2 cm, the electrodes are placed 3 cm apart, so that they run parallel to the spine over the fleshy muscle mass. It is best to place these electrodes while the patient is in a slight forward flexion. This will minimize electrode artifacts associated with skin distortions that occur during this movement (**Figure 17–48A**).

Behavioral Test: Prone extension, return from forward flexion of the trunk.

Tracing Comment: **Figure 17–48B** shows SEMG recordings from the C-4, T-1, T-12, and L-3 paraspinals during prone extension. Note the marked recruitment at the T-12 and L-3 sites (raw SEMG).

Figure 17–48C shows SEMG recordings from the C-4, T-1, T-12, and L-3 paraspinals during side bending first to the left and then to the right. Activity is seen all along the paraspinal muscles during this movement. At the initiation of the bend, one can see an ipsilateral contraction at the T-12 level as the patient goes to the left. As the patient returns to midline, both the T-12 and L-3 levels on the contralateral side show a brisk recruitment (raw SEMG).

Clinical Considerations: Surface EMG resting and recruitment patterns may be affected by several features. Attention should be paid to scoliotic curves, rotation in the rib cage, the degree of curvature in the back, leg-length discrepancies, and any antalgic postures that involve the lower and upper back.

The thoracolumbar region is of profound biomechanical significance. The floating ribs and the frontal orientation of the facet joints give the region freedom of motion that the trunk uses to flex and extend as well as to side bend. The T-11/T-12 junction provides the largest amount of vertebral rotation. In neutral standing, there is

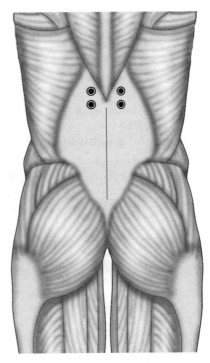

Figure 17–48A Electrode placement for the T-12 paraspinal site.
Source: Copyright © Clinical Resources, Inc.

conjoined motion of side bending and ipsilateral rotation. Normal conjunct rotation of the thoracic spine in neutral standing involves rotation and then side bending to the same side, known as *rotection*. Side bending and rotation to the opposite side is termed *latection*. Both are normal movements from a neutral posture. In flexion or extension, these joined motions are reversed, coupling side flexion and contralateral rotation. When the thoracolumbar spine is positioned in flexion, the ability of the region to shift from side flexion/ipsilateral rotation to side flexion/contralateral rotation is lost. The other transitional areas of the body (the suboccipital region, the cervicothoracic region, and, most significantly, the lumbosacral region) must compensate by moving more than they would otherwise.

Synergistic relationships with other trunk extensors—namely, the serratus posterior and the quadratus lumborum—have been described.[17] Tightness in the region has been attributed to various muscle imbalances between the overactive erector spinae, weakened gluteus muscles, and tightened hip flexors and weakened abdominals.[44]

Volume Conduction: Latissimus dorsi, lower trapezius, erector spinae.

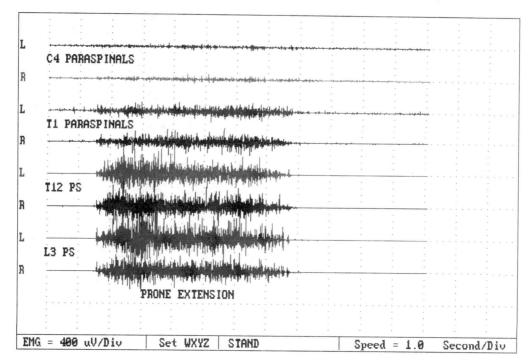

Figure 17–48B Surface EMG recordings from the cervical (C-4), T-1, T-12, and L-3 paraspinal sites during prone extension.

Source: Copyright © Clinical Resources, Inc.

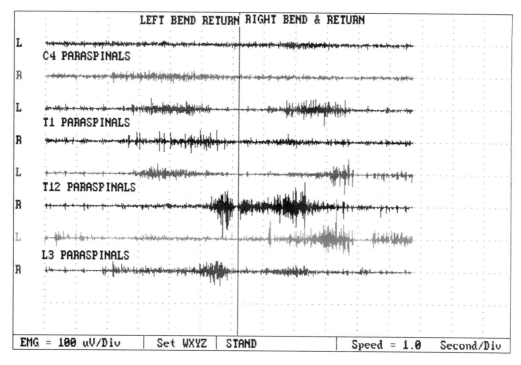

Figure 17–48C Surface EMG recordings from the C-4 paraspinals, T-1, T-12, and L-3 paraspinals during side bending first to the left and then to the right.

Source: Copyright © Clinical Resources, Inc.

Other Sites of Interest: Synergists with serratus posterior inferior and quadratus lumborum, and antagonists with rectus abdominis and abdominal obliques during flexion and extension; synergists to serratus posterior inferior and abdominal oblique during rotation.

Referred Pain Considerations: Trigger points near the spine tend to refer pain locally. As the patient moves more laterally, trigger points in the iliocostalis thoracis project pain laterally across the chest and may spill over to the anterior wall.[17]

Artifacts: Due to the degree of skin distortion experienced in the middle to lower back during certain movements, practitioners should be aware of artifacts caused by electrode slippage or popping during forward flexion and extension. ECG artifact is commonly seen on the left side. Respiration artifact is also possible.

Benchmark: Sitting quietly at midline (*N* = 104): 2.0 (±2.0) µV (RMS).

Standing quietly at midline (*N* = 104): 3.1 (±3.1) µV (RMS).

Values taken using a J&J M-501 EMG with a 100- to 200-Hz filter.[18]

LATISSIMUS DORSI PLACEMENT

Type of Placement: Specific.

Action: Medially (internally) rotates, adducts, and extends the shoulder/arm; participates in rotation, lateral bending, and extension of the torso.

Clinical Uses: Shoulder and back pain.

Muscle Insertions: This very broad muscle arises from the lower six thoracic vertebrae, the lumbodorsal fascia, the sacrum and crest of the ilium, and the last three or four ribs; it inserts, along with the teres major, on the medial edge of the humerus.

Innervation: The thoracodorsal nerve from the posterior cord of the brachial plexus via the spinal nerves of C-6, C-7, and C-8.

Joint Considerations: Related joint structures could include the spinal joints of the related motion segments (C-5/C-6, C-6/C-7, and C-7/T-1).

Additional joint structures include the shoulder complex (the scapulothoracic joint, the glenohumeral joint, and the joints of the clavicle) and the joints affecting the lumbodorsal fascia from which the latissimus arises (particularly the lower four ribs and thoracic vertebrae, the lumbar vertebrae, and the ilium).

Location: Palpate the scapula. Two active electrodes are placed (2 cm apart) approximately 4 cm below the inferior tip of the scapula, half the distance between the spine and the lateral edge of the torso. They are oriented in a slightly oblique angle of approximately 25 degrees (**Figure 17–49A**).

Behavioral Test: Extend, adduct, or medially rotate the arm.

Tracing Comment: Also see the tracings from the upper trapezius (Figure 17–19C), the suprascapular site

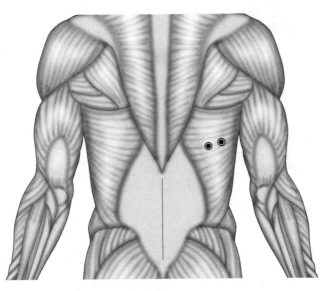

Figure 17–49A Electrode placement for the latissimus dorsi site.
Source: Copyright © Clinical Resources, Inc.

(Figure 17–23D), and the lateral low-back site (Figure 17–51B). **Figure 17–49B** shows recordings from the latissimus dorsi during shoulder extension (raw SEMG).

Clinical Considerations: Tightness in the latissimus dorsi is associated with increased thoracic kyphosis, rounded shoulders, and forward head posture. Leg-length discrepancies, unresolved lumbar lists, or any other situation that might cause lateral bending of the trunk could lead to unilateral tightness.

Volume Conduction: Teres major, lower trapezius.

Other Sites of Interest: Synergists with teres major and long head of triceps during extension, adduction, and lateral rotation; antagonists with scalene and upper trapezius during shoulder elevation.

Referred Pain Considerations: Trigger points in this region project pain to the inferior angle of the scapula and may extend to the back of the shoulder and down the medial aspect of the arm and forearm.[17]

Artifacts: ECG.

LOW-BACK (ERECTOR SPINAE) PLACEMENT AT L-3

Type of Placement: Quasi-specific.

Action: To monitor the paraspinal activity of the main trunk movers and stabilizers known as the erector spinae group.

Clinical Uses: Low-back pain.

Muscle Insertions: These electrodes are thought to record from the multifidus, rotatores, and longissimus muscle (erector spinae) groups.

Innervation: The pattern of innervation for the lumbar paraspinals is consistent with that for the thoracolumbar paraspinals. The ventral and lateral intertransversarii receive their supply from the ventral ramus of the spinal nerve; the other muscles receive their supply from the dorsal ramus of the spinal nerve. The actual muscle fibers supplied by the nerve of the given segment may be one to two segments below, as one moves more laterally from the spinous process.

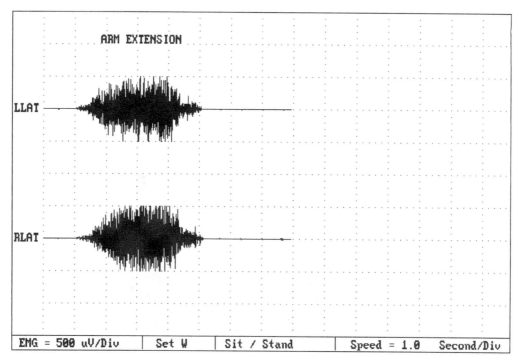

Figure 17–49B Surface EMG recordings from the latissimus dorsi during shoulder extension.
Source: Copyright © Clinical Resources, Inc.

Location: Palpate the iliac crest. Two active electrodes are placed parallel to the spine, 2 cm apart, approximately 2 cm from the spine over the muscle mass. The iliac crest may be used to determine the L-3 vertebra. The electrodes are best placed while the patient is in a slight forward flexion, hands resting on knees and supporting the torso (**Figure 17–50A**).

Behavioral Test: Forward flexion and return to midline of the torso.

Tracing Comment: **Figure 17–50B** presents SEMG recordings from the L-3 and abdominal oblique sites during forward flexion, return to midline, and extension backward. Note the flexion–relaxation phenomenon that occurs during the hang phase of this movement. The concentric contraction that occurs during the return phase is larger than the eccentric contraction that occurs during forward flexion. Both are symmetrical. Note the stabilizing activity of abdominal obliques during extension backward (raw SEMG).

Figure 17–50C shows SEMG tracings from the CA, T-1, T-12, and L-3 paraspinal muscles during forward flexion and return. A flexion–relaxation response occurs at the different spinal levels up the spine, and this response is displaced in time. Note the mildly abnormal asymmetry

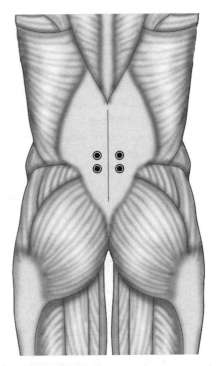

Figure 17–50A Electrode placement for the L-3 paraspinal site.

Source: Copyright © Clinical Resources, Inc.

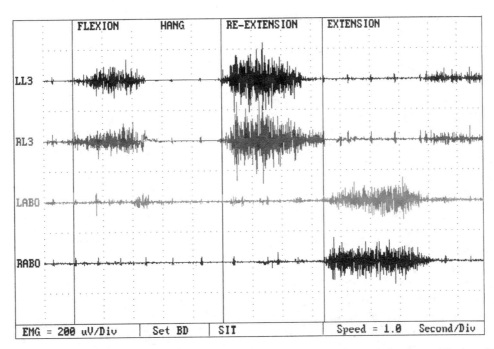

Figure 17–50B Surface EMG recordings from the L-3 paraspinal and abdominal obliques during forward flexion of the torso, return to midline, and extension of the torso.

Source: Copyright © Clinical Resources, Inc.

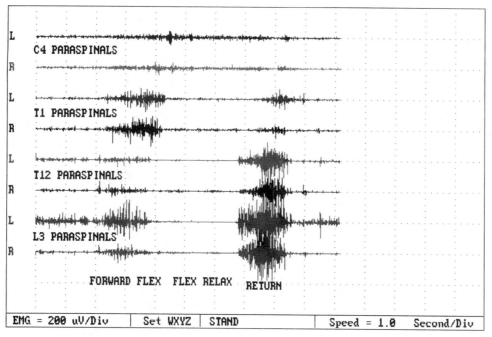

Figure 17–50C Surface EMG tracings from the C-4, T-1, T-12, and L-3 paraspinal muscles during forward flexion and return to midline. Note the flexion–relaxation phenomenon at the L-3, T-12, and T-1 sites.

Source: Copyright © Clinical Resources, Inc.

at the L-3 paraspinal site during the eccentric phase of the movement (raw SEMG).

Figure 17–50D presents tracings from the L-3 site along with the tensor fasciae latae, gluteus medius and maximus, lateral and medial hamstrings, and gastrocnemius and soleus during two types of squats. The first squat entails movement primarily at the ankle and the knees. The second squat is much deeper and entails large movements of the knee and hip. Notice how the deep squat that involves the hip strongly invokes the erector spinae at L-3.

Also see the tracings for T-12 paraspinal (Figures 17–48B and 17–48C) and lateral low-back placement (Figures 17–51B and 17–51C).

Clinical Considerations: Surface EMG resting and recruitment patterns may be affected by several features. Attention should be paid to scoliotic curves, rotation in the pelvis, the degree of curvature in the back, leg-length discrepancies, and any antalgic postures that involve the lower and upper back. Patterns are strongly influenced by postural elements. Surface EMG values are commonly lower in the sitting posture than in the standing posture.

The L-3 region is particularly sensitive to tightened hip flexors, often bilaterally, and a tightened quadratus lumborum, often unilaterally. Posture equilibrium is a model for compensation of mechanical dysfunctions. The upper lumbar region is often found to be flexed, with restricted extension, in the presence of flattened thoracic curves and/or hyperextended lumbosacral angles. The role of the abdominal muscles—particularly the obliques—in preventing this postural dysfunction should be considered.

Volume Conduction: Quadratus lumborum, gluteus maximus, latissimus dorsi.

Other Sites of Interest: Lateral low-back site (quadratus lumborum), rectus abdominis, and abdominal obliques during flexion, extension, and rotation; hamstrings and gluteus maximus during walking and trunk extension.

Referred Pain Considerations: Trigger points near the spine (i.e., multifidi) tend to refer pain locally, which may spill over to the anterior wall.[17]

Artifacts: Because of the degree of skin distortion experienced in the middle to lower back during certain

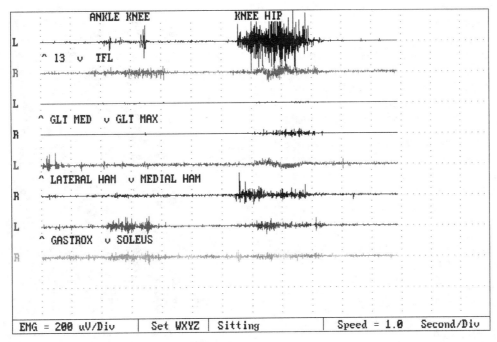

Figure 17–50D Surface EMG tracings from the L-3 site along with the tensor fasciae latae, gluteus medius and maximus, lateral and medial hamstrings, and gastrocnemius and soleus during two types of squats. The first squat entails movement primarily at the ankle and the knees; the second squat is much deeper and entails large movements of the knee and hip.

Source: Copyright © Clinical Resources, Inc.

movements, practitioners should be aware of artifacts caused by electrode slippage or popping during forward flexion and extension. ECG artifacts are commonly seen on the left side.

Benchmark: Sitting quietly at midline ($N = 104$): 1.9 (± 2.4) μV (RMS).
Standing quietly at midline ($N = 104$): 3.3 (± 3.4) μV (RMS).
Values taken using a J&J M-501 EMG with a 100- to 200-Hz filter.[18]

LATERAL LOW-BACK (QUADRATUS LUMBORUM AND EXTERNAL OBLIQUES) PLACEMENT

Type of Placement: Quasi-specific.

Action: Stabilizing the spine in general and during side bending, rotation, extension, hip hiking, and walking in particular.

Clinical Uses: Back pain.

Muscle Insertions: The quadratus lumborum is a multibellied muscle that arises from the twelfth rib and the transverse process of L-1 to L-4 and inserts on the posterior crest of the ilium. The external obliques arise from the fifth through twelfth ribs, interdigitating with the serratus anterior on the upper ribs and with the latissimus dorsi on the lower ribs, and inserting on the iliac crest and the abdominal aponeurosis at the midline. The iliocostalis lumborum extends from the sacrum, external lip of the iliac crest, the thoracolumbar fascia, and the costal process of the upper lumbar vertebrae and inserts on the sixth to ninth bottom ribs.

Innervation: The quadratus lumborum is innervated by the ventral rami of the twelfth thoracic and upper three or four lumbar spinal nerves. The abdominal obliques are innervated by the ventral rami of the lower six thoracic spinal nerves and, for the internal obliques, by the first lumbar spinal nerve as well. The iliocostalis is innervated by the lateral branch of the dorsal rami of the spinal nerves of the upper lumbar segments.

Joint Considerations: The spinal joints of the lower six thoracic vertebrae, the related costovertebral joints, and the costochondral junctions should be assessed. The lumbar spinal joints as well as those affecting the lumbodorsal fascia (the sacroiliac joints and the lumbosacral junction) also could affect the function of the muscles of this site. Possibly the most important structural component is the mobility of the eleventh and twelfth ribs and the ilium.

Location: Palpate the twelfth rib, the iliac crest, and the belly of the erector spinae muscle. Two active electrodes are placed 3 cm apart, approximately 4 cm lateral from the vertebral ridge or the belly of the erector spinae muscle, and at a slightly oblique angle at half the distance between the twelfth rib and the iliac crest (**Figure 17–51A**).

Behavioral Test: Hip hiking on the left, then the right; lateral bending; rotation.

Tracing Comment: The main muscles thought to be active in the region were monitored: the lateral low back (LLB), along with the L-3 paraspinals, latissimus dorsi, and abdominal obliques.

In **Figure 17–51B**, axial rotation is followed by side bending. During axial rotation, SEMG recruitment is

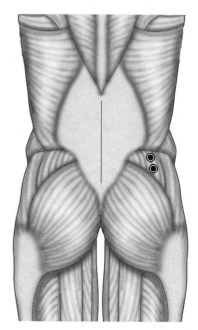

Figure 17–51A Electrode placement for the lateral low-back site.

Source: Copyright © Clinical Resources, Inc.

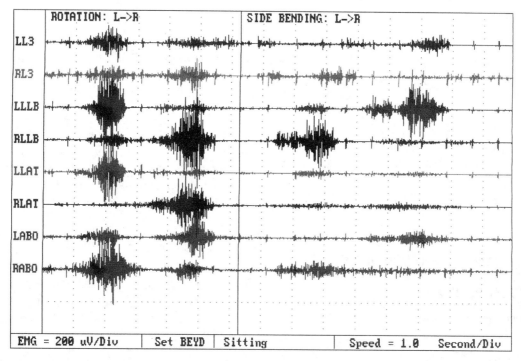

Figure 17–51B Surface EMG recordings from the L-3 paraspinals, lateral low-back (LLB), latissimus dorsi (LAT), and abdominal obliques (ABO) sites during axial rotation and side bending.

Source: Copyright © Clinical Resources, Inc.

clearly seen at all recording sites. On the ipsilateral side of the movement, the LLB site shows a large burst of recruitment, as do the latissimus dorsi and L-3 paraspinals. The abdominal obliques show a strong burst of recruitment on the side contralateral to the movement, indicating a strong rotatory component. For side bending, a large burst of recruitment is shown at the LLB site during the concentric contraction associated with the return to midline (raw SEMG).

In **Figure 17–51C**, two actions were studied: lateral bending to the left and then to the right, followed by hip hiking to the left and then to the right. During the lateral bending, notice how the LLB site contralateral to the movement provides an eccentric stabilizing function on the way down, and is a prime mover for concentric function on the way up. The contralateral abdominal oblique site also plays a role during the movement that suggests a slight axial rotation during the lateral bend. During hip hiking to the left and then to the right, both L-3 and LLB sites are strongly involved. It is entirely possible that the LLB pattern is due to volume conduction from the L-3 site or the posterior fibers of the obliques. Surface recordings do not definitively demonstrate this

relationship. Minor recruitment of the abdominal obliques can also be noted (raw SEMG).

Clinical Considerations: The resting values at this site may vary dramatically as one goes from the sitting posture to the standing posture. The degree of pelvic tilt may also moderate the resting SEMG levels. Leg-length discrepancies or scoliosis would certainly alter the horizontal axis of the pelvis, providing a basis for asymmetries at this site. The practitioner should also be alert to the possibility of antalgic postures, which could affect the resting SEMG levels and alter timing issues during dynamic movement.

The quasi-specific classification noted previously indicates that the muscle lies deep; thus attempted recordings at this site may reflect the activity of several muscles. One of the contributors at this site is the quadratus lumborum. Fine-wire recordings from the quadratus indicate EMG activity during the five following movements: lateral flexion of the spine, hip hiking, extension of the lumbar spine, forced expiration, and trunk rotation to the same side when the pelvis is fixed (e.g., sitting).[45]

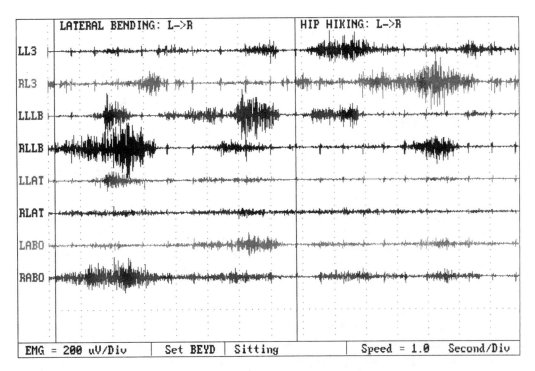

Figure 17–51C Surface EMG recordings from the L-3 paraspinals, lateral low-back (LLB), latissimus dorsi (LAT), and abdominal obliques (ABO) sites during lateral bending and hip hiking.

Source: Copyright © Clinical Resources, Inc.

The thoracolumbar junction has a tendency to become fixed into flexion. When it does so, the normal coupling of side flexion and contralateral rotation that occurs in the neutral spine becomes altered to side flexion and ipsilateral rotation. This may change the timing and amplitude of the signal seen in side flexion movements. Hyperactivity in the LLB area has been reported to be related to weakness in the gluteal muscles (Headley, personal communication). In the presence of gluteus medius weakness, lateral hip stability can be achieved via compensatory hyperactivity of the LLB and the tensor fascia latae.[17] Tight hip flexors on one side can participate in vertebral column rotation. The compensatory pelvic rotation creates an altered length of the LLB. The myofascium is lengthened on the convex side of the column.

Volume Conduction: Erector spinae, gluteus minimis, gluteus maximus, abdominals.

Other Sites of Interest: External abdominal obliques, latissimus dorsi, and erector spinae.

Referred Pain Considerations: Superficial trigger points at this site project pain posteriorly to the region of the sacroiliac joint and the lower buttock.[17]

Artifacts: ECG; electrode slippage and popping associated with severe skin distortions that occur as a function of forward flexion, extension, and, to a lesser extent, side bending.

RECTUS ABDOMINIS PLACEMENT

Type of Placement: Specific.

Action: Trunk flexion, pelvic tilt.

Clinical Uses: Abdominal and back pain.

Muscle Insertions: This multibellied muscle arises from the third through fifth ribs and the xiphoid process and inserts on the crest of the pelvic bone.

Innervation: The intercostal nerves via the ventral rami from T-5 to T-12.

Location: Palpate the abdominal wall in the area close to the umbilicus. Locate the muscle mass. A thick pad of adipose tissue may be a problem. The electrodes are placed 3 cm apart and parallel to the muscle fibers of rectus so that they are located approximately 2 cm lateral and across from the umbilicus over the muscle belly (**Figure 17–52A**).

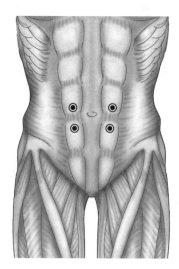

Figure 17–52A Electrode placement for the rectus abdominis site.
Source: Copyright © Clinical Resources, Inc.

Behavioral Test: From the supine posture, have the patient do a curl-up (partial sit-up). If standing, have the patient tighten the abdomen (suck it in) or do the pelvic tilt.

Tracing Comment: **Figure 17–52B** provides tracings from the rectus abdominis and abdominal obliques during a curl-up (partial sit-up) at midline from a supine position (raw SEMG).

Also see the tracings for abdominal oblique placement (Figure 17–53B).

Clinical Considerations: This site is affected by the degree of anterior versus posterior pelvic tilt. It has its greatest level of activation when the body weight is carried on the back rather than the thighs.[16] Values may differ greatly as the patient moves from the sitting to standing posture. During a sit-up, the greatest level of activation is noted during the first 45 degrees of flexion.[46]

Volume Conduction: Abdominal obliques.

Other Sites of Interest: Erector spinae muscles, latissimus dorsi.

Referred Pain Considerations: Trigger points in this multibellied muscle typically project pain to the same quadrant and occasionally to the back.[17]

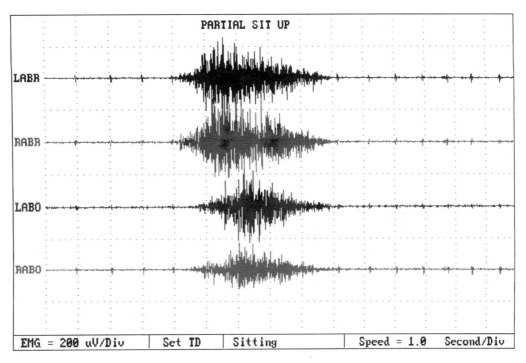

Figure 17–52B Surface EMG recordings from the rectus abdominis (ABR) and abdominal obliques (ABO) during a curl-up.
Source: Copyright © Clinical Resources, Inc.

Artifacts: Thick pad of adipose tissue; ECG.

Benchmark: Sitting quietly at midline ($N = 104$): 1.0 (± 2.5) μV (RMS).
Standing quietly at midline ($N = 104$): 1.1 (± 2.1) μV (RMS).
Values taken using a J&J M-501 EMG with a 100- to 200-Hz filter.[18]

EXTERNAL ABDOMINAL OBLIQUE PLACEMENT

Type of Placement: Quasi-specific.

Action: Flexion, rotation, and side bending of the torso.

Clinical Uses: Back pain and urinary incontinence.

Muscle Insertions: This rather broad muscle arises from the fifth through twelfth ribs, interdigitating with the serratus anterior on the upper ribs and with the latissimus dorsi on the lower ribs; it passes downward and medially inserts on the iliac crest and the abdominal aponeurosis at the midline.

Innervation: The intercostal nerve via the ventral rami from T-8 to T-12.

Location: Palpate the iliac crest and locate the anterior superior iliac spine. Two active electrodes are placed 2 cm apart, lateral to the rectus abdominis and directly above the anterior superior iliac spine, halfway between the crest and the ribs at a slightly oblique angle so that they run parallel to the muscle fibers (**Figure 17–53A**). (Note: Although this placement primarily records from the external oblique due to its superficial nature, recording from the internal obliques may be significant in some individuals; this effect probably depends on the depth of adipose tissue and movement strategy.)

Behavioral Test: Rotation of the torso, diagonal sit-up.

Tracing Comment: **Figure 17–53B** provides tracings from the rectus abdominis and external abdominal obliques during diagonal curl-ups to the left and then to the right. The rectus abdominis raises the torso, while the right and left obliques raise and rotate the torso to the left and the right, respectively. The degree of separation and specificity of recruitment of the external obliques during the diagonal sit-up vary considerably from one person to another.

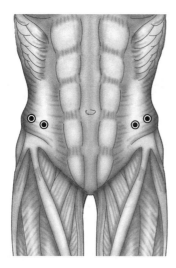

Figure 17–53A Electrode placement for the external abdominal obliques.

Source: Copyright © Clinical Resources, Inc.

Figure 17–53C shows axial rotation of the trunk during standing. Here, the muscles ipsilateral to the direction of the movement are activated. The degree of specificity and separation of the abdominal obliques vary greatly from one individual to another. In some individuals, there may exist a contralateral recruitment pattern for this movement (Figure 17–51B) (raw SEMG).

Also see the tracings from the L-3 paraspinals (Figure 17–51B) and the rectus abdominis (Figure 17–52B).

Clinical Considerations: The resting values at this site may vary dramatically as one goes from the sitting posture to the standing posture. The degree of pelvic tilt may also moderate the resting SEMG levels. Leg-length discrepancies and scoliosis would certainly alter the horizontal axis of the pelvis, providing a basis for asymmetries at this site. The practitioner should be alert to the possibility of antalgic postures that could affect the resting SEMG levels and alter timing issues during dynamic movement.

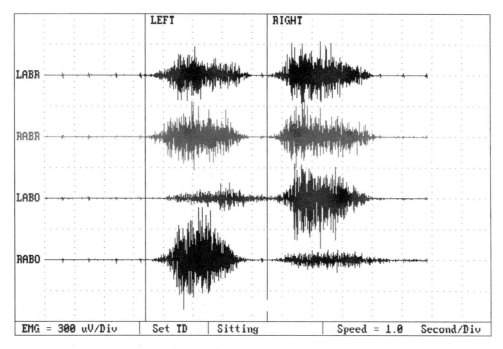

Figure 17–53B Surface EMG recordings from the rectus abdominis (ABR) and external abdominal obliques (ABO) during a diagonal curl-up.

Source: Copyright © Clinical Resources, Inc.

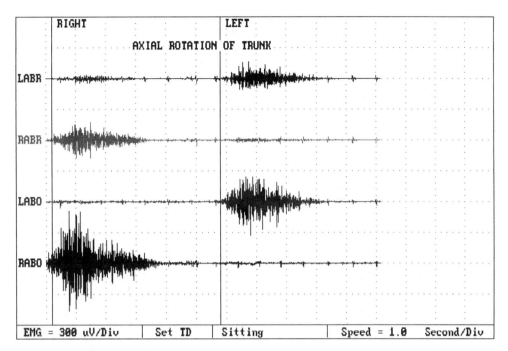

Figure 17–53C Surface EMG recordings from the rectus abdominis (ABR) and external abdominal obliques (ABO) during axial rotation while standing.

Source: Copyright © Clinical Resources, Inc.

This site has been rated as quasi-specific because the use of surface electrodes cannot differentiate between the internal and external obliques.[17] When the pelvis is fixed, the ipsilateral external obliques rotate the homolateral shoulder forward. However, most of the internal obliques rotate the homolateral shoulder backward.[29] Thus, when studying rotational movement patterns at this site, paradoxical results may be found.

Volume Conduction: Internal obliques, rectus abdominis, latissimus dorsi, and quadratus lumborum.

Other Sites of Interest: Ipsilateral aspects of serratus anterior and latissimus dorsi during rotation, and ipsilateral lateral low back (quadratus lumborum) and iliocostalis during side bending; antagonist with the contralateral homologous muscle group.

Referred Pain Considerations: Trigger points at this site may project pain down into the groin or testicles.[17]

Artifacts: Thick layers of adipose tissue may attenuate the SEMG signal.

ANKLE-TO-ANKLE (WIDE) PLACEMENT

Type of Placement: General.

Purpose: To monitor the volume-conducted muscular energy from the entire lower extremity, hips, and low back.

Clinical Uses: Assessment and treatment of lower-extremity and low-back pain.

Location: The two active electrodes are placed on the right and left ankle areas. For consistency, placement near the fibular malleolus or lateral aspect of the ankle bone is desirable. However, because this is a very general recording system, exact placement is not essential (**Figure 17–54A**).

Behavioral Test: All of the following actions will activate the SEMG recording, with the level of activation getting smaller the farther away the activating muscle is from the recording electrodes: foot flexion; foot extension; contraction of thigh, buttocks, and low-back muscles.

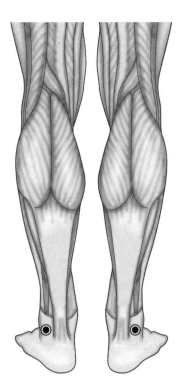

Figure 17–54A Electrode placement for the ankle-to-ankle site.

Source: Copyright © Clinical Resources, Inc.

Tracing Comment: Figure 17–54B presents a general recording from the ankle-to-ankle site, along with a wide/general recording from the rectus femoris site. Recordings on both a 100- to 200-Hz filter (narrow) and a 25- to 1000-Hz filter (wide) are displayed during systematic activation of various muscle groups in the lower extremities. The subject first tensed the foot, then the calf, then the thigh, and finally the buttocks. As the muscle activation gets farther away from the recording site, its amplitude gets smaller. Isometric contractions of the buttocks may be seen using this electrode placement. Also note that the ECG artifact usually seen under the conditions of the widely spaced electrodes and filters that go below 30 Hz is not seen in this tracing because of the extremely high resting levels (approximately 40 microvolts RMS). Recordings from the rectus femoris are always the smaller of the recruitment patterns (processed SEMG).

Clinical Considerations: Values are strongly affected by seated versus standing posture. Weight distribution and foot and toe positions during standing, and subtle changes in limb position during sitting may affect the resting SEMG levels.

One can easily demonstrate how this site monitors all of the muscles of both the lower extremities and the

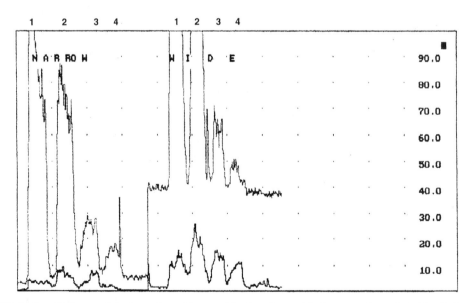

Figure 17–54B Surface EMG recordings from the ankle-to-ankle site, along with the rectus femoris (wide) during right-sided **(1)** dorsiflexion, **(2)** knee flexion, **(3)** hip flexion, and **(4)** unilateral gluteal squeeze. The left side of the tracing (narrow) is done with the 100- to 200-Hz band pass filter, while the right side of the tracing is done using the 25- to 1000-Hz band pass filter.

Source: Copyright © Clinical Resources, Inc.

lower torso by systematically asking the patient to tense and release each major muscle group of the left extremity, the gluteus maximus, the erector spinae, and the muscles of the right lower extremity.

Volume Conduction: All of the muscles of the lower extremity, hip, and low back.

Artifacts: ECG.

GLUTEUS MAXIMUS PLACEMENT

Type of Placement: Specific.

Action: Hip extender and lateral rotator.

Clinical Uses: Commonly used in the assessment and treatment of low-back pain, this muscle site is often observed to be overly inhibited (Headley, personal communication). This is also found to be true in hip dysfunction.

Muscle Insertions: This very large and broad muscle arises from the iliac crest, the ala of the ilium, the posterior superior iliac spine, the sacrum, and the coccyx. Three quarters of this muscle inserts on the iliotibial tract, while one quarter inserts on the gluteal tuberosity of the femur.

Innervation: The inferior gluteal nerve with fibers from the ventral rami of L-5 and S-1 through the dorsal division of the sacral plexus.

Joint Considerations: The spinal joints of L-4/L-5 and L-5/S-1 should be cleared of any dysfunction, if dysfunction persists at this site. The sacroiliac joint and the hip should also be assessed. Because of the contribution of the gluteus maximus to the iliotibial band, the knee and the superior tibulofibular articulation (with all the implications for lower kinetic chain interrelationships) also may play a role in the dysfunction of the gluteus maximus.

Location: Two possible locations are noted. For the upper gluteus maximus, two active electrodes (3 cm apart) are placed half the distance between the trochanter (hip) and the sacral vertebrae in the middle of the muscle on an oblique angle at the level of the trochanter or slightly above. For the lower gluteus maximus, placement is in the middle of the muscle clearly below the level of the trochanter, 1 to 2 inches above the gluteal fold (**Figure 17–55A**).

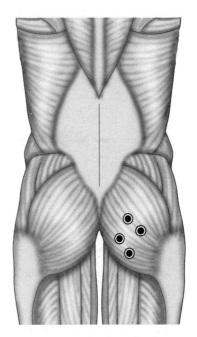

Figure 17–55A Electrode placement for the upper and lower gluteus maximus sites.

Source: Copyright © Clinical Resources, Inc.

Behavioral Test: While the patient is in the prone posture, or when he or she is standing and supported with hands on the wall, ask the patient to extend the leg back. Alternative movements include stair stepping, sit to stand, and external rotation of the thigh.

Tracing Comment: In **Figure 17–55B**, tracings for the right aspect of the L-3 (erector spinae), gluteus maximus for the upper site, and medial hamstring muscles are presented during prone hip extension. All three muscle groups work synergistically, with only a slightly larger recruitment pattern noted when the knee is flexed during this movement.

In **Figure 17–55C**, the upper and lower gluteus maximus sites are studied, along with the gluteus medius and tensor fasciae latae, during the prone leg extension. The lower gluteus maximus site reflects a larger recruitment pattern than the upper gluteus site. This may reflect differences in muscle mass, thickness of adipose tissue, or level of muscle recruitment for this individual. The decision of whether to use upper or lower placement depends on which site provides the best window to observe gluteal activity.

In **Figure 17–55D**, tracings for several of the major hip movers and stabilizers are presented while the individual is seated. Other muscle groups are known to par-

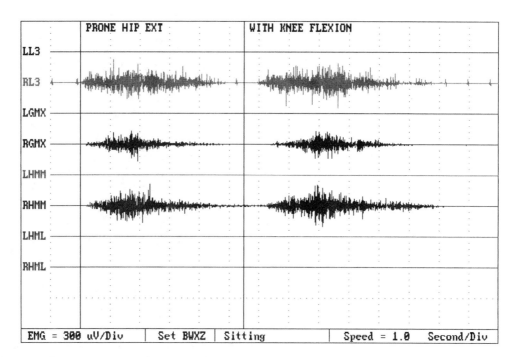

Figure 17–55B Surface EMG recordings from the right aspect of the L-3 (erector spinae), gluteus maximus (GMX) for the upper site, and medial hamstring muscles (HMM) are presented during prone hip extension with and without knee flexion.

Source: Copyright © Clinical Resources, Inc.

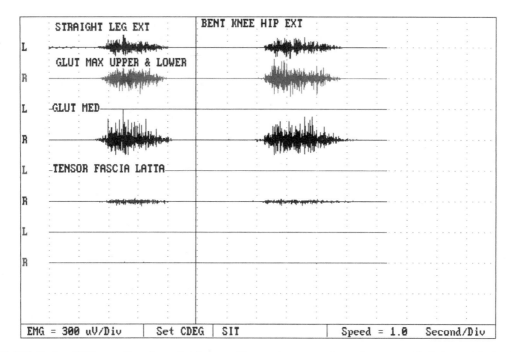

Figure 17–55C Surface EMG recordings from the upper and lower gluteus maximus sites are studied along with the gluteus medius and tensor fasciae latae during the straight leg extension and bent knee hip extension in the prone posture.

Source: Copyright © Clinical Resources, Inc.

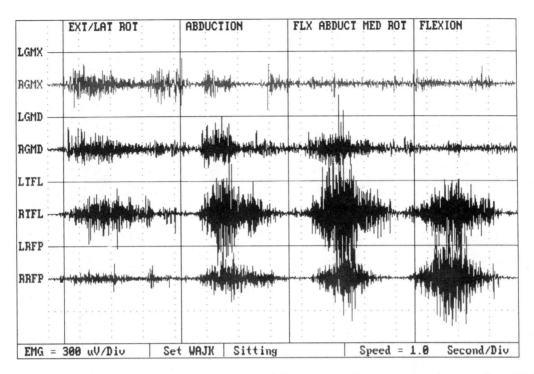

Figure 17–55D Surface EMG recordings from the right aspect of the gluteus maximus (GMX) and gluteus medius (GMD), tensor fasciae latae (TFL), and rectus femoris (RFP) are presented during external/lateral rotation; abduction; flexion, abduction, and internal rotation of the hip; and flexion of the hip. The flat lines for the left aspects of these sites reflect no SEMG input to those leads.

Source: Copyright © Clinical Resources, Inc.

ticipate in the movements described, but they are probably too deep to isolate and label. The more superficial muscles were monitored during external lateral rotation, abduction, flexion abduction and internal rotation, and flexion of the hip. The recruitment patterns of the right aspect of the gluteus maximus and gluteus medius, tensor fasciae latae, and rectus femoris are presented. The flat lines for the left aspects reflect no SEMG input to those leads. The gluteus maximus shows a burst pattern only during extension and lateral rotation of the leg. The gluteus medius appears to be active in all movements except hip flexion. The tensor fasciae latae is least active during external/lateral rotation, as is the rectus femoris. The rectus femoris is most active during hip flexion.

Also see the tracings for the hamstrings (Figures 17–64B, 17–64C, and 17–64D).

Clinical Considerations: Activity of the gluteus maximus is probably best studied during prone extension or standing postures. Leg-length discrepancy may con-

tribute to asymmetrical patterns. It may be useful to study this muscle during walking patterns, because it has been reported to fatigue easily or become easily inhibited during walking. Pronation of the foot and instability of the foot in stance and early push-off would contribute to hypoactivity of this site. An inhibited gluteus maximus is also seen in patients who stand, walk, or run with the pelvis pushed forward onto the "Y" ligaments. One can facilitate recruitment of the gluteus maximus during leg extension by having the patient engage in a pelvic tilt first.

Substitution of the trunk extensors and biceps femoris for the gluteus maximus in prone hip extension has been described[47] but not confirmed.[48] The quadratus lumborum has been proposed as a synergist capable of substituting for a hypoactive gluteus maximus. In the presence of limited hip extension, the tensor fasciae latae and gluteus maximus lose balance, with the tensor fasciae latae dominating hip motion.

Volume Conduction: Usually not a problem.

Other Sites of Interest: Erector spinae and hamstrings during extension of the trunk, particularly from the forward flexed position; the hamstrings, gluteus medius, and gluteus minimis during extension of the thigh; the rectus femoris during flexion; and the tensor fasciae latae during medial rotation.

Referred Pain Considerations: Trigger points in this muscle typically project pain locally into the buttocks.[17]

Artifacts: Thick adipose fat pad may attenuate the signal. Electrode slippage and movement artifact during walking may be a problem.

GLUTEUS MEDIUS PLACEMENT

Type of Placement: Specific.

Action: Hip abductor and stabilizer.

Clinical Uses: Low-back pain and hip rehabilitation.

Muscle Insertions: This muscle arises from the gluteal surface of the ilium and inserts on the trochanter.

Innervation: The superior gluteal nerve with fibers from L-5 and S-1 via their ventral rami and then via the dorsal branches of the sacral plexus.

Joint Considerations: The spinal joints of segments L-4 to L-5 and L-5 to S-1 could be sources of dysfunction for their myotomes, which include the gluteus medius.

The joints of origin/insertion of the gluteus medius could also create altered muscle function. These include the ilium in relation to the sacroiliac joint complex and the hip joint. Indirect contributions to gluteus medius dysfunction might include lower kinetic chain problems, particularly laxity of the longitudinal axis of the midfoot.[49] Piriformis spasm or hypertrophy might create problems at the greater sciatic foramen.

Location: Palpate the iliac crest. Two active electrodes, 2 cm apart, are placed parallel to the muscle fibers over the proximal third of the distance between the iliac crest and the greater trochanter. It is important to place the electrodes anterior to the gluteus maximus to minimize cross-talk (**Figure 17–56A**).

Behavioral Test: While the patient is side lying or standing sideways while supporting himself or herself against a wall, have the patient abduct the leg; have the patient walk.

Tracing Comment: In **Figure 17–56B**, the upper and lower gluteus maximus, the gluteus medius, and the

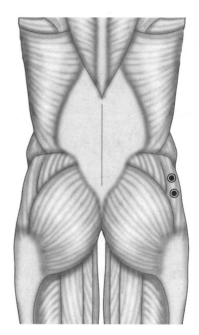

Figure 17–56A Electrode placement for the gluteus medius site.

Source: Copyright © Clinical Resources, Inc.

tensor fasciae latae are shown for the right side only. The subject is asked to stand, supporting his or her body with the left hand against a wall. Abduction of the leg is conducted in three ways: with extension, with movement in the sagittal plane, and with flexion. Note that recruitment from the gluteus medius is much smaller when abduction is conducted with flexion. To find recruitment of the gluteus medius, one must conduct this activity either in the sagittal plane or with extension.

Figure 17–56C demonstrates the same recording sites and the same posture. The subject is then asked to abduct the leg in the sagittal plane first in the neutral position, then again with internal rotation, and finally with external rotation. Here we see a clear synergy pattern, in which the tensor fasciae latae is activated during internal rotation while the recruitment from gluteus medius is augmented during external rotation.

Also see Figure 17–55D, 17–57B, and 17–57C.

Clinical Considerations: Activity of the gluteus medius is probably best studied during standing postures. Leg-length discrepancy may contribute to asymmetrical patterns. It may also be useful to study this muscle during walking patterns.

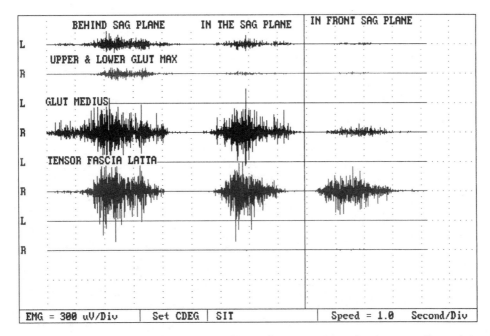

Figure 17–56B Surface EMG recordings from the upper and lower gluteus maximus, the gluteus medius, and the tensor fasciae latae are shown for the right side only. The subject is asked to stand, supporting the body with the left hand against a wall. The movement pattern of abduction of the leg is conducted in three ways: with extension, in the sagittal plane, and with flexion.

Source: Copyright © Clinical Resources, Inc.

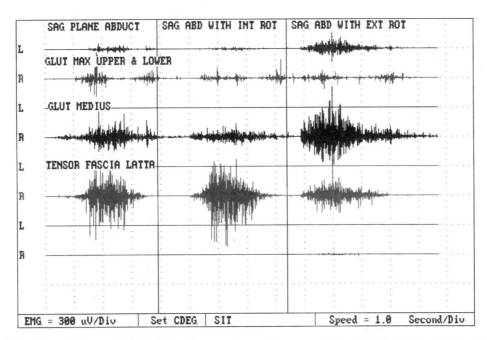

Figure 17–56C Surface EMG recordings from the upper and lower gluteus maximus, the gluteus medius, and the tensor fasciae latae are shown for the right side only. The subject is asked to stand, supporting the body with the left hand against a wall. Abduction of the leg is conducted in three ways: in neutral foot position, with internal rotation, and with external rotation.

Source: Copyright © Clinical Resources, Inc.

Indwelling electromyographic studies[16] have clearly demonstrated the gluteus medius to be the prime abductor of the thigh. The anterior portion of the gluteus medius has been demonstrated to be active during internal (medial) rotation and ambulation.[50] Carrying a load on the ipsilateral side reduced EMG recruitment, while carrying the load on the contralateral side increased EMG recruitment.[51]

The gluteus medius is prone to inhibition, particularly after injury or medical procedure. Typical substitution patterns include tensor fasciae latae and/or gait substitutions that overwork the quadratus lumborum.

Volume Conduction: Gluteus maximus, erector spinae.

Other Sites of Interest: Gluteus minimis, tensor fasciae latae during abduction.

Referred Pain Considerations: Trigger points at this site commonly project pain and tenderness along the posterior crest of the ilium, to the sacrum, and to the posterior and lateral aspects of the buttocks.[17]

TENSOR FASCIAE LATAE PLACEMENT

Type of Placement: Specific.

Action: Hip flexor, abductor, medial rotator, and knee extensor.

Clinical Uses: Hip rehabilitation.

Muscle Insertions: This muscle arises from the anterior superior iliac spine and inserts on the iliotibial tract.

Innervation: The superior gluteal nerve carrying fibers from L-4 and L-5 via their ventral rami and then via the dorsal branches of the sacral plexus.

Joint Considerations: The spinal joints of L-3 to L-4 and L-4 to L-5 should be suspected in the case of dysfunction of the tensor fasciae latae muscle. The ilium and its articulations, the sacroiliac complex, and the pubic symphysis should also be checked. The distal insertions of the iliotibial tract should be considered when ruling out articular contributions to the dysfunction seen at this site. These include the distal femur, the lateral patella, and the lateral retinaculum of the knee. The most distal insertion includes the anterolateral tibia and the head of the fibula.

Location: Palpate just below the anterior superior iliac spine of the iliac crest while the leg is extended. Two active electrodes, 2 cm apart, are placed parallel to the muscle fibers approximately 2 cm below the anterior superior iliac spine (**Figure 17–57A**).

Behavioral Test: Standing on one leg; abduction of leg with internal rotation; walking.

Tracing Comment: **Figure 17–57B** presents recordings from the right side of the body only during a unilateral stance on the right leg for the gluteus maximus, gluteus medius, tensor fasciae latae, and rectus femoris (proximal). The tensor fasciae latae shows the predicted burst pattern that stabilizes the hip and knee. The slight activation at the gluteus medius site could represent crosstalk or a minimal synergistic contraction.

In **Figure 17–57C**, abduction of the leg is conducted behind the sagittal plane, in the sagittal plane, and behind the sagittal plane while side lying. This tracing differs from tracings from the same movements during standing (Figure 17–56B) in that the tensor fasciae latae is more clearly active in all three planes of movement, while the gluteus medius shows most of its activation during abduction with extension.

Also see tracings for gluteus maximus (Figures 17–55C and 17–55D) and gluteus medius (Figures 17–56B and 17–56C).

Clinical Considerations: Activity of the tensor fasciae latae is probably best studied during a standing or side-lying posture. Leg-length discrepancy may contribute to asymmetrical patterns. It may be useful to study this muscle during walking patterns.

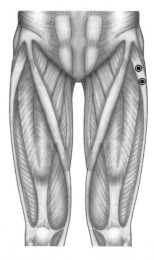

Figure 17–57A Electrode placement for the tensor fasciae latae site.

Source: Copyright © Clinical Resources, Inc.

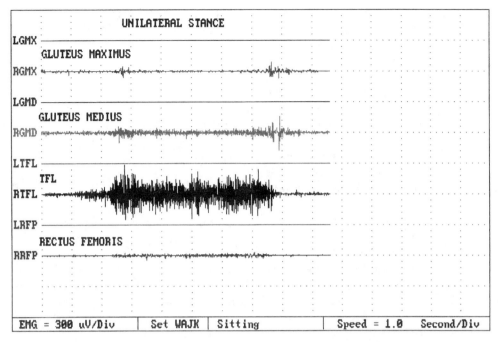

Figure 17–57B Surface EMG recordings from the right leg for the gluteus maximus, gluteus medius, tensor fasciae latae, and rectus femoris (proximal) during unilateral stance on the right leg.

Source: Copyright © Clinical Resources, Inc.

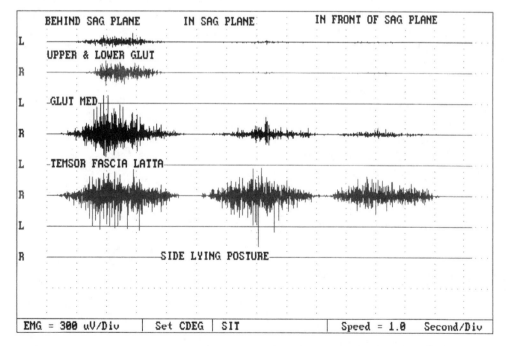

Figure 17–57C Surface EMG recordings from the upper and lower gluteus maximus, the gluteus medius, and the tensor fasciae latae are shown for the right side only while in the side lying position. The movements are abduction with extension, abduction, and abduction with flexion.

Source: Copyright © Clinical Resources, Inc.

Fine-wire studies of this muscle demonstrate that different aspects of it are active during different aspects of lower extremity use (i.e., anteromedial fibers are always active during flexion and abduction of the thigh, and posterolateral fibers are always active during medial rotation[52]). Using surface electrodes, one would not be able to separate out these different sections and movements. Instead, one would expect the tensor fasciae latae to be active across the entire range of motion noted using fine-wire techniques. It has been observed that the tensor fasciae latae is active during hip flexion, abduction, and unilateral stance.

Pelvic inclination as compensation for the limited hip extension from a tight tensor fasciae latae and/or tight hip flexors has been proposed[53,54] but also refuted.[55] Economy in gait may also be affected by tight hip flexors.[54] Inability to get the center of the body over the middle of the foot in stance will allow the tensor fasciae latae to remain tight.[49] A long leg ipsilateral to the iliotibial band can increase the tension on the iliotibial band, and presumably the stretch on the tensor muscle. External tibial torsion, rear foot eversion, and fore foot pronation can also be related to iliotibial band tightness.[56]

The lateral line of body that incorporates the quadratus lumborum, the origin of the oblique abdominals, and the latissimus dorsi can carry fascial restrictions that hide dysfunctions in multiple layers of compensatory adaptations. The substitution of the tensor fasciae latae for a weak gluteus medius is common. A lifestyle that includes excessive sitting can perpetuate tightness in the tensor fasciae latae and weakness in the gluteus medius. Trochanteric bursitis, as well as problems with lateral migration of the patella, is frequently associated with this condition.

Volume Conduction: If electrodes are placed too far lateral, volume conduction from the gluteus medius may be a problem.

Other Sites of Interest: Rectus femoris and sartorius during flexion of the hip; gluteus maximus.

Referred Pain Considerations: Trigger points at this site project pain to the anterolateral thigh over the greater trochanter and extending down the thigh toward the knee.[17]

FEMORAL TRIANGLE (ILIOPSOAS) PLACEMENT

Type of Placement: Quasi-specific.

Action: Hip flexion.

Clinical Uses: Hip rehabilitation.

Muscle Insertions: The iliopsoas arises from the first to fifth lumbar and the inner surface of the ilium and inserts on the lesser trochanter of the femur.

Innervation: The lumbar plexus via spinal nerves at L-1 to L-4.

Location: Palpate the proximal/medial/anterior aspect of the thigh just below the pelvis for the femoral triangle. Locate the femoral pulse. Go lateral to this point, yet medial to the quadriceps femoris and inferior to the inguinal ligament. Two active electrodes, 2 cm apart, are placed parallel to the muscle fibers. It is important to stay proximal to avoid cross-talk with the rectus femoris (**Figure 17–58A**).

Behavioral Test: In quadrupedal stance (on hands and knees), flex hip.

Tracing Comment: **Figure 17–58B** shows SEMG recordings from the right aspect of the tensor fasciae latae, iliopsoas, rectus femoris, and sartorius sites during hip flexion. Hip flexion was conducted in the three

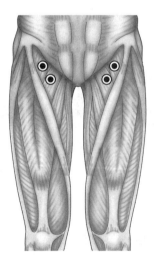

Figure 17–58A Electrode placement for the femoral triangle (iliopsoas) site.

Source: Copyright © Clinical Resources, Inc.

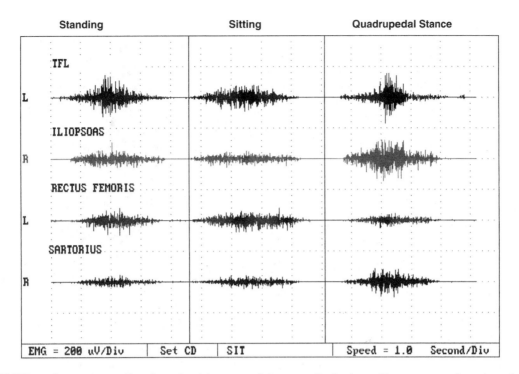

Figure 17–58B Surface EMG recordings from the right aspect of the tensor fasciae latae, iliopsoas, rectus femoris, and sartorius sites are presented during hip flexion.

Source: Copyright © Clinical Resources, Inc.

postures of standing, sitting, and quadrupedal stance. Hip flexion recruitment patterns are not clearly seen at the iliopsoas site in the two postures of standing and sitting. Only during the quadrupedal stance, where the rectus femoris is in the shortened position, is robust flexor action observed at this site. The tensor fasciae latae site is active during all three positions of hip flexion.

Clinical Considerations: This site is considered quasi-specific because of the depth of this muscle. Without fine-wire recordings, it is difficult to know with certainty that the iliopsoas muscle is making the major contribution to the surface EMG signal. However, the iliopsoas is well known for its role in hip flexion,[16] and this site is a good one wherein to study hip flexion activities. Hip flexion studies may be done in many positions: supine, sitting, standing, or quadrupedal stance.

The recruitment pattern may differ depending on the position. In addition, studies have shown that using an open versus a closed kinetic chain may affect the recording.

Volume Conduction: Sartorius, rectus femoris, adductor magnus.

Other Sites of Interest: Tensor fasciae latae, rectus femoris, sartorius, gluteus medius, and gluteus maximus.

Referred Pain Considerations: Trigger points at this site tend to project pain downward onto the anterior portion of the thigh.[17]

HIP FLEXOR (SARTORIUS) PLACEMENT

Type of Placement: Quasi-specific.

Action: Hip flexion and external (lateral) rotation during flexion of the knee.

Clinical Uses: Rehabilitation.

Muscle Insertions: This muscle arises from the superior aspect of the iliac spine and inserts distally on the medial surface of the upper tibia.

Innervation: The femoral nerve via spinal nerves at L-2 and L-3.

Location: Palpate the proximal aspect of the thigh. Two active electrodes, 2 cm apart, are placed parallel to the muscle fibers, approximately 4 cm distal from the anterior superior iliac spine, obliquely on the anterior surface of the thigh. It is important to stay in a proximal position in an attempt to minimize cross-talk with the rectus femoris (**Figure 17–59A**).

Behavioral Test: From the supine posture, flex and externally rotate the thigh while flexing the knee.

Tracing Comment: **Figure 17–59B** shows SEMG recording from the right aspect of tensor fasciae latae, iliopsoas, rectus femoris, and sartorius sites during tailor (cross-legged) sitting and external rotation of the hip while in a quadrupedal stance (on hands and knees). While activity is noted at the sartorius site, it is difficult to see any isolation of recruitment during these movements.

Clinical Considerations: This site is considered quasi-specific due to the potential for cross-talk when using

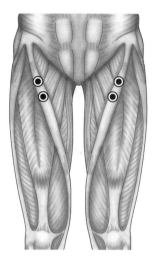

Figure 17–59A Electrode placement for the hip flexor (sartorius) site.
Source: Copyright © Clinical Resources, Inc.

surface electrodes to record here. Like the femoral triangle (iliopsoas) site, this site is a good one for monitoring

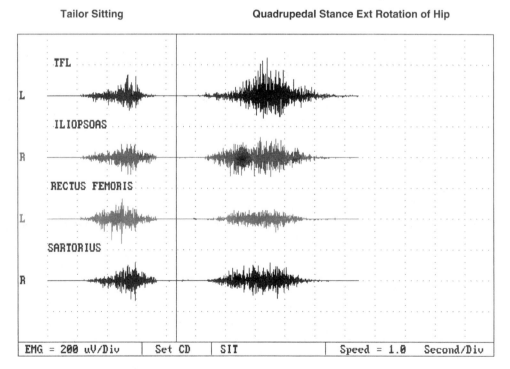

Figure 17–59B Surface EMG recordings from the right aspect of the tensor fasciae latae, iliopsoas, rectus femoris, and sartorius sites during tailor (cross-legged) sitting and external rotation of the hip while in a quadrupedal stance.
Source: Copyright © Clinical Resources, Inc.

hip flexion and hip flexion with external rotation, even though it is difficult to identify the specific muscle contributing to the SEMG signal. Hip flexion and external rotation studies may be done in many positions: supine, sitting, standing, or quadrupedal stance. The recruitment pattern may differ depending on the position.

Volume Conduction: Rectus femoris, iliopsoas, adductor magnus.

Other Sites of Interest: Rectus femoris, femoral triangle (iliopsoas), and tensor fasciae latae in hip flexion; gluteus maximus and hamstrings.

Referred Pain Considerations: Trigger points at this site project pain locally along the course of the muscle itself.[17]

RECTUS FEMORIS PLACEMENT

Type of Placement: Specific.

Action: Knee extensor and hip flexor.

Clinical Uses: Hip and knee rehabilitation.

Muscle Insertions: This muscle arises from the anterior ridge of the iliac crest and inserts on the upper border of the patella via the quadriceps tendon.

Location: This muscle is located on the center of the anterior surface of the thigh, approximately half the distance between the knee and the iliac spine. The two active electrodes are placed 2 cm apart, parallel to the muscle fibers (**Figure 17–60A**, right leg).

> *Variations:* The electrodes may be placed with a wide spacing (10 to 15 cm apart) to monitor from the quadriceps in general (Figure 17–60A, left leg).

Behavioral Test: While the patient is seated, ask him or her to extend the knee. While the patient is standing, ask him or her to squat slightly.

Tracing Comment: In **Figure 17–60B**, the rectus femoris is presented during hip flexion and knee extension, along with straight leg raising. As can be seen, a strong burst pattern is present for both hip flexion and knee extension. Supine straight leg raising, however, brings about the largest level of recruitment.

In **Figure 17–60C**, the vastus medialis oblique, the vastus lateralis, and the rectus femoris are compared to

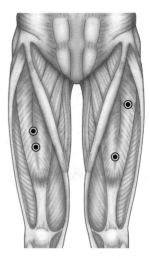

Figure 17–60A Electrode placement for the rectus femoris site (left side) and quadriceps muscles in general (right side).

Source: Copyright © Clinical Resources, Inc.

the medial hamstring and the lateral hamstring during isometric flexion and extension of the knee. Note the strong and isolated contractions of the anterior and posterior compartments of the thigh during these efforts (raw SEMG).

Also see the tracings from the gluteus maximus (Figure 17–55D), the tensor fasciae latae (Figure 17–57B), the femoral triangle (Figure 17–58B), and the hip flexor (Figure 17–59B).

Clinical Considerations: Recordings of resting tone and recruitment patterns at this site are affected by isometric efforts versus weight-bearing movements. Surface EMG monitoring and feedback training for rectus femoris have been used in the rehabilitation of patients with anterior cruciate ligament dysfunctions and repair.[57,58]

Volume Conduction: Vastus lateralis, vastus medialis, vastus intermedius, sartorius, adductor longus, and adductor brevis.

Other Sites of Interest: Vastus lateralis and vastus medialis during knee extension, sartorius and tensor fasciae latae during hip flexion, hamstring.

Referred Pain Considerations: Trigger points in the proximal aspect of this muscle project pain down to the knee.[17]

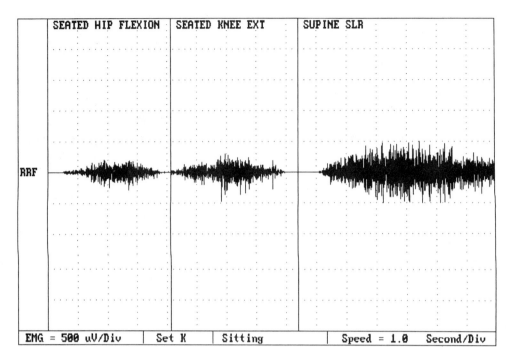

Figure 17–60B Surface EMG recordings from the rectus femoris site during hip flexion, knee extension, and supine straight leg raising.

Source: Copyright © Clinical Resources, Inc.

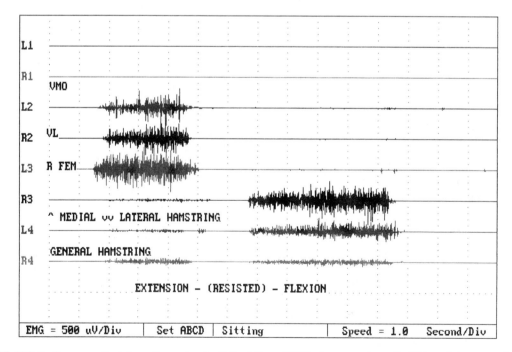

Figure 17–60C Surface recordings from the vastus medialis oblique (VMO), the vastus lateralis (VL), and the rectus femoris (R FEM) are compared to the medial hamstring and lateral hamstring during isometric flexion and extension of the knee.

Source: Copyright © Clinical Resources, Inc.

VASTUS LATERALIS PLACEMENT

Type of Placement: Specific.

Action: Extensor muscles of the knee.

Clinical Uses: General knee rehabilitation; patellofemoral pain.

Muscle Insertions: This muscle arises from the lateral surface of the greater trochanter, the intertrochanteric line, the gluteal tuberosity, and the lateral lip of the linea aspera. It inserts on the superior rim of the patella via the patella tendon.

Innervation: This muscle is innervated via the femoral nerve carrying fibers from the L-2, L-3, and L-4 spinal nerves. The femoral nerve is formed by the ventral rami of the spinal nerves as they pass down along and through the psoas major, then pass under the inguinal ligament where the femoral nerve separates into anterior and posterior branches. The vastus lateralis receives its innervation in the distal portion of the muscle.

Joint Considerations: The L-2/L-3 and L-3/L-4 joints need to be cleared of problems in the presence of abnormal activity in this region. The patellofemoral joint is central to the role of the vastus lateralis. It is usually symptomatic in the presence of quadriceps imbalance or dysfunction. A symptomatic patellofemoral joint can be the cause of quadriceps dysfunction; at other times, it may result from quadriceps dysfunction.

Location: Two active electrodes, 2 cm apart, are placed approximately 3 to 5 cm above the patella, on an oblique angle just lateral to midline (**Figure 17–61A**).

Behavioral Test: Have the patient extend the knee while seated, or squat while standing.

Tracing Comment: **Figure 17–61B** presents the tensor fasciae latae, adductor magnus, rectus femoris, vastus medialis oblique, vastus lateralis, medial hamstring, and the long head and lateral hamstring for the right leg during two squats. Note the strong recruitment in the vastus lateralis and vastus medialis oblique as they stabilize the knee in both movements, and in the rectus femoris during its eccentric contractions. The hamstrings are quiet in this individual, but this may not always be the case (raw SEMG).

Also see the tracings in Figure 17–60C.

Clinical Considerations: Recordings of resting tone and recruitment patterns at this site are affected by isometric efforts versus weight-bearing movements. The rela-

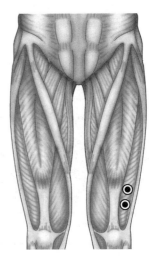

Figure 17–61A Electrode placement for the vastus lateralis site.
Source: Copyright © Clinical Resources, Inc.

tionship between the vastus lateralis and the vastus medialis oblique has been studied extensively; these muscles are relatively balanced in timing and magnitude during knee extension.[16,59] The ratio of vastus medialis oblique to vastus lateralis has been found to be 1.10 ($\pm$0.27) for normalized SEMG.[60]

Femoral anteversion or tibial torsion can change the orientation of the fibers. Poor functional alignment of the lower extremity can create chronic excitation of the vastus lateralis secondary to the dysfunctional pull; such alignment causes the muscle to affect the path of the patella.

Tightness in the iliotibial band as a result of ilial torsion or as a result of conditions related to lower kinetic chain dysfunction can alter the line of pull of the lateral quadriceps or the length tension of the muscle, thereby affecting vastus lateralis function.

Gait is a fundamental function of the quadriceps muscle. Idiosyncratic gaits can mask weakness in the hip flexors or hip stabilizers, placing more burden on the quadriceps for preventing collapse at heel strike through midstance. Collapse of the longitudinal arch at mid- to late stance limits the lateral sway of the pelvis and keeps the lateral structures from thoroughly stretching. It could be that iliotibial band tightness from this or other sources creates patellar tracking problems that lead to vastus medialis oblique dysfunction and vastus lateralis hyperactivity. Alternatively, medialis oblique dysfunction may lead to iliotibial band tightness.

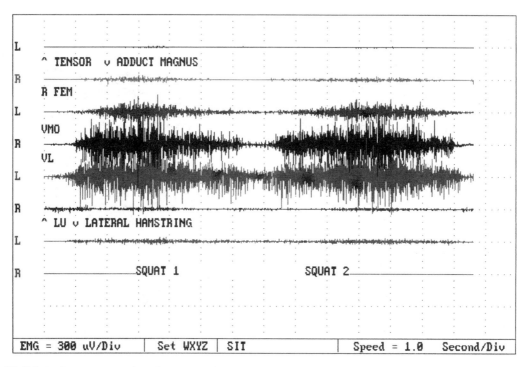

Figure 17–61B Surface EMG recordings from the tensor fasciae latae, adductor magnus, rectus femoris (R FEM), vastus medialis oblique (VMO), vastus lateralis (VL), medial hamstring, and lateral hamstring for the right leg only during two bilateral squats.

Source: Copyright © Clinical Resources, Inc.

Volume Conduction: Rectus femoris and vastus intermedius.

Other Sites of Interest: Rectus femoris and vastus medialis oblique during extension of the knee; hamstrings.

Referred Pain Considerations: Trigger points at this site tend to project pain along the lateral aspect of the thigh and knee.[17]

VASTUS MEDIALIS (OBLIQUE) PLACEMENT

Type of Placement: Specific.

Action: Assists in the medial tracking of the patella by stabilizing the patella in the trochlear groove.

Type of Placement: General knee rehabilitation, patellofemoral pain.

Muscle Insertions: The vastus medialis arises from the entire length of the posteromedial aspect of the shaft of the femur, to the lower half of the intertrochanteric line, the medial lip of the linea aspera, and the tendons of the adductor longus and magnus. It inserts on the

patella via the tendon. The oblique aspect of the vastus medialis also inserts on the medial patella retinaculum.

Innervation: This muscle is innervated by the femoral nerve, carrying fibers from the L-2, L-3, and L-4 spinal nerves. The femoral nerve is formed by the ventral rami of the spinal nerves as they pass down along and through the psoas major, then pass under the inguinal ligament where the femoral nerve separates into anterior and posterior branches. The vastus medialis is innervated by a portion of the deep branch of the femoral nerve after it passes through the adductor tunnel and goes to the middle portion of the muscle.

Joint Considerations: The L-2/L-3 and L-3/L-4 joints need to be cleared of problems in the presence of abnormal activity in this region. The patellofemoral joint has a strong influence on the vastus medialis. It is usually symptomatic in the presence of quadriceps imbalance or dysfunction. A symptomatic patellofemoral joint can be the cause of quadriceps dysfunction; at other times, it may result from quadriceps dysfunction. Additionally, the pubic symphysis should be checked, as dysfunctions there can negatively affect the adductor origins of the vastus medialis.

Location: The placement for vastus medialis oblique is done using 2-cm spacing, with the electrodes placed at an oblique angle (55 degrees), 2 cm medially from the superior rim of the patella. Palpate for the muscle during extension of the knee. It is somewhat easier to palpate toward the end of the range of motion. The electrodes are placed on the distal third of the vastus medialis (**Figure 17–62**).

Behavioral Test: Ask the patient to extend his or her knee while seated, or to partially squat during standing.

Tracing Comment: Refer to the tracing for the vastus lateralis site (Figure 17–61B).

Clinical Considerations: Recordings of resting tone and recruitment patterns at this site are affected by isometric efforts versus weight-bearing movements. The relationship between the vastus lateralis and the vastus medialis oblique has been studied extensively; these muscles are relatively balanced in timing and magnitude during knee extension.[16,59] The ratio of vastus medialis to vastus lateralis has been found to be 1.10 ($\pm$ 0.27) for normalized SEMG.[60] It is probably best to study these relationships in a closed kinetic chain (i.e., squats and isometrics). Several authors have suggested the use of SEMG feedback therapy in the treatment of patellofemoral pain.[61, 62] In general, the SEMG biofeedback therapies attempt to selectively recruit and uptrain the vastus medialis oblique. For a review of the research in this area, see *Clinical Applications in Surface Electromyography* by Kasman, Cram, and Wolf.[63]

Femoral anteversion or tibial torsion can change the orientation of the fibers. Poor functional alignment of the lower extremity can create chronic excitation of the vastus medialis secondary to the dysfunctional stretch such alignment causes the muscle. Tightness in the iliotibial band as a result of ilial torsion or as a result of conditions related to lower kinetic chain dysfunction can alter the line of pull of the lateral quadriceps or the length tension of the muscle, thereby affecting the medial portion's functional efficiency.

Gait is a fundamental function of the quadriceps muscle. Idiosyncratic gaits can mask weakness in the hip flexors, hip stabilizers, or hip adductors, placing more burden on the lateral quadriceps for preventing collapse at heel strike through midstance. This can lead to tightness and imbalance between the lateral and medial quadriceps functions.

Collapse of the longitudinal arch at mid- to late stance limits the lateral sway, and keeps the lateral structures from thoroughly stretching. Iliotibial band tightness from this or other sources can create patellar tracking problems and lead to medial quadriceps dysfunction, which appears as relative vastus medialis hypoactivity.

Volume Conduction: Rectus femoris, adductor longus and magnus.

Other Sites of Interest: Vastus lateralis and rectus femoris; hamstring and adductor magnus.

Referred Pain Considerations: Trigger points at this site refer pain to the medial and anterior aspects of the knee.[17]

HIP ADDUCTOR (ADDUCTOR LONGUS/GRACILIS) PLACEMENT

Type of Placement: Quasi-specific.

Action: Adduction of the leg.

Clinical Uses: Rehabilitation of cerebral palsy scissors gait.

Muscle Insertions: The adductor longus muscle arises from the superior ramus of the pubis and inserts on the middle third of the medial lip of the linea aspera. The gracilis originates from the inferior half of the symphysis pubis and the medial margin of the inferior ramus of

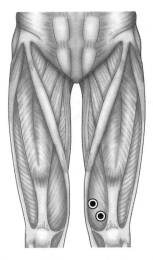

Figure 17–62 Electrode placement for the vastus medialis oblique site.

Source: Copyright © Clinical Resources, Inc.

the pubic bone. It inserts on the proximal part of the medial surface of the tibia.

Innervation: The obturator nerve via the spinal nerves at L-2 to L-4.

Location: Two active electrodes, 2 cm apart, are placed on the medial aspect of the thigh in an oblique direction 4 cm from the pubis. Palpate the area while the patient conducts an isometric adduction. Avoid placing electrodes close to the midline of the thigh so as to avoid cross-talk from the rectus femoris (**Figure 17–63A**).

Behavioral Test: Pressing the knees together to adduct the legs; walking.

Tracing Comment: **Figure 17–63B** presents the tensor fasciae latae, adductor magnus, rectus femoris, vastus medialis oblique, vastus lateralis, long head, and medial hamstrings during an isometric adduction and abduction of the leg. The largest recruitment patterns occur at the tensor fasciae latae and adductor magnus sites.

Clinical Considerations: Recordings of resting tone and recruitment patterns at this site are affected by isometric efforts versus weight-bearing movements. This muscle is active during ambulation, and fine-wire studies

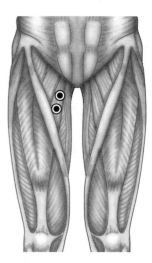

Figure 17–63A EMG electrode placement for the adductor longus site.

Source: Copyright © Clinical Resources, Inc.

have demonstrated that it is most active before, during, and slightly after toe off.[50,64,65]

Volume Conduction: Rectus femoris, vastus medialis, and adductor magnus.

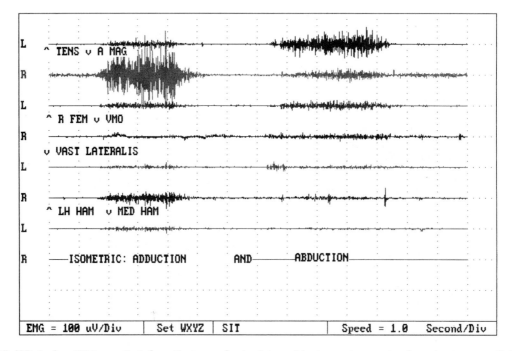

Figure 17–63B Surface EMG recordings from the tensor fasciae latae, adductor magnus, rectus femoris, vastus medialis, vastus lateralis, and long head and medial aspects of the hamstrings during isometric adduction and abduction of the leg.

Source: Copyright © Clinical Resources, Inc.

Other Sites of Interest: Adductor brevis and magnus, gracilis, gluteus medius, gluteus minimis, and tensor fasciae latae muscles.

Referred Pain Considerations: Trigger points at this site project pain upward toward the groin and downward to the knee and shin.[17]

MEDIAL AND LATERAL HAMSTRING PLACEMENT

Type of Placement: Specific and general.

Action: Flexion of the knee, medial or lateral rotation and extension of the hip.

Clinical Uses: Knee, hip, and back pain.

Muscle Insertions: Two muscles, the biceps femoris (lateral) and the semitendinosus (medial), arise from the ischial tuberosity and insert on the lateral and medial heads of the tibia, respectively. The semimembranosus arises from the ischial tuberosity and inserts on the posterior medial tibial condyle.

Innervation: The tibial nerve via L-4, L-5, and S-1.

Location: For general recordings, two electrodes, 3 to 4 cm apart, may be placed parallel to the muscle in the center of the back of the thigh, approximately half the distance from the gluteal fold to the back of the knee (**Figure 17–64A**, right leg).

For specific recording of the biceps femoris, the two active electrodes are placed 2 cm apart, parallel to the muscle fibers on the lateral aspect of the thigh, two-thirds of the distance between the trochanter and the back of the knee. Palpate for the muscle while manually muscle testing with the knee at 90 degrees and the thigh in a slight lateral rotation. The semitendinosus may be monitored by placing the electrode on the medial aspect of the thigh, located approximately 3 cm from the lateral border of the thigh and approximately half the distance from the gluteal fold to the back of the knee. Palpate this area while manually muscle testing with the knee at 90 degrees and the thigh in the midline position (Figure 17–64A, left leg).

Behavioral Test: With the patient in a prone position, ask him or her to flex the knee against resistance. In the standing position, have the patient flex his or her knee.

Tracing Comment: In **Figure 17–64B**, the L-3 paraspinals, tensor fasciae latae, gluteus medius and maximus, lateral and medial hamstrings, and gastrocne-

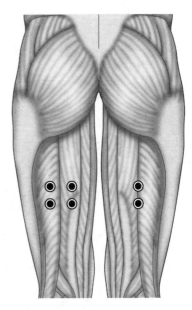

Figure 17–64A Electrode placement for the lateral and medial hamstrings (left) and a general placement (right).
Source: Copyright © Clinical Resources, Inc.

mius and soleus are monitored during forward flexion of the torso. The L-3 site shows the flexion–relaxation response. However, the hamstring and soleus are placed on stretch and become quite active. The medial aspect of the hamstring in this patient is abnormally active (raw SEMG).

In **Figure 17–64C**, the L-3 paraspinals, tensor fasciae latae, gluteus medius and maximus, and lateral and medial hamstrings are monitored during flexion, abduction, and extension of the hip while standing. Hip flexion brought about a strong recruitment pattern for the tensor fasciae latae. Abduction also strongly activated the tensor fasciae latae. Extension activated all of the muscle groups; it was the only movement that activated the hamstrings (raw SEMG).

In **Figure 17–64D**, the same muscles are monitored as in Figure 17–64C, but this time the posture is prone, and the movements are all extensions with different angles of rotation of the leg. This is a particularly interesting recording, showing that the tensor fasciae latae no longer participates in extension when the leg is laterally rotated. The lumbar paraspinals, in contrast, become more active when the leg is laterally rotated during extension. Of course, the lateral hamstring becomes more active during extension as the leg is laterally rotated.

Also see the tracings for the rectus femoris (Figure 17–60C).

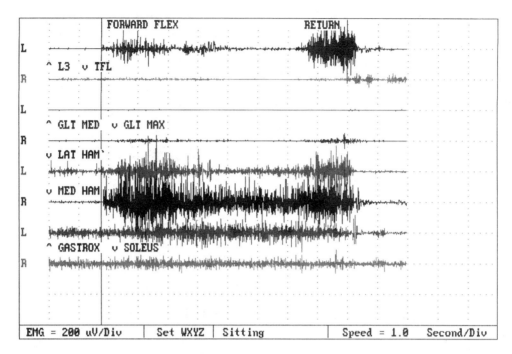

Figure 17–64B Surface EMG readings for the L-3 paraspinals, tensor fasciae latae, gluteus medius and maximus, lateral and medial hamstrings, and gastrocnemius and soleus during forward flexion of the torso.

Source: Copyright © Clinical Resources, Inc.

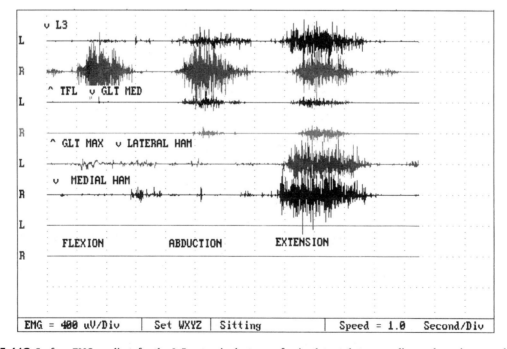

Figure 17–64C Surface EMG readings for the L-3 paraspinals, tensor fasciae latae, gluteus medius and maximus, and lateral and medial hamstrings during flexion, abduction, and extension of the hip while standing.

Source: Copyright © Clinical Resources, Inc.

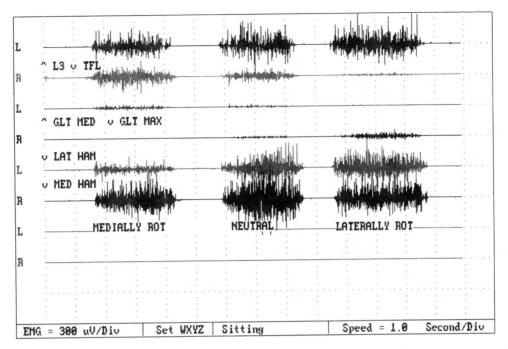

Figure 17–64D Surface EMG readings for the L-3 paraspinals, tensor fasciae latae, gluteus medius and maximus, and lateral and medial hamstrings during prone extension of the leg while it is medially rotated, neutral, and laterally rotated.

Source: Copyright © Clinical Resources, Inc.

Clinical Considerations: Recordings of resting tone and recruitment patterns at this site are affected by isometric efforts versus weight-bearing movements, along with the initial angle of the knee.

The hamstrings are known to be electrically silent when standing in neutral,[16] but active when the trunk is flexed while standing and when the arms are extended.[44] In walking, the hamstrings are most active just before or at heel strike.[16] The long head of the biceps femoris shows activity beginning at midswing and lasting through the period of heel strike.[66] The tendency for the hamstring muscle to become tight and hyperactive is associated with a corresponding tendency for the gluteus maximus to become lax and inhibited. Finally, an interesting review of the firing pattern of hip muscles during prone extension has been published by Pierce and Lee.[48]

Volume Conduction: Lateral and medial hamstrings, quadriceps.

Other Sites of Interest: Gluteus maximus for hip extension; sartorius, gastrocnemius, and plantaris during knee flexion; femoral triangle (iliopsoas), tensor fasciae latae, and rectus femoris during extension of the hip; knee flexion for quadriceps femoris.

Referred Pain Considerations: Trigger points in the semitendinosus project pain up to the gluteal fold, while the biceps femoris projects pain down to the back of the knee.[17]

ANKLE DORSIFLEXOR (TIBIALIS ANTERIOR) PLACEMENT

Type of Placement: Quasi-specific.

Action: Dorsiflexors of the foot.

Clinical Uses: Used in the treatment of the swing-through phase of gait training for patients following a stroke.

Muscle Insertions: Several different muscle groups are potentially monitored from this site: tibialis anterior, extensor hallucis longus, and extensor digitorum longus. The tibialis anterior is the largest and most superficial muscle group and contributes the most to the SEMG signal.

Location: Two active electrodes, 2 cm apart, are placed parallel to and just lateral to the medial shaft of the tibia (shin), at approximately one-quarter to one-third the distance between the knee and the ankle. Palpate the area while the patient dorsiflexes the foot. Place the electrode over the largest muscle mass (**Figure 17–65A**).

Behavioral Test: Dorsiflex the foot.

Tracing Comment: Two tracings are presented. **Figure 17–65B** depicts recordings from the soleus, gastrocnemius, anterior tibialis, and rectus femoris for the left leg. The right aspect was not monitored, and the flat lines represent no input. With the patient supported in some way and both feet flat on the ground, the patient is asked to lean or sway forward and then backward. The soleus and gastrocnemius stabilize the individual during the forward sway, while the anterior tibialis and rectus femoris stabilize the patient during the backward sway. The rectus femoris comes into play only as a hip flexor, and as the patient sways far enough back to invoke this action.

    Figure 17–65C shows recordings from the anterior tibialis, general gastrocnemius, medial gastrocnemius,

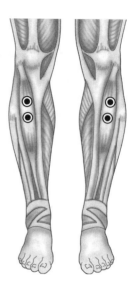

Figure 17–65A Electrode placement for the ankle dorsiflexor (tibialis anterior) site.

Source: Copyright © Clinical Resources, Inc.

lateral gastrocnemius, lateral soleus, and medial soleus of the right leg during standing on toes (plantar flexion) versus standing on heels (dorsiflexion). All aspects of

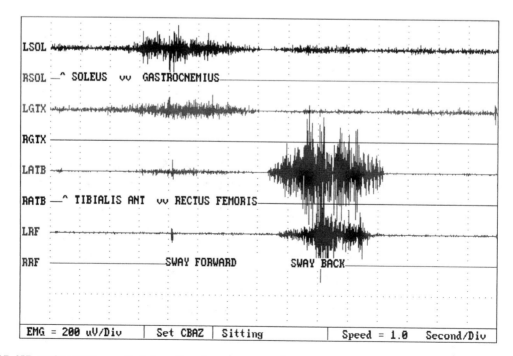

Figure 17–65B Surface EMG recordings from the soleus, gastrocnemius, anterior tibialis, and rectus femoris for the left leg during an anterior sway and a posterior sway. The right aspect was not monitored, and the flat lines represent no input.

Source: Copyright © Clinical Resources, Inc.

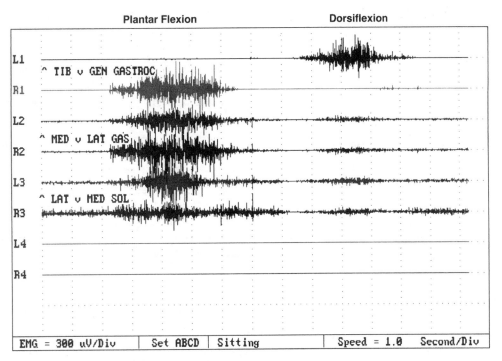

Figure 17–65C Surface EMG recordings from the anterior tibialis, general gastrocnemius, medial gastrocnemius, lateral gastrocnemius, lateral soleus, and medial soleus of the right leg during standing on toes (plantar flexion) versus standing on heels (dorsiflexion).

Source: Copyright © Clinical Resources, Inc.

the posterior compartment are active during toe standing, while only the anterior compartment is active during heel standing.

Clinical Considerations: This site is rated as quasi-specific because of the close proximity of, and potential for cross-talk from, surrounding muscles. It is an excellent site, however, for monitoring and providing feedback during dorsiflexion. It serves different functions when the muscle is weighted versus not weighted. When not weight bearing, this site dorsiflexes the foot; when weight bearing, it shifts the postural weight back.[16]

During walking, this muscle is most active at heel strike and primarily serves to prevent "foot slap." It also assists the toes in clearing the floor during the swing phase of gait.[16] For this reason, it is a useful site in rehabilitation of foot drop.

This site is also used to monitor the tibialis anterior while retraining foot position. The tibialis posterior is necessary to create the arch/neutral foot position. Often, however, people "cheat"—that is, they use the

tibialis anterior in an attempt to lift the arch. Surface EMG monitoring of the tibialis anterior can be used to downtrain unnecessary substitution patterns.

This site is also used to examine the tibialis anterior for excessive recruitment in patients with shin splints. Often, insufficient dorsiflexion is noted in these patients' range of motion, and downtraining can be nicely coupled with a stretching program.

With maximal squatting with the heels flat on the floor, the tibialis anterior was found to be at 60% of its maximum voluntary contraction.[67]

Volume Conduction: Potential contributions from extensor hallucis, extensor digitorum longus, and soleus.

Other Sites of Interest: Gastrocnemius, soleus, rectus femoris, medial hamstrings.

Referred Pain Considerations: Trigger points in the tibialis anterior tend to project pain downward to the great toe.[17]

GASTROCNEMIUS PLACEMENT

Type of Placement: Specific and general.

Action: Plantar flexor (of the foot); knee flexion.

Clinical Uses: Gait retraining.

Muscle Insertions: The muscle crosses two joints, with the medial and lateral heads of this muscle arising from just above the femoral condyles. It inserts on the calcaneus via the Achilles tendon (heel).

Innervation: Tibial nerve via S-1 and S-2.

Location: General recordings from this muscle may be obtained by placing the two active electrodes proximally so that one electrode resides on each muscle (**Figure 17–66**, right leg). Cross-talk from the dorsiflexors would be expected.

Specific recordings from the medial or lateral aspect may be obtained by placing active electrodes 2 cm apart, running parallel to the muscle fibers, just distal from the knee and 2 cm medial or lateral to midline (Figure 17–66, left leg).

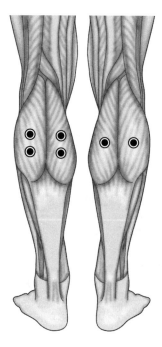

Figure 17–66 Electrode placement for the gastrocnemius site. The right side represents the general placement. The left side represents the more specific placement.

Source: Copyright © Clinical Resources, Inc.

Behavioral Test: While standing, lean forward. In an open kinetic chain, plantar flex the foot (point the toe); in a closed kinetic chain, stand on the toes.

Tracing Comment: See the tracings for the hamstrings (Figure 17–64B) and the tibialis anterior for postural sway off the central axis of gravity (Figure 17–65B) and for dorsiflexion and plantar flexion (Figure 17–65C).

Clinical Considerations: This muscle assists in plantar flexion in the controlling of the forward movement of the leg over the fixed foot during ambulation.[17]

This site is affected by the position of the body over the center of gravity. It is quiet in the neutral posture; the more forward the body is over its axis, the more active this muscle becomes. It is most active when one is standing on the toes.[67] Knee position changes the strength of the recording. As the knee becomes flexed, it becomes less effective as a plantar flexor.

Volume Conduction: Soleus, extensor hallucis, and extensor digitorum longus.

Other Sites of Interest: Soleus for plantar flexion; tibialis anterior; hamstring for knee flexion; quadriceps.

Referred Pain Considerations: Trigger points in this muscle may project pain to the insole of the foot and locally to the calf area.[17]

SOLEUS PLACEMENT

Type of Placement: Quasi-specific.

Action: Plantar flexor and inverter of the foot.

Clinical Uses: Gait training.

Muscle Insertions: This muscle arises from the posterior head and upper third of the fibula, the middle of the tibia, and the tendinous arch, and joins the gastrocnemius to insert on the Achilles tendon.

Innervation: The tibial nerve via L-5, S-1, and S-2.

Location: Two electrodes, 2 cm apart, are placed parallel to the muscle fibers on the inferior and lateral aspects of the leg, clearly below the belly of gastrocnemius (**Figure 17–67A**).

Behavioral Test: Forward leaning while standing or dorsiflexion of the foot.

Tracing Comment: **Figure 17–67B** shows recordings from the anterior tibialis site, general gastrocnemius site, medial gastrocnemius site, lateral gastrocnemius

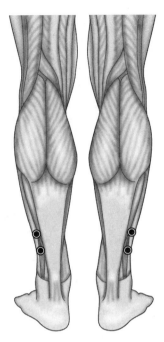

Figure 17–67A Electrode placement for the soleus site.

Source: Copyright © Clinical Resources, Inc.

site, lateral soleus site, and medial soleus site of the right leg during inversion and eversion of the foot. The possibility of cross-talk from the peroneus and tibialis posterior entering the SEMG signal must be considered (raw SEMG).

Also see the tracings in Figure 17–65B for postural sway off the central axis of gravity and Figure 17–65C for dorsiflexion and plantar flexion.

Clinical Considerations: This site was rated as quasi-specific because Perry, Easterday, and Antonelli's systematic study of the selectivity of surface sensors indicated that only 36% of the amplified signal comes from the soleus.[68] The remaining 64% of the amplified signal represents cross-talk from neighboring muscles (primarily the gastrocnemius).

The soleus muscle is commonly studied during ambulation. Its primary purpose is thought to be stabilizing the knee during the stance phase of gait.[16] It is also known to provide ankle stability and restrain the forward movement of the tibia over the fixed foot.

The soleus, along with tibialis anterior, is well known for its role in maintaining upright posture.[16] As the body

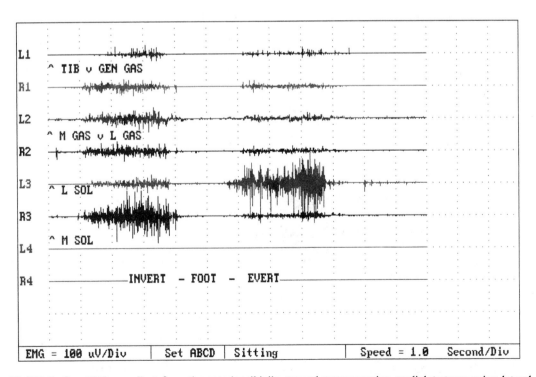

Figure 17–67B Surface EMG recordings from the anterior tibialis, general gastrocnemius, medial gastrocnemius, lateral gastrocnemius, lateral soleus, and medial soleus of the right leg during inversion and eversion of the foot.

Source: Copyright © Clinical Resources, Inc.

sways forward over the center of gravity, the soleus becomes more active. High heels tend to activate the soleus group.[69]

Volume Conduction: Gastrocnemius, peroneus longus, posterior tibialis, flexor hallicus longus, and flexor digitorum longus.

Other Sites of Interest: Gastrocnemius during planter flexion; tibialis anterior.

Referred Pain Considerations: Trigger points at this site tend to project pain down to the heel or up into the calf. They are also known to project pain up to the sacroiliac joint.[17]

EXTENSOR DIGITORUM BREVIS PLACEMENT

Type of Placement: Specific.

Action: Dorsiflexion of the toes and eversion of the foot.

Clinical Uses: Neurologic rehabilitation, gait training.

Muscle Insertions: These muscles arise from the calcaneus and insert on the tendons of the dorsal aponeurosis of the second to fourth digits.

Innervation: The peroneal nerve via the spinal nerves at L-5 and S-1.

Location: Two active electrodes, 2 cm apart, are placed parallel to the muscle fibers (same direction of the

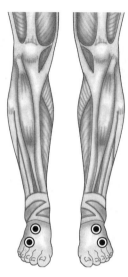

Figure 17–68A Electrode placement for the extensor digitorum brevis site.

Source: Copyright © Clinical Resources, Inc.

metatarsal bones) on the dorsal, lateral aspect of the foot, half the distance from the ankle to the base of the toes (**Figure 17–68A**).

Behavioral Test: Dorsiflexion of the toes.

Tracing Comment: In **Figure 17–68B**, the extensor digitorum brevis is presented during dorsiflexion of the toes (raw SEMG).

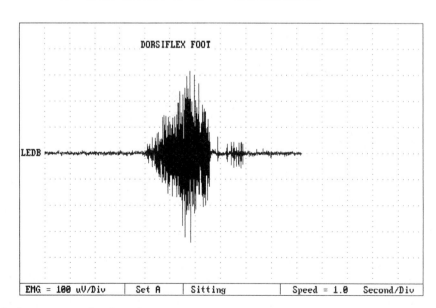

Figure 17–68B Surface EMG recording from the extensor digitorum brevis site during dorsiflexion of the toes and foot.

Source: Copyright © Clinical Resources, Inc.

Clinical Considerations: The primary function of this muscle is to extend the second, third, and fourth toes. It is usually not included in a discussion regarding gait. A novel use of this site is to monitor and provide feedback during the swing phase of gait to assist the patient in dorsiflexion.[70]

Volume Conduction: Extensor hallucis brevis.

Other Sites of Interest: Extensor digitorum longus, extensor hallucis longus, and abductor hallucis during gait.

Referred Pain Considerations: Trigger points at this site project pain locally over the dorsum of the foot.[17]

PERIVAGINAL AND PERIRECTAL PLACEMENT

Type of Placement: Quasi-specific.

Purpose: Monitors from the levator ani and transversus perinei profundus. The sphincter ani externus contributes heavily to recordings using the rectal sensor; the bulbospongiosus contributes heavily to recordings using the vaginal sensor. These placement sites monitor the general support offered by the pelvic floor.

Clinical Uses: Urinary and fecal incontinence, urogenital pain (vestibulitus/vulvodynia and prostatitis).

Muscle Insertions: The levator ani arises from the pubic bone, the tendinous arch of the levator ani muscle, and the ischial spine. Its fibers are divisible into the puborectalis, prerectal, pubococcygeal, and iliococcygeal muscles. The deeper iliococcygeal muscle of the levator ani forms a hammock across the pelvic floor. The sphincter ani externus encircles the anus. In the male, the bulbospongiosus muscle arises from the perineal body and inserts into the corpus spongiosis and corpus cavernosus that it encloses. In the female, the bulbospongiosus muscle also arises from the perineal body and then surrounds the vagina on its way to the corpora cavernosa clitoridis.

Location: The vaginal sensor is inserted into the vagina, and the rectal sensor is inserted into the rectum. A cross-sectional view of this electrode placement may be seen in **Figure 17–69A**. Comparison of recordings from this type of sensor and fine-wire EMG recording has shown very high correlations.[71,72]

In addition, surface electrodes may be placed near or on the labia of the vagina, as shown in **Figure 17–69B**. This electrode placement is found to correlate quite well

A

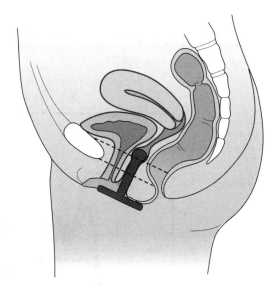

Figure 17–69A Cross-sectional view of an SEMG sensor inserted into the vagina.

Source: Copyright © Marek Jantos, PhD.

B

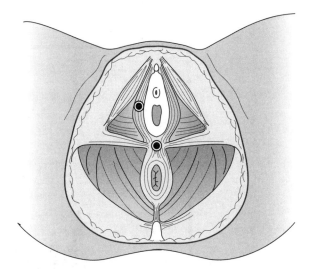

Figure 17–69B Electrode placements for the perivaginal and perirectal sites are near the vagina and anus, respectively.

Source: Adapted from: Kahle, Leonhardt, and Plaatzer, *Color Atlas and Textbook of Human Anatomy,* Vol. 1, © 1978, Georg Thieme Verlag.

($r > 0.95$) (Jantos, personal communication). An example of this correlation is seen in the simultaneous recording from a vaginal sensor and an external surface electrode in **Figure 17–69D**. Finally, external perianal surface recordings may be conducted using the placement shown in **Figure 17–69E**.[73]

Behavioral Test: Kegel exercise; tense or flick pelvic floor.

Tracing Comment: **Figure 17–69C** presents an intravaginal SEMG recording. Its normalcy is reflected by (1) the low resting baseline, (2) the good recruitment with clear demarcation between rest and contraction, (3) a strong contraction without any fatigue, (4) the abrupt fall from

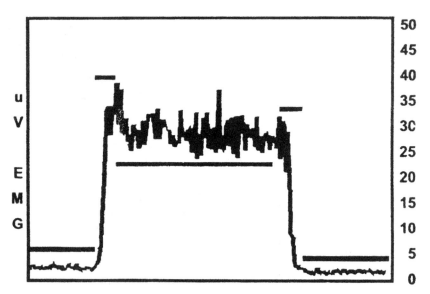

Figure 17–69C Intravaginal SEMG recording with a baseline, contraction, and return to baseline.
Source: Copyright © Marek Jantos, PhD.

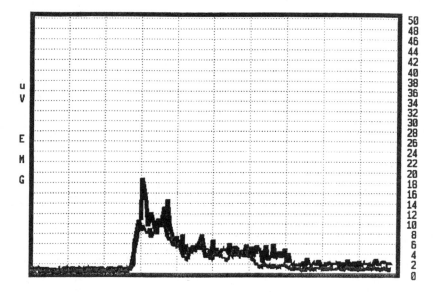

Figure 17–69D Simultaneous time series recordings from intravaginal (Figure 17-69A) and external (Figure 17-69B) electrode placement. Note the high correlation between the two.
Source: Copyright © Marek Jantos, PhD.

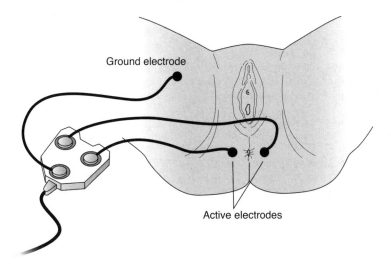

Ground electrode

Active electrodes

Figure 17–69E Electrode placement for perianal recordings using an external placement strategy.

Source: Reprinted with permission from J. Coracos, S. Drew, and L. West, "Urinary and Fecal Incontinence," *Electromyography: Applications in Physical Therapy*, © 1992, Thought Technology.

contraction to resting baseline, and (5) a low resting baseline with good muscle stability (i.e., low variance) post contraction.

Clinical Considerations: Effects may change as a function of prone, sitting, or standing postures. They may be affected by squats, coughs, sneezes, and exertional lifts.

Volume Conduction: Gluteus maximus, abdominals, adductors of the thigh.

Referred Pain Considerations: Trigger points in the levator ani can refer pain to the sacral region.[17]

Benchmark: Resting baseline: 2.0 ($\pm$ 0.2) μV (RMS). Strong contraction: 17.5 μV (RMS).
Values taken using a Thought Technology EMG with a 25- to 1000-Hz filter.

REFERENCES

1. Lader MH, Mathews AM. A physiological model of phobic anxiety and desensitization. *Behav Res Ther.* 1968;6: 411–421.
2. Malmo RB, Shagass C. Physiologic studies of reaction to stress in anxiety and early schizophrenia. *Psychosomatic Med.* 1949;11:9–24.
3. Goldstein B. Electromyography: A measure of skeletal muscle response. In: Greenfield S, Sternbach R, eds. *Handbook of Psychophysiology.* New York, NY: Holt, Rinehart & Winston; 1972.
4. Munro RR. Electromyography of the muscles of mastication. In: Griffin CJ, Harris R, eds. *The Temporomandibular Joint Syndrome.* Basel, Switzerland: S. Darger; 1975. *Monographs in Oral Sciences*, vol. 4.
5. Schwartz M, ed. *Biofeedback: A Practitioner's Guide.* New York, NY: Guilford; 1987.
6. Andrasik F, Blanchard EB. Biofeedback treatment of muscle contraction headache. In: Hatch JP, Fischer JG, Rugh J, eds. *Biofeedback: Studies in Clinical Efficacy.* New York, NY: Plenum Press; 1987.
7. Donaldson S, Skubick D, Donaldson M. *Electromyography, Trigger Points and Myofascial Syndromes.* Calgary, Alberta: Behavioral Health Consultants; 1991.
8. Hudzynski L, Lawrence G. Significance of EMG surface electrode placement models and headache findings. *Headache.* 1988;28:30–35.
9. Zemach-Berson D, Zemach-Berson K, Reese M. *Relaxercise.* San Francisco, CA: Harper; 1990.
10. Schneider C, Wilson E. Special considerations for EMG biofeedback training. In: *Foundations of Biofeedback Practice.* Wheat Ridge, CO: Biofeedback Society of America; 1985.
11. Bryant M. Biofeedback in the treatment of selected dysphagic patients. *Dysphagia.* 1991;6:140–144.
12. Curtis D, Braham SL, Karr S, Holborow G, Worman D. Identification of unopposed intact muscle pair actions affecting swallowing: potential for rehabilitation. *Dysphagia.* 1987;3:57–64.
13. Ettare D, Ettare R. Muscle learning therapy: a treatment protocol. In: Cram JR, ed. *Clinical EMG for Surface*

Recordings, II. Nevada City, CA: Clinical Resources; 1990:197–234.

14. Cahn T, Cram JR. Muscle scanning: support for the back. *Perceptual Motor Skills.* 1990;70:851–857.

15. Peper E, Wilson V, Taylor W, et al. Repetitive strain injury. *Phys Ther Prod.* September 1994:17–22.

16. Basmajian JV, DeLuca C. *Muscles Alive.* 5th ed. Baltimore, MD: Williams & Wilkins; 1985.

17. Travell J, Simons D. *Myofascial Pain and Dysfunction: A Trigger Point Manual, I and II.* Baltimore, MD: Williams & Wilkins; 1983.

18. Cram JR. EMG muscle scanning and diagnostic manual for surface recordings. In: Cram JR, ed. *Clinical EMG for Surface Recordings, II.* Nevada City, CA: Clinical Resources; 1990:1–142.

19. Staling LM, Fetcher P, Vorro J. Premature occlusal contact influence on mandibular kinesiology. In: Komi PV, ed. *Biomechanics, V-A.* Baltimore, MD: University Park Press; 1976.

20. Cacioppo JT, Tassinary G, Fridlund AJ. The skeletalmotor system. In: Cacioppo JT, Tassinary G, eds. *Principles of Psychophysiology.* New York, NY: Cambridge University Press; 1990.

21. Bennett H, Kornhauser S. Assessment of general anesthesia by facial muscle electromyography (FACE). *Am J Electromed.* June 1995:94–97.

22. Ekman P, Friesen WV. *Unmasking the Human Face.* Englewood Cliffs, NJ: Prentice Hall; 1972.

23. Sackeim HA, Gur RC, Saucy MC. Emotions are expressed more intensely on the left side of the face. *Science.* 1978;202:434–436.

24. Worth DR. Movements of the cervical spine in modern manual therapy of the vertebral column. In: Grieve G, ed. *Modern Manual Therapy of the Vertebral Column.* New York, NY: Churchill Livingstone; 1986.

25. Carstensen B. Indications and contraindications for manual therapy for temporomandibular joint dysfunction. In: Grieve G, ed. *Modern Manual Therapy of the Vertebral Column.* New York, NY: Churchill Livingstone; 1986.

26. Upledger J, Vredevoogd JD. *CranioSacral Therapy.* Seattle, WA: Eastland Press; 1983.

27. Campbell EJM. Accessory muscles. In: Campbell EJM, Agostini E, Davis JN, eds. *The Respiratory Muscles: Mechanics and Neural Control.* Phildelphia, PA: W.B. Saunders; 1970.

28. Kendall FP, Kendall E, McCreary BA. *Muscles, Testing and Function.* 3rd ed. Baltimore, MD: Williams & Wilkins; 1983.

29. Gray H. *Anatomy of the Human Body.* 29th ed. Goss CM, ed. Phildelphia, PA: Lea & Febiger; 1973.

30. Cook EE, Gray, VL, Savinar-Nogue E, Madeiros J. Shoulder antagonistic strength ratios: a comparison between college-level baseball pitchers and non-pitchers. *J Orthop Sports Phys Ther.* March 1987:451–461.

31. Duchenne GB. *Physiologie des Mouvement.* Kaplan EB, trans. Phildelphia, PA: W.B. Saunders; 1949.

32. Rasch PI, Burke RK. *Kinesiology and Applied Anatomy.* Phildelphia, PA: Lea & Febiger; 1978.

33. Taylor W. Dynamic EMG biofeedback in assessment and treatment using a neuromuscular re-education model. In: Cram JR, ed. *Clinical EMG for Surface Recordings, Volume 2.* Nevada City, CA: Clinical Resources; 1990:175–196.

34. Hollingshead WH. *Functional Anatomy of the Limbs and Back.* Phildelphia, PA: W.B. Saunders; 1976.

35. Bao S, Mathiassen SE, Winkel J. Normalizing upper trapezius EMG amplitude: comparison of different procedures. *J Electromyogr Kinesiol.* 1995;5:251–257.

36. McConnell JS. *Treatment of the Unstable Shoulder: Course Manual.* Marina Del Rey, CA: McConnell Seminars; 1993.

37. Lundervold AJS. Electromyographic investigations of position and manner of working in typewriting. *Acta Physiol Scand.* 1951;24:84.

38. Skubick D, Clasby R, Donaldson CCS, Marshall W. Carpal tunnel syndrome as an expression of muscular dysfunction in the neck. *J Occup Rehab.* 1993;3:31–41.

39. Singh M, Karpovich PV. Isotonic and isometric forces of forearm flexors and extensors. *J Applied Physiol.* 1966;21:1435.

40. Sullivan WE, Mortensen OA, Miles M, Green LS. Electromyographic studies of m. biceps brachii during normal voluntary movement at the elbow. *Anat Rec.* 1950;107:243–251.

41. Travill AA. Electromyographic study of the extensor apparatus of the forearm. *Anat Rec.* 1962;144:373–376.

42. Mortimer JT, Kerstein MD, Magnusson R, Petersen H. Muscle blood flow in the human biceps as a function of developed muscle force. *Arch Surg.* 1971;103:376–377.

43. McMahon T, Pianta R, Couch L, Wolf S, Segal R, Mason L. Normalized electromyographic activity patterns in human extensor carpi radialis longus and flexor carpi radialis muscles: differential activity. In: Anderson PA, Hobart DJ, Danoff N, eds. *Electromyographical Kinesiology.* Amsterdam: Elsevier; 1991:39–42.

44. Joseph J, Williams PL. Electromyography of certain hip muscles. *J Anat.* 1957;91:286–294.

45. Simons D. Functions of the quadratus lumborum muscle and relation of its myofascial trigger points to low back pain. *Pain Abstracts, I.* Montreal: Second World Congress on Pain; August 1978.

46. Flint MM. An electromyographic comparison of the function of the iliacus and rectus abdominis muscles. *J Am Phys Ther Assoc.* 1965;45:248–253.

47. Jull G, Janda V. Muscles and motor control in low back pain: assessment and management. In: Twomey L, Taylor J, eds. *Physical Therapy of the Low Back.* New York, NY: Churchill Livingstone; 1987.

48. Pierce M, Lee W. Muscle firing order during active prone hip extension. *J Orthop Sports Phys Ther.* 1990; 12:2–9.

49. Jackson R. Functional relations of the lower half. Unpublished data, 1996.

50. Greenlaw RK. *Function of Muscles about the Hip during Normal Level Walking.* Thesis, Queen's University, Kingston, Ontario.

51. Neumann DA, Cook TM. Effect of load and carrying position on the electromyographic activity of the gluteus medius muscle during walking. *Phys Ther.* 1985;65:305–311.

52. Pere EB, Stem JT, Schwartz JM. Functional differentiation within the tensor fasciae latae. *J Bone Joint Surg Am.* 1981;63:1457–1471.

53. Godges J, et al. The effects of two stretching procedures on hip range of motion and gait economy. *J Orthop Sports Phys Ther.* March 1989:350–357.

54. Godges J, McRae P, Engelkey K. Effects of exercise on hip range of motion, trunk muscle performance and gait economy. *Phys Ther.* 1993;73:468–477.

55. Godges J, Heino J, Carter C. Relationship between hip extension range of motion and postural alignment. *J Orthop Sports Phys Ther.* 1990;12:243–247.

56. Gose J, Schweizer P. Iliotibial band tightness. *J Orthop Sports Phys Ther.* April 1989:399–407.

57. Draper V. Electromyographic biofeedback and recovery of quadriceps femoris muscle function following anterior cruciate ligament reconstruction. *Phys Ther.* 1990; 69:11–17.

58. Draper V, Ballard L. Electrical stimulation versus electromyographic biofeedback in the recovery of quadriceps femoris muscle function following anterior cruciate ligament surgery. *Phys Ther.* 1991;71:455–463.

59. Basmajian N, Harden TP, Regenos EM. Integrated action of the four heads of the quadriceps femoris: an electromyographic study. *Anat Rec.* 1972;172:15–20.

60. Souza DR, Gross MT. Comparison of vastus medialis oblique: vastus lateralis muscle integrated electromyographic ratios between healthy subjects and patients with patellofemoral pain. *Phys Ther.* 1991;71:310–320.

61. Felder CR, Lesson MA. The use of electromyographic biofeedback for training the vastus medialis oblique in patients with patellofemoral pain. *Physical Ther Prod.* March 1990:49–52.

62. McConnell JS. *McConnell Patellofemoral Treatment Plan: Course Manual.* Marina Del Rey, CA: McConnell Seminars; 1991.

63. Kasman G, Cram J, Wolf S. *Clinical Applications in Surface Electromyography.* Gaithersburg, MD: Aspen; 1997.

64. Close JR. *Motor Function in the Lower Extremity.* Springfield, IL: Charles C. Thomas; 1964.

65. Green DL, Morris JM. Role of adductor longus and adductor magnus in postural movements and in ambulation. *Am J Phys Med.* 1970;49:223–240.

66. Murray MP, Mollinger LA, Gardner GM, et al. Kinematic and EMG patterns during slow, free and fast walking. *J Orthop Res.* 1984;2:272–280.

67. Okada M. An electromyographic estimation of the relative muscular load in different human postures. *J Hum Ergol.* 1972;1:75–93.

68. Perry J, Easterday CS, Antonelli DJ. Surface versus intramuscular electrodes for electromyography of superficial and deep muscles. *Phys Ther.* 1981;61:7–15.

69. Campbell KM, Biggs NL, Blanton PL, et al. Electromyographic investigation of the relative activity among four components of the triceps surae. *Am J Phys Med.* 1973;52:30–41.

70. Wolf S. *Anatomy and Electrode Placement: Upper Extremities; Face and Back; Lower Extremities* [video]. Nevada City, CA: Clinical Resources; 1991.

71. Maizels M, Pirlit CF. Pediatric urodynamics: a clinical comparison for surface versus needle pelvic floor/external sphincter electromyography. *J Urol.* 1979;122:518–522.

72. Nygaard I, et al. Exercise and incontinence. *Obstet Gynecol.* 1983;75:848–851.

73. Corocos J, Drew S, West L. *Urinary and Fecal Incontinence: Electromyography Applications in Physical Therapy.* Montreal: Thought Technology; 1992.

CHAPTER QUESTIONS

1. As a general rule, the depth of an SEMG recording is directly proportionate to:
   a. the size of the muscle below
   b. the type of the muscle fiber below
   c. the interelectrode distance
   d. the shape of the electrode

2. The quasi-specific site designation is offered when:
   a. the intended muscle for recording lies beneath another muscle
   b. the intended muscle for recording is superficial
   c. the intended muscle for recording lies close to other muscles
   d. either a or c

3. The location for an electrode placement needs to be verified by:
   a. muscle testing with the electrode attached
   b. knowledge of muscle origin and insertions
   c. knowledge of muscle function
   d. all of the above

4. The SEMG tracings presented in the atlas are:
   a. based on normative groups
   b. samples reflecting one individual subject's performance
   c. examples of an ideal recruitment pattern
   d. none of the above

5. Benchmark values presented in the atlas:
   a. are based on normative data
   b. are useful for resting baseline comparisons only
   c. are useful for resting tone and dynamic movement peaks
   d. are based on normalized values
   e. both a and b

6. Abduction reflects:
   a. movement toward the body
   b. movement away from the body
   c. movement of an upward nature
   d. movement of a downward nature

7. In the upper extremities, *supination* is:
   a. the palm-up position
   b. the palm-down position
   c. the neutral position
   d. none of the above
8. Which of the following is *not* one of the attributes of the lower extremities?
   a. side bending
   b. flexion
   c. extension
   d. abduction
   e. adduction
9. The frontal (wide) placement is best used:
   a. to monitor stress
   b. to reach general relaxation
   c. to monitor negative emotions
   d. both a and b
   e. all of the above
10. Using the temporal mastoid (wide) placement, it is possible to observe recruitment during:
    a. eyebrow flashes
    b. head rotation
    c. ear wiggling
    d. both a and b
    e. all of the above
11. If SEMG recruitment at the temporalis site is associated with elevation of the mandible, which site would you monitor to see jaw opening?
    a. zygomaticus
    b. suprahyoid
    c. masseter
    d. none of the above
12. When using the cervical trapezius placement, ECG artifact:
    a. will contaminate the left lead
    b. will contaminate the right lead
    c. will contaminate both leads
    d. is a problem only if you are using a 100- to 200-Hz filter
13. Which pattern of muscle recruitment would one expect to see during cervical rotation to the left?
    a. right sternocleidomastoid, right C-4 paraspinals
    b. right sternocleidomastoid, left C-4 paraspinals
    c. left sternocleidomastoid, right C-4 paraspinals
    d. left sternocleidomastoid, left C-4 paraspinals
14. During a deep inspiration, one would expect to see the scalene muscles:
    a. show a symmetrical recruitment pattern
    b. show an asymmetrical recruitment pattern
    c. not be involved in respiratory patterns
    d. recruit four times more than the upper trapezius
15. The posterior deltoid should recruit most heavily during:
    a. shoulder elevation
    b. external rotation
    c. extension of the arm
    d. a, b, and c tend to recruit at the same level

16. The ratio of the peak contraction between upper and lower trapezius during abduction of the arms to 90 degrees should be approximately:
    a. 3:1
    b. 1:1
    c. 1:3
    d. 10:1
17. Recruitment patterns for serratus anterior are greatest during:
    a. a wall push-up
    b. a kneeling push-up
    c. a floor push-up
    d. forward flexion of the arms
18. Which of the deltoids is most heavily recruited during forward flexion of the arms?
    a. anterior deltoid
    b. middle deltoid
    c. posterior deltoid
    d. both b and c
19. The widely spaced extensor–flexor site on the forearm will show activation during:
    a. extension
    b. flexion
    c. making a fist
    d. both a and c
    e. all of the above
20. During elbow flexion in the pronated position, one would expect the biceps:
    a. to fire briskly along with the brachioradialis
    b. not to recruit
    c. to fire briskly without the brachioradialis
    d. to fire only during the first 30 degrees of arc
21. When placing electrodes on the triceps, the arm:
    a. should be flexed at 90 degrees
    b. should be fully extended
    c. should be in the position the practitioner plans to train in
    d. can be in any convenient position
22. The extensor carpi ulnaris tends to show the least amount of recruitment during:
    a. resisted radial deviation
    b. resisted ulnar deviation
    c. resisted wrist extension
    d. none of the above
23. Placement for extensor digitorum should be:
    a. over the belly of the muscle
    b. at the distal end of the muscle belly
    c. at the proximal end of the muscle
    d. none of the above
24. During forward flexion of the torso, a flexion–relaxation response should be seen:
    a. at the L-3 site only
    b. at the L-3 and T-12 sites only
    c. at the L-3, T-12, and T-1 sites only
    d. at the L-3, T-12, T-1, and C-4 sites

25. During axial rotation of the trunk, do the abdominal muscles play a role?
    a. definitely yes
    b. definitely no
    c. only at the extreme end of the range of motion
    d. only during the first 15 degrees of arc
26. During a diagonal sit-up to the left, which electrode placements on the abdominal muscles seem to recruit heavily?
    a. right rectus and left oblique
    b. left rectus and right oblique
    c. left and right rectus and left oblique
    d. left and right rectus and right oblique
27. Which action would you expect to recruit the gluteus medius most heavily?
    a. abduction of the leg with internal rotation
    b. abduction of the leg with external rotation
    c. abduction of the leg in the neutral position
    d. a, b, and c would recruit equally
28. Which action would you expect to recruit the tensor fasciae latae the least?
    a. abduction of the leg with internal rotation
    b. abduction of the leg with external rotation
    c. abduction of the leg in the neutral position
    d. a, b, and c would recruit equally
29. Which of the statements is correct about the flexors of the hip (femoral triangle site and hip flexor site/sartorius and iliopsoas) sites?
    a. They are easily isolated.
    b. They are quasi-specific sites.
    c. They are specific sites.
    d. They are general sites.

30. The relative balance between the vastus lateralis (VL) and the vastus medialis oblique (VMO) has been indicated as beng important in patellofemoral pain. What should the normal ratio of the peak VMO:VL be?
    a. 1:3
    b. 3:1
    c. a little greater than 1:1
    d. a little less than 1:1
31. The level of recruitment during prone leg extension of the tensor fasciae latae is reduced when the leg is laterally rotated. Which position would reduce the recruitment of lateral hamstrings during leg extension?
    a. medial rotation
    b. neutral position
    c. lateral rotation
    d. a, b, and c would recruit equally
32. The tibialis anterior placement site is:
    a. a specific site
    b. a quasi-specific site
    c. a general site
    d. a linear site
33. Which of the following characteristics of the recruitment pattern for the pelvic floor is not one of its normal attributes?
    a. low resting baseline
    b. good demarcation between rest and contraction
    c. strong contraction with minimal fatigue
    d. high variance during the postcontraction period

Glossary

abduction: Movement away from midline of the sagittal plane.

abrasion of the skin: A procedure by which the oils and horny layer of skin are removed by rubbing the skin with a rough texture. It is used to reduce impedance and to improve recording quality.

acoustic startle: A reflex response to sudden changes in sound.

active electrode: An electrode design that incorporates the EMG preamplifier in an adjacent housing directly at the recording site. It commonly uses a very high input impedance, rendering it less sensitive to the impedance of the electrode interface.

active range of motion: Joint motion produced by muscle contraction.

adduction: Movement toward the midline of the sagittal plane.

adipose tissue: The subcutaneous fat layer between the surface of the skin and the muscle. This tissue is known to attenuate the source EMG as it travels to the surface. The greater the thickness of the adipose tissue, the greater the attenuation. It is recommended that the thickness be measured prior to SEMG recordings.

adjunct procedure: A technique combined with surface EMG feedback, such as progressive relaxation or visualization.

agonist muscle group: The muscle group that initiates a contraction of movement.

alpha motor system: The part of the central nervous system that activates the extrafusal muscle fibers.

amplitude probability distribution function: A graphical representation of the variability of SEMG activity. Here the amplitude of the SEMG signal for a specified epoch of time is plotted as a histogram, with amplitude plotted along the x-axis and the frequency of a given amplitude plotted along the y-axis. This may be used to inspect for the presence of interspersed rest during a work task.

ankle-to-ankle recordings: A procedure in which the recording electrodes are placed on the right and left ankles. This procedure is used to teach systemic relaxation to the lower extremities, hips, and low-back region.

antagonist muscle group: A muscle group that provides a negative, stabilizing force during a contraction or movement.

antalgic posture: Adoption of a postural stance that occurs in response to pain.

autogenic training: A technique developed by Wolfgang Luthe in Germany in the 1950s for verbally relaxing the muscles and other physiological systems.

ballistic contraction: Movement that is executed in the fastest possible speed.

band pass filter: A filter that defines the lower and upper frequency limits (expressed in Hertz) of the energy of the SEMG signal that is passed on for further amplification. Some SEMG amplifiers use a very narrow

100- to 200-Hz band-pass filter, allowing only about 20% of the SEMG spectrum to be processed. Others use a wider 15- to 500-Hz band pass filter, allowing 98% of the SEMG to be processed.

bilateral electrode placement: A technique in which each of the recording electrodes from a differential amplifier is placed on the right and left aspects of a muscle group.

bracing: The habitual and inappropriate use of postural muscles.

cathode ray oscilloscope: A laboratory instrument that displays voltage signals from muscles.

cerebral palsy: A condition characterized by hypertonic and/or hypotonic muscle tone. It is often caused by brain injury during birth.

Cinderella motor units: Low-threshold motor units that are recruited first and whose activity levels do not decrease until the muscle fully relaxes.

cocontraction: The tendency of agonist and antagonist muscle groups to become activated simultaneously. It is commonly expressed as percent asymmetry for normalized SEMG.

common mode rejection: A characteristic of a differential amplifier, in which the signal that is common to both recording electrodes in reference to ground is eliminated from further amplification. It reduces the environmental noise that might otherwise contaminate the signal. It is mathematically defined as a common mode rejection ratio (CMRR) and should be 90 dB or better.

concentric contraction: The activation of a muscle that is associated with the shortening of its length.

contracture: An electrically silent, involuntary state of maintained muscle shortness due to decreased extensibility (i.e., increased stiffness) of the passive elastic properties of the connective tissue. The elasticity of the muscle should be concurrently determined through palpation, and the muscle length and joint angle should be reported along with the SEMG levels.

contralateral walk: A gait in which the shoulders move in opposite directions to the legs.

corollary discharge: The process that the brain uses to prepare for upcoming movements and to decrease sensory feedback from the person's own movements that might disrupt the intended movement.

corticospinal tract: A voluntary motor tract originating in the motor and sensory cortices.

cortisol: A hormone produced by the adrenal cortex that has been associated with stress.

derecruitment: Training in the reduction of SEMG activity. It is commonly associated with teaching the patient to turn off a recruitment pattern once the movement is completed.

differential amplification: A characteristic of the SEMG amplifier, in which the biological potential reaching both recording electrodes is compared to that of the reference electrode, and only the energy that is different is passed on for further amplification. Also see *common mode rejection*.

diffuse muscular coactivation (DMC): A term developed by Donaldson et al. to describe "an increase from resting levels (tonus) in the electrical activity of any muscle during movement which does not involve that muscle and is not a part of the agonist-antagonist unit" [Donaldson CCS, MacInnes AL, Snelling LS, Sella GE, Mueller HH. Characteristics of diffuse muscular coactivation (DMC) in persons with fibromyalgia: part 2. *NeuroRehabilitation*. 2002;17(1):41–48].

direct contact electrode: Surface EMG that makes contact with the skin.

discrimination training: Surface EMG biofeedback training procedure in which the subject learns to associate a specific root mean square (RMS) microvolt level with proprioceptive sensations. Extrinsic feedback is withdrawn as the subject comes to discriminate different levels of muscle tension.

downtraining: Training in the reduction of SEMG activity. It is commonly associated with relaxation training.

dynamic equinus deformity: A condition in which the foot is plantar flexed.

dynamic SEMG evaluation: The use of single-site or multisite SEMG recordings for the study of recruitment patterns of muscles during movement. The record is examined for stereotypic SEMG events as a function of the range of motion arc—such as symmetry of recruitment, cocontractions, synergies, substitution patterns, and irritability (differentiated from needle EMG findings).

dyspareunia: A condition marked by painful intercourse.

dysponesis: Literally "bad effort." In the context of SEMG, it implies an inappropriate site or intensity of muscle activation.

dystonia: A movement disorder characterized by chronically contracted muscles and difficulty controlling the muscles.

eccentric contraction: Muscle contraction generated as a muscle increases in length.

electroencephalograph (EEG): An instrument that measures brain wave patterns. The brain wave is produced by comparing the electrical potential difference between two electrode placements on the scalp or on the scalp and a nonactive site across time.

electomyography (EMG): The sum of the energy from all muscle action potentials detected by the recording electrode.

endopelvic fascia: Connective tissue consisting of elastin (distensible tissue), collagen (noncompliant, less distensible soft tissue), and smooth muscle.

epinephrine: A hormone produced by the adrenal medulla associated with sympathetic nervous system activation.

erythema: An increase in blood to an area resulting in a reddening of the skin.

fascia: A sheet of fibrous tissue that encapsulates muscles and groups of muscles and separates muscle layers or groups.

fast-twitch muscle fibers: Muscle fibers that are pale in color; they rely on anaerobic metabolism.

Feldenkrais Method: An approach to movement reeducation developed by Moshe Feldenkrais. It includes "Awareness Through Movement" (floor exercises) and "Functional Integration" (individual hands-on table work).

female orgasmic disorder: Persistent and recurrent difficulty in achieving an orgasm.

flexion cross-extension reflex: A polysynaptic reflex that excites the flexor group and inhibits the extensor group on the ipsilateral side of pain, while simultaneously exciting the extensor group and inhibiting the flexor group on the contralateral side.

flexion–relaxation: A phenomenon commonly seen in the lumbar paraspinal muscles during forward flexion of the neck or torso. At the end range of motion, there is a reduction in signal amplitude of SEMG as the body moves out onto ligament support.

floating electrode: Surface EMG electrode that is recessed above the skin and uses an electrolytic medium to bridge between the electrode and the skin.

free nerve ending: The sensory apparatus in the muscle that is sensitive to pain. It senses pain when the internal environment is too acidotic or when swelling and edema are present.

frontal EMG: Surface EMG biofeedback procedure in which the recording electrodes are placed on the frontalis muscle directly above each eye. It is used for systemic relaxation training.

Functional Integration: A hands-on technique developed by Moshe Feldenkrais for enabling the person to move more easily and comfortably.

functional magnetic resonance imaging (fMRI): A magnetic resonance imaging technique that measures the brain during function.

gain: How much larger an amplifier makes the biological signal. The amount of gain or amplification determines how large or small the SEMG appears on the visual display.

gait: The pace and sequence of walking.

gamma motor system: The part of the central nervous system that is known to activate the intrafusal muscle fibers associated with the muscle spindle.

generalization: Applying specific learning to everyday life situations.

Golgi tendon organ: Part of the sensory system of muscle, this tissue is located at the tendon/muscle junction, is in series with the muscle, and informs the central nervous system of the strength of contraction or effort made by the muscle.

green light reflex: An assertive and active posture with back arched and arms and legs extended that was described by Thomas Hanna.

hypothalamic–pituitary–adrenal (HPA) axis: A set of structures (part of the neuroendocrine system) that are responsive to stress. Its activity is frequently measured using salivary cortisol.

integral average (μV/s): A method for quantifying SEMG in which the absolute value of each SEMG data point is obtained, the data are simply summed, and an average is calculated. The following formula is used:

$$I[|m(t)|] = 1/T\int_t^{t+T}|m(t)|dt$$

interelectrode distance: The distance between the two recording electrodes (differential amplification). The closer the electrodes, the more circumscribed the area of effective recording. The farther apart the electrodes, the more general the SEMG recording.

interstitial cystitis (IC): A chronic and debilitating bladder syndrome of unknown etiology.

ipsilateral walk: A gait in which the shoulder and leg on the same side move forward simultaneously.

isometric contraction: A muscle contraction in which the muscle length, and thus joint angle, is kept constant.

isotonic contraction: A muscle contraction in which the tension of the muscle is kept constant through regulation of external forces.

Kegel exercises: A protocol for improving the tone of pelvic floor muscles developed by Arnold Kegel.

kinetic chain: Movement in which the distal segment is fixed, such as during weight bearing of the lower limb. Movement at one joint induces movement at another joint.

lactic acid: The by-product of muscle function that exceeds the supply of available oxygen.

ligament: A band or sheet of fibrous tissue connecting bones, cartilage, or other structures.

magnetic resonance imaging (MRI): A technique used to create images of the internal structures of the body.

maximum voluntary contraction (MVC): The greatest amount of effort an individual can put forth with volitional activation of a particular muscle or muscle group.

mechanomyography: The use of a piezoelectric accelerometer to measure muscle activity.

motor unit: The alpha motor neuron, its axon, the neuromuscular junction, and the muscle fibers it innervates (from 3 to 2000). It is the smallest motor unit under voluntary control.

motor unit action potential (MUAP): The electrical recording of the neuron output to muscle fibers.

movement-related cortical potential (MRCP): A waveform recorded by the electroencephalograph during movement.

muscle action potential (MAP): The transmembrane voltage wave associated with the depolarization of muscle fibers. MAPs of a single motor unit may be detected by nearby electrodes residing in the muscle. Populations of MAPs may be detected by SEMG electrodes.

muscle irritability: The persistence of SEMG activity following the cessation of voluntary contraction of a muscle (differentiated from the irritability seen with needle EMG findings).

muscle scanning: A clinical procedure in which multiple sites are evaluated using surface electrodes set at a fixed distance and held in place by hand.

muscle spasm: Reflexive increase in SEMG activity in muscle (with or without shortening). The activity cannot be stopped voluntarily.

muscle spindle: Part of the sensory system of muscle, this tissue is located in the muscle itself, is parallel to the muscle fibers, and informs the central nervous system of the instantaneous length and velocity of change of muscle fibers. It also represents the "stretch receptor." When the muscle is stretched, the output of the muscle spindle provides an excitatory influence on the lower motor neuron that innervates the muscle of origin.

myofascial release (MFR): An approach, associated with John Barnes, that seeks to release distortions and tension of the fascia.

myofascial trigger point: A hyperirritable spot, usually with a taut band of skeletal muscle or in the muscle fascia, that is painful on compression and gives rise to characteristic referred pain patterns, tenderness, and autonomic phenomena.

myotatic unit: A group of agonist and antagonist muscles that function together as a unit because they share a common spinal reflex response.

neuromuscular reeducation: Clinical use of SEMG biofeedback for the treatment of specific neuromuscular disorders.

nocioceptors: Receptors that are responsive to noxious stimuli.

normative data: Quantitative description of the behavior of the muscles under controlled conditions for a representative sample of healthy subjects. It may include means and standard deviations of raw data or consist of standardized/normalized scores.

orienting reflex: The physiological responses of the organism to new stimuli.

palpation: A technique using the fingers for assessing muscle tonicity and other physiological features.

pandiculation: A term popularized by A. F. Fraser to label the full-body contractions and slow release of muscles used by animals. It looks superficially like stretching.

passive range of motion: Joint motion produced by external force and without voluntary assistance by the subject.

patellofemoral pain syndrome: A pain associated with the tracking and misalignment of the patella.

peak to peak: The unit of measurement associated with raw SEMG recordings.

pelvic floor: Several layers of muscle tissue and supporting fasciae that span the pelvic cavity forming a strong horizontally oriented platform [DeLancey J. Functional anatomy of the pelvic floor and urinary continence mechanisms. In: Schussler B, Laycock J, Norton P, Stanton S, eds. *Pelvic Floor Re-education: Principles and Practice.* London, Springer-Verlag; 1994:9–27].

playing-related musculoskeletal complaints (PRMCs): Muscle complaints reported by musicians in response to their playing.

processed SEMG: A mathematically derived presentation of the SEMG signal. Common methods include integral, root mean square (RMS), and spectral analysis representations.

progressive relaxation: A technique introduced by Edmund Jacobson in 1934 for systematically relaxing the skeletal muscles.

protective guarding: The learned motor response in which the individual favors an injured area by substituting other muscle groups for its use. For example, the patient may learn to redistribute a weight-bearing load toward the side opposite the injury. At the same segmental level, typically the SEMG activation pattern is located on the side opposite that of the reported pain.

psychophysiology: The study of physiological responses to psychological events.

raw SEMG: A peak-to-peak oscilloscopic display of the SEMG signal. The signal is not processed; there are no rectification, no time constants, and no conversions or transformations of the SEMG data.

red light reflex: A posture reflecting the withdrawal response from perceived stress or danger characterized by bending forward with knees bent; it was described by Thomas Hanna.

reticulospinal tract: A motor tract originating in the brain stem that contributes to voluntary movements and increased muscle tone.

root mean square (RMS): A method for quantifying SEMG in which each SEMG value is first squared, then summed and averaged, and finally the root of the product is derived. The following formula is used:

$$RMS = [|m(t)|] = 1/T \left[\int_t^{t+T} m^2(t)\, dt \right]^{1/2}$$

Rosen Method: A technique developed by Marion Rosen to deal with forgotten emotions and memories "stored in the body."

rubrospinal tract: A motor tract originating in the brain stem that innervates neurons of the flexor muscles of the limbs.

Ruffini endings: Mechanoreceptors that inform the brain of the relationship of angles of the bones.

sarcomere: The basic anatomical unit of muscle fiber, consisting of a single unit of overlapping myosin and actin filaments extending from one Z line to the next Z line.

scratch reflex: A polysynaptic suprasegmental reflex in which the stimulus evokes a motor response several segments away, whose action is directed toward eradicating the stimulation of the original segment.

self-efficacy: A term popularized by Albert Bandura regarding self-perceived ability.

sensory-motor amnesia (SMA): A term developed by Thomas Hanna to describe chronic muscle contractions and the loss of awareness and control.

slow-twitch muscle fibers: Muscle fibers that are generally small in diameter and red in color; they rely on aerobic metabolism.

somatic psychotherapy: Body-oriented psychotherapy.

somatics: A term coined by Thomas Hanna to label the mind–body integration field.

somatics disciplines: Eastern and Western approaches to the mind–body disciplines that bring the psychological dimension into body work.

spasmodic torticollis: A movement disorder characterized by abnormal turning of the head and other postural distortions.

spectral analysis: A type of analysis in which the SEMG signal is recorded and submitted for a decomposition of the energy into its frequency components, typically using a fast Fourier transform (FFT). It may be used to verify that the SEMG is "clean" of 60-Hz noise, and to assess muscle fatigue.

splinting: The phenomenon whereby muscles reflexively contract around an injured joint to provide a protective stability (immobility) to that joint. These activation patterns are found on the same side of the injury and are associated with increased SEMG activity for the muscles that cross that joint. Also referred to as *acute reflexive spasm.*

static SEMG evaluation: The use of multisite SEMG recordings at rest (neutral postures), for the study of patterns of muscle activity. The record is examined for splinting, protective guarding, antalgia, and chronic bracing.

stretch reflex: A monosynaptic reflex that occurs when a muscle is stretched.

Structural Integration (Rolfing): A method of releasing the myofascial system, thereby reestablishing flexibility and ease of movement in the body.

submaximal contraction: Contraction of the muscle below the maximum voluntary contraction.

substitution pattern: A situation in which the muscle action of a primary mover or stabilizer is consistently replaced by a muscle that would not normally perform that action.

surface electromyography (SEMG): The use of surface electrodes for the recording of electrical potentials from the underlying musculature. It is used in the study of posture, movement, and emotional expression. The record is typically inspected for evidence of the following: emotional lability, antalgic postures, splinting, guarding, cocontractions, symmetries and asymmetries, flexion–relaxation, and other recruitment patterns.

symmetry: The degree of parity between the right and left aspects of a given muscle group. It may be assessed during rest, or the peak activity may be assessed for symmetry during the eccentric or concentric phase of a contraction.

synergistic muscle: A muscle group that participates in an additive fashion with other muscles to create a smooth, coordinated movement.

systemic relaxation training: Surface EMG biofeedback training procedure in which feedback is given from the frontal region or other larger regions.

tectospinal tract: A motor tract originating in the brain stem that innervates the muscles of the neck in reflex responses to changes in the visual field.

time constant: A characteristic of a resistor compactor (RC) circuit used in amplifiers to smooth out the SEMG signal. The larger the time constant, the smoother the variations of recording from the SEMG signal.

Trager Approach: An approach developed by Milton Trager to communicate with the unconscious and reeducate the nervous system toward a more relaxed way of being. It includes wiggling and jiggling different parts of the body and becoming more aware of the changes.

trauma reflex: A posture that develops as a result of an accident, surgery, or repetitive use and that leads to an asymmetrical posture: side bending and rotations. It was first described by Thomas Hanna.

unilateral electrode placement: A technique in which the recording electrodes of a differential amplifier are placed on one side (right or left) of a homologous muscle pair.

uptraining: Surface EMG biofeedback training procedure in which feedback is used to increase the recruitment of a specific muscle group.

urinary incontinence (UI): Defined by the International Continence Society as "any involuntary leakage of urine."

vaginismus: An involuntary spasm of the muscles surrounding the outer third of the vagina when penetration is attempted.

vestibulospinal tract: A motor tract originating in the brain stem that enables the resistance to gravity through contraction of the extensor muscles.

volume conduction: The spread of electrical or magnetic activity through biological tissues.

vulvodynia: Unexplained vulvar discomfort.

withdrawal reflex: A fixed action pattern in which the muscles automatically move a body part away from the source of a painful stimulus.

wrist-to-wrist recording: A procedure in which the recording electrodes of a differential amplifier are placed on the right and left wrists. This procedure is used to teach systemic relaxation of the upper extremities, torso, neck, and head.

Answers to Chapter Questions

Chapter 2. Anatomy and Physiology

1a, 2b, 3d, 4c, 5b, 6b, 7a, 8b, 9c, 10a, 11b, 12a, 13b, 14b, 15c, 16c, 17a, 18d, 19a, 20b, 21d, 22d, 23a, 24d, 25b, 26b, 27c, 28a, 29b, 30c, 31a, 32a, 33d, 34b, 35b

Chapter 3. Instrumentation

1b, 2d, 3b, 4c, 5c, 6c, 7c, 8c, 9b, 10a, 11b, 12a, 13b, 14b, 15c, 16a, 17d, 18c

Chapter 4. Electrode and Site Selection Strategies

1b, 2c, 3c, 4d, 5a, 6a, 7b, 8e, 9a, 10d, 11e, 12d

Chapter 5. General Assessment Considerations

1c, 2b, 3b, 4a, 5b, 6b, 7d

Chapter 6. Static Assessment and Clinical Protocol

1e, 2b, 3d, 4d, 5b, 6d, 7d, 8e

Chapter 7. Emotional Assessment and Clinical Protocol

1a, 2b, 3a, 4d, 5c, 6d

Chapter 8. Dynamic Assessment

1d, 2b, 3b, 4d, 5b, 6a, 7c, 8d, 9b, 10c, 11b, 12a, 13e

Chapter 9. Treatment Considerations and Protocols

1c, 2a, 3d, 4b, 5a, 6a, 7b, 8c, 9b, 10a, 11d, 12c, 13a, 14e, 15c, 16c, 17d, 18a

Chapter 10. Documentation

1b, 2b, 3a, 4b

Chapter 11. The History of Muscle Dysfunction and Surface Electromyography

1d, 2c, 3d, 4a, 5d, 6c, 7b, 8a, 9d, 10a, 11d, 12d, 13a, 14d, 15c, 16c

Chapter 12. Somatics and Surface Electromyography

1d, 2c, 3a, 4d, 5b, 6b, 7d, 8c, 9d, 10d

Chapter 13. Electromyographic Assessment of Female Pelvic Floor Disorders

1e, 2e, 3e, 4c, 5b, 6b&c, 7d, 8f, 9e, 10f, 11f

Chapter 17. Electrode Placements

1c, 2d, 3d, 4b, 5e, 6b, 7a, 8a, 9e, 10e, 11b, 12a, 13b, 14c, 15c, 16b, 17c, 18a, 19e, 20b, 21c, 22b, 23b, 24d, 25a, 26d, 27b, 28b, 29b, 30c, 31a, 32b, 33d

Index

Italicized page locators indicate a photo/figure; tables are denoted with a *t*.